SPEECH ENHANCEMENT

Theory and Practice

Second Edition

Supplementary Resources Disclaimer

Additional resources were previously made available for this title on DVD. However, as DVD has become a less accessible format, all resources have been moved to a more convenient online download option.

You can find these resources available here: www.routledge.com/9781466504219

Please note: Where this title mentions the associated disc, please use the downloadable resources instead.

SPEECH ENHANCEMENT

Theory and Practice

Second Edition

Philipos C. Loizou

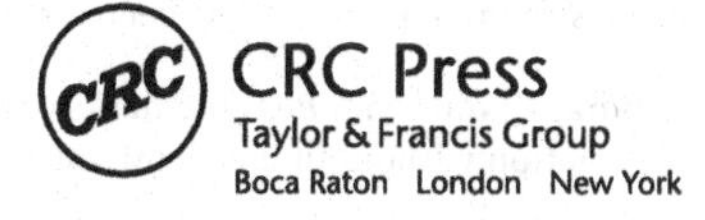

CRC Press is an imprint of the
Taylor & Francis Group, an **informa** business

CRC Press
Taylor & Francis Group
6000 Broken Sound Parkway NW, Suite 300
Boca Raton, FL 33487-2742

First issued in paperback 2017

Version Date: 20130109

ISBN 13: 978-1-138-07557-3 (pbk)
ISBN 13: 978-1-4665-0421-9 (hbk)

Visit the Taylor & Francis Web site at
http://www.taylorandfrancis.com

and the CRC Press Web site at
http://www.crcpress.com

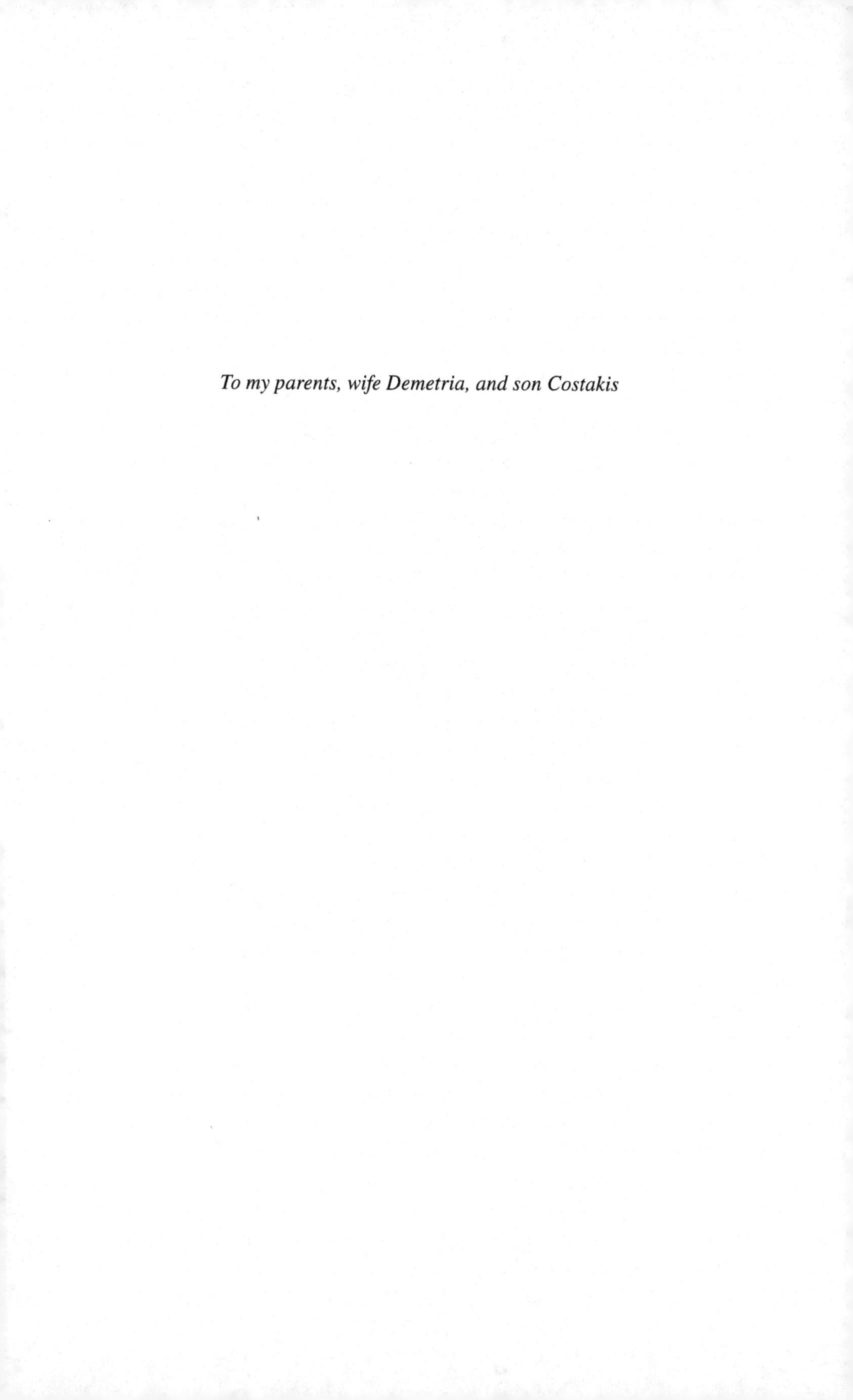

To my parents, wife Demetria, and son Costakis

Contents

PART I Fundamentals

PART II Algorithms

PART III Evaluation

PART IV Future Steps

Preface to the Second Edition

The second edition of this text not only revises the first edition but also expands it. In particular, it includes two new chapters. Chapter 11 provides a thorough coverage of objective intelligibility measures and Chapter 13 covers algorithms that *can* improve speech intelligibility. The feedback I received from most readers about the first edition is that much of the focus of the text has been placed on algorithms that can improve speech quality rather than speech intelligibility. The second edition comes in response to those readers. With the proliferation of mobile devices and hearing devices (hearing aids and cochlear implants), there is a growing and pressing need to design algorithms that can improve speech intelligibility without sacrificing quality. The inclusion of a chapter on intelligibility measures, which can predict reliably speech intelligibility, is absolutely necessary in order to understand why the algorithms described in Chapter 13 *do* improve speech intelligibility. Secondly, having a good understanding of some of the commonly used intelligibility metrics can assist us in the design of novel noise reduction algorithms that derive statistical estimators that maximize/minimize such metrics. This stands in contrast with the conventional estimators that aim to minimize the mean-square error (MSE), a metric that is "speech ignorant" and not motivated by any known facts about how human listeners are able to perceive speech in complex listening situations. It is the opinion of this author that our obsession with the MSE metric delayed progress in the field of noise reduction.

The contents of the DVD-ROM have also been updated to include (1) MATLAB® code with the implementation of some of the intelligibility measures described in Chapter 11, (2) MATLAB code and C/C++ code with the implementation of the algorithms described in Chapter 13, and (3) real-world noise recordings. In addition, it includes the implementation of the wideband-version of the PESQ measure for assessing the quality of speech sampled at rates higher than 8 kHz.

I wish to express my sincere thanks to all my graduate students who contributed in some way to the writing of the second edition. In particular, I would like to thank my postdoctorate students, Drs. Kamil Wójcicki, Jianfen Ma, and Fei Chen, who wrote many of the MATLAB algorithms included in the updated DVD-ROM. Many thanks also go to Oldooz Hazrati and Dr. Kostas Kokkinakis. Thanks also go to Jacky Gao, Yi Gao, Li Xiao, and Fang Deng who, in the course of translating the first edition to Chinese, found many errors and typos. I am also thankful to Nora Konopka, editor at Taylor & Francis Group, for providing the support and encouragement for this book.

Finally, I would like to express my deepest gratitude to my wife Demetria for her understanding and undying support throughout this project.

Philipos C. Loizou
University of Texas at Dallas
Dallas, Texas

Preface to the First Edition

This text is, in part, an outgrowth of my graduate course on speech signal processing, which I have been teaching at the University of Texas at Dallas since the fall of 1999. It is also, in part, a product of my own research in the area. The fact that no textbook existed at the time on speech enhancement, other than a few edited books suitable for the experts, made it difficult to teach the fundamental principles of speech enhancement in a graduate-level course. It must be equally frustrating for new students or speech scientists interested in getting into the field of speech enhancement without having access to a tutorial review or introductory paper (the last review paper was published in the *Proceedings of IEEE* in 1979 by Lim and Oppenheim). That work provided the initial motivation to write this book. My interest in this area stems from my research to develop noise reduction algorithms that can be used to help hearing-impaired listeners (cochlear implant listeners) better communicate in noisy environments.* Crucial to the development of such noise reduction algorithms is the basic understanding of the limitations and potential of existing enhancement algorithms, which I believe this book provides.

The textbook consists of 11 chapters, which are outlined in detail in Chapter 1 (Introduction). It is divided into three main parts. Part I presents the digital-signal processing and speech-signal fundamentals needed to understand speech enhancement algorithms. Part II presents the various classes of speech enhancement algorithms proposed over the past two decades, and Part III presents the methods and measures used to evaluate the performance of speech enhancement algorithms.

The text body is supplemented with examples and figures designed to help the reader understand the theory. The book is accompanied by a DVD-ROM, which contains a speech corpus appropriate for quality and intelligibility evaluation of processed speech, and MATLAB® code with the implementation of major speech enhancement algorithms. It is my strong belief that having access to MATLAB code and a common speech database against which to evaluate new speech enhancement algorithms is crucial and necessary in order to move the field forward. Appendix C provides a detailed description of the contents of the DVD-ROM.

The book can be used as a textbook for a one-semester graduate-level course on speech enhancement. Necessary prerequisites for such a course would be a course on digital signal processing and fundamental knowledge of probability theory, random variables, and linear algebra. This book can also be used as a supplement to an introductory course on speech processing. In this case, Chapters 4 through 8 could be covered along with a select set of sections from Chapters 9 and 10.

I wish to express my sincere thanks to the many colleagues and graduate students who contributed in some way to the writing of this book. I would like to thank Professors Patrick Wolfe, Kuldip Paliwal, Peter Assmann, John Hansen, and

* This work is supported by the National Institutes on Deafness and Other Communication Disorders, NIH.

Jim Kaiser for reviewing chapters of this book and providing valuable feedback. Thanks also go to my graduate students who wrote many of the MATLAB algorithms included in the DVD-ROM. In particular, I would like to thank Sundarrajan Rangachari, Sunil Kamath, Yang Lu, Ning Li, and Yi Hu. Special thanks go to Yi Hu who contributed immensely to this project in the form of ideas for new speech enhancement algorithms (many of which are described in this book) and in terms of implementing those ideas in MATLAB and allowing me to include his code. I would also like to thank Professor John Hansen for allowing me to include some of his MATLAB codes on objective measures and to David Pearce for allowing me to use the noise recordings from the AURORA database. Thanks go to Chaitanya Mamidipally and Jessica Dagley for all their help with the recordings of the noisy speech corpus. I am also thankful to B.J. Clark, acquisitions editor at Taylor & Francis Group, for providing the support and encouragement for this book.

Finally, I would like to express my deepest gratitude to my wife Demetria for her understanding and undying support throughout this project.

Publisher's Note

We were very saddened by Philip's death—such a highly accomplished, intelligent, and gracious man.

Philip passed before he could review the proofs for this book or provide the final files for the DVD. It is with our greatest thanks to Dr. John H.L. Hansen, department head and professor in the Department of Electrical Engineering at The University of Texas at Dallas for diligently reviewing and correcting the page proofs; and to Dr. Kamil Wójcicki for modifying, enhancing, and testing the software that accompanies this book.

Nora Konopka
Publisher of Engineering and Environmental Sciences
CRC Press, Boca Raton, Florida

In Memoriam

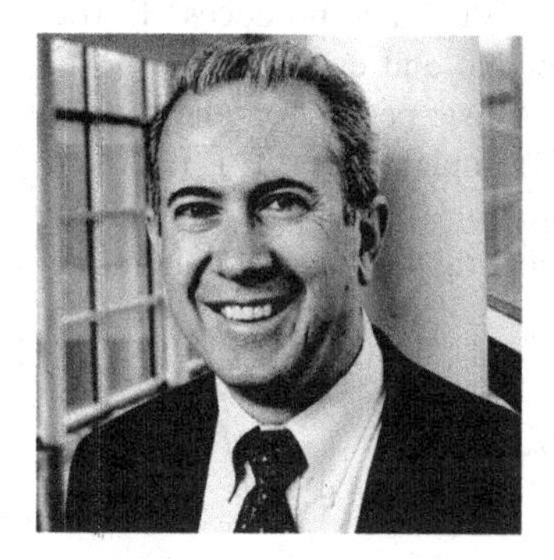

It is with sadness that the Department of Electrical Engineering, University of Texas at Dallas (USA) reports that Professor Philipos Loizou, a professor of Electrical Engineering and pioneer in the fields of hearing aids and speech enhancement, and whose work has helped restore partial hearing to countless people, passed away on Sunday, July 22, 2012 due to cancer. He was 46, and is survived by his wife and 11 year old son.

Philipos C. Loizou received the BS, MS, and PhD degrees from Arizona State University (ASU), Tempe, AZ, in 1989, 1991, and 1995, respectively, all in electrical engineering. From 1995 to 1996, he was a postdoctoral fellow in the Department of Speech and Hearing Science, ASU, where he was involved in research related to cochlear implants. From 1996 to 1999, he was an assistant professor at the University of Arkansas at Little Rock, Little Rock, AR. He later moved to join the Department of Electrical Engineering, University of Texas at Dallas, Richardson, TX, where he helped co-found the Center for Robust Speech Systems (CRSS) in the Jonsson School and directed the Speech Processing and Cochlear Implant Labs within CRSS. He served as professor of Electrical Engineering and held the Cecil and Ida Green chair in Systems Biology Science at UT Dallas.

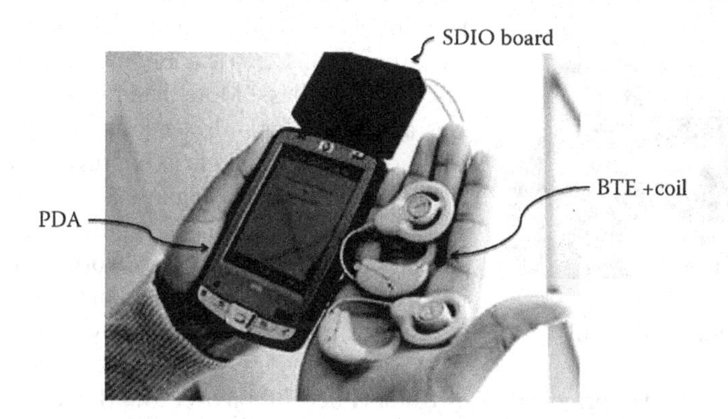

Dr. Loizou was an internationally known leader in signal and speech processing, speech perception and cochlear implant research. He formulated advancements in both signal processing and cochlear implant devices for electrical stimulation of the inner ear of profoundly deaf people. His algorithms also helped improve the performance of cochlear implants by programming the device to operate more effectively in diverse listening environments. More recently, he developed a research platform that enables smartphones and personal digital assistants (PDAs) to interact with cochlear implants and optimize users' listening experience by controlling stimulation parameters using touch screen user interface. Smartphone application processes the acoustic signal using novel sound processing algorithms and produces electric stimuli in real-time. This has lead to quick development and evaluation of novel research ideas and algorithms for noise suppression, music perception and speech enhancement resulting in better listening experience for implant users. This interface was approved by the U.S. Food and Drug Administration (FDA), and Dr. Loizou was overseeing a clinical trial on the interface with more than a dozen collaborating universities, medical centers, and laboratories.

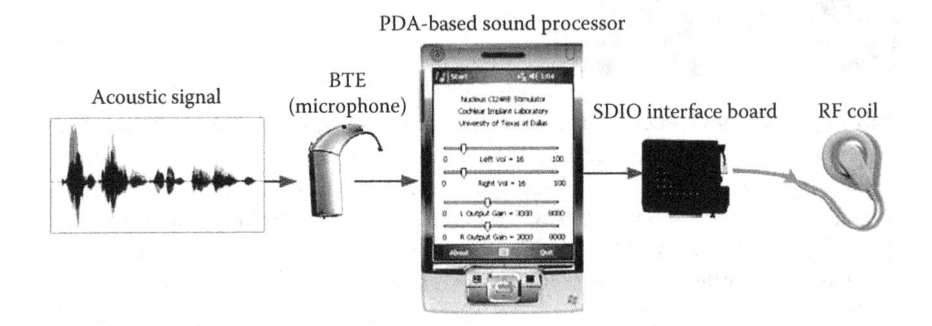

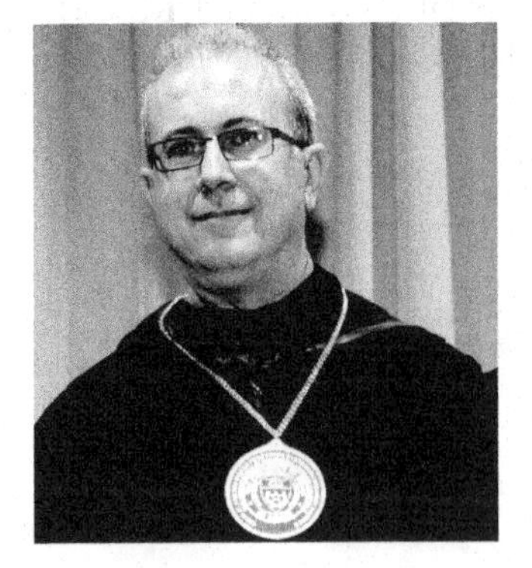

"He was one of the first persons to explore specific speech enhancement algorithms that directly improve intelligibility—previously believed not to be possible," said Dr. John Hansen, head of the Department of Electrical Engineering, University of Texas at Dallas. "More than his research, Philip was a true scholar—always looking to make contributions which would help improve the quality of life of people with hearing loss."

Loizou attributed much of his success to his students. "I've had very hardworking and dedicated students," he said earlier this year. "Without them, I find it's difficult for me to progress in my research so I owe a lot of praise to them."

He has served as principal investigator (PI/co-PI) on over $9.4M in external funding in his career from U.S. National Institutes of Health, U.S. National Science Foundation, Texas Instruments, Cochlear Corporation, U.T. Southwestern Medical Center, U.S. Air Force, Starkey Corp., Advanced Bionics Corp., and collaborated with many groups, having received the NIH Shannon Award in 1998. He was known for mentoring his students and helping mentor other faculty members in their quest to obtain research support from the NIH.

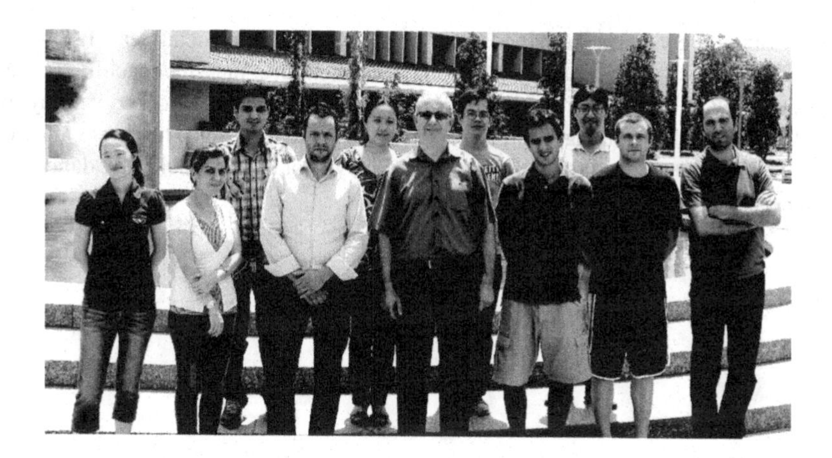

"He sought out collaborations which would later become some of the most profound contributions in the field," Hansen said. "In addition to his work, he was a valued colleague, mentor and academic citizen. In true Philip style, he always brought a careful, thoughtful approach to all he did and made all around him better."

"There is a lot of research one can do to make cochlear implants more natural for patients, and easier for them to use", was another comment Philip shared with his collaborator Nasser Kehtarnavaz (Professor, Electrical Engineering).

During his career, he graduated 8 PhD and 15 MSEE students. He has published 93 journal papers (primarily in *The Journal of the Acoustical Society of America* and IEEE journals as well as in other journals such as: *Ear and Hearing; American Journal of Audiology; Speech Communication; and Hearing Research*), 54 peer-reviewed conference papers, 5 book chapters, and 3 textbooks including: *Speech Enhancement: Theory and Practice*, Taylor & Francis, Boca Raton, FL (2007); *An Interactive Approach to Signals and Systems Laboratory* (Austin, TX: National Instruments), with co-authors Kehtarnavaz, N. and Rahman, M. (2008); and *Advances in Modern Blind Signal Separation Algorithms: Theory and Applications*, Morgan & Claypool Publishers (with co-author Kokkinakis, K. (2010)).

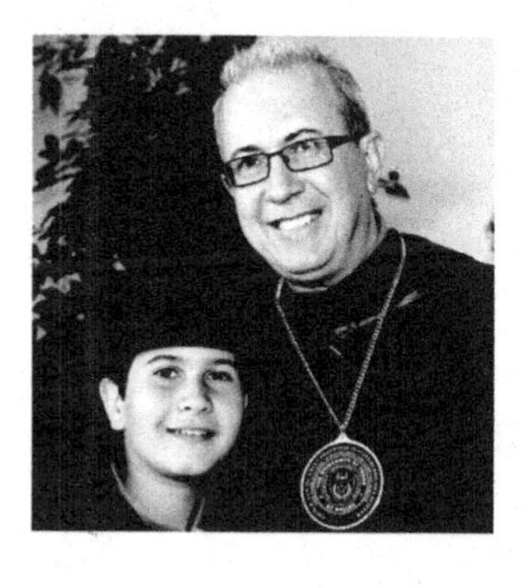

Dr. Loizou was an elected member of the IEEE Speech-Language Technical Committee (SLTC) (2006–09) for the IEEE Signal Processing Society, and served as member of the Organizing Committee for IEEE ICASSP-2010 (Dallas, TX; USA) overseeing Tutorials. He also served as associate editor during his career for *IEEE Signal Processing Letters* (2006–08), *IEEE Trans. on Speech and Audio Processing* (1999–02), and most recently *IEEE Trans. Biomedical Engineering* and *International Journal of Audiology*. He was elected to the grade of Fellow of the Acoustical Society of America for his work on cochlear implants and speech enhancement.

Dr. Loizou grew up on the Island of Cyprus in the Mediterranean Sea. He enjoyed outdoor activities with his family including hiking, nature, playing/coaching soccer, and especially fishing with his 11-year-old son, Costakis. He is also survived by his wife, Demetria whose background is also in speech and hearing. They were married for 18 years and treasured their common Greek Cypriot culture including dance and regular trips to visit family and friends in Cyprus.

1 Introduction

Speech enhancement is concerned with improving some perceptual aspect of speech that has been degraded by additive noise. In most applications, the aim of speech enhancement is to improve the quality and intelligibility of degraded speech. The improvement in quality is highly desirable as it can reduce listener fatigue particularly in situations where the listener is exposed to high levels of noise for long periods of time (e.g., manufacturing). Speech enhancement algorithms reduce or suppress the background noise to some degree and are sometimes referred to as *noise suppression* algorithms.

The need to enhance speech signals arises in many situations in which the speech signal originates from a noisy location or is affected by noise over a communication channel. There are a wide variety of scenarios in which it is desired to enhance speech. Voice communication, for instance, over cellular telephone systems typically suffers from background noise present in the car, restaurant, etc. at the transmitting end. Speech enhancement algorithms can therefore be used to improve the quality of speech at the receiving end. That is, they can be used as a preprocessor in speech coding systems employed in cellular phone standards (e.g., [1]). If the cellular phone is equipped with a speech recognition system for voice dialing, then recognition accuracy will likely suffer in the presence of noise. In this case, the noisy speech signal can be preprocessed by a speech enhancement algorithm before being fed to the speech recognizer. In an air–ground communication scenario, speech enhancement techniques are needed to improve quality, and preferably intelligibility, of the pilot's speech that has been corrupted by extremely high levels of cockpit noise. In this, as well as in similar communication systems used by the military, it is more desirable to enhance the intelligibility rather than the quality of speech. In a teleconferencing system, noise sources present in one location will be broadcast to all other locations. The situation is further worsened if the room is reverberant. Enhancing the noisy signal prior to broadcasting it will no doubt improve the performance of the teleconferencing system. Finally, hearing impaired listeners wearing hearing aids (or cochlear implant devices) experience extreme difficulty communicating in noisy conditions, and speech enhancement algorithms can be used to somehow preprocess or "clean" the noisy signal before amplification.

The foregoing examples illustrate that the goal of speech enhancement varies depending on the application at hand. Ideally, we would like speech enhancement algorithms to improve both quality and intelligibility. It is possible to reduce the background noise, but at the expense of introducing speech distortion, which in turn may impair speech intelligibility. Hence, the main challenge in designing effective speech enhancement algorithms is to suppress noise without introducing any perceptible distortion in the signal. Thus far, most speech enhancement algorithms have been found to improve only the quality of speech. The last chapter included in the second edition provides future steps that can be taken to develop algorithms that can improve speech intelligibility.

The solution to the general problem of speech enhancement depends largely on the application at hand, the characteristics of the noise source or interference, the relationship (if any) of the noise to the clean signal, and the number of microphones or sensors available. The interference could be noise-like (e.g., fan noise) or speech-like such as an environment (e.g., restaurant) with competing speakers. Acoustic noise could be additive to the clean signal or convolutive if it originates from a highly reverberant room. Furthermore, the noise may be statistically correlated or uncorrelated with the clean speech signal. The number of microphones available can influence the performance of speech enhancement algorithms. Typically, the larger the number of microphones, the easier the speech enhancement task becomes. Adaptive cancellation techniques can be used when at least one microphone is placed near the noise source.

This book focuses on enhancement of speech signals degraded by statistically uncorrelated (and independent) additive noise. The enhancement algorithms described in this book are not restricted to any particular type of noise, but can be generally applied to a wide variety of noise sources (more on this later). Furthermore, it is assumed that only the noisy signal, containing both the clean speech and additive noise, is available from a single microphone for speech enhancement. This situation constitutes one of the most challenging problems in speech enhancement since it assumes no access to a reference microphone that picks up the noise signal.

1.1 UNDERSTANDING THE ENEMY: NOISE

Prior to designing algorithms to combat additive noise, it is crucial to understand the behavior of various types of noise, the differences between the noise sources in terms of temporal and spectral characteristics, and the range of noise levels that may be encountered in real life.

1.1.1 Noise Sources

We are surrounded by noise wherever we go. Noise is present, for instance, in the street (e.g., cars passing by, street construction work), in the car (e.g., engine noise, wind), the office (e.g., PC fan noise, air ducts), the restaurant (e.g., people talking in nearby tables), and the department stores (e.g., telephone ringing, sales representatives talking). As these examples illustrate, noise appears in different shapes and forms in daily life..

Noise can be stationary, that is, does not change over time, such as the fan noise coming from PCs. Noise can also be nonstationary, such as the restaurant noise, that is, multiple people speaking in the background mixed in some cases with noise emanating from the kitchen. The spectral (and temporal) characteristics of the restaurant noise are constantly changing as people carry on conversations in neighboring tables and as the waiters keep interact and converse with people. Clearly, the task of suppressing noise that is constantly changing (nonstationary) is more difficult than the task of suppressing stationary noise.

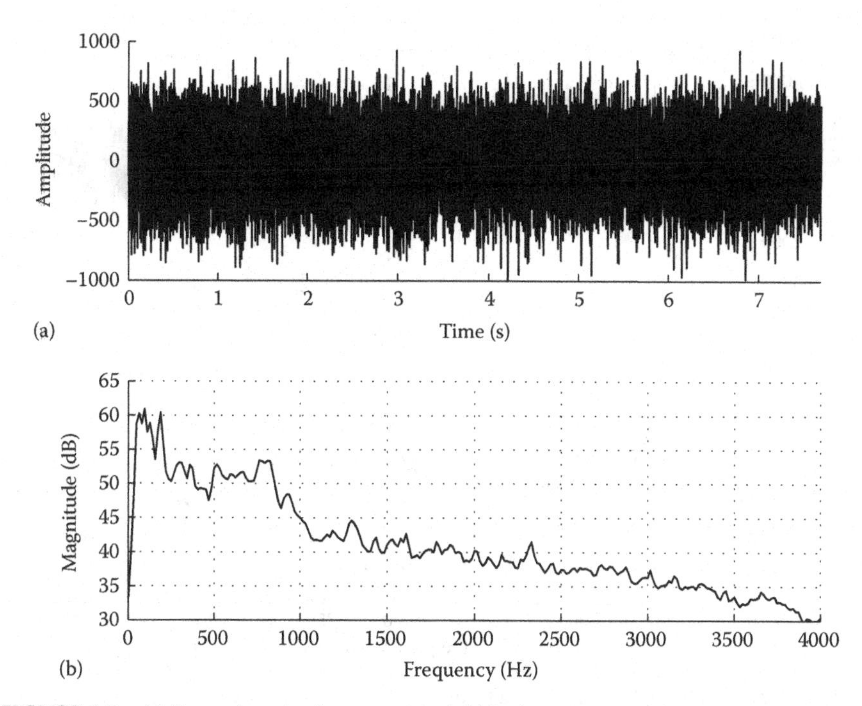

FIGURE 1.1 (a) Example noise from a car and (b) its long-term average spectrum.

Another distinctive feature of the various types of noise is the shape of their spectrum, particularly as it relates to the distribution of noise energy in the frequency domain. For instance, the main energy of wind noise is concentrated in the low frequencies, typically below 500 Hz. Restaurant noise, on the other hand, occupies a wider frequency range. Figures 1.1 through 1.3 show example time waveforms of car noise, train noise, and restaurant noise (noise sources were taken from the NOIZEUS corpus [2], which is included in the DVD of this book). The corresponding long-term average spectra of these noise sources are also shown. In these three example noise sources, the car noise (Figure 1.1) is relatively stationary but the train and restaurant noises are not. It is clear from Figures 1.1 through 1.3 that the differences between these three types of noise sources are more evident in the frequency domain rather than the time domain. Most of energy of the car noise is concentrated in the low frequencies, that is, it is low-pass in nature. The train noise, on the other hand, is more broadband as it occupies a wider frequency range.

1.1.2 Noise and Speech Levels in Various Environments

Critical to the design of speech enhancement algorithms is knowledge of the range of speech and noise intensity levels in real-world scenarios. From that, we can estimate the range of signal-to-noise ratio (SNR) levels encountered in realistic environments. This is important since speech enhancement algorithms need to be effective in suppressing the noise and improving speech quality within that range of SNR levels.

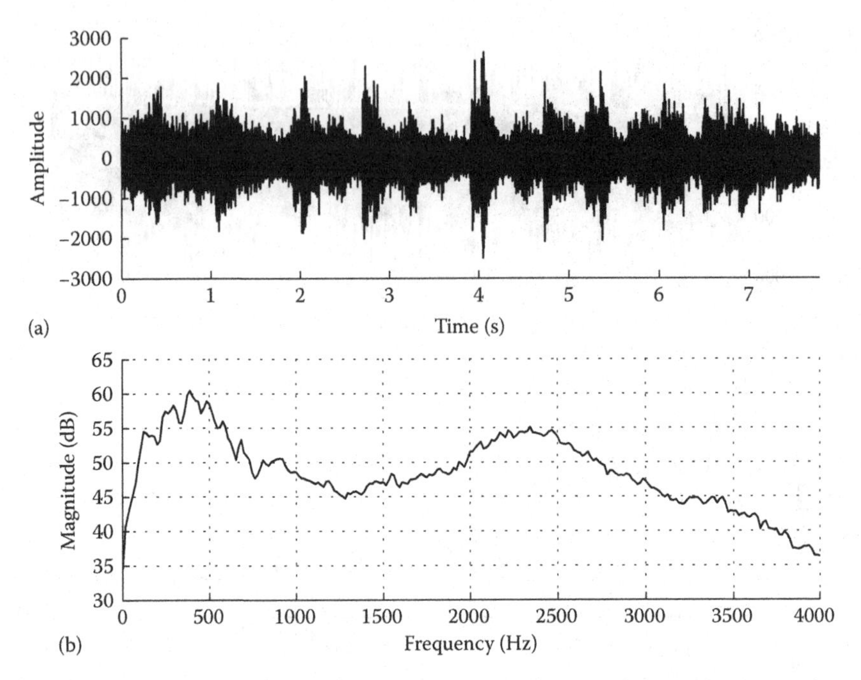

FIGURE 1.2 (a) Example noise from a train and (b) its long-term average spectrum.

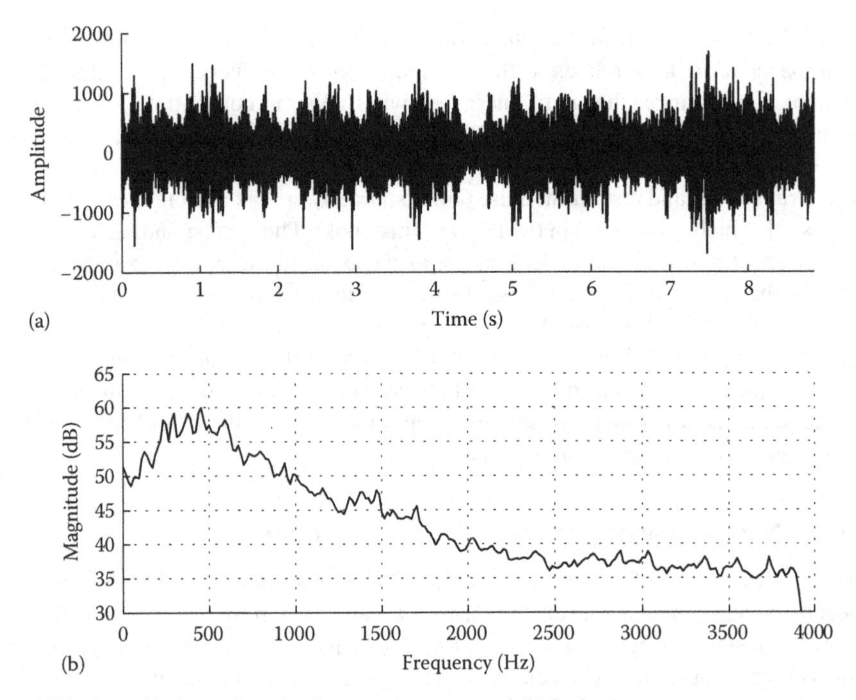

FIGURE 1.3 (a) Example noise from a restaurant and (b) its long-term average spectrum.

A comprehensive analysis and measurement of speech and noise levels in real-world environments was done by Pearsons et al. [3]. They considered a variety of environments encountered in daily life, which included classrooms, urban and suburban houses (inside and outside), hospitals (nursing stations and patient rooms), department stores, trains, and airplanes. The speech and noise levels were measured using sound level meters. The measurements were reported in dB sound pressure level (SPL) (dB SPL is the relative pressure of sound in reference to 0.0002 dynes/cm^2, corresponding to the barely audible sound pressure). As the distance between the speaker and the listener can affect the sound intensity levels, measurements were made with the microphone placed at different distances. Typical distance in face-to-face communication is one meter, and for every doubling of that distance, the sound level is reduced by 6 dB [4]. In certain scenarios (e.g., in transportation vehicles such as trains and airplanes), the distance in face-to-face communication may be reduced to 0.4 m [3].

Figure 1.4 summarizes the average speech and noise levels measured in various environments. Noise levels are the lowest in the classroom, hospital, inside the house, and in the department stores. In these environments, noise levels range between 50 and 55 dB SPL. The corresponding speech levels range between 60 and 70 dB SPL. This suggests that the effective SNR levels in these environments range between 5 and 15 dB. Noise levels are particularly high in trains and airplanes, averaging about 70–75 dB SPL. The corresponding speech levels are roughly the same, suggesting that the effective SNR levels in these two environments are near 0 dB. In classrooms, the effective SNR for students closest to the teacher are most favorable (Figure 1.4), but for those sitting in the back of the classroom it is quite unfavorable as the SNR may approach 0 dB. Noise levels are also high in restaurants and in most cases exceed 65 dB SPL [4]. Generally, it is rare to find a quiet restaurant, as the architectural design of restaurants focuses more on the aesthetics rather than on the acoustics of the interior walls [4]. The study in [5] measured the noise levels in 27 San Francisco Bay Area restaurants and found a median noise level of 72 dBA SPL. The range in noise levels varied across different types of restaurants from a low of

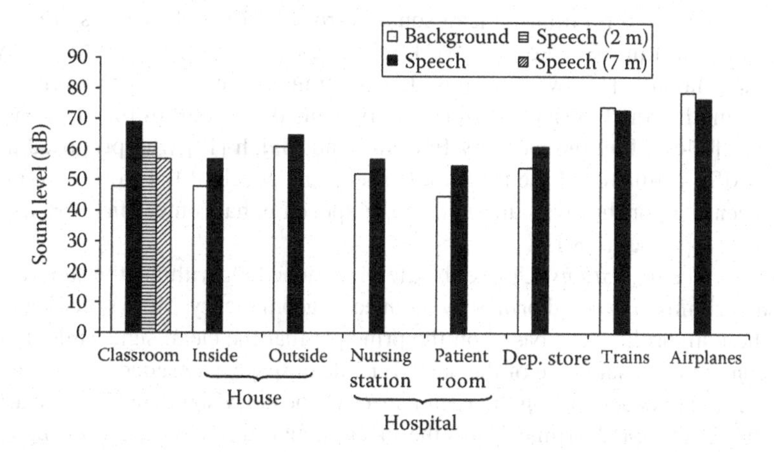

FIGURE 1.4 Average noise and speech levels (measured in dB SPL) in various environments.

59 dBA SPL (family restaurant) to a high of 80 dBA SPL (bistro). In food courts of shopping malls, the range of noise levels varied from 76 to 80 dBA SPL [6].

Note that the speech levels increase in extremely high background noise levels (Figure 1.4). Generally, when the noise level goes beyond 45 dB SPL, people tend to raise their voice levels, a phenomenon known as Lombard effect [7]. The speech level tends to increase with the background level by about 0.5 dB for every 1 dB increase in background level [3]. People stop raising their voice when the ambient noise level goes beyond 70 dB SPL (Figure 1.4). The raising of the voice level is a simple, and efficient, technique that most people use to improve their "listening SNR" whenever in extremely noisy environments.

In brief, for the speech enhancement algorithm to be employed in a practical application it needs to operate, depending on the vocal effort (e.g., normal, raised), within a range of signal-to-noise levels (–5 to 15 dB).

1.2 CLASSES OF SPEECH ENHANCEMENT ALGORITHMS

A number of algorithms have been proposed in the literature for speech enhancement (for an old review of enhancement algorithms, see [8]) with the primary goal of improving speech quality. These algorithms can be divided into three main classes:

1. *Spectral subtractive algorithms*: These are, by far, the simplest enhancement algorithms to implement. They are based on the basic principle that as the noise is additive, one can estimate/update the noise spectrum when speech is not present and subtract it from the noisy signal. Spectral subtractive algorithms were initially proposed by Weiss et al. [9] in the correlation domain *and* later by Boll [10] in the Fourier transform domain.
2. *Statistical-model-based algorithms*: The speech enhancement problem is posed in a statistical estimation framework. Given a set of measurements, corresponding say to the Fourier transform coefficients of the noisy signal, we wish to find a linear (or nonlinear) estimator of the parameter of interest, namely, the transform coefficients of the clean signal. The Wiener algorithm and minimum mean square error (MMSE) algorithms, among others, fall in this category. Work in this area was initiated by McAulay and Malpass [11] who proposed a maximum-likelihood approach for estimating the Fourier transform coefficients (spectrum) of the clean signal, followed by the work by Ephraim and Malah [12] who proposed an MMSE estimator of the magnitude spectrum. Much of the work with the Wiener algorithm was initiated in the speech enhancement field by Lim and Oppenheim [8,13].
3. *Subspace algorithms*: Unlike the aforementioned algorithms, the subspace algorithms are rooted primarily on linear algebra theory. More specifically, these algorithms are based on the principle that the clean signal might be confined to a subspace of the noisy Euclidean space. Consequently, given a method of decomposing the vector space of the noisy signal into a subspace that is occupied primarily by the clean signal and a subspace occupied primarily by the noise signal, one could estimate the clean signal simply by

nulling the component of the noisy vector residing in the "noise subspace." The decomposition of the vector space of the noisy signal into "signal" and "noise" subspaces can be done using well-known orthogonal matrix factorization techniques from linear algebra and, in particular, the singular value decomposition (SVD) or the eigenvector–eigenvalue factorization. Work in this area was initiated by Dendrinos et al. [14] who proposed *the u*se of SVD on a data matrix containing time-domain amplitude values and later on by Ephraim and Van Trees [15] who proposed the use of eigenvalue decomposition of the signal covariance matrix.

The aforementioned algorithms have been shown to improve speech quality and reduce listener fatigue, but failed in as far improving speech intelligibility. Recently, a new class of algorithms based on the time-frequency binary mask has been explored and evaluated for noise reduction applications (the binary mask algorithms were originally developed for computational auditory scene analysis and automatic speech recognition applications). The binary mask algorithms are the only algorithms that have been proven to improve speech intelligibility, and constitute the fourth class of algorithms described in this book.

4. *Binary mask algorithms*: Unlike the algorithms in Classes 1–3, which for the most part make use of smooth gain functions for noise suppression, the binary mask algorithms make use of binary gain functions. This amounts to selecting a subset of frequency bins (or channels) from the corrupted speech spectra, while discarding the rest. The selection of those bins is done according to a prescribed rule or criterion. The selection criterion is not unique, and when applied to corrupted speech spectra, can produce large gains in speech intelligibility. Work in this area originated in the field of computational auditory scene analysis [16,17], and for the most part, binary mask algorithms have been utilized in ASR applications [18] rather than for noise reduction. Under ideal conditions (where *a priori* access to the clean *signal* and noise are assumed), the binary mask algorithms can improve speech intelligibility at any SNR level and for any type of background noise. The first demonstration that binary mask algorithms can indeed improve speech intelligibility in binaural conditions was presented in [19] and the first demonstration that binary mask algorithms can improve speech intelligibility in monaural conditions (i.e., where only access to single-microphone noisy observations is available) was presented in [20].

A different chapter is dedicated in this book for each of the aforementioned four classes of algorithms. MATLAB® implementations of representative algorithms from each class are provided in the accompanying DVD.

1.3 BOOK ORGANIZATION

The main goal of this book is to introduce the reader to the basic problems of speech enhancement and the various algorithms proposed to solve these problems. The book is organized into four main parts: "Fundamentals," "Algorithms," "Evaluation," and "Future Steps."

Part I (Fundamentals) consists of Chapters 2 through 4. These chapters provide the fundamentals needed to understand speech enhancement algorithms.

Chapter 2 provides a review of the fundamentals of discrete-time signal processing including discrete-time signals, linear-time invariant systems, z-transform, and Fourier transform representations. Emphasis is placed on the short-time Fourier representation of speech signals, needed to understand many of the speech enhancement algorithms described in later chapters.

Chapter 3 provides a brief overview of the speech production process, properties and acoustic characteristics of speech signals, and the various acoustic cues used by listeners for speech perception. Fundamental knowledge about speech perception is important for designing algorithms capable of improving intelligibility (and quality) in noisy environments.

Chapter 4 presents an overview of the literature on speech perception in noise. It focuses on cues used by human listeners to communicate in highly adverse conditions particularly in situations where multiple talkers are speaking in the background. Understanding the strategies and acoustic cues used by human listeners to segregate speech from other signals in adverse conditions is important as it would help us design better speech enhancement algorithms that would mimic listening strategies used by humans. Such algorithms would hold promise in improving speech intelligibility in noise.

Part II (Algorithms) includes Chapters 5 through 9 and covers all major enhancement algorithms as well as noise estimation algorithms.

Chapter 5 describes the spectral subtractive algorithms for speech enhancement. These algorithms are simple to implement, but suffer for the most part by a so-called musical noise distortion. This chapter describes the many methods proposed to reduce musical noise.

Chapter 6 describes the Wiener filtering approach to speech enhancement. It describes the many variations of Wiener filtering that includes iterative and noniterative methods, and the methods derived from constrained and unconstrained optimization of various error criteria.

Chapter 7 describes statistical-model-based algorithms for speech enhancement. The problem of estimating the spectrum of the clean signal in noisy environments is posed using a statistical estimation framework. This chapter presents various probabilistic-based estimators of the signal spectrum including the maximum likelihood estimator, MMSE, and maximum *a posteriori* estimators.

Chapter 8 describes subspace algorithms for speech enhancement. These algorithms are rooted in linear algebra theory and are based on the principle that the vector space of the noisy signal can be decomposed into "signal" and "noise" subspaces. The decomposition can be done using either the SVD of a Toeplitz-structured data matrix or the eigenvalue decomposition (EVD) of a covariance matrix. This chapter presents SVD-based and EVD-based algorithms for speech enhancement.

Chapter 9 presents noise-estimation algorithms. All speech enhancement algorithms require an estimate of the noise spectrum, and noise estimation algorithms can be used to provide such an estimate. Unlike voice activity detection (VAD) algorithms, noise estimation algorithms estimate and update the noise spectrum continuously, even during speech activity. As such, noise-estimation algorithms are more suited for speech-enhancement applications operating in highly nonstationary environments.

Part III (Evaluation) consists of Chapters 10 through 12. It provides a description of the measures used to assess the performance (quality and intelligibility) of enhancement algorithms as well as the evaluation results obtained from a comparison between several algorithms.

Chapter 10 provides an overview of the various subjective listening tests used to evaluate speech enhancement algorithms in terms of quality and intelligibility. Human listeners, with normal hearing, participate in these types of tests.

Chapter 11 provides a thorough description of objective quality and intelligibility measures. It also provides the correlation of these measures with human listener's judgments of quality (quality measures) and listener's intelligibility scores (intelligibility measures).

Chapter 12 provides a comprehensive evaluation and comparison of representative speech enhancement algorithms taken from each chapter of this book. It reports on both subjective quality and intelligibility evaluation of speech processed by enhancement algorithms. The quality evaluation is done using subjective listening tests, in which listeners are asked to rate the quality of speech on a five-point scale. The intelligibility evaluation is done with listening tests, wherein listeners are presented with enhanced speech and asked to identify the words spoken.

Part IV (Future Steps) consists of Chapter 13. Under ideal conditions, the algorithms presented in this chapter can improve substantially speech intelligibility, and this chapter provides guidance for future steps that can be taken to realize the full potential of these algorithms under realistic conditions.

Chapter 13 provides a thorough presentation of binary mask algorithms in the context of noise reduction. The full potential of these algorithms is demonstrated in ideal conditions where *a priori* access to the speech and/or noise is assumed. The first steps in implementing these algorithms in realistic conditions are also presented. Given the large benefits in speech intelligibility obtained with these algorithms in various listening conditions, including reverberant conditions, future work is warranted to pursue realistic implementations of binary mask algorithms.

The book is accompanied by a DVD containing speech and noise databases appropriate for evaluation of quality and intelligibility of speech processed by enhancement algorithms. The DVD also contains MATLAB implementations of representative enhancement algorithms taken from each chapter of the book. Detailed description of the DVD contents is provided in Appendix C.

REFERENCES

1. Ramabadran, T., Ashley, J., and McLaughlin, M. (1997), Background noise suppression for speech enhancement and coding, *Proceedings of IEEE Workshop on Speech Coding for Telecommunications*, Pocono Manor, PA, pp. 43–44.
2. Hu, Y. and Loizou, P. (2006), Subjective comparison of speech enhancement algorithms, *Proceedings of IEEE International Conference on Acoustic, Speech, Signal Processing*, Vol. I, Toulouse, France, pp. 153–156.

3. Pearsons, K., Bennett, R., and Fidell, S. (1977), Speech levels in various noise environments, Technical Report EPA-600/1-77-025, U.S. Environmental Protection Agency, Washington, DC.
4. Long, M. (2005), Dinner conversation (an oxymoron?), *Acoust. Today*, 1(1), 25–27.
5. Lebo, C., Smith, M., Mosher, E., Jelonek, S., Schwind, D., Decker, K., Krusemark, H., and Kurz, P. (1994), Restaurant noise, hearing loss, and hearing aids, *West J. Med.*, 161(1), 45–49.
6. Porto, M., Navarro, N., and Pimentel, R. (2007), Speech interference in food courts of shopping centers, *Appl. Acoust.*, 68, 364–375.
7. Lombard, E. (1911), Le signe de l'élévation de la voix, *Ann. Mal. Oreil. Larynx.*, 37, 101–119.
8. Lim, J. and Oppenheim, A. V. (1979), Enhancement and bandwidth compression of noisy speech, *Proc. IEEE*, 67(12), 1586–1604.
9. Weiss, M., Aschkenasy, E., and Parsons, T. (1974), Study and development of the INTEL technique for improving speech intelligibility, Technical Report NSC-FR/4023, Nicolet Scientific Corporation, Northvale, NJ.
10. Boll, S. F. (1979), Suppression of acoustic noise in speech using spectral subtraction, *IEEE Trans. Acoust. Speech Signal Process.*, ASSP-27(2), 113–120.
11. McAulay, R. J. and Malpass, M. L. (1980), Speech enhancement using a soft-decision noise suppression filter, *IEEE Trans. Acoust. Speech Signal Process.*, ASSP-28, 137–145.
12. Ephraim, Y. and Malah, D. (1984), Speech enhancement using a minimum mean-square error short-time spectral amplitude estimator, *IEEE Trans. Acoust. Speech Signal Process.*, ASSP-32(6), 1109–1121.
13. Lim, J. and Oppenheim, A. V. (1978), All-pole modeling of degraded speech, *IEEE Trans. Acoust. Speech Signal Process.*, ASSP-26(3), 197–210.
14. Dendrinos, M., Bakamides, S., and Carayannis, G. (1991), Speech enhancement from noise: A regenerative approach, *Speech Commun.*, 10, 45–57.
15. Ephraim, Y. and Van Trees, H. L. (1993), A signal subspace approach for speech enhancement, *Proceedings of IEEE International Conference on Acoustic, Speech, Signal Processing*, Vol. II, Minneapolis, MN, pp. 355–358.
16. Brown, G. and Cooke, M. (1994), Computational auditory scene analysis, *Comput. Speech Lang.*, 8, 297–336.
17. Weintraub, M. (1985), A theory and computational model of auditory monaural sound separation, PhD thesis, Stanford University, Stanford, CA.
18. Cooke, M., Green, P., Josifovski, L., and Vizinho, A. (2001), Robust automatic speech recognition with missing and uncertain acoustic data, *Speech Commun.*, 34, 267–285.
19. Roman, N., Wang, D., and Brown, G. (2003), Speech segregation based on sound localization, *J. Acoust. Soc. Am.*, 114, 2236–2252.
20. Kim, G., Lu, Y., Hu, Y., and Loizou, P. (2009), An algorithm that improves speech intelligibility in noise for normal-hearing listeners, *J. Acoust. Soc. Am.*, 126(3), 1486–1494.

Part I

Fundamentals

2 Discrete-Time Signal Processing and Short-Time Fourier Analysis

We start with a review of the fundamentals of discrete-time signal processing. Emphasis is placed on the short-time Fourier representation of speech signals, which is needed to understand many of the speech enhancement algorithms described in later chapters. A more thorough coverage of discrete-time signal processing principles can be found in [1,2].

2.1 DISCRETE-TIME SIGNALS

Given a continuous-time (analog) signal, $x_a(t)$, the discrete-time signal $x(n)$ can be obtained by sampling the analog signal at time nT_s, that is,

$$\begin{aligned} x(n) &= x_a(t)\big|_{t=nT_s} \qquad -\infty < n < \infty \\ &= x_a(nT_s) \end{aligned} \tag{2.1}$$

where
  n is an integer
  T_s is the sampling period (s)

The reciprocal of T_s is known as the *sampling frequency*, $F_s = 1/T_s$, expressed in hertz. For perfect signal reconstruction [from discrete $x(n)$ to continuous $x_a(t)$], the Nyquist–Shannon sampling theorem [1] requires that the sampling frequency must be at least twice the highest frequency in the signal.

There are four simple discrete-time signals that are often used as building blocks for constructing more complicated signals. These are the discrete impulse, unit step, exponential, and discrete sinusoid sequences.

The *unit sample* or *discrete impulse* is denoted by $\delta(n)$ and is defined by

$$\delta(n) = \begin{cases} 1 & n = 0 \\ 0 & \text{else} \end{cases} \tag{2.2}$$

The discrete impulse is used as a building block for forming arbitrary discrete-time signals. More specifically, any discrete-time signal can be represented as a sum of weighted and shifted impulses as follows:

$$x(n) = \sum_{k=-\infty}^{\infty} x(k)\delta(n-k) \tag{2.3}$$

For example, the discrete-time signal $x(n) = \{1, 0, \underset{\uparrow}{2}, -1, 0, 0, 5\}$, where the arrow indicates the time origin ($n = 0$), can be expressed as

$$x(n) = \delta(n+2) + 2 \cdot \delta(n) - \delta(n-1) + 5 \cdot \delta(n-4) \tag{2.4}$$

The discrete *unit step* function, $u(n)$, is defined by

$$u(n) = \begin{cases} 1 & n \geq 0 \\ 0 & \text{Otherwise} \end{cases} \tag{2.5}$$

and is related to $\delta[n]$ by

$$u(n) = \sum_{k=0}^{\infty} \delta(n-k) \tag{2.6}$$

Note that Equation 2.6 is derived from Equation 2.3, because $x(n) = 1$ for $n \geq 0$. Multiplication of any discrete sequence by $u(n)$ creates a new sequence that is nonzero for $n \geq 0$. Such sequences are called *right-sided* sequences, as they are nonzero in the right-hand side of the time origin. Similarly, multiplication of any discrete sequence by $u(-n)$ creates a new sequence that is nonzero for $n \leq 0$. These sequences are called *left-sided* sequences.

The discrete exponential sequence has the form

$$x(n) = Ca^n \tag{2.7}$$

where C and a are arbitrary constants. The right-sided exponential sequence is given by $x(n) = Ca^n u(n)$ and the left-sided exponential by $x(n) = Ca^n u(-n)$.

Finally, the *discrete-time sinusoid* is given by

$$x(n) = A\cos(2\pi fn + \theta) \quad -\infty < n < \infty \tag{2.8}$$

where

A is the amplitude of the sinusoid
θ is the initial phase
f is the *normalized frequency* and takes values in the range of $-0.5 < f < 0.5$

The discrete-time sinusoid is derived by sampling the continuous (analog) sinusoid as follows:

$$\begin{aligned} x(n) &= A\cos(2\pi Ft+\theta)\big|_{t=nT_s} \\ &= A\cos\left(2\pi\frac{F}{F_s}n+\theta\right) \\ &= A\cos\left(2\pi fn+\theta\right) \end{aligned} \tag{2.9}$$

where

F is the *frequency* in Hz

f is the *normalized* frequency

It is clear from Equation 2.9 that the two frequencies (F and f) are related by

$$f=\frac{F}{F_s} \tag{2.10}$$

where F_s is the sampling frequency in Hz. Figure 2.1 shows example plots of $\delta(n)$, $u(n)$, $2.5(0.8)^n u(n)$, and $2\cos(2\pi 0.1n)u(n)$.

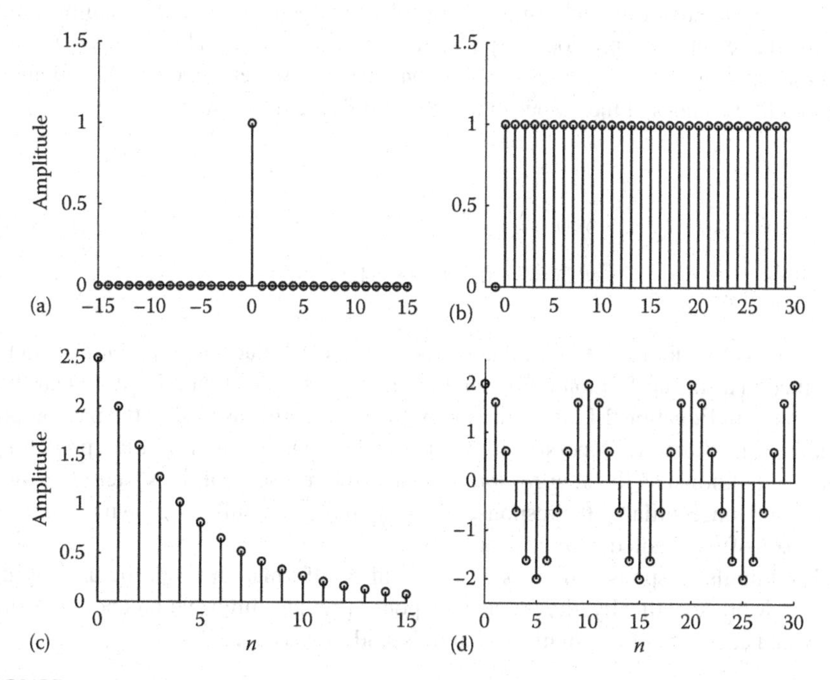

FIGURE 2.1 Example of basic discrete-time signals: (a) $\delta(n)$, (b) $u(n)$, (c) $2.5(0.8)^n u(n)$, and (d) $2\cos(2\pi 0.1n)$.

2.2 LINEAR TIME-INVARIANT DISCRETE-TIME SYSTEMS

Discrete-time systems can be viewed as mathematical transformations that map an input discrete-time signal $x(n)$ into an output discrete-time signal $y(n)$. We denote these transformations by

$$y(n) = T\{x(n)\} \tag{2.11}$$

where the mapping function $T\{\cdot\}$ can be linear or nonlinear. In this chapter, we restrict ourselves to systems that are both linear and time invariant (LTI). Linear systems satisfy the superposition principle, and time-invariant systems possess the following property: $T\{x(n-m)\} = y(n-m)$; that is, a system is said to be time invariant if a shift in the input signal by m samples [i.e., $x(n-m)$] results in a shift in the output by m samples [i.e., $y(n-m)$].

2.2.1 Difference Equations

LTI systems are often described in terms of difference equations. For instance, the following difference equation describes the relationship between the discrete-time input $x(n)$ and the output signal $y(n)$:

$$y(n) = 2x(n) + 0.7y(n-1) \tag{2.12}$$

The output signal at time index n is obtained by multiplying the input signal by 2 and adding the result to the previous output value, which is multiplied by 0.7. If we assume that the input signal is a discrete step function, that is, $x(n) = u(n)$, then we can compute the first three values of the output signal $y(n)$, $n = 0, 1, 2$ as follows:

$$\begin{aligned} &y(0) = 2 && n = 0 \\ &y(1) = 2 + 0.7 \cdot 2 = 3.4 && n = 1 \\ &y(2) = 2 + 0.7 \cdot (3.4) = 4.38 && n = 2 \end{aligned} \tag{2.13}$$

assuming zero initial conditions, that is, $y(n) = 0$, $n < 0$. Values of $y(n)$ for $n > 2$ can be obtained in a similar fashion following the recursion in Equation 2.12. It is clear that the system in Equation 2.12 is a function of the input signal as well as the past output signals. It is, therefore, recursive in nature. The output signal $y(n)$ in the preceding example is known as the *step response*, as it is the response of the system to a step input function. Similarly, the response of a system to an impulse is known as *impulse response*, often denoted by $h(n)$; that is, $h(n) = T\{\delta(n)\}$.

The impulse response provides a great deal of information about the underlying system. More specifically, the impulse response provides information about the stability and causality of a system. A system is said to be *causal* if

$$h(n) = 0, \quad n < 0 \tag{2.14}$$

In a causal system, the output at time n depends only on the present and the past and does not depend on future samples. Causal systems are desirable as they are amenable to real-time implementation. A discrete-time system is *stable* if

$$\sum_{n=-\infty}^{\infty} |h(n)| < \infty \tag{2.15}$$

That is, the impulse response has to be absolutely summable.

The general equation describing LTI systems is given by

$$y(n) = \sum_{k=0}^{M-1} b_k x(n-k) + \sum_{k=1}^{N} a_k y(n-k) \tag{2.16}$$

It is clear that the difference equation in Equation 2.12 is a special case of Equation 2.16, with $b_0 = 2$ and $a_1 = 0.7$.

Systems with $a_k = 0$ ($k = 1, 2, \ldots, N$) in Equation 2.16 are known as *finite impulse response* (FIR) systems, and systems with $b_k \neq 0$ and $a_k \neq 0$ (for all k) are known as *infinite impulse response* (IIR) systems. FIR systems have finite-duration impulse responses, whereas IIR systems have infinite-duration impulse responses.

2.2.2 Linear Convolution

The general equation relating the output of an LTI system to a given input sequence $x(n)$ is given by the convolution sum:

$$y(n) = \sum_{k=-\infty}^{\infty} x(k)h(n-k) \tag{2.17}$$

where $h(n)$ is the impulse response of the system. For simplicity, we often use the following notation for the convolution:

$$y(n) = x(n) * h(n) \tag{2.18}$$

where $*$ denotes the convolution operator. The convolution operation is commutative, associative, and distributive over addition [1]. The convolution operation distributes over addition such that

$$x(n) * [h_1(n) + h_2(n)] = x(n) * h_1(n) + x(n) * h_2(n) \tag{2.19}$$

where $h_1(n)$ and $h_2(n)$ are impulse responses. This property suggests that a system connected in parallel with impulse responses $h_1(n)$ and $h_2(n)$ is equivalent to a single system whose impulse response is the sum of the individual impulse responses.

2.3 z-TRANSFORM

The z-transform is an extremely valuable tool that can be used to analyze discrete-time signals and systems. The z-transform of a sequence $x(n)$ is defined by

$$X(z) = \sum_{n=-\infty}^{\infty} x(n) z^{-n} \tag{2.20}$$

where z is a complex variable. The set of z values for which $X(z)$ converges is called the *region of convergence* (ROC). The ROC and $X(z)$ are both required to uniquely determine the sequence $x(n)$.

2.3.1 Properties

The z-transform has a number of properties that are often used in the analysis of discrete-time signals and systems. We list in the following text a few of those properties. Table 2.1 shows the other properties of the z-transform. We denote the relationship between the sequence $x(n)$ and its z-transform $X(z)$ by

$$x(n) \overset{Z}{\Leftrightarrow} X(z) \tag{2.21}$$

or equivalently $X(z) = Z[x(n)]$, where $Z[\cdot]$ denotes the z-transformation. The time-shifting and convolution properties are widely used in the analysis of discrete-time signals and are described in the following text.

Let $x(n)$ be a sequence defined only for $n \geq 0$, then

$$Z[x(n - n_0)] = z^{-n_0} X(z) \tag{2.22}$$

where n_0 corresponds to the time delay in samples. This property is called the *time-shifting* property of the z-transform, which is often used to convert difference

TABLE 2.1
Properties of the z-Transform

Property	Sequence	z-Transform
Linearity	$a_1x_1(n) + a_2x_2(n)$	$a_1X_1(z) + a_2X_2(z)$
Time shift	$x(n - n_0)$	$z^{-n_0}X(z)$
Frequency scaling	$a^n x(n)$	$X\frac{z}{a}$
Multiplication by n	$nx(n)$	$-z\frac{d}{dz}X(z)$
Convolution	$x_1(n)*x_2(n)$	$X_1(z)X_2(z)$

equations in the z-domain. For instance, the difference equation in Equation 2.12 can be converted in the z-domain using the shifting property (Equation 2.22) and the linearity property as follows:

$$Y(z) = 2X(z) + 0.7z^{-1}Y(z) \tag{2.23}$$

The convolution property relates the convolution of two sequences in terms of their z-transforms. Let $x_1(n)$ and $x_2(n)$ be two sequences with the following z-transforms and ROCs:

$$\begin{aligned} x_1(n) &\overset{Z}{\Leftrightarrow} X_1(z) \quad \text{ROC} = R_1 \\ x_2(n) &\overset{Z}{\Leftrightarrow} X_2(z) \quad \text{ROC} = R_2 \end{aligned} \tag{2.24}$$

where R_1 and R_2 are the ROCs of $x_1(n)$ and $x_2(n)$, respectively. Then, the z-transform of the convolution of the two sequences is given by

$$x_1(n) * x_2(n) \overset{Z}{\Leftrightarrow} X_1(z) \cdot X_2(z) \tag{2.25}$$

and the resulting ROC is given by the intersection of the individual ROCs, that is, $R_1 \cap R_2$. Hence, convolution in the time domain is equivalent to multiplication in the z-domain. For that reason, it is sometimes easier, and preferred, to operate in the z-domain than in the time domain.

2.3.2 *z*-Domain Transfer Function

Making use of the convolution property of the z-transform, we can analyze LTI systems in the z-domain. More specifically, the relationship between the input sequence $x(n)$ and output sequence $y(n)$ in Equation 2.18 can be expressed as

$$Y(z) = H(z)X(z) \tag{2.26}$$

where $Y(z)$, $H(z)$, and $X(z)$ are the z-transforms of the output sequence, impulse response, and input sequence, respectively. $H(z)$ is known as the discrete-time *system function* or *transfer function* as it relates the output to the input.

We can derive the transfer function of the general constant-coefficient difference equation (Equation 2.16) by using the linearity and shifting properties:

$$Y(z) = X(z)\sum_{k=0}^{M-1} b_k z^{-k} + Y(z)\sum_{k=1}^{N} a_k z^{-k} \tag{2.27}$$

Solving Equation 2.27 for $H(z) = Y(z)/X(z)$, we get

$$H(z) = \frac{\sum_{k=0}^{M-1} b_k z^{-k}}{1 - \sum_{k=1}^{N} a_k z^{-k}} \tag{2.28}$$

After computing the roots of the polynomials in the numerator and denominator, we can express Equation 2.28 in factored form as

$$H(z) = b_0 \frac{\prod_{k=1}^{M-1} \left(1 - c_k z^{-1}\right)}{\prod_{k=1}^{N-1} \left(1 - p_k z^{-1}\right)} \tag{2.29}$$

where

c_k are the roots [also called the *zeros* of $H(z)$] of the numerator polynomial
p_k are the roots [also called *poles* of $H(z)$] of the denominator polynomial

This form of the transfer function is often used to check for system stability. If the poles are inside the unit circle, that is, $|p_k| < 1$, then the system is bounded-input bounded-output stable, otherwise it is considered unstable.

As an example, we consider the system given in Equation 2.12. From Equation 2.23, we can compute the system transfer function as

$$H(z) = \frac{Y(z)}{X(z)} = \frac{2}{1 - 0.7z^{-1}} \tag{2.30}$$

From the preceding equation, we can see that $H(z)$ has a pole at $z = 0.7$ and a zero at $z = 0$. Because the pole is smaller than one, the system is stable. Note that the impulse response of the system, that is, $h(n)$, can be computed using the inverse z-transform of $H(z)$. After making use of the following z-transform pair [2]

$$a^n u(n) \overset{Z}{\leftrightarrow} \frac{1}{1 - az^{-1}} \quad \text{ROC:} |z| > a \tag{2.31}$$

we get

$$h(n) = 2(0.7)^n u(n) \tag{2.32}$$

for the impulse response of the system given in Equation 2.12.

2.4 DISCRETE-TIME FOURIER TRANSFORM

The discrete-time Fourier transform (DTFT) of a sequence $x(n)$ is given by

$$X(\omega) = \sum_{n=-\infty}^{\infty} x(n) e^{-j\omega n} \tag{2.33}$$

It is easy to show that $X(\omega) = X(\omega + 2\pi)$, that is, $X(\omega)$ is periodic with a period of 2π. Given $X(\omega)$, we can recover the sequence $x(n)$ using the inverse DTFT:

$$x(n) = \frac{1}{2\pi} \int_{-\pi}^{\pi} X(\omega) e^{j\omega n} \, d\omega \tag{2.34}$$

In general, the DTFT is a complex-valued function of ω and can be represented in polar form as

$$X(\omega) = |X(\omega)| e^{j\phi_x(\omega)} \tag{2.35}$$

where

$|X(\omega)|$ is the *magnitude spectrum*

$\phi_x(\omega)$ is the *phase spectrum*

For real discrete sequences, $X(\omega)$ is conjugate symmetric. This means that the magnitude spectrum is an even function of ω, that is, $|X(\omega)| = |X(-\omega)|$, and the phase spectrum is an odd function of ω, that is, $\phi_x(\omega) = -\phi_x(-\omega)$.

The DTFT, $X(\omega)$, is generally complex for real-valued signals that have no symmetry. If, however, a signal $x(n)$ is even [i.e., $x(n) = x(-n)$], then $X(\omega)$ is purely real (see Example 2.1). If a signal $x(n)$ has odd symmetry [$x(n) = -x(-n)$], then $X(\omega)$ is purely imaginary.

Example 2.1: Compute the DTFT of the Signal:

$$x(n) = \begin{cases} 1 & -M \le n \le M \\ 0 & \text{Otherwise} \end{cases} \tag{2.36}$$

Using the DTFT definition (Equation 2.33), we get

$$\begin{aligned} X(\omega) &= \sum_{n=-M}^{M} e^{-j\omega n} \\ &= \sum_{n=-M}^{-1} e^{-j\omega n} + \sum_{n=0}^{M} e^{-j\omega n} \end{aligned} \tag{2.37}$$

These summations can be evaluated in closed form using the following identity:

$$\sum_{n=0}^{N} a^n = \frac{1 - a^{N+1}}{1 - a} \tag{2.38}$$

Using Equation 2.38 in Equation 2.37 and after some manipulation, we get

$$X(\omega) = \frac{e^{j\omega} - e^{j\omega(M+1)}}{1-e^{j\omega}} + \frac{1-e^{-j\omega(M+1)}}{1-e^{-j\omega}}$$

$$= \frac{\sin\left[\left(M+\frac{1}{2}\right)\omega\right]}{\sin(\omega/2)} \tag{2.39}$$

Note that $X(\omega)$ is real because $x(n)$ has even symmetry. The magnitude and phase spectra are given by

$$|X(\omega)| = \left|\frac{\sin\left[\left(M+\frac{1}{2}\right)\omega\right]}{\sin(\omega/2)}\right|$$

$$\theta_x(\omega) = \begin{cases} 0 & \text{if } X(\omega) > 0 \\ \pi & \text{if } X(\omega) < 0 \end{cases} \tag{2.40}$$

The magnitude and phase spectra given in the preceding text are plotted in Figure 2.2.

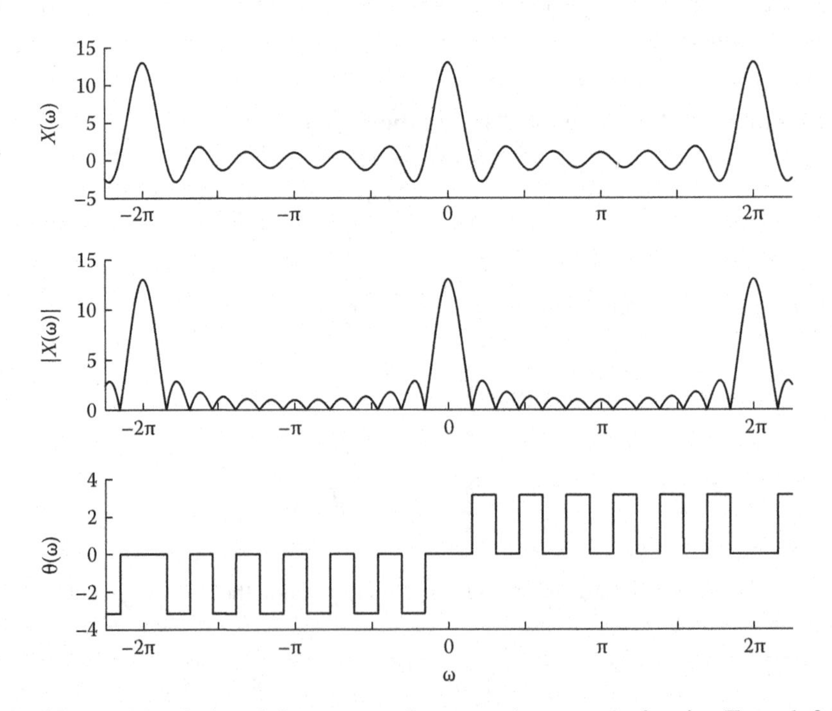

FIGURE 2.2 Magnitude and phase spectra of a symmetric rectangular function (Example 2.1).

2.4.1 DTFT Properties

The DTFT has a number of properties, a few of which we list in the following text. Table 2.2 lists some additional properties of the DTFT. We denote the relationship between the sequence $x(n)$ and its DTFT by

$$x(n) \overset{DTFT}{\Leftrightarrow} X(\omega) \tag{2.41}$$

The *time-shifting* property states that if

$$x(n) \overset{DTFT}{\Leftrightarrow} X(\omega) \tag{2.42}$$

then

$$x(n-n_0) \overset{DTFT}{\Leftrightarrow} e^{-j\omega n_0} X(\omega) \tag{2.43}$$

where n_0 is an integer corresponding to the delay in samples.

The *modulation property* states that multiplying a sequence by a complex exponential corresponds to shifting its DTFT in the frequency domain, that is,

$$e^{j\omega_0 n} x(n) \overset{DTFT}{\Leftrightarrow} X(\omega-\omega_0) \tag{2.44}$$

The *multiplication property* states that multiplication of two sequences results in a periodic convolution of their DTFTs. That is, if

$$\begin{aligned} x(n) &\overset{DTFT}{\Leftrightarrow} X(\omega) \\ w(n) &\overset{DTFT}{\Leftrightarrow} W(\omega) \end{aligned} \tag{2.45}$$

TABLE 2.2
Properties of DTFT

Property	Sequence	DTFT Transform
Linearity	$a_1x_1(n) + a_2x_2(n)$	$a_1X_1(\omega) + a_2X_2(\omega)$
Time shift	$x(n - n_0)$	$e^{-j\omega n_0}X(\omega)$
Modulation	$e^{-j\omega_0 n}x(n)$	$X(\omega - \omega_0)$
Multiplication	$x_1(n)x_2(n)$	$\frac{1}{2\pi}\int_{-\pi}^{\pi} X_1(\theta)X_2(\omega-\theta)d\theta$
Convolution	$x_1(n)*x_2(n)$	$X_1(\omega)X_2(\omega)$

then

$$x(n)w(n) \overset{DTFT}{\Leftrightarrow} \frac{1}{2\pi}\int_{-\pi}^{\pi} X(\theta)W(\omega-\theta)\,d\theta \tag{2.46}$$

The *convolution property* states that the convolution of two sequences results in multiplication of the corresponding DTFTs. For the two sequences given in Equation 2.45, we have

$$x(n) * w(n) \overset{DTFT}{\Leftrightarrow} X(\omega)W(\omega) \tag{2.47}$$

In the context of LTI systems, if $h(n)$ is the impulse response of the system, its DTFT, that is,

$$H(\omega) = \sum_{n=-\infty}^{\infty} h(n)e^{-j\omega n} \tag{2.48}$$

is known as the *frequency response* of the LTI system.

Finally, *Parseval's theorem* relates the total energy in the sequence to its DTFT. It states that the total energy of the sequence $x(n)$, defined as $\Sigma_n|x(n)|^2$, is related to its DTFT according to

$$\sum_{n=-\infty}^{\infty} |x(n)|^2 = \frac{1}{2\pi}\int_{-\pi}^{\pi} |X(\omega)|^2 d\omega \tag{2.49}$$

2.4.2 Discrete Fourier Transform

The DTFT of a discrete-time sequence is a continuous function of frequency ω (see Equation 2.33). In practice, the sequence $x(n)$ is finite in duration (e.g., consisting of N samples), and we can sample the DTFT at N uniformly spaced frequencies, that is, at $\omega_k = 2\pi k/N$, $k = 0, 1, \ldots, N-1$. This sampling yields a new transform referred to as the *discrete Fourier transform* (DFT). The DFT of $x(n)$ is given by

$$X(k) = \sum_{n=0}^{N-1} x(n)e^{-j\frac{2\pi kn}{N}} \quad 0 \le k \le N-1 \tag{2.50}$$

Given $X(k)$, we can recover $x(n)$ from its DFT, using the inverse DFT (IDFT):

$$x(n) = \frac{1}{N}\sum_{k=0}^{N-1} X(k)e^{j\frac{2\pi kn}{N}} \quad 0 \le n \le N-1 \tag{2.51}$$

Many of the properties of the DFT are similar to those of the DTFT. The main distinction is that many of the operations with the DFT are done modulo N. This is largely due to the implicit periodicity of the sequence $x(n)$ [1, Chapter 5].

We will consider the convolution properties of the DFT (a list of other properties of the DFT can be found in [1, Chapter 5]). We saw earlier (see Equation 2.46) that multiplication of two signals corresponds to a convolution of the individual DTFTs. In the DFT domain, however, multiplication of the two discrete-time sequences does not correspond to *linear convolution* but *circular convolution* of the individual DFTs. That is,

$$x(n)w(n) \overset{DFT}{\Leftrightarrow} X(k) \otimes W(k) = \frac{1}{N}\sum_{m=0}^{N-1} X(m)W((k-m)_N) \tag{2.52}$$

where $\otimes$ denotes circular convolution, $X(k)$ and $W(k)$ are the N-point DFTs of $x(n)$ and $w(n)$, respectively, and the notation $(i)_j$ indicates integer i modulo integer j.

Multiplication of the DFTs of two sequences does not correspond to linear convolution but circular convolution of the two sequences, that is,

$$x(n) \otimes w(n) = \sum_{m=0}^{N-1} x(m)W((n-m)_N) \overset{DFT}{\Leftrightarrow} X(k)W(k) \tag{2.53}$$

Therefore, we cannot use the inverse DFT of $X(k)W(k)$ to obtain the linear convolution of $x(n)$ with $w(n)$. In other words, $IDFT\{X(k)W(k)\} \neq x(n) * w(n)$, where $IDFT\{\cdot\}$ denotes the inverse DFT operation (Equation 2.51).

It is possible, however, to use the DFT to compute the linear convolution of two sequences provided we properly pad the two sequences with zeros. Suppose that $x(n)$ is nonzero over the interval $0 \leq n \leq M-1$ and $w(n)$ is nonzero over the interval $0 \leq n \leq L-1$. If we choose an N-point DFT such that $N \geq M + L - 1$, the circular convolution will be equivalent to linear convolution; that is, $IDFT\{X(k)W(k)\} = x(n) * w(n)$. The requirement that $N \geq M + L - 1$ comes from the fact that the length of the output sequence resulting from linear convolution is equal to the sum of the individual lengths of the two sequences minus one [1, Chapter 2].

Figure 2.3 shows an example of circular convolution of two discrete-time sequences, a triangle sequence $x(n)$, $n = 0, 1, \ldots, 9$ (Figure 2.3a) and a truncated ramp sequence $h(n)$, $n = 0, 1, \ldots, 15$ (Figure 2.3b). Figure 2.3c shows the output of the circular convolution of the two sequences obtained by computing the IDFT of $X(k)H(k)$, where $X(k)$ denotes the 16-point DFT of the triangle sequence, and $H(k)$ denotes the 16-point DFT of the truncated ramp sequence. Figure 2.3d shows the output of the linear convolution of the two sequences obtained by computing the IDFT of $X_p(k)H_p(k)$, where $X_p(k)$ denotes the 25-point DFT of the triangle sequence, and $H_p(k)$ denotes the 25-point DFT of the truncated ramp sequence. $X_p(k)$ was obtained by padding the triangle sequence with 15 zeros, whereas $H_p(k)$ was obtained by padding the truncated ramp sequence with 9 zeros. The circular convolution effects are evident when comparing the outputs shown in Figure 2.3c and d.

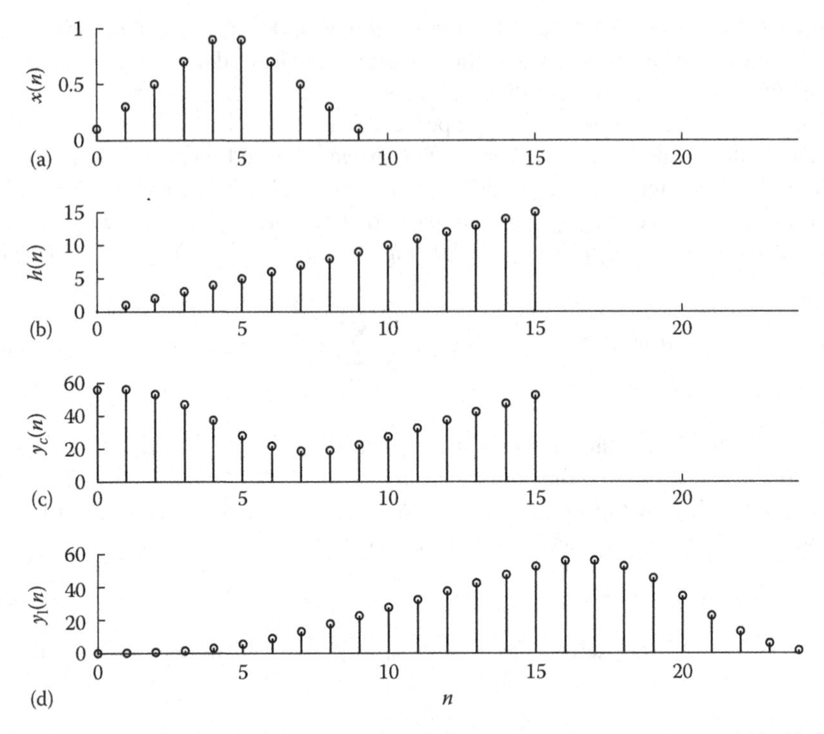

FIGURE 2.3 (a) A triangle sequence $x(n)$ and (b) a truncated ramp sequence $h(n)$. (c) The circular convolution of $x(n)$ and $h(n)$ and (d) the linear convolution of the two sequences.

2.4.3 Windowing

The definition of the DTFT (Equation 2.33) assumes knowledge of the values of $x(n)$ for all n. In practice, we only observe $x(n)$ for a finite duration, say, for N samples. Mathematically, this is equivalent to truncating $x(n)$ via the use of a finite-duration function, which we call a *window*. The signal truncation can be expressed mathematically as

$$x_W(n) = x(n)w(n) \tag{2.54}$$

where

$w(n)$ denotes the window function
$x_W(n)$ denotes the truncated signal

One simple window function to use is the *rectangular function* defined as

$$w(n) = \begin{cases} 1 & 0 \le n \le L-1 \\ 0 & \text{otherwise} \end{cases} \tag{2.55}$$

As we will see shortly, the windowing operation in Equation 2.54 affects the spectrum of $x(n)$ in many ways, depending on the shape of the window function. To demonstrate this, we consider in the following example the DTFT of a truncated sinusoid.

Example 2.2:

Suppose that the discrete-time signal $x(n)$ is a single sinusoid given by

$$x(n) = 2\cos(\omega_0 n) \tag{2.56}$$

where $\omega_0 = 2\pi 0.1$. Compute the DTFT of $x_W(n)$ given in Equation 2.54, where $w(n)$ denotes the window function given in Equation 2.55.

Using Euler's formula, we can express $x(n)$ as

$$x(n) = e^{j2\pi 0.1n} + e^{-j2\pi 0.1n} \tag{2.57}$$

After multiplying $w(n)$ in Equation 2.55 by the exponentials given in the preceding text and using the modulation property (Equation 2.44) of the DTFT, we obtain the DTFT of the windowed signal $x_W(n)$ as follows:

$$X_W(\omega) = W(\omega - \omega_0) + W(\omega + \omega_0) \tag{2.58}$$

where $W(\omega)$ is the DTFT of $w(n)$. Using the result from Example 2.1 along with the time-shifting property, we can compute $W(\omega)$ as follows:

$$W(\omega) = e^{-j\omega(L-1)/2}\left[\frac{\sin(\omega L/2)}{\sin(\omega/2)}\right] \tag{2.59}$$

Note that the first zero crossing of $W(\omega)$ occurs at $\omega = 2\pi/L$, which is regarded as the effective bandwidth of $W(\omega)$ (see Figure 2.4). Figure 2.5 shows the magnitude spectrum, $|X_W(\omega)|$, obtained by computing the N-point DFT of $x_W(n)$, where $N > L$, and L is the duration of the window. Figure 2.5 shows the magnitude spectrum using $N = 1024$ and different values of L, that is, $L = 100$, 300, and 500. As can be seen, $|X_W(\omega)|$ has a single peak at the frequency of the sinusoid, that is, at $f_0 = 0.1$. The spectrum, however, is not narrowband or localized near the signal frequency but, rather, it is spread out over the entire frequency range ($-0.5 < f < 0.5$). This phenomenon, caused by the windowing, is called *spectral leakage*, as information from the signal frequency leaks out to other frequencies. Note that the true magnitude spectrum of a discrete sinusoid defined over $-\infty < n < \infty$ consists of two discrete impulses at the signal frequency, that is,

$$X(\omega) = \delta(\omega - \omega_0) + \delta(\omega + \omega_0) \tag{2.60}$$

The true magnitude spectrum is thus completely localized at the signal frequency. From Figure 2.5, we can see that as L gets larger (i.e., window gets longer in duration), the spectrum gets more localized, resembling that of two discrete impulses (Equation 2.60). This is because the effective bandwidth of $W(\omega)$ (Equation 2.59) becomes smaller as L becomes larger.

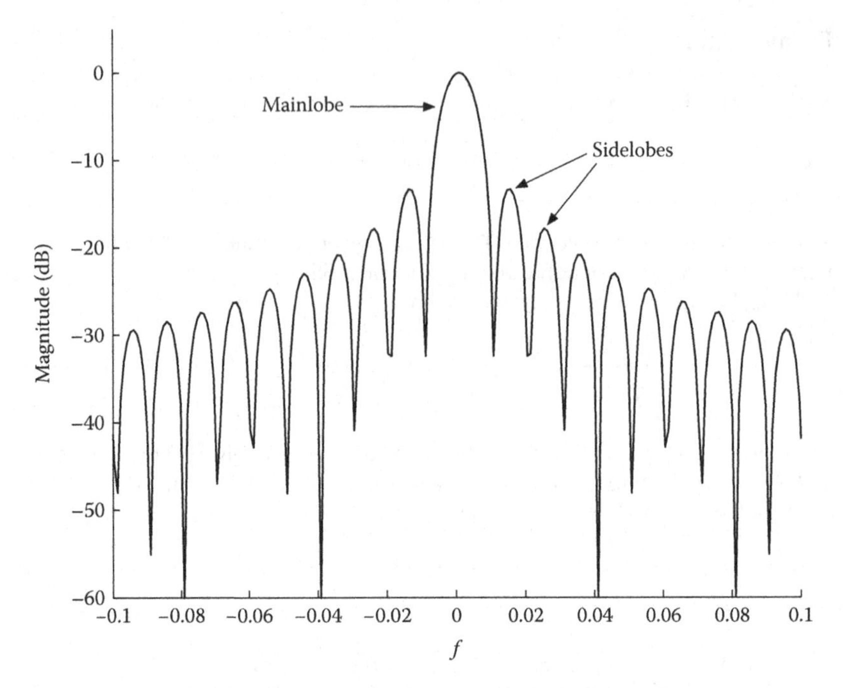

FIGURE 2.4 Magnitude spectrum of a rectangular window of length L.

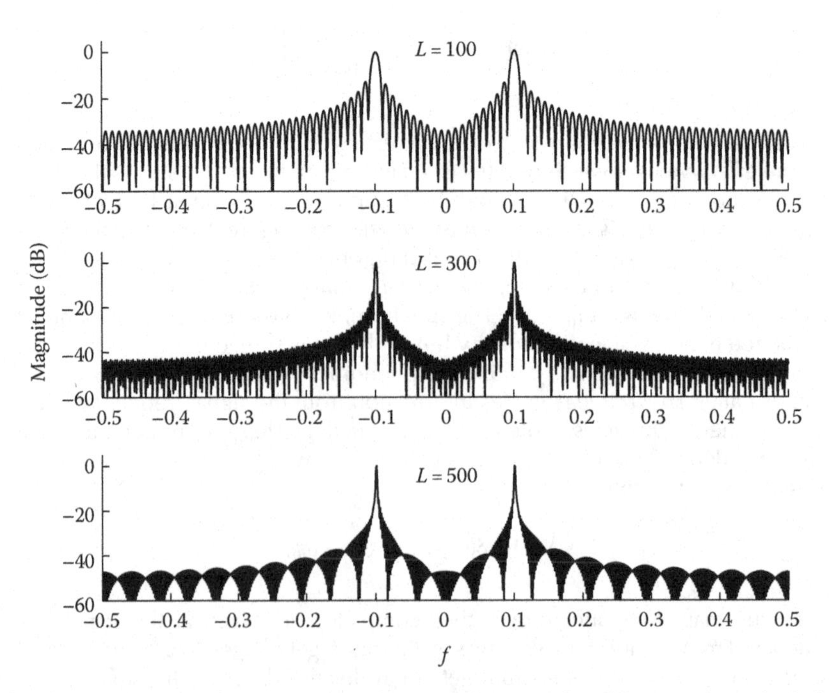

FIGURE 2.5 Spectra of a rectangular-windowed sine wave for different values of window length L.

The example given in the preceding text considered a rectangular window (Equation 2.55). A different picture emerges when a *Hamming window* is used. The Hamming window is defined as

$$w(n) = \begin{cases} 0.54 - 0.46\cos\left(\frac{2\pi n}{L-1}\right) & 0 \le n \le L-1 \\ 0 & \text{Otherwise} \end{cases} \tag{2.61}$$

Figure 2.6 shows the magnitude spectrum of the Hamming-windowed signal for different values of L. Compared to Figure 2.5, the spectral peak is broader (i.e., less localized); however, the spectral sidebands (also called *sidelobes*) are smaller. In fact, the bandwidth of the spectrum of the Hamming window is twice that of the rectangular window [3, p. 44]. This is more evident with $L = 500$. Hence, from Figures 2.5 to 2.6 we see that the spectrum of windowed signals is greatly affected by the shape of the windowing function.

Windowing not only alters the shape of the spectrum owing to the leakage effect, but also reduces the spectral resolution. The leakage effect reduces the ability to resolve or detect a weak (in amplitude) sine wave in the presence of a dominant (large-amplitude) sine wave. To illustrate this problem, we consider the following signal consisting of two sine waves

$$x(n) = 2\cos(\omega_1 n) + 0.1\cos(\omega_2 n) \tag{2.62}$$

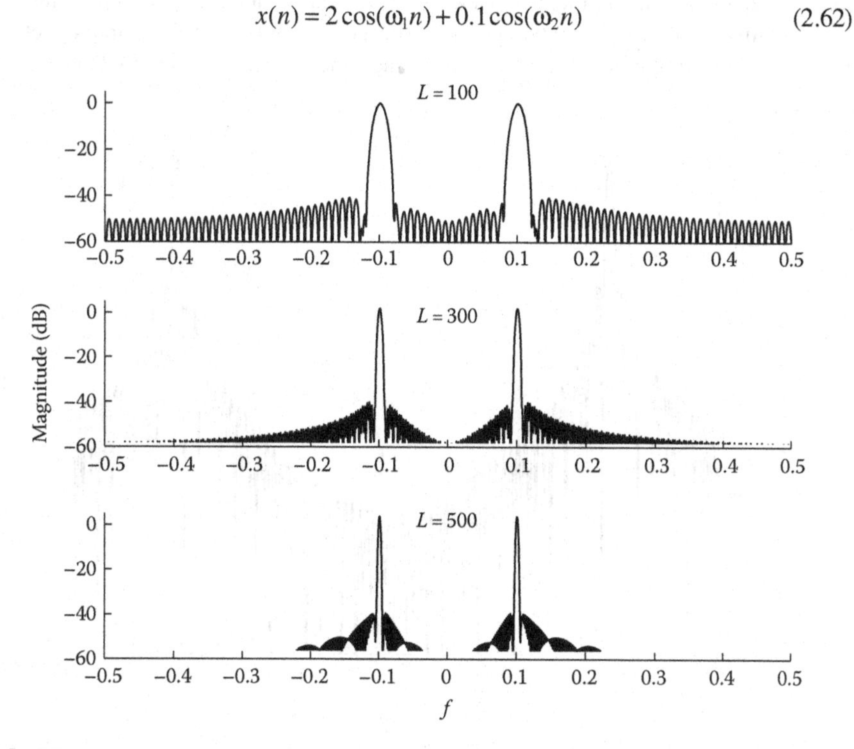

FIGURE 2.6 Spectra of a Hamming-windowed sine wave for different values of window length L.

where $\omega_1 = 0.1\pi$ and $\omega_2 = 0.11\pi$. The spectrum of the windowed sequence, truncated to L samples, is given by

$$X_W(\omega) = W(\omega - \omega_1) + W(\omega + \omega_1) + \frac{0.1}{2}[W(\omega - \omega_2) + W(\omega + \omega_2)] \quad (2.63)$$

Figure 2.7 shows the magnitude spectrum $|X_W(\omega)|$ obtained using a rectangular window, and Figure 2.8 shows the spectrum obtained using a Hamming window for $L = 300$. In theory, there should be two distinct spectral lines centered at ω_1 and ω_2. However, as shown in Figure 2.7, the two spectral lines for the sequence truncated with a rectangular window are not distinguishable. In contrast, the two spectral lines are resolvable for the sequence truncated with the Hamming window. This is because the second spectral line is "buried" under the sidelobe of the rectangular window but remains above the first sidelobe of the Hamming window. Note that the first sidelobe of the spectrum of the rectangular window is −13 dB below the peak [3, p. 44]. However, the amplitude of the weak sine wave is −26 dB (=20 log (0.1/2)) below the peak and is therefore not detectable.

In brief, the windowing function needs to be chosen carefully, depending on the application. The selection of the window should be based on the trade-off between spectral smearing and leakage effects. For the previous example in which we considered the detection of a dominant sinusoid in the presence of a weak amplitude sinusoid, the Hamming windowing function proved to be a better choice. Aside from the rectangular and Hamming windows, other windowing functions can be used [3, Chapter 2].

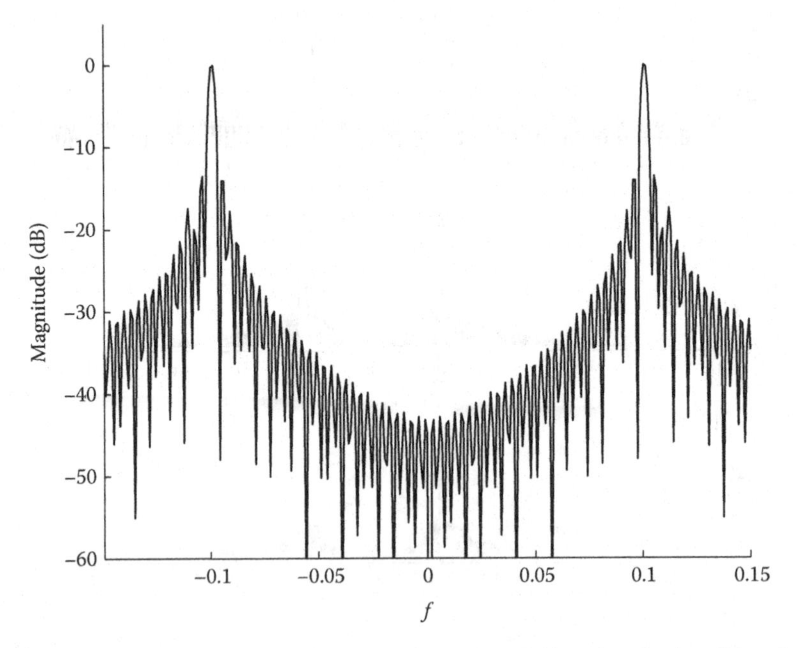

FIGURE 2.7 Spectrum of the sum of two sine waves [$x(n) = 2\cos(\omega_1 n) + 0.1\cos(\omega_2 n)$] truncated using a rectangular window.

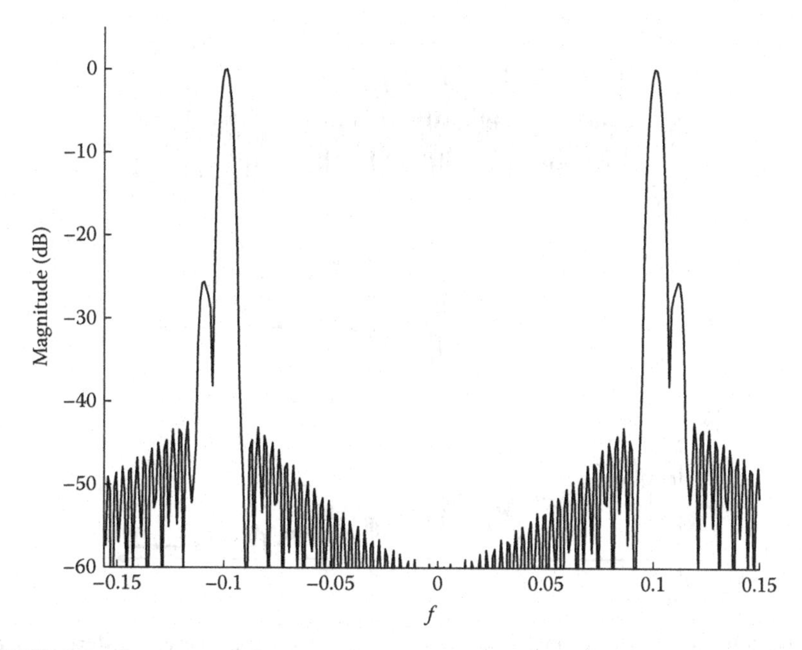

FIGURE 2.8 Spectrum of the sum of two sine waves [$x(n) = 2\cos(\omega_1 n) + 0.1\cos(\omega_2 n)$] truncated using a Hamming window.

2.5 SHORT-TIME FOURIER TRANSFORM

In the previous section, we presented the DTFT. This Fourier transform representation is more appropriate for stationary or deterministic signals and not necessarily for speech signals with temporal and spectral characteristics changing markedly over time. The DTFT representation is, however, applicable to speech processing, provided we consider analysis of short segments (10–30 ms) of speech, during which the properties of speech do not change much.

In this section, we introduce a time-varying Fourier representation that reflects the time-varying properties of the speech waveform. In-depth coverage of the short-time Fourier transform (STFT) can be found in [4, Ch. 7; 5, Ch. 6; 6].

2.5.1 Definition

The STFT is given by

$$X(n,\omega) = \sum_{m=-\infty}^{\infty} x(m)w(n-m)\, e^{-j\omega m} \tag{2.64}$$

where $x(m)$ is the input signal and $w(m)$ is the analysis window, which is time-reversed and shifted by n samples (see example in Figure 2.9). The STFT is a function of two variables: the discrete-time index, n, and the (continuous) frequency variable, ω. To obtain $X(n + 1, \omega)$, we slide the window by one sample, multiply it with $x(m)$, and

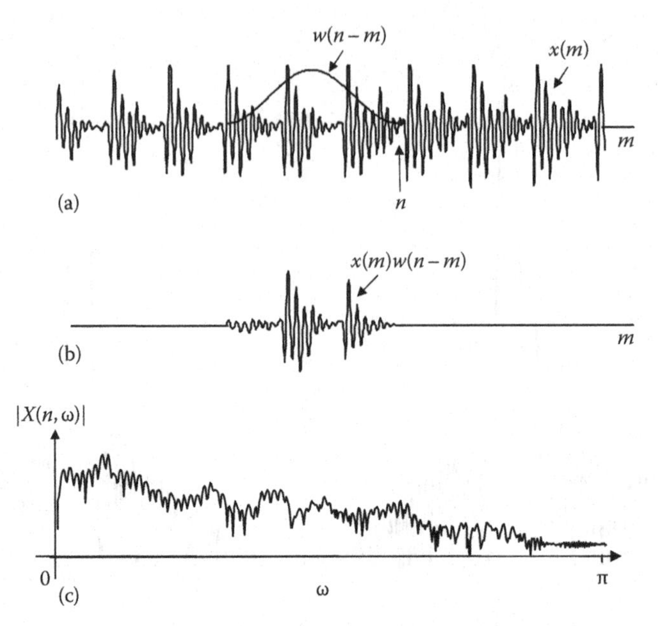

FIGURE 2.9 Steps involved in the computation of the short-time Fourier transform, $X(n, \omega)$: (a) the window (Hamming window, in this example) shifted by n samples, (b) the windowed signal, and (c) the magnitude spectrum of the windowed signal.

compute the Fourier transform of the windowed signal. Continuing this way, we generate a set of STFTs for various values of n until we reach the end of the signal $x(m)$. Note that the two-dimensional function $|X(n, \omega)|^2$ provides the so-called spectrogram of the speech signal—a two-dimensional display of the power spectrum of speech as a function of time. This is a widely used tool employed for studying the time-varying spectral and temporal characteristics of speech (more on this in Section 2.6).

Figure 2.9 shows the steps involved in the computation of the STFT, $X(n, \omega)$. Figure 2.9a shows the window (Hamming window, in this example) shifted by n samples, Figure 2.9b shows the windowed signal, and Figure 2.9c shows the magnitude spectrum of the windowed signal.

Similar to the discrete Fourier transform derivation, one can obtain a discrete version of the STFT by sampling the frequency variable ω at N uniformly spaced frequencies, that is, at $\omega_k = 2\pi k/N$, $k = 0, 1, \ldots, N-1$. The resulting discrete STFT is defined as

$$X(n,\omega_k) \triangleq X(n,k) = \sum_{m=-\infty}^{\infty} x(m)w(n-m)\, e^{-j\frac{2\pi}{N}km} \tag{2.65}$$

The STFT $X(n, \omega)$ can be interpreted in two distinct ways, depending on how we treat the time (n) and frequency (ω) variables. If, for instance, we assume that n is fixed but ω varies, then $X(n, \omega)$ can be viewed as the Fourier transform of a windowed sequence. If we assume that ω is fixed and the time index n varies, a filtering interpretation emerges.

2.5.2 Interpretations of the STFT

We begin with the Fourier transform interpretation in which the time index n is held fixed. When comparing the equation of the DTFT (Equation 2.33) with the equation of the STFT (Equation 2.64) for a fixed value of n, we observe that $X(n, \omega)$ is the normal DTFT of the sequence $x(n-m)w(m)$. As such, $X(n, \omega)$ has the same properties as the DTFT.

The STFT can also be viewed as the output of a filtering operation. For this interpretation, we fix the value of ω at, say, ω_k and vary the time index n. We can rewrite Equation 2.64 as the convolution of two sequences:

$$\begin{aligned} X(n,\omega_k) &= \sum_{m=-\infty}^{\infty}\left[x(m)e^{-j\omega_k m}\right]\cdot w(n-m) \\ &= \left[x(n)e^{-j\omega_k n}\right] * w(n) \end{aligned} \tag{2.66}$$

The STFT at frequency ω_k can be viewed as the output of a system with input $x(n)e^{-j\omega_k n}$ and impulse response $w(n)$. The analysis window $w(n)$ plays here the role of the filter's impulse response and is sometimes called the *analysis filter*. The signal $x(n)$ is first multiplied by $e^{-j\omega_k n}$ (corresponding to a shift in the frequency domain by ω_k), and the output signal is passed through a filter whose impulse response is $w(n)$ (see Figure 2.10). After making use of the modulation (Equation 2.44) and convolution (Equation 2.47) properties of the DTFT, we can express Equation 2.66 in the frequency domain in terms of the individual DTFTs of the two signals, that is,

$$X(n,\omega_k) = X(\omega+\omega_k)W(\omega) \tag{2.67}$$

where

$W(\omega)$ is the DTFT of $w(n)$

$X(\omega)$ is the DTFT of $x(n)$

This filtering operation is shown graphically in Figure 2.10.

Yet another interpretation of the STFT can be obtained as follows. Letting $m' = n - m$ in Equation 2.64 and changing the summation indices accordingly, we can express $X(n, \omega)$ as follows:

$$\begin{aligned} X(n,\omega) &= \sum_{m=-\infty}^{\infty} x(n-m)w(m)\, e^{-j\omega(n-m)} \\ &= e^{-j\omega n}\sum_{m=-\infty}^{\infty} x(n-m)w(m)\, e^{j\omega m} \end{aligned} \tag{2.68}$$

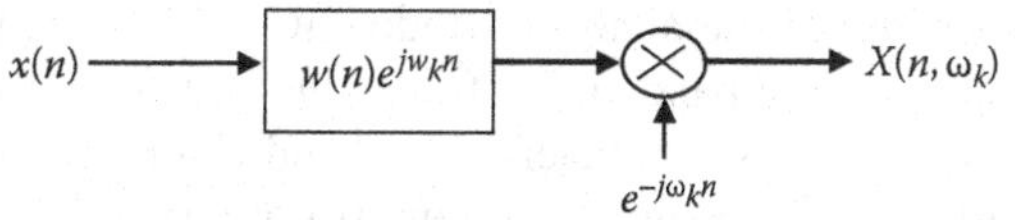

FIGURE 2.10 Variant filtering interpretation of the short-time Fourier transform.

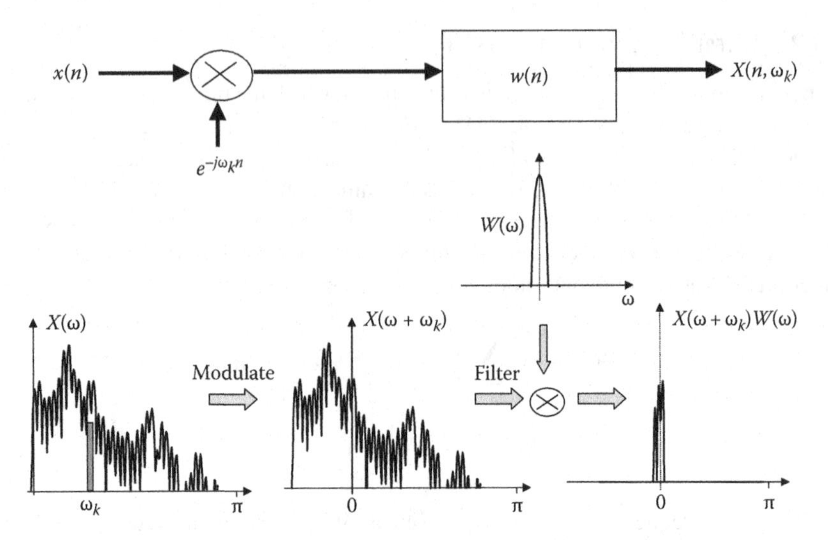

FIGURE 2.11 Filtering interpretation of the short-time Fourier transform.

Realizing that the summation term in the previous equation is nothing but the convolution of the signal $x(n)$ with $w(n)e^{-j\omega_k n}$, we can express $X(n, \omega)$ at $\omega = \omega_k$ as

$$X(n,\omega_k) = e^{-j\omega_k n}\left[x(n) * w(n)e^{j\omega_k n}\right] \tag{2.69}$$

This filtering operation is depicted in Figure 2.11.

2.5.3 Sampling the STFT in Time and Frequency

The STFT $X(n,\omega)$ is a two-dimensional function of time n and frequency ω. In principle, $X(n,\omega)$ can be evaluated for each value of n; however, in practice, $X(n,\omega)$ is decimated in time due partly to the heavy computational load involved and partly to the redundancy of information contained in consecutive values of $X(n,\omega)$ (e.g., between $X(n,\omega)$ and $X(n + 1^{®}\omega)$). Hence, in most practical applications $X(n,\omega)$ is not evaluated for every sample but for every R sample, where R corresponds to the decimation factor, often expressed as a fraction of the window length. The sampling, in both time and frequency, has to be done in such a way that $x(n)$ can be recovered from $X(n,\omega)$ without aliasing.

We first consider the sampling of $X(n,\omega)$ in time. For that, we will use the filtering interpretation of the STFT. It is clear from Equation 2.67 and Figure 2.10 that the bandwidth of the sequence $X(n,\omega_k)$ (along n, for a fixed frequency ω_k) is less than or equal to the bandwidth of the analysis window $w(n)$. This suggests that $X(n,\omega_k)$ has to be sampled at twice the bandwidth of the window $w(n)$ to satisfy the Nyquist sampling criterion. If, for instance, the effective bandwidth of the analysis window is B Hz, then according to the Nyquist theorem $X(n,\omega_k)$ has to be sampled at a rate of $2B$ samples/second.

Let us consider, for example, the L-point Hamming window, which has an effective bandwidth of [3, p. 44]

$$B = \frac{2F_s}{L}\,\text{Hz} \tag{2.70}$$

where F_s is the sampling frequency. For this window, $X(n, \omega_k)$ has to be sampled in time at a minimum rate of $2B$ samples/second = $4F_s/L$ samples/second to avoid time aliasing. The corresponding sampling period is $L/(4F_s)$ second or $L/4$ samples. This means that for an L-point Hamming window, $X(n, \omega_k)$ needs to be evaluated at most every $L/4$ samples, corresponding to a minimum overlap of 75% between adjacent windows. This rather strict requirement on the minimum amount of overlap between adjacent windows can be relaxed if we allow zeros in the window transform [4, Ch. 7]. In speech enhancement applications, it is quite common to use a 50% rather than 75% overlap between adjacent windows. This implies that $X(n, \omega_k)$ is evaluated every $L/2$ samples; that is, it is decimated by a factor of $L/2$, where L is the window length.

The sampling requirement in the frequency domain can be derived using the Fourier transform interpretation of the STFT. We know that the STFT $X(n, \omega_k)$ (for fixed n) is the DTFT of the windowed sequence $w(m)x(n-m)$. Hence, to recover the windowed sequence $w(m)x(n-m)$ with no aliasing, we require that the frequency variable ω be sampled at N ($N \geq L$) uniformly spaced frequencies, that is, at $\omega_k = 2\pi k/N$, $k = 0, 1, \ldots, N-1$.

2.5.4 Short-Time Synthesis of Speech

Given $X(n, \omega)$, it is necessary to reconstruct the time sequence $x(n)$. This is represented mathematically by a *synthesis equation* that expresses $x(n)$ in terms of its STFT. Consider, for example, the Fourier transform interpretation of the STFT. The fact that $X(n, \omega)$ is the DTFT of the windowed sequence $w(n-m)x(m)$ (for a fixed value of n) implies that the sequence $w(n-m)x(m)$ can be recovered exactly via the use of the inverse DTFT, that is,

$$w(n-m)x(m) = \frac{1}{2\pi}\int_{-\pi}^{\pi} X(n,\omega)e^{j\omega n}\, d\omega \tag{2.71}$$

Assuming $w(0) \neq 0$ and after evaluating Equation 2.71 at $m = n$, we obtain

$$x(m) = \frac{1}{2\pi w(0)}\int_{-\pi}^{\pi} X(m,\omega)e^{j\omega m}\, d\omega \tag{2.72}$$

This equation clearly demonstrates that it is possible to recover $x(n)$ exactly from its STFT. Equation 2.72 represents one of many synthesis equations for the STFT. This equation is inefficient, however, in that it requires that the analysis window slides one sample at a time. In practice, more efficient methods can be used, which impose certain constraints on the properties of the windows as well as the time and frequency sampling resolution of $X(n, \omega)$.

We describe next two classical methods, the filterbank summation method and the overlap-add method [7–9], for short-time synthesis of speech. Of the two methods, the overlap-add method is typically used in speech enhancement. Other methods based on least-squares estimates of $x(n)$ from its STFT were proposed in [10].

2.5.4.1 Filterbank Summation for Short-Time Synthesis of Speech

This synthesis method is based on the filterbank interpretation of the STFT. From Equation 2.68, we have

$$X(n,\omega_k) = e^{-j\omega_k n} \sum_{m=-\infty}^{\infty} x(n-m) w_k(m) e^{j\omega_k m} \tag{2.73}$$

where $w_k(m)$ denotes the window applied at frequency ω_k. Defining $h_k(n)$ as

$$h_k(n) = w_k(n) e^{j\omega_k n} \tag{2.74}$$

we can write Equation 2.73 as

$$\begin{aligned} X(n,\omega_k) &= e^{-j\omega_k n} \sum_{m=-\infty}^{\infty} x(n-m) h_k(m) \\ &= e^{-j\omega_k n} y_k(n) \end{aligned} \tag{2.75}$$

where $y_k(n)$ is defined as follows:

$$y_k(n) = \sum_{m=-\infty}^{\infty} x(n-m) h_k(m) \tag{2.76}$$

We observe from Equation 2.76 that $y_k(n)$ can be viewed as the output of a system with impulse response $h_k(n)$ at frequency ω_k (see Figure 2.12). From Equation 2.75, $y_k(n)$ can also be expressed as

$$y_k(n) = X(n,\omega_k) e^{j\omega_k n} \tag{2.77}$$

and the reconstructed signal is formed as

$$\begin{aligned} y(n) &= \sum_{k=0}^{N-1} y_k(n) \\ &= \sum_{k=0}^{N-1} X(n,\omega_k) e^{j\omega_k n} \end{aligned} \tag{2.78}$$

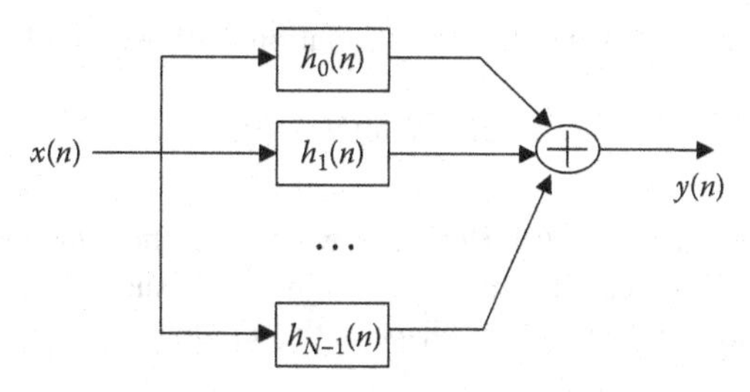

FIGURE 2.12 Filtering interpretation of the filterbank summation method for short-time speech synthesis.

where N is the number of uniformly spaced frequencies. The filtering interpretation of Equation 2.78 is shown in Figure 2.12. Note that Equation 2.78 gives the equation of the inverse discrete Fourier transform of $X(n, \omega_k)$ provided that $X(n, \omega_k)$ is properly sampled in frequency at N uniformly spaced frequencies, that is, at $\omega_k = 2\pi k/N$, $k = 0, 1, \ldots, N-1$, where $N \geq L$, and L is the window duration.

To find the relationship between $x(n)$ and $y(n)$, we consider the filtering operation in Figure 2.12 in the frequency domain. From Figure 2.12 and after using the distributive property of the convolution (Equation 2.19), we have

$$\begin{aligned} Y(\omega) &= X(\omega)H(\omega) \\ &= X(\omega)\cdot\sum_{k=0}^{N-1} H_k(\omega_k) \end{aligned} \tag{2.79}$$

where $H_k(\omega)_k$ is the frequency response of the filter $h_k(n)$.

From Equation 2.74 we see that if $w_k(n)$ is the impulse response of a low-pass filter with cutoff frequency ω_c, then the frequency response of the filter $h_k(n)$ will be (due to the modulation property) that of a band-pass filter with center frequency ω_k and bandwidth $2\omega_c$. If we consider N such band-pass filters, then we will be able to cover the entire signal bandwidth. The frequency response of the kth band-pass filter, $H_k(\omega)$, is then given by

$$H_k(\omega) = W_k(\omega - \omega_k) \tag{2.80}$$

where $W_k(\omega)$ is the Fourier transform of $w_k(n)$. Hence, $H_k(\omega)$ is equal to the frequency response of the low-pass filter $W_k(\omega)$ shifted at frequency ω_k (the shift comes from the modulation property of the Fourier transform). If we assume that the same window $w_k(n)$ is used for all frequencies, that is, $w_k(n) = w(n)$ for all k, and that $W(\omega)$ is properly sampled in frequency (i.e., $N \geq L$, where L is the time duration of the window), then it can be shown that [5, p. 269]

$$\frac{1}{N}\sum_{k=0}^{N-1} W(\omega - \omega_k) = w(0) \tag{2.81}$$

Substituting Equations 2.80 and 2.81 into Equation 2.79, we finally get

$$Y(\omega) = X(\omega)N \cdot w(0) \tag{2.82}$$

or equivalently, $y(n) = x(n)N \cdot w(0)$. Hence, provided that the window $w(n)$ has a finite duration L (and $N \geq L$), we can reconstruct the signal $x(n)$ exactly from its STFT $X(n, \omega)$. This can be done independently of the shape of the window $w(n)$.

2.5.4.2 Overlap-and-Add Method for Short-Time Synthesis

An alternative method for reconstructing $x(n)$ from its STFT is the overlap-and-add method, which is widely used in speech enhancement.

Assume that the STFT $X(n, \omega)$ is sampled in time every R samples. We denote this sampling in the time dimension by $X(rR, \omega)$. The overlap-and-add method is motivated by the discretized version of Equation 2.72 and is based on the following equation [4, p. 325; 5, p. 275]:

$$y(n) = \sum_{r=-\infty}^{\infty} \left[\frac{1}{N} \sum_{k=0}^{N-1} X(rR, \omega_k) e^{j\omega_k n} \right] \tag{2.83}$$

The term in brackets (see also Equation 2.78) is an inverse discrete Fourier transform yielding for each value of r the sequence

$$y_r(n) = x(n)w(rR - n) \tag{2.84}$$

and therefore, Equation 2.83 can be expressed as

$$y(n) = \sum_{r=-\infty}^{\infty} y_r(n) = x(n) \sum_{r=-\infty}^{\infty} w(rR - n) \tag{2.85}$$

From Equation 2.85 we see that the signal $y(n)$ at time n is obtained by summing all the sequences $y_r(n)$ that overlap at time n. Provided that the summation term in Equation 2.85 is constant for all n, we can recover $x(n)$ exactly (within a constant) as

$$y(n) = C \cdot x(n) \tag{2.86}$$

where C is a constant. It can be shown that if $X(n, \omega)$ is sampled properly in time, that is, R is small enough to avoid time aliasing (see Section 2.5), then C is equal to [5, p. 275]

$$C = \sum_{r=-\infty}^{\infty} w(rR - n) = \frac{W(0)}{R} \tag{2.87}$$

independent of the time n. Equations 2.86 and 2.87 indicate that $x(n)$ can be reconstructed exactly (within a constant) by adding overlapping sections of the windowed sequences $y_r(n)$. The constraint imposed on the window is that it satisfies Equation 2.87; that is, the sum of all analysis windows shifted by increments of R samples adds up to a constant. Furthermore, R needs to be small enough to avoid time aliasing. For an L-point Hamming window, R has to be set to, $R = L/4$ suggesting that adjacent windows overlap by 75%. According to Equation 2.85, if $R = L/4$ the signal $y(n)$ consists of four terms:

$$y(n) = x(n)w(R-n)+x(n)w(2R-n)+x(n)w(3R-n)+x(n)w(4R-n) \quad (2.88)$$

where $0 \leq n \leq R - 1$. With $R = L/2$ (i.e., 50% window overlap), which is most commonly used in speech enhancement, the signal $y(n)$ consists of two terms:

$$y(n) = x(n)w(R-n)+x(n)w(2R-n) \quad (2.89)$$

for $0 \leq n \leq R - 1$. Figure 2.13 shows how the overlap addition is implemented for an L-point Hamming window with 50% overlap ($R = L/2$). In the context of speech enhancement, the enhanced output signal in frame t consists of the sum of the windowed signal [with $w(R - n)$] enhanced in the previous frame ($t - 1$) and the windowed signal [with $w(2R - n)$] enhanced in the present frame (t).

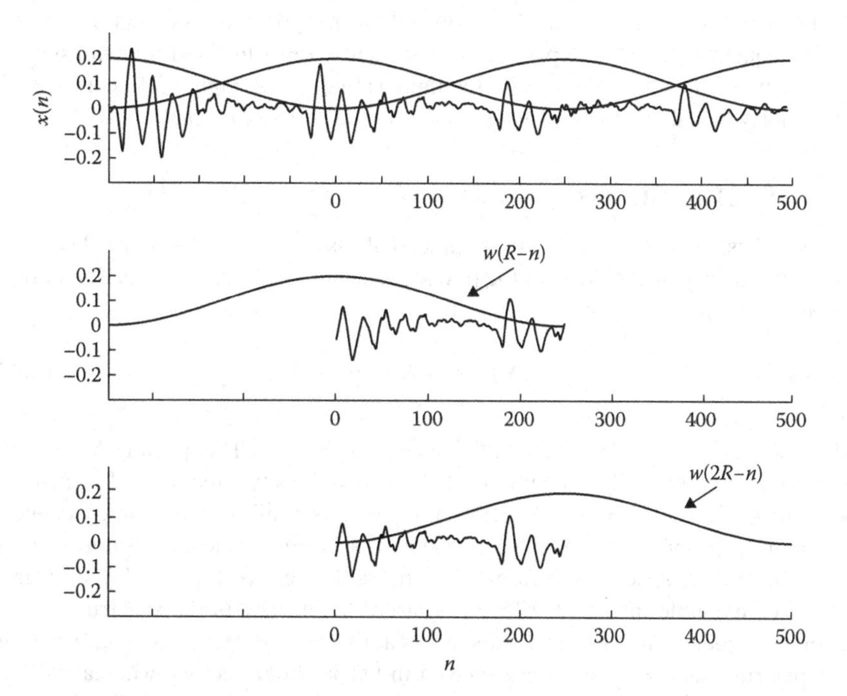

FIGURE 2.13 Example of reconstruction procedure for overlap-and-add method with 50% overlap. Window length is 500 samples ($L = 500$) and $R = L/2$.

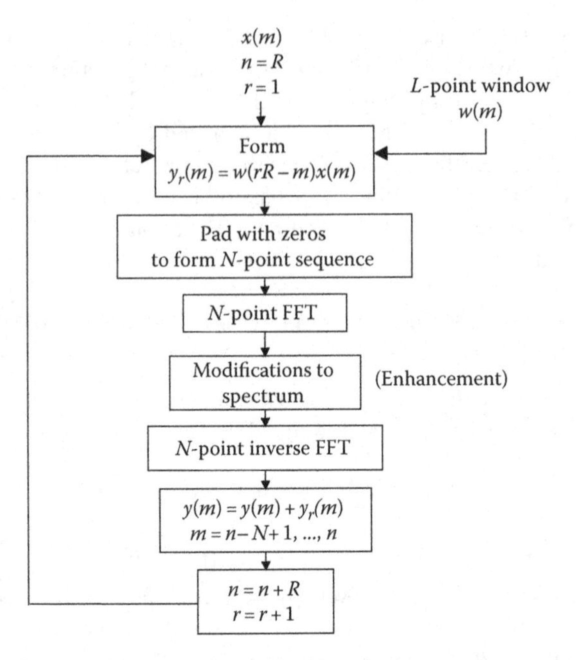

FIGURE 2.14 Flow diagram of overlap-and-add method.

Figure 2.14 shows the flow diagram of the overlap-and-add method, which can be used in any frequency domain speech enhancement algorithm. Note that the L-point signal sequence needs to be padded with sufficient zeros to avoid time aliasing. In the context of speech enhancement, the input signal $x(n)$ in Figure 2.13 corresponds to the noisy signal and the output signal $y(n)$ to the enhanced signal.

2.6 SPECTROGRAPHIC ANALYSIS OF SPEECH SIGNALS

The STFT is often used for spectrographic analysis of the speech signals. The *spectrogram* is a graphical display of the power spectrum of speech as a function of time and is given by

$$S(n, \omega) = |X(n, \omega)|^2 \tag{2.90}$$

where $X(n, \omega)$ denotes the STFT of the speech signal $x(n)$. The quantity $S(n, \omega)$ can be viewed as a two-dimensional "power-spectral density," the second dimension being time. The spectrogram describes the speech signal's relative energy concentration in frequency as a function of time and, as such, it reflects the time-varying properties of the speech waveform. Spectrograms are typically displayed in gray scale (see example in Figure 2.15). The larger the energy in the spectrum is at a specific frequency, the darker the display is at that frequency. Large magnitudes in the spectrum such as peaks are displayed in black or dark colors, whereas valleys are displayed in white colors (see example in Figure 2.15). Values falling between peaks and valleys are displayed using different shades of gray.

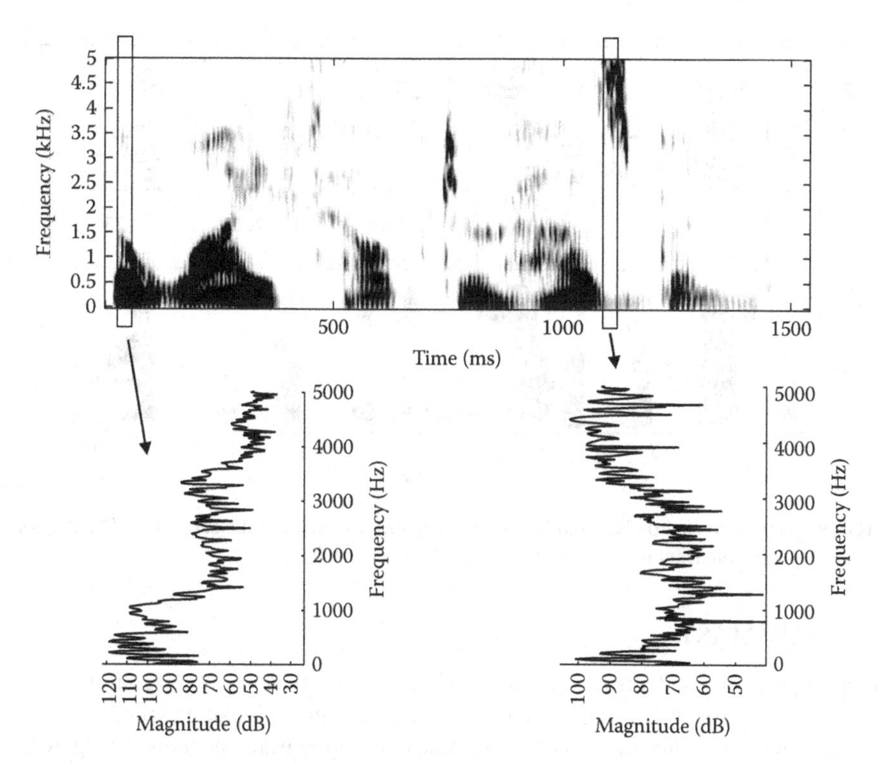

FIGURE 2.15 Spectrogram of the sentence "The wife helped her husband" produced by a male speaker. Bottom panels show the magnitude FFT spectrum obtained at two instances in time enclosed by the rectangles in the spectrogram.

Two kinds of spectrograms, *narrowband* and *wideband,* can be produced, depending on the window length used in the computation of $S(n, \omega)$. A long-duration window (at least two pitch periods long) is typically used in the computation of the narrowband spectrogram and a short window in the computation of the wideband spectrogram. The narrowband spectrogram gives good frequency resolution but poor time resolution. The fine frequency resolution allows the individual harmonics of speech to be resolved. These harmonics appear as horizontal striations in the spectrogram (see example in Figure 2.16a). The main drawback of using long windows is the possibility of temporally smearing short-duration segments of speech, such as the stop consonants. The wideband spectrogram uses short-duration windows (less than a pitch period) and gives good temporal resolution but poor frequency resolution. The main consequence of the poor frequency resolution is the smearing (in frequency) of individual harmonics in the speech spectrum, yielding only the spectral envelope of the spectrum (see example in Figure 2.16b). The wideband spectrogram provides good temporal resolution, making it suitable for analysis and examination of all sounds in the English language. The wideband spectrogram is an invaluable tool for speech analysis, and we will be using it throughout the text.

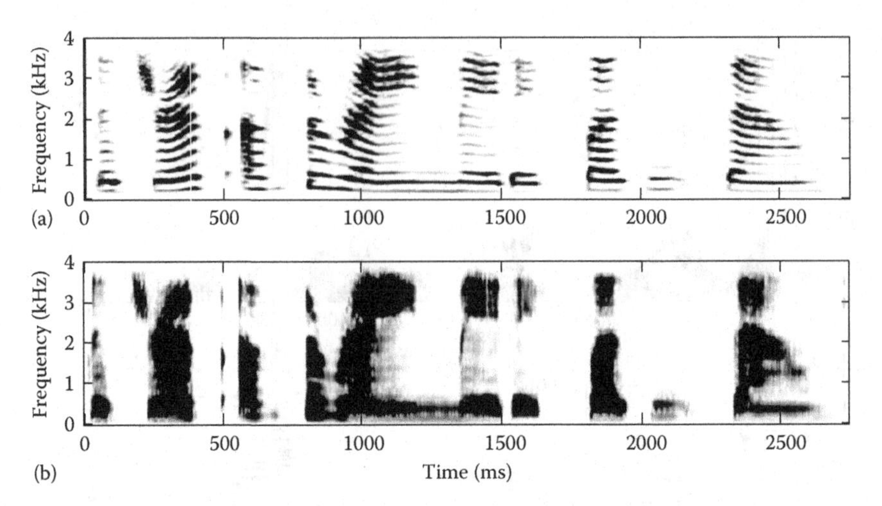

FIGURE 2.16 (a) Narrowband and (b) wideband spectrograms of the sentence "The drip of the rain made a pleasant sound" produced by a female speaker.

2.7 SUMMARY

This chapter provided a review of the fundamentals of discrete-time signal processing (a more thorough coverage of signal processing principles can be found in [1,2]). We reviewed discrete-time signals and linear time-invariant systems, along with their z-transform and Fourier transform representations. The concept of windowing was covered, as most enhancement algorithms operate on a frame-by-frame basis rather than on a sample-by-sample basis. We introduced the STFT as a more suitable tool for representing the speech signal with temporal and spectral characteristics changing markedly over time. We mentioned that the DTFT representation is still applicable to speech processing provided we consider analysis of short segments (10–30 ms) of speech, during which the properties of speech do not change much. We presented the overlap-and-add method as a common synthesis approach used by nearly all speech enhancement algorithms. Lastly, we introduced the spectrogram (derived from the STFT) as a valuable tool that can be used to obtain a time-frequency representation of speech.

REFERENCES

1. Proakis, J. and Manolakis, D. (1996), *Digital Signal Processing*, 3rd ed., Upper Saddle River, NJ: Prentice Hall.
2. Oppenheim, A., Schafer, R., and Buck, J. (1999), *Discrete-Time Signal Processing*, 2nd ed., Upper Saddle River, NJ: Prentice Hall.
3. Stoica, P. and Moses, R. (1997), *Introduction to Spectral Analysis*, Upper Saddle River, NJ: Prentice Hall.
4. Quatieri, T. (2002), *Discrete-Time Speech Signal Processing*, Upper Saddle River, NJ: Prentice Hall.
5. Rabiner, L. and Schafer, R. (1978), *Digital Processing of Speech Signals*, Englewood Cliffs, NJ: Prentice Hall.

6. Nawab, S. and Quatieri, T. (1987), Short-time Fourier transform, in Lim, J. and Oppenheim, A. (Eds.), *Advanced Topics in Signal Processing*, Englewood Cliffs, NJ: Prentice Hall.
7. Allen, J. and Rabiner, L. (1977), A unified theory of short-time spectrum analysis and synthesis, *Proc. IEEE*, 65(11), 1558–1564.
8. Portnoff, M. (1980), Time-frequency representation of digital signals and systems based on short-time Fourier analysis, *IEEE Trans. Acoust. Speech Signal Process.*, 28(1), 55–69.
9. Crochiere, R. E. (1980), A weighted overlap-add method of short-time Fourier analysis/synthesis, *IEEE Trans. Acoust. Speech Signal Process.*, 28(1), 99–102.
10. Griffin, D. and Lim, J. (1984), Signal estimation from modified short-time Fourier analysis/synthesis, *IEEE Trans. Acoust. Speech Signal Process.*, 32(2), 236–243.

3 Speech Production and Perception

Before beginning to describe speech enhancement algorithms, it is important that we become acquainted with the speech signal, the speech production process, and the various acoustic cues used by listeners for speech perception. In doing so, we will gain an understanding of the properties and characteristics of the speech signal, and particularly the elements of the speech signal that need to be preserved (or at least preferentially enhanced) to maintain high quality and intelligibility in noisy environments.

3.1 SPEECH SIGNAL

The speech signal is a highly nonstationary signal in that its second-order statistics (power spectrum) change over time. When examined closely, however, over a sufficiently short period of time (10–30 ms), its spectral characteristics are fairly stationary. Figure 3.1 shows an example time waveform of the sentence "The wife helped her husband." The signal waveform can be broken into a number of segments or events corresponding to different sounds/words spoken. As shown in Figure 3.1, some speech segments are quasi-periodic, for instance, during the syllable "er" in "h<u>er</u>." Other segments are aperiodic and noiselike, for instance, during the production of the consonant/f/in "wi<u>f</u>e." Other segments may contain brief silence gaps even amid the sentence (see arrow in Figure 3.1). Some segments have large intensity (e.g., sound "i" in "w<u>i</u>fe"), whereas other segments have low intensity (e.g., consonant/f/). In general, the duration, intensity, and spectrum of each segment will be highly variable between speakers and across different utterances.

The preceding types of speech segments—periodic, noiselike, and silence—are commonly found in fluent speech with variable intensities, durations, and spectral characteristics. Next, we describe how these segments of the speech signal are produced by the human speech production system.

3.2 SPEECH PRODUCTION PROCESS

Figure 3.2 shows a cross-sectional view of the anatomy of speech production. As shown, speech production involves a number of organs and muscles and includes the lungs, the larynx, and the vocal tract.

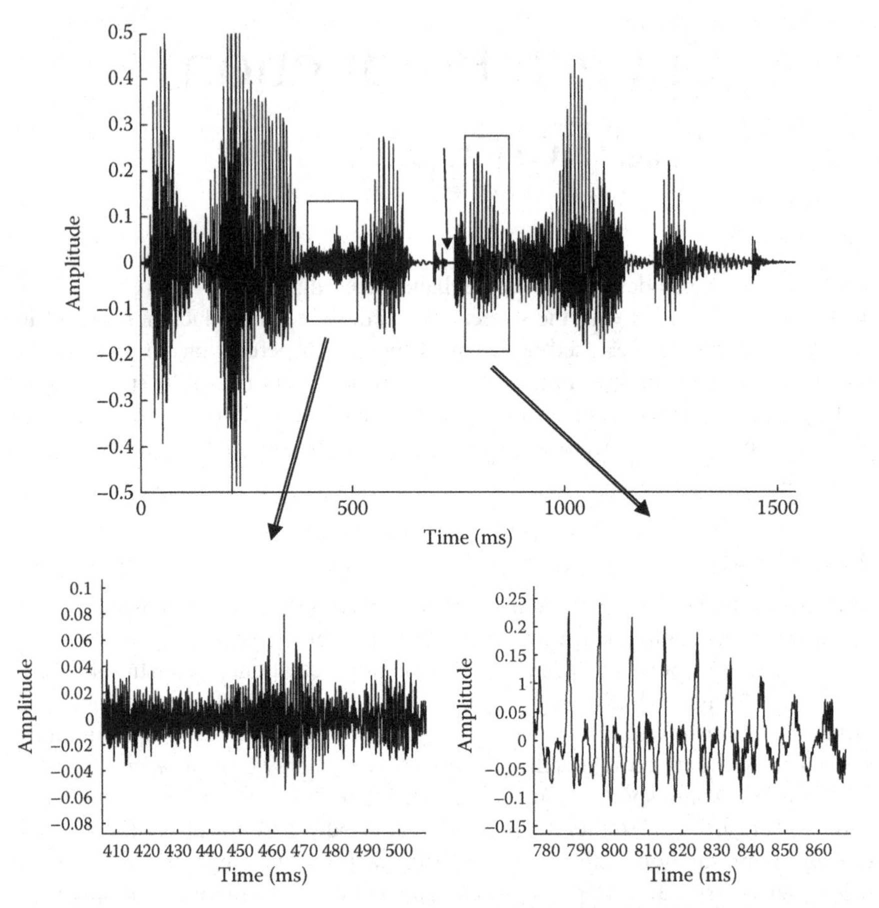

FIGURE 3.1 Time waveform of the sentence "The wife helped her husband" produced by a male speaker. Bottom zoomed-in plots show the waveform of the vocalic segment "er" in "h<u>er</u>" and the consonant "f" in "wi<u>f</u>e." Note that the vocalic segment is quasi-periodic, whereas the other segment is noiselike. The arrow in the middle of the waveform points to a brief silent gap occurring during the production of "p" in "helped."

3.2.1 Lungs

The lungs, which are used for the purpose of oxygenating the blood by inhalation and exhalation of air, provide the main source of excitation in speech production. When inhaling air, the chest cavity is enlarged (by expanding the rib cage and lowering the diaphragm), which in turn lowers the air pressure in the lungs and causes air to go through the vocal tract, down the trachea (also called *windpipe*) and into the lungs. When exhaling air, the volume of the chest cavity is reduced (by contracting the rib cage muscles), which in turn causes the lung air pressure to increase. This increase in pressure causes air to flow through the trachea into the larynx.

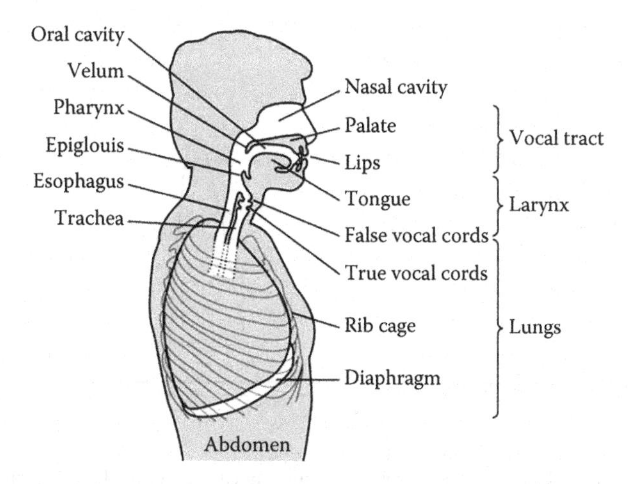

FIGURE 3.2 Cross section of the anatomy of speech production. (Reprinted from Quatieri, T., *Discrete-Time Speech Signal Processing*, Prentice Hall, Upper Saddle River, NJ, 2002. With permission.)

3.2.2 Larynx and Vocal Folds

The larynx, composed of muscles, ligaments, and cartilages, controls the function of the *vocal folds* (or *vocal cords*). The vocal folds are two masses of ligament and muscle stretching from the posterior to the anterior of the larynx. The *glottis* is the opening between the two folds. The posterior ends of the folds are attached to two arytenoid cartilages that move laterally along with the cricoid cartilage (Figure 3.3).

The vocal folds can assume three states: breathing, voiced, and unvoiced. In the breathing state, the air from the lungs flows freely through the glottis (which is wide open) with no notable resistance from the vocal folds. In the voicing state, as during the production of a vowel (e.g., /aa/), the arytenoid cartilages move toward one another, bringing the vocal folds closer together (see Figure 3.3). An increase and decrease of tension of the folds, together with a decrease and increase in pressure at the glottis,

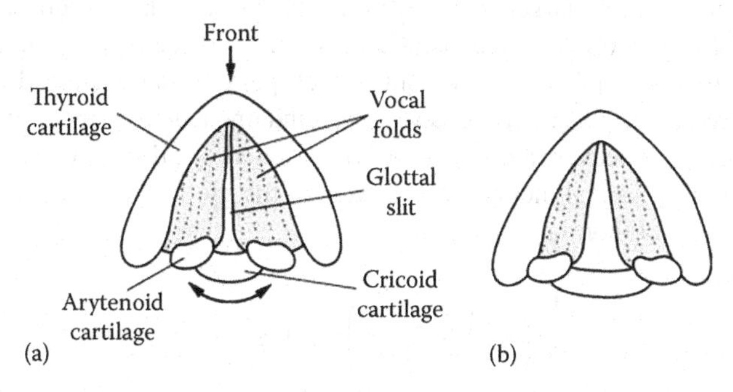

FIGURE 3.3 Sketch of vocal folds, looking down the larynx, in two states: (a) voicing and (b) breathing. (Reprinted from Quatieri, T., *Discrete-Time Speech Signal Processing*, Prentice Hall, Upper Saddle River, NJ, 2002. With permission.)

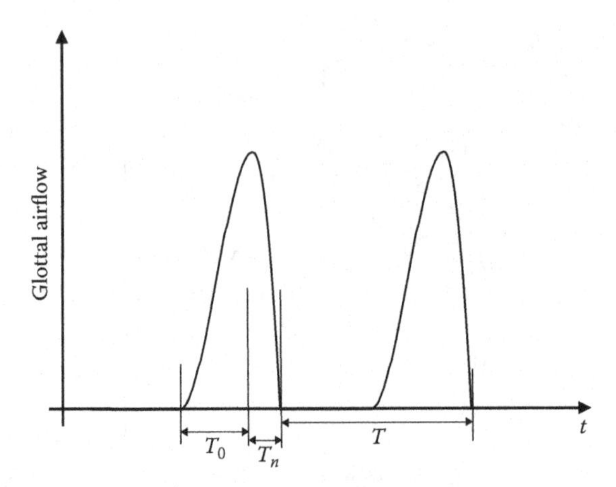

FIGURE 3.4 Glottal airflow waveform. The pitch period is labeled T. The ratios T_0/T and T_n/T controlling the shape of the glottal pulse were set to 0.4 and 0.16, respectively, as per [3]. (From Rosenberg, A., *J. Acoust. Soc. Am.*, 49(2), 583, 1971.)

cause the folds to open and close periodically. This periodic opening and closing of the folds can be explained using Bernoulli's fluid dynamic principle [1, p. 80]. Two aerodynamic forces are responsible for the vibration of the vocal folds: (a) the air pressure that is applied to the lower part of the folds forcing them apart and (b) the negative pressure that occurs as air passes between the folds (Bernoulli effect).

If we were to measure the airflow velocity at the glottis as a function of time, we would obtain a waveform similar to that shown in Figure 3.4. When the folds are shut, the airflow begins slowly, builds up to a maximum, and then suddenly decreases to zero, at which point the folds close. When the folds are closed, no airflow goes to the vocal tract, and this phase is referred to as the glottal *closed phase*. The period during which the vocal folds are open is referred to as the glottal *open phase*. The time duration of one glottal cycle is known as the *pitch period*, and the reciprocal of the pitch period is known as the *fundamental frequency* (expressed in Hz). The rate at which the vocal folds oscillate (i.e., the pitch frequency) is influenced primarily by the elasticity and mass of the folds. If the folds' mass is large, then they will be sluggish and, consequently, the pitch period will be longer (or the fundamental frequency will be lower). Males typically have a lower fundamental frequency (longer pitch period) than females because their vocal folds are longer and more massive. The fundamental frequency range is about 60–150 Hz for male speakers and 200–400 Hz for females and children [2].

A simple mathematical model for one cycle of the glottal flow waveform is given by the following polynomial relationship [3]:

$$g(n) = \begin{cases} 3\left(\dfrac{n}{T_0}\right)^2 - 2\left(\dfrac{n}{T_0}\right)^3 & 0 \le n \le T_0 \\ 1 - \left(\dfrac{n - T_0}{T_N}\right)^2 & T_0 < n \le T_0 + T_N \end{cases} \tag{3.1}$$

where

T_0 is the interval between the end of the closed phase and the peak of the open phase (see Figure 3.4)

T_N is the time interval between the peak of the open phase and the end of the open phase

The preceding glottal waveform has been used successfully in speech synthesizers to yield high-quality speech [4].

Example 3.1:

Determine the Fourier transform of the glottal waveform shown in Figure 3.4 assuming that (a) the glottal waveform is infinitely long and (b) the waveform has finite duration.

Assuming that the glottal waveform is infinitely long (i.e., no window is applied), it can be expressed mathematically as

$$g_M(n) = g(n) * p(n) \tag{3.2}$$

where $p(n)$ is an impulse train, that is, $p(n) = \sum_{k=-\infty}^{\infty} \delta(n - kT)$, and T is the pitch period. Using the convolution property (Equation 2.47) of the Fourier transform and the impulse property, we can compute the Fourier transform of $g_M(n)$ as follows:

$$\begin{aligned} G_M(\omega) &= G(\omega) \cdot \frac{2\pi}{T} \sum_{k=-\infty}^{\infty} \delta\left(\omega - \frac{2\pi}{T}k\right) \\ &= \frac{2\pi}{T} \sum_{k=-\infty}^{\infty} G(\omega)\delta\left(\omega - \frac{2\pi}{T}k\right) \\ &= \frac{2\pi}{T} \sum_{k=-\infty}^{\infty} G\left(\frac{2\pi}{T}k\right)\delta\left(\omega - \frac{2\pi}{T}k\right) \end{aligned} \tag{3.3}$$

where $G(\omega)$ is the Fourier transform of $g(n)$. As indicated by the preceding equation, $G_M(\omega)$ consists of a sequence of impulses in the frequency domain, and the impulses are spaced $2\pi/T$ apart. Hence, $G_M(\omega)$ has a harmonic spectrum and the individual harmonics are spaced $2\pi/T$ apart. The amplitudes of the impulses are determined by the envelope of $G(\omega)$.

We now consider the case that the glottal waveform is defined over a few pitch periods, that is, it is windowed in time. The windowed signal is given by $g_W(n) = g_M(n)w(n)$, where $w(n)$ is the windowing function. Using the multiplication property of the Fourier transform (Equation 2.46), we can compute the Fourier transform of $g_W(n)$ as follows:

$$G_W(\omega) = \frac{1}{2\pi} W(\omega) \otimes \frac{2\pi}{T} \sum_{k=-\infty}^{\infty} G(\omega_k)\delta(\omega - \omega_k)$$

$$= \frac{1}{T} \sum_{k=-\infty}^{\infty} G(\omega_k) W(\omega - \omega_k) \tag{3.4}$$

where

$\omega_k = (2\pi/T)k$

$\otimes$ denotes periodic convolution

$W(\omega)$ is the Fourier transform of the windowing function

The Fourier transform of most windowing functions has the shape of a sinc-type function (Chapter 2), and therefore according to Equation 3.4, $G_W(\omega)$ consists of a sequence of shifted sinc-type functions spaced $2\pi/T$ apart in frequency. The amplitudes of the sinc functions are determined by the envelope of $G(\omega)$.

The Fourier transform of the glottal waveform (computed as per Equation 3.4) is shown in Figure 3.5b. As demonstrated in Example 3.1, the Fourier transform of the glottal waveform is characterized by harmonics. The first harmonic occurs at the fundamental frequency, which is denoted by F0, and the other harmonics occur

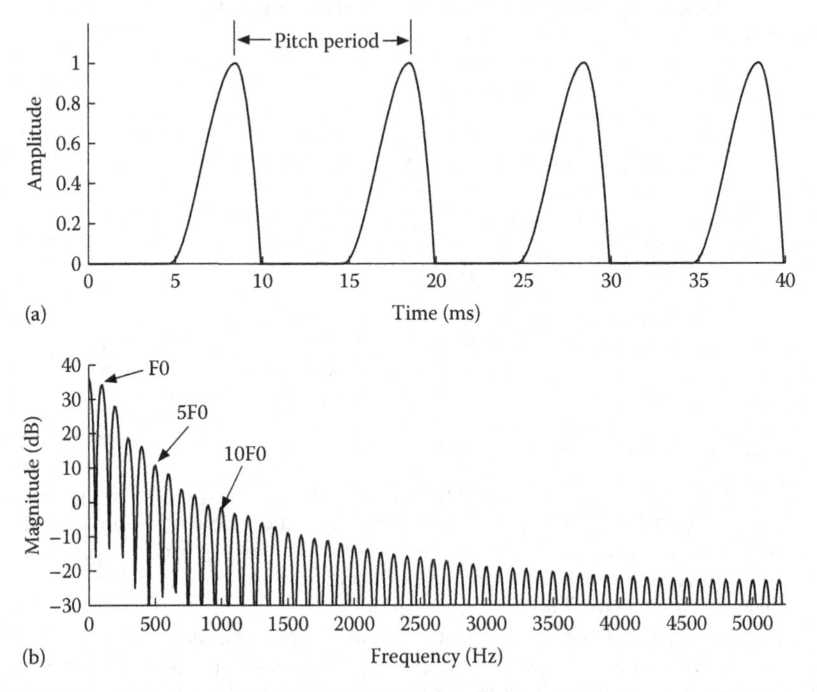

FIGURE 3.5 (a) An example of glottal airflow waveform and (b) its spectrum. In this example, the pitch period is 10 ms and the fundamental frequency (F0) is 100 Hz.

at integer multiples of the fundamental frequency. The spectral envelope has on the average a −12 dB/octave roll-off (observe the difference in magnitude between the 5th harmonic at 500 Hz and the 10th harmonic at 1000 Hz). This roll-off depends on the shape of the glottal wave, particularly whether the glottal closure is abrupt (shallower roll-off) or gradual (sharper roll-off).

As mentioned earlier, when the vocal folds are in the voicing state, vowels such as /aa/, /iy/, /uw/, etc., are produced. For this reason, vowels are also known as *voiced* sounds. A different class of sounds, called *unvoiced* (or voiceless) sounds, is generated when the vocal folds are in the *unvoicing* state. This state is similar to the breathing state in that the vocal folds do not vibrate. The folds, however, are tenser and come closer together, thus allowing the air stream to become turbulent as it flows through the glottis. This air turbulence is called the *aspiration*. Aspiration occurs in normal speech when producing sounds like /h/, as in "house" or when whispering. Turbulence can also be created when the articulators (e.g., tongue, lips) form constrictions and occlusions within the vocal tract. Sounds like /s/ and /t/ are produced by such constrictions in the vocal tract. The sounds produced when the folds are in the unvoicing state are called *unvoiced* sounds and include the majority of the consonants (e.g., /s/, /f/, /h/).

3.2.3 Vocal Tract

The vocal tract (Figure 3.2) consists of the oral cavity that extends from the larynx to the lips, and the nasal cavity, which is coupled to the oral cavity via the velum. The oral cavity can take on different shapes with different cross-sectional areas, depending on the position of the tongue, teeth, lips, and jaws, which are known collectively as the *articulators*. The average length of the male oral tract is 17 cm and is shorter in females.

As mentioned in the previous section, the input to the vocal tract is the airflow wave (see Figure 3.5) coming via the vocal folds. The vocal tract acts as a physical linear filter that spectrally shapes the input wave to produce distinctly different sounds. The characteristics of the filter (e.g., frequency response) change depending on the position of the articulators, that is, the shape of the oral tract.

The vocal tract is often viewed as an acoustic resonator because it resonates in response to sounds containing frequencies that match the natural resonant frequencies of the volume of air. During vowel production, the vocal tract can be approximated as a tube closed at one end and open at the other as the vocal folds are almost closed during phonation and the speaker's mouth is open. It is known that the lowest frequency that such a tube resonates has a wavelength (λ) four times the length of the tube. Given that the male vocal tract is approximately 17 cm long, we can calculate the lowest resonant frequency of such a tube using the following equation:

$$f = \frac{c}{\lambda} = \frac{34{,}400 \text{ cm/s}}{4 \times 17 \text{ cm}} = 506 \text{ Hz} \tag{3.5}$$

where c is the speed of sound expressed in cm/s. The tube will also resonate at odd multiples of that frequency, that is, at approximately 1500 Hz, 2500 Hz, and so on. The frequency response of the neutral vocal tract, approximated as a tube closed at

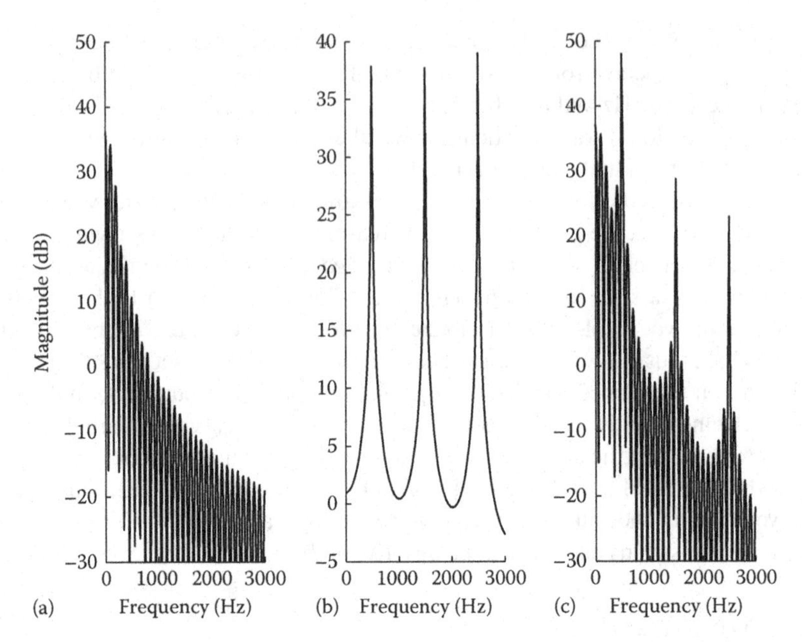

FIGURE 3.6 (a) Spectrum of the glottal pulse waveform, (b) the frequency response of the vocal tract for a uniform (neutral) tube configuration, and (c) the spectrum of the output speech.

one end and open at the other, is shown in Figure 3.6b. It has three peaks at the corresponding resonant frequencies.

When the input to the vocal tract is the periodic glottal source waveform, the resulting output speech spectrum can be obtained as the product of the glottal source spectrum (Figure 3.6a) and the vocal tract's frequency response (Figure 3.6b). The output speech spectrum is shown in Figure 3.6c. It resembles the spectrum of the vowel /aa/ as in "uh." Note that the speech spectrum has the same harmonic structure as the sound at the source, but the amplitudes of the harmonics have been shaped according to the frequency response of the vocal tract. Different sounds can thus be produced simply by changing the shape of the vocal tract, that is, its frequency response.

The preceding resonant frequencies (500, 1500, and 2500 Hz) are appropriate for a neutral tubelike configuration of the vocal tract, as when a speaker says the vowel in "uh." This simplistic neutral tube configuration assumes no constriction at any other point in the oral cavity. Most common vocal tract shapes assumed in speech production, however, have constrictions in certain parts of the tube. This alters the oral cavity size and, consequently, the resonant frequencies. The vocal tract is a time-varying resonator, and as its shape changes over time, the resonances change in frequency to produce different sounds.

The vocal tract resonances are known as *formants*, and the frequencies at which they resonate are called *formant frequencies*. The first formant, denoted as

F1, is associated with changes in mouth opening. Sounds requiring small mouth openings have low-frequency first formants (F1) and those requiring a wide mouth opening have high-frequency F1s. Contrast, for example, the vowel /i/, requiring a small mouth opening, to the vowel /aa/, requiring a wider mouth opening. The F1 of the vowel /iy/ is about 200 Hz, whereas the F1 of the vowel /aa/ is about 700 Hz. The second formant, denoted F2, is associated with changes in the oral cavity such as tongue position and lip activity. Finally, the third formant, denoted F3, is associated with front vs. back constriction in the oral cavity.

Figure 3.7 shows the Fourier magnitude spectrum (computed using the fast Fourier transform [FFT]) of the vowel /eh/ (as in "head") and its spectral envelope. The vowel was produced by a female speaker (F0 = 225 Hz). The spectral envelope of /eh/ was determined using linear prediction techniques (more on this in Chapter 6). The formant frequencies of the vowel /eh/ can be determined from its spectral envelope and not from its FFT magnitude spectrum. In contrast, the harmonics can be determined by the FFT magnitude spectrum and not from the spectral envelope. The first three formants (F1–F3) correspond to the first three peaks of the spectral envelope (see Figure 3.7b). Note that the formant frequencies may or may not coincide with one of the harmonics. Observe that F3 falls between two high-frequency harmonics.

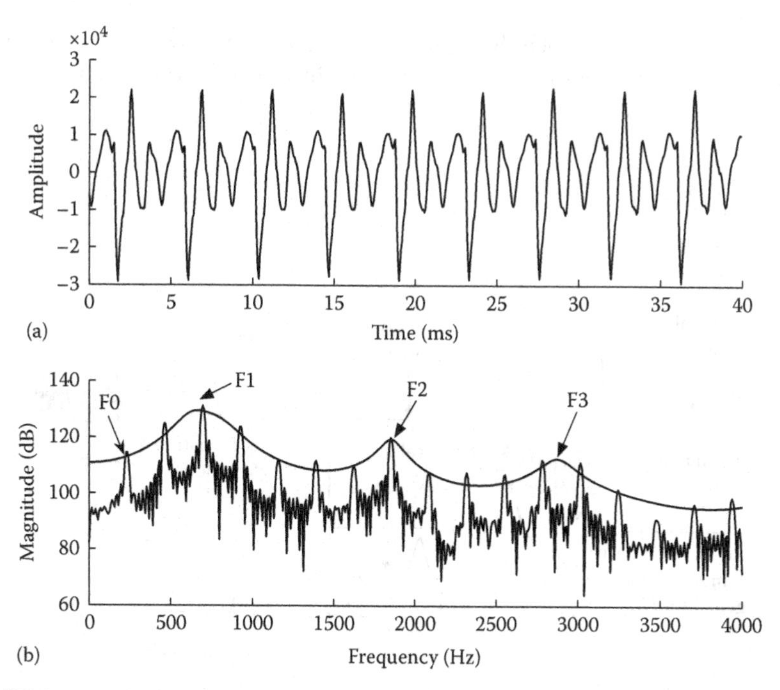

FIGURE 3.7 (a) Time waveform and (b) spectrum of the vowel /eh/ (as in "head"). Vowel was produced by a female speaker with F0 = 228 Hz. The formant frequency values were F1 = 719 Hz, F2 = 1800 Hz, and F3 = 2875 Hz.

3.3 ENGINEERING MODEL OF SPEECH PRODUCTION

We mentioned earlier that the vocal tract can be viewed as a filter that spectrally shapes the flow wave coming from the vocal folds to produce various sounds. The vocal folds provide the excitation to the vocal tract, and that excitation can be periodic or aperiodic, depending on the state of the vocal folds. Voiced sounds (e.g., vowels) are produced when the vocal folds are in the voicing state (and vibrate), whereas unvoiced sounds (e.g., consonants) are produced when the vocal folds are in the unvoicing state. These facts about the roles of the vocal tract and vocal folds led researchers to develop an engineering model of speech production (see Figure 3.8). In this model, the vocal tract is represented by a quasi-linear system that is excited by either a periodic or aperiodic source, depending on the state of the vocal folds. The output of this model is the speech signal, which is the only signal that we can measure accurately.

The fact that the vocal folds can assume one of two states (ignoring the breathing state) is modeled by a switch. The vocal tract is modeled by a time-invariant linear filter, and the parameters (e.g., filter coefficients) of the vocal tract model can be obtained using linear prediction analysis techniques (to be discussed later in Chapter 6). The output of the vocal tract filter is fed to another filter that models the effect of sound radiation at the lips. A filter of the form $R(z) = 1 - z^{-1}$ is typically used for the sound radiation block, introducing about a 6 dB/octave high-pass boost.

For the voiced case, when the input is a periodic glottal airflow sequence (e.g., Figure 3.5), the z-transform at the output of the lips can be written as a product of

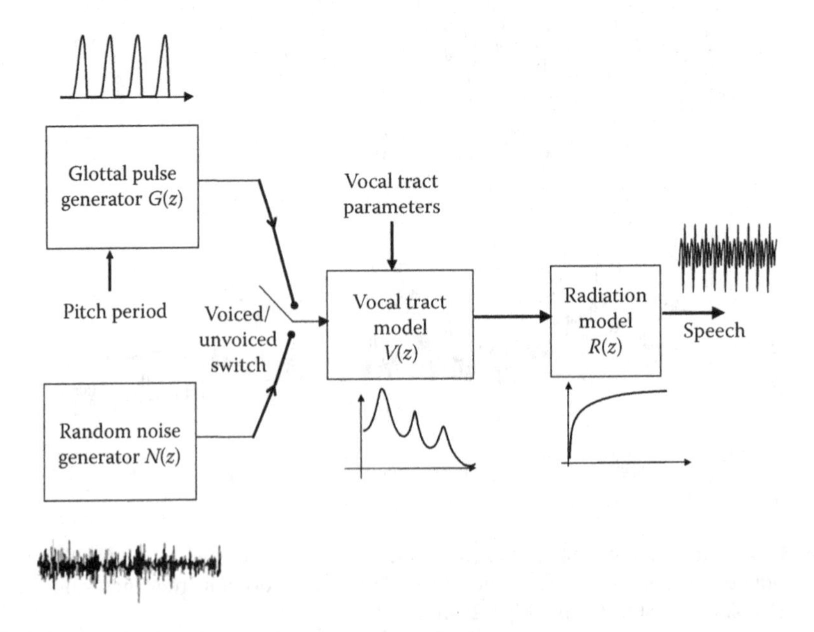

FIGURE 3.8 Engineering model of speech production.

three transfer functions modeling the glottal source ($G(z)$), the vocal tract ($V(z)$), and the lip radiation ($R(z)$):

$$X(z) = G(z)V(z)R(z) \tag{3.6}$$

For the unvoiced case, when the source is noise, as during the production of consonants (e.g., /s/), a random sequence is used, typically, with a flat spectrum, that is, white noise, and the z-transform at the output of the lips can be written as

$$X(z) = N(z)V(z)R(z) \tag{3.7}$$

where $N(z)$ is the z-transform of the noise sequence.

The speech production model shown in Figure 3.8, also known as the *source/filter* model, is ideal for transmission of speech over narrow-band channels as it requires only three sets of parameters for transmission: the fundamental frequency, voicing state, and vocal tract parameters. For that reason, this model has been used extensively for low-bit-rate speech coding applications (e.g., [5]).

It is worth noting that the aforementioned source/filter model is a rather simplistic linear model of speech production in that it assumes that the source is independent of the vocal tract system and that the relationship between pressure and volume velocity is linear. In reality, the coupling between the glottal source and the vocal tract system is far more complex and nonlinear, and there are aeroacoustic [6, p. 562] contributions to sound generation from the vocal tract that are not accounted for by the source/filter model. The interested reader can find more information in [6, p. 562] [7,8]. The source/filter approach to speech production, despite its limitations, underlies virtually all the speech recognition, analysis, and synthesis systems in use today.

3.4 CLASSES OF SPEECH SOUNDS

We are now in a position to classify and describe all the sounds of the English language. The sounds are described in terms of the nature of the source: periodic, noisy, or a combination of the two. They are also described in terms of the place and manner of articulation, determined primarily by the placement of the tongue in the oral cavity and the associated degree of constriction in the vocal tract.

Sounds are typically written in terms of *phonemes*, the smallest distinctive unit of a language. For example, the word "tan" consists of three phonemes, each belonging to a different class of sounds. The first phoneme "t" belongs to the stop consonant (also called *plosives*) class, the second phoneme "a" belongs to the vowel class, and the third phoneme "n" belongs to the nasals. Phonetically, the word "tan" is written as /t ae n/ using the ARPABET phonetic symbols (see Table 3.1).

There are a total of 40 phonemes in the American English language. The classification of the 40 phonemes in various subgroups is shown in Figure 3.9. Phonemes are written using the ARPABET phonetic symbols. Example words are given in Table 3.1 for all phonemes. The 40 phonemes in English can be broadly classified into eight groups: vowels, diphthongs, semivowels, nasals, fricatives, affricates, stops, and whispers (see Figure 3.9).

TABLE 3.1
Phonetic Symbols of American English

Class	ARPABET Phonetic Symbol	Example Word	Class	ARPABET Phonetic Symbol	Example Word
Vowels	iy	beat	Nasals	m	mom
	ih	bit		n	none
	eh	bet		ng	sing
	ae	bat	Stops	b	bet
	aa	Bob		d	dad
	er	bird		g	get
	ax	about		p	pet
	ah	but		t	Tom
	ao	bought		k	kite
	uw	boot	Fricatives	v	vet
	uh	book		dh	that
	ow	boat		z	zebra
Diphthongs	ay	buy		zh	azure
	oy	boy		f	five
	aw	down		th	thing
	ey	bait		s	Sam
Semivowels	w	wet		sh	shoe
	l	lid	Affricates	jh	judge
	r	red		ch	chew
	y	yet	Whispers	h	hat

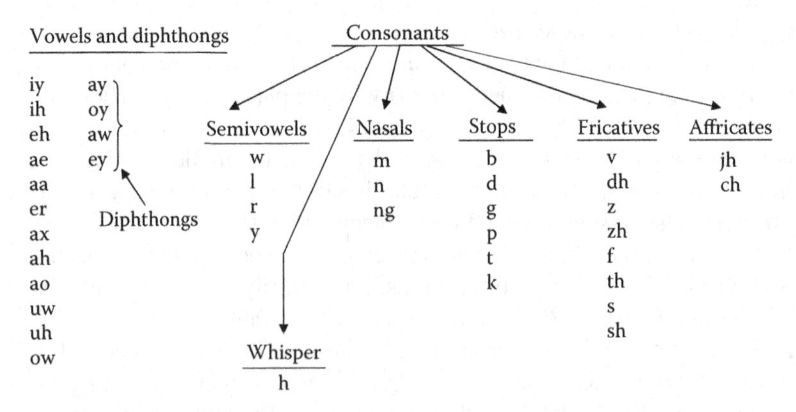

FIGURE 3.9 Classification of the phonemes of American English in broad sound classes.

3.5 ACOUSTIC CUES IN SPEECH PERCEPTION

Next, we describe the acoustic cues that are essential in phoneme identification. These are perceptual cues used by the auditory system to discriminate between and among the various classes of speech sounds. Each class of sounds, as we will see shortly, possesses certain acoustic properties that make them unique and easily discriminable from other classes. Preserving these acoustic cues is critically important, particularly in noise, as it can affect the identification of individual phonemes and, consequently, speech intelligibility.

3.5.1 Vowels and Diphthongs

Vowels are voiced and are relatively high in intensity (and energy) compared to the other classes of sounds. The most important cues to the perception of vowels are the formant frequencies, particularly the first three formants (F1, F2, and F3). In the seminal study by Peterson and Barney [2], 76 speakers, including men, women, and children, produced all English vowels in /h V d/ format (e.g., "heed"), and the vowels were analyzed in terms of their formant frequencies and durations. When the first two formant frequencies, F1 and F2, were plotted on an F1–F2 plane, an interesting pattern emerged. The majority of the F1 and F2 values of the same vowel produced by the various speakers fell within an ellipse. The variability in the formant frequencies obtained for the same vowel was not surprising given the differences in vocal tract size among the speakers. More interesting was the fact that there was little overlap between the ellipses of the various vowels. This finding provided an initial view and a simple model for vowel perception based on the formant frequencies extracted at the steady-state segment (center) of the vowel.

The preceding study was replicated 40 years later by Hillenbrand et al. [9]. Contrary to what Peterson and Barney reported, Hillenbrand et al. noted a large overlap between the ellipses of adjacent vowels (see Figure 3.10). Yet, the listeners identified the spoken vowels with over 95% accuracy, suggesting that a single time slice of F1–F2 information extracted from the steady-state segment of the vowels cannot explain the high identification accuracy. The difference in outcomes between the studies in [2] and [9] was attributed partly to the differences in the dialect of the speakers used in the two studies. This dialect difference might have contributed to the difference in the way the two groups of speakers produced the vowels after a passage of 40 years. Discriminant analysis performed in [9] showed that classification performance was modest when a single F1–F2 value was used for each vowel, but improved significantly when vowel duration and spectral change were incorporated.

Average values of F1 and F2 for a subset of the vowels recorded by Hillenbrand et al. [9] are given in Table 3.2. From this table it is clear that the formant frequency values of women and children are higher than that of male speakers. For instance, the average F2 value of the vowel /iy/ (as in "heed") produced by 19 girls is 3158 Hz, whereas the average F2 value of /iy/ produced by 36 men is 2322 Hz. This pattern is consistent across all vowels and for F1 values as well.

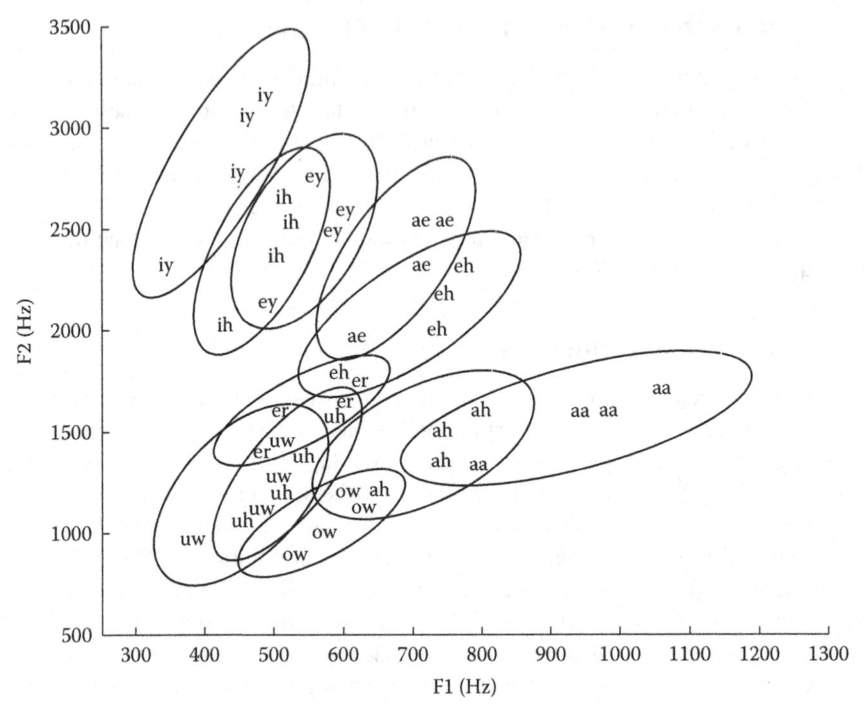

FIGURE 3.10 Average values of F1 and F2 for 11 vowels produced by 36 men, 36 women, 25 boys, and 19 girls. The vowels were used in [10] and were taken from the database in [9]. Each phonetic symbol (see Table 3.1) within each ellipse denotes the average F1–F2 value for each of the four speaker groups (men, women, boys, and girls). The highest formant frequency values correspond to the children's vowels and the lowest values correspond to the male speakers' vowels. (From Hillenbrand, J. et al., *J. Acoust. Soc. Am.*, 97(5), 3099, 1995; Loizou, P. et al., *J. Acoust. Soc. Am.*, 103(2), 1141, 1998.)

TABLE 3.2
Average Values (in Hz) of F1 and F2 for 11 Vowels Produced by 36 Men (M), 36 Women (W), 25 Boys (B), and 19 Girls (G)

		Heed /iy/	Hid /ih/	Hayed /ey/	Head /eh/	Had /ae/	Hod /aa/	Hoed /ow/	Hood /uh/	Who'd /uw/	Hud /ah/	Heard /er/
F1	M	333	418	488	579	606	789	512	462	364	637	468
	W	438	492	567	720	699	929	554	503	469	726	508
	B	452	513	589	723	698	970	611	551	488	720	589
	G	478	503	545	759	719	1046	588	564	491	776	603
F2	M	2322	2022	2117	1826	1971	1351	894	1099	971	1188	1386
	W	2782	2364	2490	2001	2322	1600	1004	1156	1116	1382	1623
	B	3056	2529	2593	2176	2540	1603	1130	1377	1238	1518	1706
	G	3158	2652	2759	2314	2541	1712	1181	1547	1435	1644	1708

The appealing notion that steady-state formant frequencies are the only cues used for vowel perception was challenged by many researchers (see review in [11, Chapter 5]). For one thing, such a proposal fails to account for the dynamic variation of formant frequencies in the context of other sounds. The formant pattern of a vowel produced in isolation differs from the pattern of the same vowel produced in different contexts. More specifically, the F2 frequency of vowels produced in, say, a consonant–vowel–consonant (CVC) syllable often does not reach the "target" value determined from the isolated vowel [12]. Furthermore, the rate of articulation as well as linguistic stress can influence the formant pattern.

In addition to vowel formant frequencies, listeners often use duration as a cue to identify vowels. The vowel /ih/ (e.g., "hid"), for instance, is shorter in duration than the vowel /iy/ (e.g., "heed"). Dynamic information presented in terms of formant transitions into and out of a vowel also plays an important role in vowel perception [13]. In fact, in several experiments it was shown that vowels in context can be identified with high accuracy even when *only* the transitional segments were presented, that is, after the steady-state segments were removed [14].

The effect of noise on the vowel's formant frequencies was examined in [15] using acoustic analysis and listening tests. The F1 and F2 formant frequencies of 11 vowels were measured and compared before and after adding noise (multitalker babble and stationary speech-shaped noise). Results indicated that the F1 frequency was affected the least by the noise, whereas the F2 values were affected the most. This outcome suggests that in noise, listeners must have access to relatively reliable information about F1, but perhaps coarse or vague information about F2 (more on this in Chapter 4).

In brief, although it is generally accepted that the steady-state formant frequencies are the primary (and necessary) cues to vowel perception, they are not the only ones. Additional cues (e.g., duration and spectral change) are often used (and needed) by listeners for accurate vowel identification.

Vowels are also called monophthongs, a Greek word meaning a single (*mono-*) voiced sound (*phthong*). A related class of sounds is the diphthongs, meaning two (*di-*) voiced sounds. There are four diphthongs in the English language all of which can be found in the sentence "H<u>ow</u> J<u>oe</u> l<u>i</u>kes tr<u>ai</u>ns!" The sound "ow" in "How" is not considered as two consecutive vowels but as the diphthong /aw/. Diphthongs are similar to the vowels in the way they are produced, that is, they are produced with a relatively open vocal tract. Unlike vowels, however, diphthongs are more dynamic in nature and cannot be characterized by a single vocal tract shape or a single formant pattern. Diphthongs' formant pattern changes slowly during the sound's production.

3.5.2 Semivowels

The sounds /y/, /w/, /r/, and /l/ are called *semivowels* because their formant pattern is similar to that of vowels and diphthongs. Semivowels are classified as consonants, despite their vowel-like characteristics (see example waveform in Figure 3.11), because they occur at the onset or offset of syllables as do other consonants. Also, unlike the formants in vowels, semivowels' formants do not reach steady state. Semivowels are often subclassified as glides (/y/ and /w/) and liquids (/l/ and /r/).

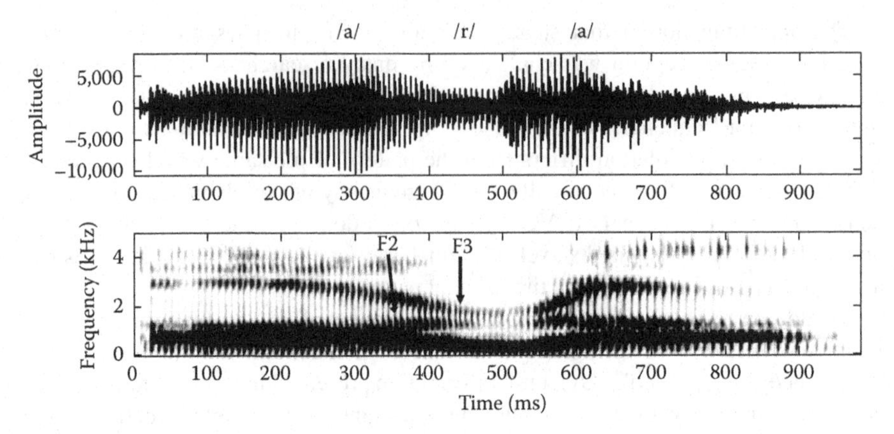

FIGURE 3.11 Time waveform and spectrogram of the syllable /a r a/.

The most important acoustic cues to semivowel perception are the formant transitions. The frequency changes in F2 and F3 are especially important. It is the second formant (F2) that distinguishes /w/ from /y/, and it is the third formant (F3) that distinguishes /r/ from /l/. The liquid /r/ is characterized by a low F3 (see example in Figure 3.11). In the example shown in Figure 3.11, the F3 value decreased from roughly 3 kHz during the vowel /aa/ to less than 2 kHz during the semivowel /r/.

3.5.3 Nasals

During the production of nasal consonants /m, n, and ng/, the velum is low, leaving the entrance to the nasal cavity open while obstructing the entrance to the oral cavity. The inclusion of the nasal cavity in the vocal tract creates a larger and longer resonator, which is associated with a lower resonant frequency. For this reason, the nasal consonants are characterized by a low-frequency resonance in the range of 200–500 Hz, called the nasal "murmur." As the nasals are produced with a complete occlusion of the oral cavity, it is not surprising to observe antiresonances (i.e., deep valleys) in their spectra. As a result, the higher formants are heavily attenuated (see example in Figure 3.12). In brief, two features distinguish nasals from other classes of speech sounds. The first is the suppressed intensity of the higher-frequency formants, and the second is the presence of a low-frequency resonance (<500 Hz). The most effective cues to the identification of nasals are the formant transitions preceding and following the nasals.

3.5.4 Stops

The sounds we considered so far—vowels, semivowels, and nasals—are characterized by a relatively free flow of air from the vocal folds. We now turn our attention to sounds such as stops and fricatives, which are characterized by a restricted, and in some cases obstructed, airflow.

With respect to other classes of sounds, the stops (also called *plosives*) possess two unique characteristics. First, during the production of stops there is a

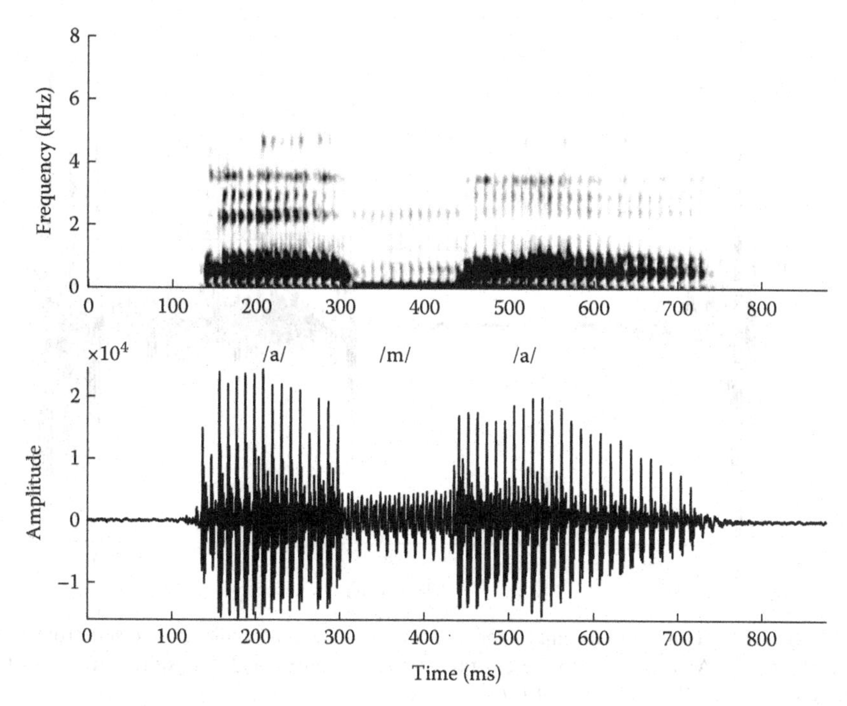

FIGURE 3.12 Spectrogram and time waveform of the syllable /a m a/.

complete occlusion of the vocal tract and thus a brief blockage of airflow, which manifests itself as silence in the acoustic signal (see example in Figure 3.13). This silence is called the *closure* period and is a very robust and distinctive cue to stops. Inserting, for instance, silence between /s/ and /l/ in "slit" will make the word to be heard as "split." Second, following the occlusion of air and pressure buildup, the air is released and heard as a transient burst of noise (Figure 3.13). Noise, called *aspiration*, follows the burst. Both the closure and the presence of a release burst are considered to be the two main acoustic cues to the stop consonants as a class.

Stops are subclassified into voiceless (/p, t, k/) and voiced (/b, d, g/). Voiced stops differ from unvoiced ones in the characteristics of their closure and duration. In unvoiced stops, there is no flow of air out of the vocal tract during the closure. In voiced stops, a low-intensity periodic signal (at the fundamental frequency) may pass through during all or part of the duration of the closure. This low-intensity periodic signal is called the *voice bar* and appears as a constant low-frequency signal on the spectrogram (see Figure 3.14b). Voiced stops are on average shorter in duration than voiceless ones. The voiced onset time (VOT), that is, the time interval between the release of the burst and the onset of vocal fold vibrations, is about 10–20 ms for the voiced stops and 40–100 ms for the unvoiced ones [16]. Finally, the release burst, which shows in spectrograms as a vertical stripe following the silent gap (closure), is more intense in the voiceless stops than in the voiced ones (see example in Figure 3.14).

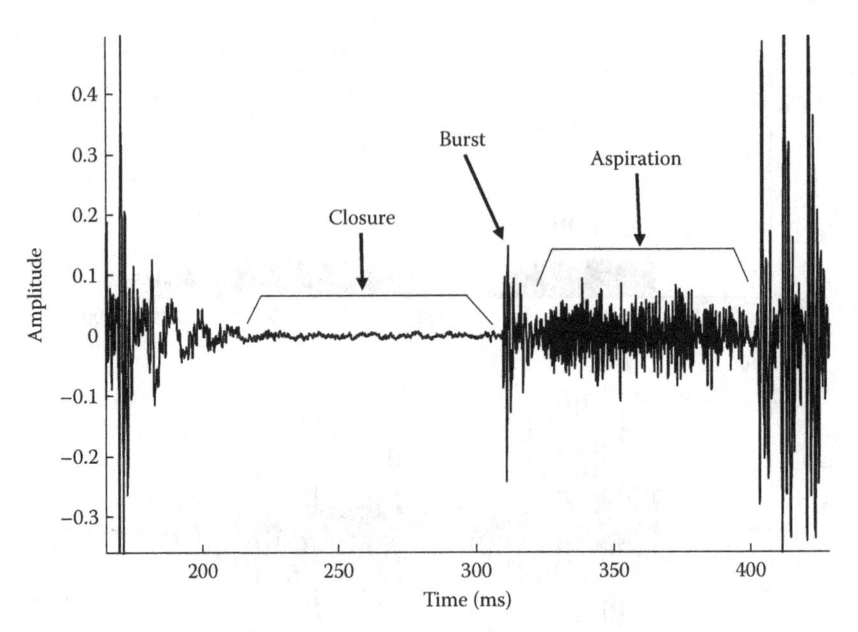

FIGURE 3.13 Time-domain characteristics of the stop consonant /k/ excised from the syllable /a k a/. Arrows point to the closure period, the burst, and the aspiration segments occurring during the production of /k/.

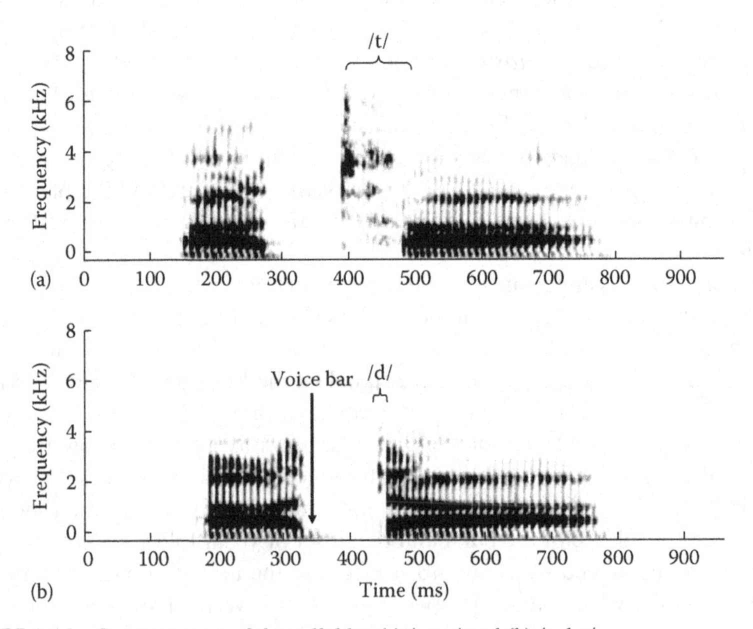

FIGURE 3.14 Spectrograms of the syllables (a) /a t a/ and (b) /a d a/.

Cues to voicing include the presence or absence of a voice bar during the stop closure, the presence or absence of aspiration (noise) following the stop release and the onset frequency of F1. Early experiments [17] showed that after a certain degree of "cutting back" the F1 transition present in the /ba/ stimulus, listeners reported hearing /pa/ instead of /ba/—that is, the presence of the F1 transition made the synthetic syllable /ba/ sound voiced. The F1 cue to voicing has been found to be robust to the presence of noise [18].

The stops are marked by rapid formant transitions preceding or following vowels. These rapid transitions are caused by sudden changes to the vocal tract shape as the articulators quickly move from the position of a consonant to that for a vowel or *vice versa*.

Stops are also classified in terms of their place of articulation into labials (/b, p/), alveolars (/d, t/), and velars (/k, g/). This classification is based on the location of the occlusion formed by the lips or tongue within the oral cavity. For the labial stops, the occlusion is in the lips; for the alveolar stops, it is in the alveolar ridge; and for the velar stops, it is in the back of the vocal tract, near the velum. The major cues to place of articulation are the formant transitions, particularly frequency changes in F2, between the stop consonants and the steady-state portions of the following (or preceding) vowels. The difference between /d a/ and /b a/, for instance, lies in the slope of the F2 transition. In the /d a/ syllable, the slope of the F2 transition is falling, whereas in the /b a/ syllable the slope is rising.

The cues to the manner of articulation for stops, namely, the closure and the release burst, are more resistant to the masking effects of additive noise than the acoustic cues to place of articulation (formant transitions) [19]. In an extensive study, Miller and Nicely [19] analyzed the effect of noise on consonants and found that listeners were able to identify the stops as a class (i.e., manner of articulation) even when the place cues were masked.

3.5.5 Fricatives

Similar to the stop consonants, fricatives are produced when the articulators form narrow constrictions and occlusions in part of the vocal tract. These occlusions and constrictions produce noise as the airflow passes through them and are subsequently shaped by the vocal tract. The fricative /f/, for instance, is produced by forming a narrow constriction near the lips. Depending on the place of the constriction, fricatives are classified according to their place of articulation as labiodental (/f, v/), linguadental (/th, dh/), alveolar (/s, z/), and palatal (/sh, zh/). The fricatives are also classified into *stridents* (/s, z, sh, zh/) and *non-stridents* (/f, v, th, dh/).

Unlike stops, fricatives are continuants in that they can be prolonged. The main acoustic cue to the fricatives as a class (i.e., manner of articulation) is the presence of a relatively long segment of aperiodic noise (frication). The duration of fricative noise in /s/ is influenced by context, and can vary from 50 ms in consonant clusters to 200 ms in phrase-final position.

There are three main cues to the place of articulation of fricatives. The first cue is the intensity of the fricative noise. Fricatives /s, z, sh, zh/ are characterized by higher intensity and higher energy than the fricatives /th, dh, f, v/. The second cue is the shape of the fricative spectra. Fricatives /s, z, sh, zh/ are characterized by the presence of high-frequency spectral peaks, whereas /th, dh, f, v/ are characterized by flat spectra (see example in Figure 3.15). The low intensity and flat spectra of the fricatives /th, dh, f, v/

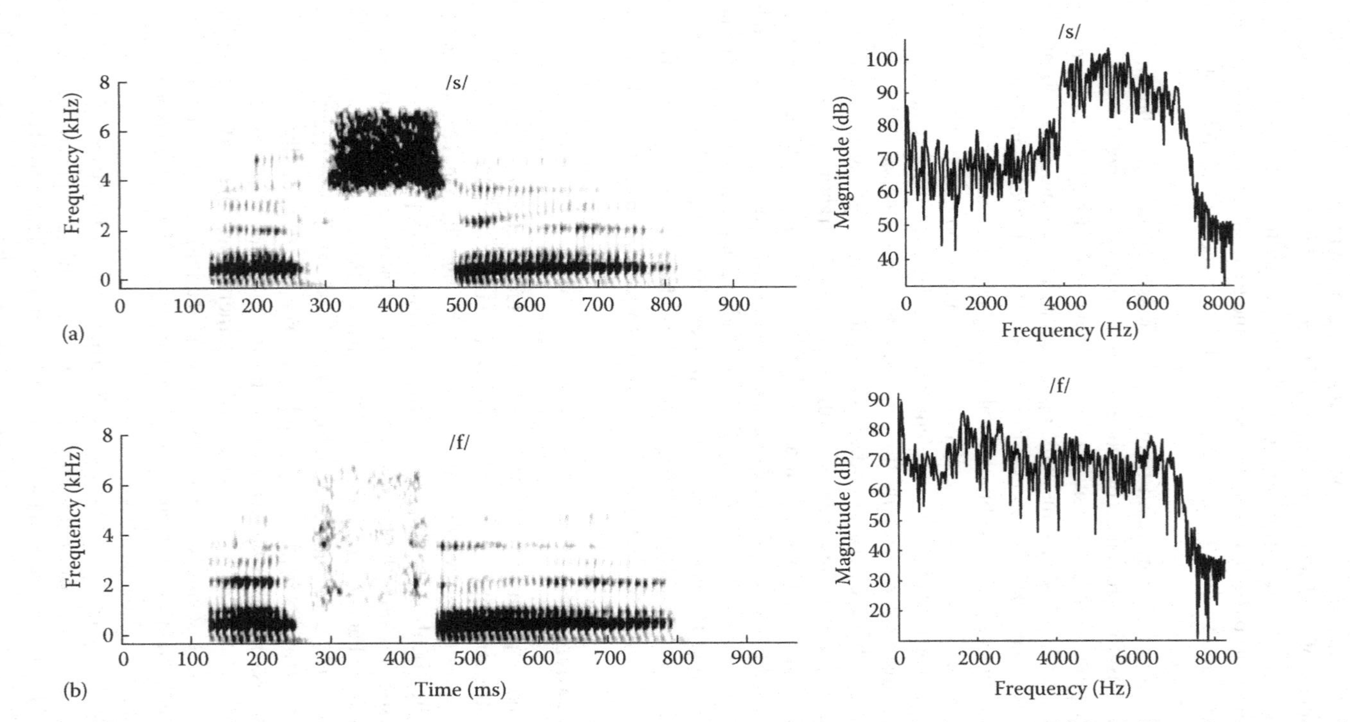

FIGURE 3.15 Spectrograms of the syllables (a) /a s a/ and (b) /a f a/. Sample Fourier transform magnitude spectra of /s/ and /f/ are shown on the right. The syllables were band-limited to 7.5 kHz and sampled at 16 kHz.

make it extremely difficult to differentiate them from low-level background noise. The spectral peaks of /sa, z/ (located at around 4 kHz) are typically higher in frequency than the spectral peaks of /sh, zh/ (located at around 2.5 kHz). Example spectra of /s/ and /f/ are shown in Figure 3.15. The third cue to place of articulation is the F2 and F3 formant transitions of voiced sounds preceding and/or following them. Compared to the stops, however, the formant transition cues are less important in the perception of place of articulation of fricatives. This was confirmed in splicing experiments in which the noise segment of one strident fricative was combined with the formant transitions of another fricative [20]. Results indicated that fricative identification was unaffected by this manipulation, suggesting that the noise spectrum of each fricative is highly distinctive.

3.6 SUMMARY

This chapter introduced the speech signal and briefly described the speech production process. It presented an engineering model of speech production, a model that is often used by speech coding algorithms and some speech enhancement algorithms. The chapter described the broad classes of speech sounds in the English language and presented the acoustic cues used by human listeners in perceiving sounds from each class of sounds. Knowledge of these acoustic cues is important in the design of effective noise suppression algorithms. Speech enhancement algorithms need to preserve the perceptually important acoustic cues present in the signal to maintain high quality and intelligibility in noisy environments.

REFERENCES

1. Borden, G., Harris, K., and Raphael, L. (1994), *Speech Science Primer*, 3rd ed., Baltimore, MD: Williams & Wilkins.
2. Peterson, G. and Barney, H. (1952), Control methods used in a study of the vowels, *J. Acoust. Soc. Am.*, 24(2), 175–184.
3. Rosenberg, A. (1971), Effect of glottal pulse shape on the quality of natural vowels, *J. Acoust. Soc. Am.*, 49(2), 583–588.
4. Klatt, D. and Klatt, L. (1990), Analysis, synthesis and perception of voice quality variations among female and male talkers, *J. Acoust. Soc. Am.*, 87(2), 820–857.
5. Tremain, T. (1982), The government standard linear predictive coding algorithm: LPC-10, *Speech Technol.*, 4, 40–49.
6. Quatieri, T. (2002), *Discrete-Time Speech Signal Processing*, Upper Saddle River, NJ: Prentice Hall.
7. Teager, H. and Teager, S. (1990), Evidence for non-linear sound production mechanisms in the vocal tract, in Hardcastle, W. and Marchal, A. (Eds.), *Speech Production and Speech Modeling*, Boston, MA: Kluwer Academic Publishers, pp. 241–262.
8. Kaiser, J. (1983), Some observations on vocal tract operation from a fluid flow point of view, in Titzer, R. and Scherer, R. (Eds.), *Vocal Fold Physiology: Biomechanics, Acoustics and Phonatory Control*, Denver, CO: The Denver Center for the Performing Arts, pp. 358–386.
9. Hillenbrand, J., Getty, L., Clark, M., and Wheeler, K. (1995), Acoustic characteristics of American English vowels, *J. Acoust. Soc. Am.*, 97(5), 3099–3111.
10. Loizou, P., Dorman, M., and Powell, V. (1998), The recognition of vowels produced by men, women, boys, and girls by cochlear implant patients using a six-channel CIS processor, *J. Acoust. Soc. Am.*, 103(2), 1141–1149.

11. Kent, R. and Read, C. (1992), *The Acoustic Analysis of Speech*, San Diego, CA: Singular Publishing Group.
12. Lindblom, B. (1963), Spectrographic study of vowel reduction, *J. Acoust. Soc. Am.*, 35, 1773–1781.
13. Strange, W. (1987), Evolving theories of vowel perception, *J. Acoust. Soc. Am.*, 85, 2081–2087.
14. Jenkins, J., Strange, W., and Edman, T. (1983), Identification of vowels in "vowelless" syllables, *Percept. Psychophys.*, 34, 441–450.
15. Parikh, G. and Loizou, P. (2005), The influence of noise on vowel and consonant cues, *J. Acoust. Soc. Am.*, 118(6), 3874–3888.
16. Lisker, L. and Abramson, A. (1964), A cross-language study of voicing in initial stops: Acoustic measurements, *Word*, 20, 384–422.
17. Liberman, A., Delattre, P., and Cooper, F. (1958), Some rules for the distinction between voiced and voiceless stops in initial position, *Lang. Speech*, 1, 153–167.
18. Jiang, J., Chen, M., and Alwan, A. (2006), On the perception of voicing in syllable-initial plosives in noise, *J. Acoust. Soc. Am.*, 119(2), 1092–1105.
19. Miller, G. and Nicely, P. (1955), An analysis of perceptual confusions among some English consonants, *J. Acoust. Soc. Am.*, 27(2), 338–352.
20. Harris, K. (1958), Cues for discrimination of American English fricatives in spoken syllables, *Lang. Speech*, 1, 1–17.

4 Noise Compensation by Human Listeners

In many everyday situations, we are surrounded by sounds originating from a variety of sources. These sounds might include a number of people speaking in the background, a car passing by, music playing on the radio, a telephone ringing, the wind blowing, and so on. The signals from each source are mixed together when they enter the two ears to form a composite waveform. The frequency components of each source are not constrained within an isolated region of the spectrum but overlap with frequency components of other sources. The problem of sorting out which components belong to which sound source is highly complex, but it is a task that the brain performs effortlessly, at least by listeners with normal hearing. In the context of signal processing, this task is equivalent to solving a blind source separation problem: given a mixture of signals recorded with multiple microphones, identify the target signal. How does the brain solve this blind source separation problem?

The purpose of this chapter is to review the literature investigating the cues used by human listeners when communicating in highly adverse conditions, particularly in situations where multiple talkers are speaking in the background. Understanding the strategies and acoustic cues used by human listeners to segregate speech from other signals in adverse conditions is important for several reasons. For one, such knowledge would tell us which spectral and temporal characteristics of the speech signal need to be preserved by speech enhancement algorithms. Second, it would help us design better speech enhancement algorithms that would mimic listening strategies used by humans. Such algorithms would hold promise in improving speech intelligibility in noise.

Research in this area was triggered by the seminal paper of Cherry [1] in the early 1950s on the intelligibility of speech in multiple-talker conditions. He referred to this listening task as the "cocktail party" problem, simply formulated as: How do we understand what one person is saying when others are speaking at the same time? The more general problem of segregating speech in the presence of multiple noise sources (not necessarily speech) is commonly referred to as the "auditory scene analysis" problem [2].

This chapter is organized into four sections. The first section reviews the research on speech intelligibility in multiple-talker conditions. The remaining sections focus on the various factors influencing speech segregation, including the properties of the speech signal itself that shield information from distortion. The perceptual strategies used by listeners for speech recognition in noisy environments are discussed in the last section.

4.1 INTELLIGIBILITY OF SPEECH IN MULTIPLE-TALKER CONDITIONS

The intelligibility of speech in adverse conditions is greatly influenced by the spectral and temporal characteristics of the noise, specifically, whether the noise is stationary or nonstationary, narrowband or wideband, modulated or continuous (steady-state), and whether it is presented monaurally or binaurally [3]. In this section, we focus on intelligibility of speech in the presence of single or multiple talkers presented monaurally or binaurally. Because the interfering signal in multiple-talker listening conditions is speech, we will use the term *masker* to differentiate the interfering signal from the voice of interest, also called the *target* voice.

4.1.1 Effect of Masker's Spectral/Temporal Characteristics and Number of Talkers: Monaural Hearing

Several studies have demonstrated that the intelligibility of speech (presented monaurally) in multiple-talker conditions (e.g., in a restaurant) is greatly affected by the number of competing talkers present as well as by the temporal characteristics of the noise [4]. In an early study, Miller [4] obtained articulation scores—percent correct identification scores of monosyllabic words as a function of the intensity of the masker—for speech in the presence of one, two, four, six, and eight competing voices. The target voice was male, and the interfering voices consisted of equal number of male and female talkers. Results indicated that word identification in the presence of two voices was significantly more difficult than word identification in the presence of a single voice. Word identification became progressively worse as the number of voices increased, with only a small change in identification scores when the number of voices increased from four to eight. When a large number of voices are present, the masker waveform becomes nearly continuous, leaving no silent gaps in the waveform. As we will discuss in Section 4.3.2, these gaps or dips in the waveform produce high-SNR segments in the signal that enable the listeners to "hear out" (glimpse) segments of the target voice.

Evidence of the idea that normal-hearing listeners are exploiting the gaps or dips present in speech waveforms corrupted by a single competing voice comes from several studies. These studies compared speech intelligibility in the presence of steady-state continuous noise, amplitude-modulated noise, and single interfering voice. Results were reported in terms of the speech reception threshold (SRT), defined as the SNR (dB) at which 50% of the words are reliably identified (see Chapter 10 for more details on how to measure the SRT). Several studies confirmed that it is more difficult to identify words in the presence of steady-state noise than in the presence of a single competing speaker. The difference in SRT (50% intelligibility level) can range from 6 dB [5] to 10 dB [4]; that is to say, listeners can identify words in steady-state noise or in the presence of a single competing talker with the same accuracy (50% correct) even when the SNR of the competing-talker sentences is 6–10 dB lower. The interfering voice is therefore a much less effective masker than steady-state noise when presented at the same level. The intelligibility advantage gained by using a single (or a small number) competing talker instead of steady-state noise as the interfering signal is described in the literature as *masking release* [6,7].

Studies that investigated the effect of the masker's temporal fluctuations showed that the difference in SRT between stationary noise and modulated noise was 4–6 dB [5,7,8]. Some studies used noise that was modulated by the envelope fluctuations of the speech signal, whereas others used noise constructed to have the same long-term spectrum as speech. The latter noise was used to eliminate or reduce spectral difference cues between the target and interfering signals. Other studies included time-reversed speech (i.e., speech played backward) as maskers. These maskers were used to assess whether the difference in performance (with competing speech maskers) can be attributed to differences in temporal fluctuations or to the distractive linguistic contents of the interfering sentence. A large release of masking (5 dB) was obtained with speech-modulated maskers, suggesting that the temporal fluctuations in the interfering signal can have a significant effect on speech intelligibility in noise despite the similarities in the spectra of the signal and interfering noise. Masking release (of about 7 dB) was also obtained when time-reversed speech was used as the masker [5,8]. These findings provide evidence that the release of masking can be attributed solely to the temporal fluctuations of the interfering signal rather than to spectral differences between the masker and target signals.

Aside from the temporal fluctuations of the interfering signal, other factors can potentially influence intelligibility of speech in the presence of a single competing talker. These include gender differences and similarities in information content of the target and masker speech. As one would expect, recognition is easier when the talkers are of different sexes than when they are of the same sex [9]. Similarities in the information content of the target and masker sentences can also influence recognition, contributing to the so-called "informational masking" [10]. Generally, it is believed that the difficulty that normal-hearing listeners experience with single-talker maskers is attributed to a combination of (1) "energetic masking," resulting from overlap of the target and masker in the auditory periphery and (2) "informational masking," resulting from competition between the target and masker at more central stages of auditory processing [10]. Energetic masking is considered to be a peripheral masking phenomenon occurring when the energy from two (or more) sounds overlap both spectrally and temporally, making signal recovery difficult. Teasing out the contributions of energetic and informational masking has been a challenging task [10].

When the number of maskers or the number of voices increases beyond four, the temporal fluctuations average out, and the composite masker approximates a steady-state signal. Figure 4.1 (bottom panel) shows an example time waveform of eight-talker babble resembling that of stationary white noise. Unlike the waveform of a single competing talker, the waveform of the eight-talker babble does not contain any dips or gaps, at least in the time domain. Consequently, listeners are not able to take advantage of any silent periods in the masker to hear out the target signal.

As demonstrated earlier, normal-hearing listeners benefit a great deal from the temporal fluctuations present in the interfering signal. In contrast, hearing-impaired listeners receive little benefit. Whereas normal-hearing listeners gain about 6–10 dB when steady-state noise is replaced by interfering speech or modulated noise, hearing-impaired listeners gain no more than 0–2 dB [5]. This reduced release of

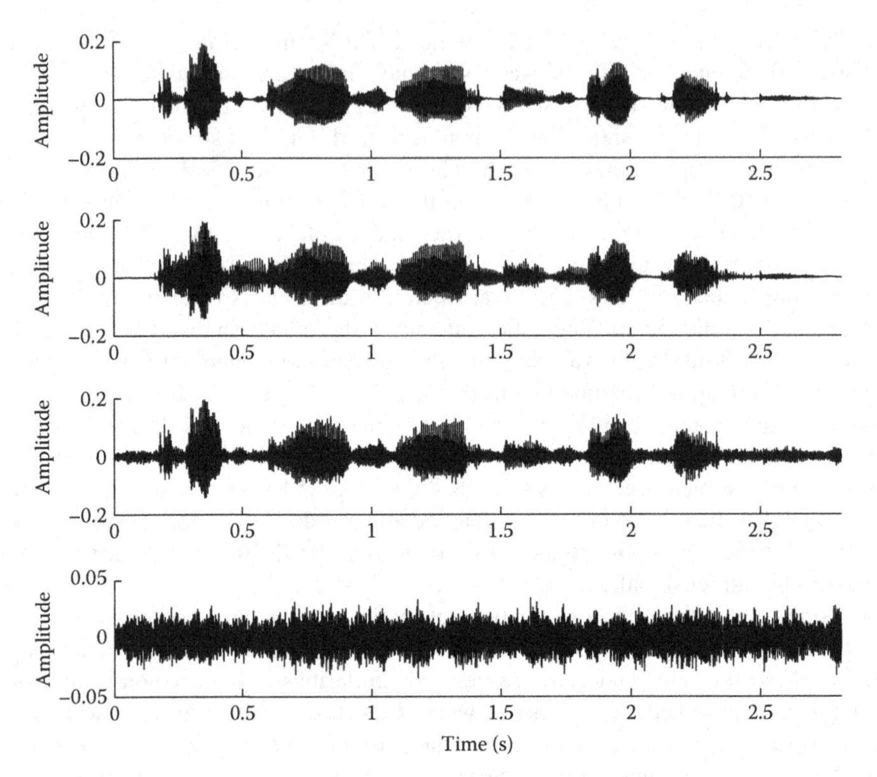

FIGURE 4.1 Time waveforms of the sentence "The birch canoe slid on the smooth planks" corrupted by a single-talker interferer (second panel from top) and eight-talker babble (third panel from top) at +5 dB S/N. Top panel shows the sentence in quiet and bottom panel shows the time waveform of eight-talker babble.

masking is partly responsible for the difficulty that hearing-impaired listeners experience in understanding speech in noisy situations.

So far, we have considered intelligibility of speech in the presence of multiple talkers when presented monaurally, as for instance, through telephones; that is, listeners had to rely exclusively on monaural cues to recognize the target signal. The situation becomes more complicated when speech is presented binaurally, as the spatial locations of the signal and noise sources, among other factors, can significantly affect speech recognition. The latter situation is more realistic as it reflects everyday listening situations.

4.1.2 Effect of Source Spatial Location: Binaural Hearing

In real-world listening scenarios, competing voices (along with other types of noise) typically originate from different locations in space. Consequently, each ear receives a slightly different signal. The signals emanating from various sources reach the two ears at different times and with different amplitudes owing to the attenuation from the mass of the head, often called *head shadow*. The differences in amplitude level due to head shadow are called interaural level differences (ILDs), and the differences in time of arrival are called interaural time differences (ITDs). Both ILDs and ITDs provide cues to sound localization and also contribute to binaural intelligibility of speech under noisy conditions.

It is reasonable to expect that binaural speech intelligibility is affected by the spatial distribution of the noise sources (i.e., their location with respect to the listener) and the number of sources. Several studies demonstrated large intelligibility benefit when the noise source was moved spatially away from the target along the horizontal plane [11–13]. In these studies, speech was presented from the front (0° azimuth), whereas the noise (single interfering noise source) was presented from various angles (azimuths) in the horizontal plane. Results indicated that the largest benefit (10–12 dB) in terms of SRT improvement occurred when the interfering sound source was located at 110–120° azimuth. This binaural benefit—often called *spatial release of masking*—is attributed to two components: one caused by head shadow, that is, access to a "better" ear with more favorable SNR, and the other caused by interaural time delays (ITDs) [14]. To better understand the head shadow advantage, consider, for instance, the situation where the noise source is at 90° azimuth and the target signals come from the front of the listener. The ear contralateral to the noise source will receive a better SNR signal owing to head shadow, thus making it easier for the listener to identify the words spoken by the target speaker. The difference between the SRT obtained using the better ear (i.e., ear contralateral to the noise source) vs. the worse ear (ear closest to the noise source) can be as large as 8 dB when there is only a single masker present and the target signal comes from the front [11]. This difference, however, gradually disappears as the number of noise sources increases and the noise sources get distributed around the head [11].

When multiple noise sources are present, the spatial configuration of the sources has a large impact on speech intelligibility. More specifically, the spatial separation of the sources and the distribution of the sources around the listener play a critical role in speech intelligibility [11,12,15,16].

To illustrate this, we will consider the data collected in [12], in which target sentences were presented from the front and one to three interfering speakers were presented from different locations. To evaluate the benefit incurred by listening with two ears (binaural hearing) vs. listening with one ear (monaural hearing), data were collected for both binaural and monaural listening conditions. The various spatial configurations considered were simulated by convolving anechoic head-related impulse responses [17] (for different positions and the left and right ears) with the speech material. The "virtual" stimuli were presented binaurally to the listeners through headphones. The results are plotted in Figure 4.2 for a single interfering speaker and in Figure 4.3 for three interfering speakers. These results are expressed in terms of SRT (dB), for recognition of IEEE sentences [18]. A 10 dB SRT improvement was obtained simply by moving the noise sources (three talkers) at 90° azimuth. A smaller improvement (5 dB) was obtained when the three interfering speakers were located at (30°, 60°, 90°). Data from monaural listening are shown in right panel for comparison. In the monaural condition, the left ear was used as it was considered to be the "better" ear for the majority of the noise configurations (see Figure 4.3). Clearly, better performance is obtained with binaural than with

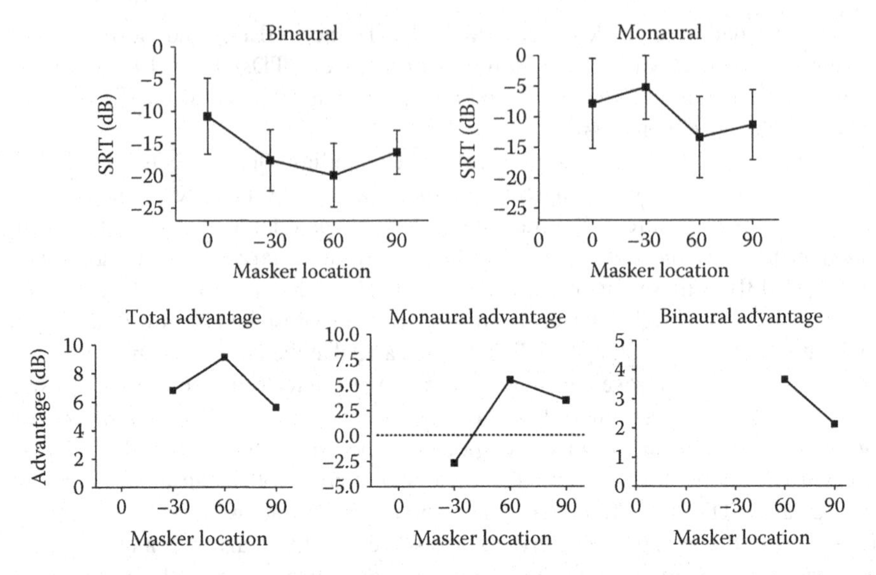

FIGURE 4.2 Binaural and monaural speech intelligibility (top two panels) as a function of masker (single talker) position expressed in degrees. Target signal was coming from the front of the listener, that is, from 0°. Masker location of 0° indicates the front direction, positive angles indicate directions from the right of the listener, and negative angles indicate directions from the left of the listener. Masker was a single talker. Bottom panels show the advantage (in dB) gained when listening with two ears (see text for explanation).

monaural hearing, even when listening through the "better" ear—the ear farthest from the noise sources. As expected, the configuration (−30°, 60°, 90°) is least favorable for monaural hearing as the noise sources (interfering talkers) are distributed on both sides (left and right) of the listener.

The bottom panels in Figures 4.2 and 4.3 summarize the results in terms of the total advantage, gained by the mere fact that the noise sources are spatially separated (total spatial release of masking), and its two additive components: monaural advantage and binaural advantage (also called *binaural squelch*). The monaural advantage is defined as the difference in SRT between each monaural (best-ear listening) condition where the noise and target are spatially separated and the unseparated condition (both speech and noise come from the front). The binaural advantage is defined as the part of the total spatial release advantage that is not accounted for by the monaural advantage. The binaural advantage reflects the true benefit obtained when listening with two ears over listening with just the better monaural ear. The total advantage is greatly affected by the noise spatial configuration, with the largest benefit obtained at (90°, 90°, 90°), where the noise sources were locally isolated.

The monaural advantage is also affected by the spatial configuration and disappears once the interfering sources are spatially distributed on the right and left of the listener. This finding suggests that the head shadow plays a minor role in realistic listening environments when competing noise sources (e.g., speakers) surround the listener. Unlike the monaural advantage, the binaural advantage is more robust to spatial configurations. The data in [12] showed that the binaural

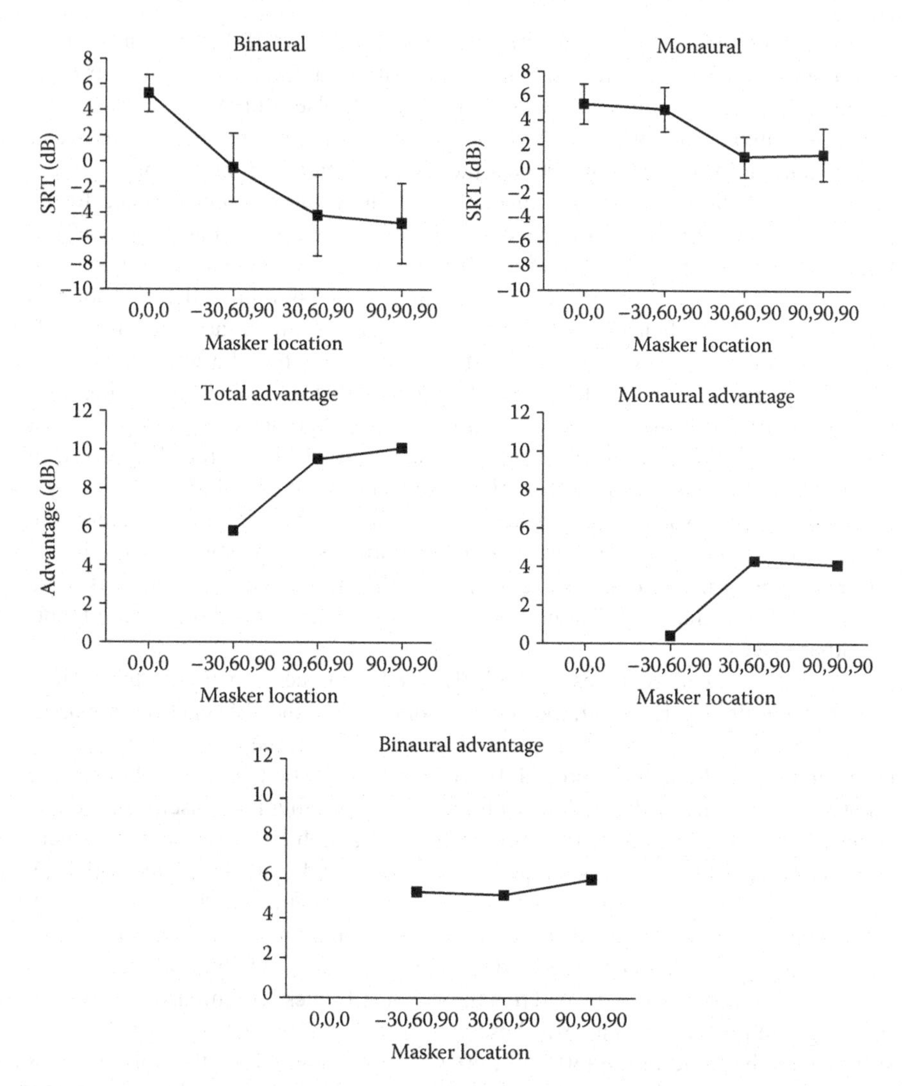

FIGURE 4.3 Binaural and monaural speech intelligibility (top two panels) as a function of the position of three different interfering talkers (maskers). The spatial configuration (30°, 60°, 90°), for instance, indicates that the three interfering talkers were located at 30°, 60°, and 90°, respectively. Target signal was coming from the front of the listener, that is, from 0°. Bottom panels show the advantage (in dB) gained when listening with two ears (see text for explanation).

advantage increased as the number of interfering talkers increased from 1 to 3, varying from a low of 3 dB (one interfering talker) to 7 dB (three interfering talkers) improvement in SRT. The temporal properties of the interfering sound can affect the binaural advantage, with larger benefits obtained with multiple speech maskers [12,13,19] than with multiple noiselike maskers (e.g., continuous and speech-modulated). For the latter maskers, a limited 3 dB binaural advantage was maintained in [11], independent of the spatial configuration (symmetric vs. asymmetric) and the number of speech-modulated noise sources.

As indicated earlier, when multiple noise sources are present, the importance of spatial configuration increases. In fact, the effect of spatial configuration is greater than that of adding or removing one source; that is, one can compensate for an additional interfering noise source simply by choosing a more favorable configuration [15]. In the study by Yost et al. [16], the scores for correct identification of words, letters, and numbers presented simultaneously from three different sources increased by 30% when the angle between adjacent sources increased from 30° to 90°. In contrast, the scores increased only by 10% when the number of noise sources was reduced from 3 to 2. The study concluded that binaural hearing does provide significant benefit when there are more than two noise sources present. It should be noted that a "divided attention" task was used in the preceding study, in that listeners were asked to identify all active sound sources rather than identify a particular source, as is typically done in most studies. The latter task is referred to as *selective attention* task because the listener attends to one source while ignoring other competing sources. Some argue that the selective attention task is more reflective of "cocktail party" situations, where we attend to one voice while ignoring other voices.

As mentioned earlier, access to both ILD and ITD cues contributes to binaural speech intelligibility. However, the contributions of ITD and ILD cues are not additive and depend on the spectral content of the speech material as well as the spatial configuration of the noise sources [20,21]. The benefits of ITD and ILD cues are known to be frequency dependent, with the ITD cues being more useful in the low frequencies and ILD cues being more useful in the high frequencies. This dependence is due to the fact that low frequencies are diffracted around the head with little attenuation, while high frequencies (>4 kHz) are heavily attenuated.

Several studies investigated the individual contributions of ILD and ITD cues by creating stimuli that contained either ILD cues alone, ITD cues alone, or both [20,21]. Results from [21] indicated that the use of ILD cues is dominated by best-ear listening (see Figure 4.4). This was based on the fact that intelligibility of ILD-only stimuli was the same in the (30°, 60°, 90°) configuration, where the noise sources were spatially separated from speech, as it was in the (0°, 0°, 0°) configuration, where the noise sources were coincident with speech. From Figure 4.4, it is clear that the use of ILD cues is heavily influenced by the location of the noise sources. Performance in the (–30°, 60°, 90°) configuration, for instance, was significantly worse than performance in other configurations because the noise sources were distributed across the two hemifields. In contrast, the use of ITD cues is relatively more robust (see Figure 4.4) to the location of noise sources, suggesting that the binaural system is able to exploit ITDs even in complex listening situations where multiple speakers might be present.

Considerable effort has been made to find ways to predict the binaural benefit from spatial release of masking [14,22]. One simple formula that was found to work quite well in predicting binaural intelligibility data is the one proposed in [14]. For speech presented from the front, the release of masking due to spatial separation

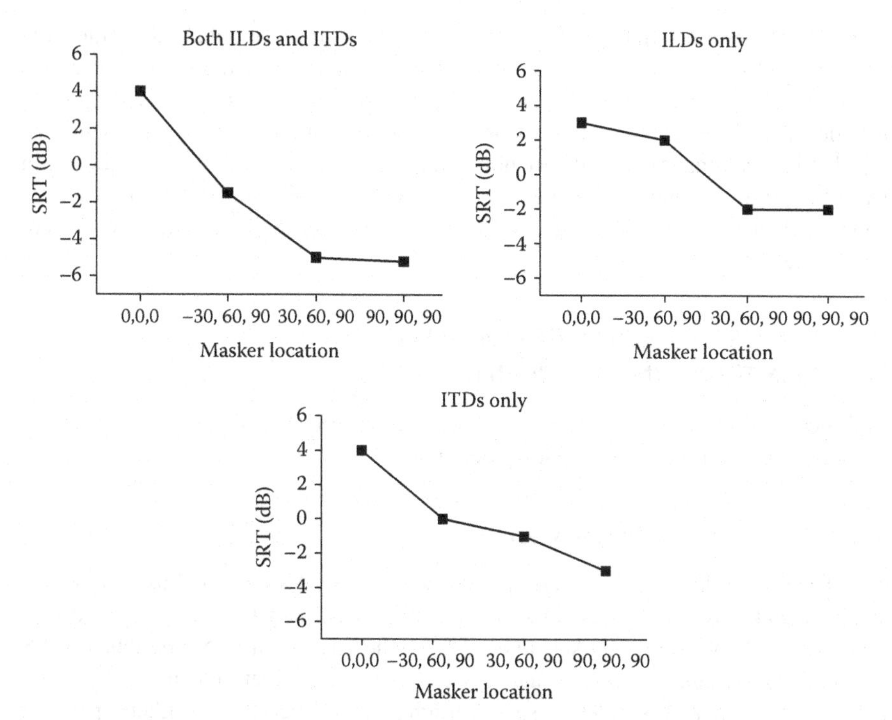

FIGURE 4.4 Binaural speech intelligibility as a function of the position of three different interfering talkers (maskers). Signals were processed so as to contain both ITD and ILD cues (left panel), or ILD cues only (right panel), or ITD cues only (bottom panel). The target signal was coming from the front of the listener, that is, from 0°.

(i.e., the difference in SRT for speech and noise presented from the front vs. speech and noise being spatially separated) is given by

$$R = C\left[\alpha\left(1 - \frac{1}{N}\sum_{i=1}^{N}\cos\theta_i\right) + \beta\frac{1}{N}\left|\sum_{i=1}^{N}\sin\theta_i\right|\right] \quad (4.1)$$

where

- R is the predicted release from masking
- C is a constant ($C = 0.85 - 1$) used to account for differences in speech material
- α and β are constants
- N is the number of noise sources
- θ_i is the azimuth of the ith noise source

Good fits with experimental data were found with $\alpha = 1.38$ and $\beta = 8.02$. The cosine term in Equation 4.1 estimates the average displacement contribution between the target (coming from the front) and each of the N noise sources, and the sine term estimates the symmetry contribution of the noise sources. The sine term assumes a smaller value when the noise sources are symmetrically located.

It should be noted that all the data discussed so far were obtained in anechoic conditions, that is, in the absence of reverberation. In realistic environments there might be reverberation in the room, and speech intelligibility will deteriorate because (1) the contribution of head shadow will be reduced, causing in turn a reduction in binaural release of masking, and (2) there will be a smaller gain from temporal fluctuations of the noise sources. A small number of studies were conducted in realistic listening conditions where reverberation might be present (e.g., [23,24]).

4.2 ACOUSTIC PROPERTIES OF SPEECH CONTRIBUTING TO ROBUSTNESS

The speech signal itself possesses a number of properties that shield it from external distortion. These properties are described next.

4.2.1 Shape of the Speech Spectrum

The shape of the long-term average speech spectrum (LTASS) can tell us a great deal about which frequency regions of the spectrum are most likely to be affected by distortion and which ones are most likely to be affected the least. Figure 4.5 shows the LTASS obtained from a large number of native speakers of 12 different languages [25]. The LTASS was estimated by filtering speech through 25 1/3-octave-wide filters spanning the range of 63–16,000 Hz, and computing the root-mean-square (rms) level within each band. The 1/3-octave analysis was performed using 125 ms segments of speech and averaged over a 1 min recorded passage. Figure 4.5 shows separately the LTASS spectra obtained for male and female speakers. As one would expect, the difference between the male and female LTASS is most prominent in the very-low-frequency region, reflecting the lower fundamental frequency of male speakers. Most of the speech energy lies below 1 kHz, with a peak at 500 Hz. Speech energy gradually decreases starting at 500 Hz.

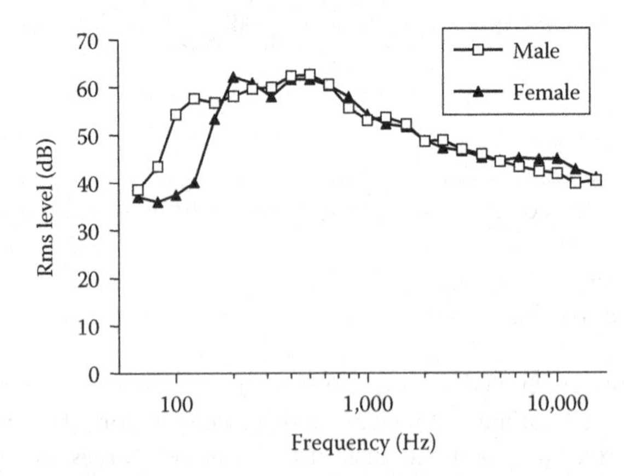

FIGURE 4.5 LTASS from 10 adult males (open squares symbols) and 10 adult females (filled triangles symbols) for 12 different languages.

It is clear from Figure 4.5 that the LTASS has a low-frequency dominance. This low-frequency emphasis of the LTASS shields speech information from distortion and noise for several reasons:

1. With decreasing S/N levels, the low-frequency region is the last to be masked by noise. Generally, the low-frequency region will be masked to a lesser degree than the high-frequency region (see example in Figure 4.6). This holds for both white and pink-type of input noise. The effect, however, is more evident with white noise.
2. As a direct consequence of the aforementioned reason, listeners will have access to reliable F1 and partial F2 information [26]. Such information is critically important for vowel identification and stop-consonant perception.
3. Speech harmonics falling in the low frequencies will be affected less than the high-frequency harmonics. Listeners will therefore have access to relatively reliable F0 cues needed for segregating speech from competing voices.
4. Neural phase-locking provides an effective means of temporally coding information pertaining to the lower formant frequencies [27], and is known to be preserved at the auditory nerve level up to 4–5 kHz.
5. Auditory frequency selectivity is sharpest in low frequencies and decreases at high frequencies [28]. This enables listeners to make fine F0 distinctions, important for segregating speech in multitalker environments.

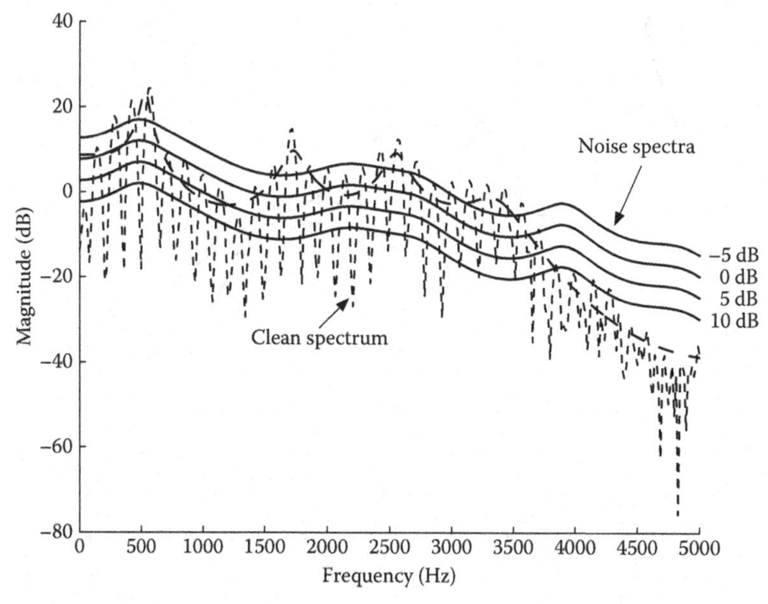

FIGURE 4.6 LPC spectra of the vowel /eh/ (male speaker, F0 = 144 Hz) overlaid with the LPC spectra of multitalker babble scaled at different S/N ratios. The LPC spectra of the noise are shown prior to addition of the clean vowel at the indicated S/N ratios. Dashed lines show the clean FFT- and LPC-magnitude spectra.

Each of the preceding factors contributes to the robustness of speech information in noisy conditions.

4.2.2 Spectral Peaks

The low-frequency spectral peaks are more likely to be preserved in noise than the spectral valleys [26]. This is illustrated in Figure 4.7, which shows the linear predictive coding (LPC) spectra of the vowel /eh/ (as in "head") corrupted in 5–10 dB multitalker babble. As can be seen, the frequency locations of the first three peaks, corresponding to the lower three formants (F1–F3), do not change much after adding noise. For this particular example, the F1 peak location appears to shift from 691 Hz in quiet to 633 Hz in 0 dB, whereas the F2 peak location appears to change from 1879 Hz in quiet to 1726 Hz in 0 dB. As one might expect, the effect of noise on the location of the spectral peaks will depend on the spectral characteristics of the noise, and this is demonstrated in Figure 4.8, which shows the LPC spectra of the vowel /eh/ corrupted in white noise at +5 and 0 dB S/N. As can be seen, white noise reduced the dynamic range and spectral contrast (peak-to-valley ratio) of the vowel, possibly to a greater extent as compared to babble. However, the frequency location of the first peak corresponding to F1 did not change by much even at 0 dB.

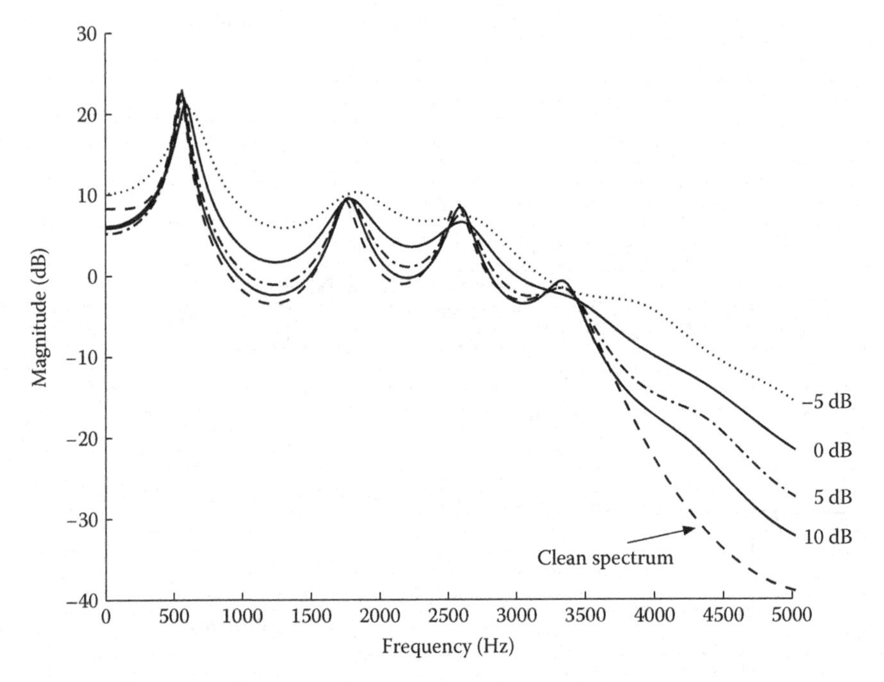

FIGURE 4.7 LPC spectra of the vowel /eh/ (same as in Figure 4.6) corrupted by multitalker babble at −5 to 10 dB S/N.

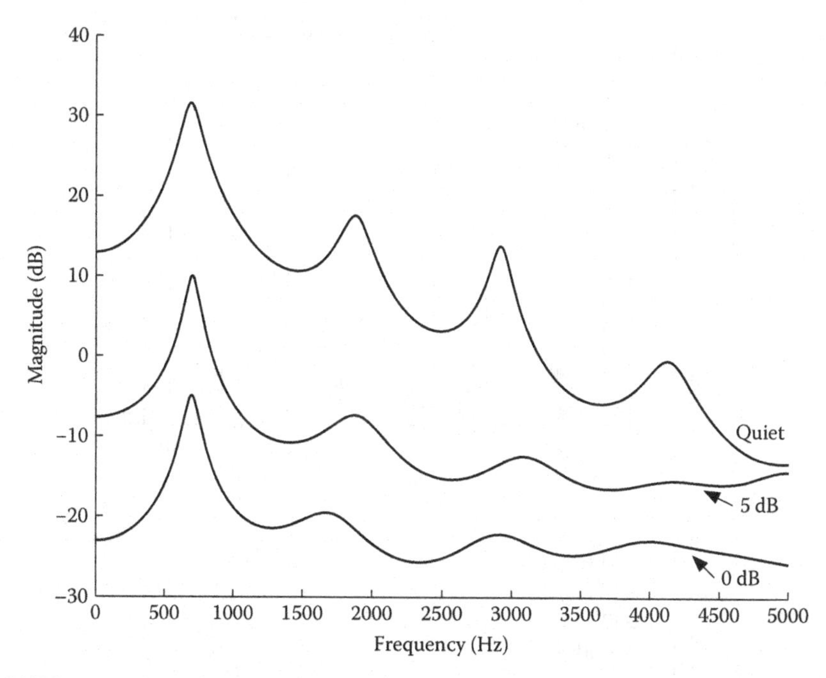

FIGURE 4.8 LPC spectra of the vowel /eh/ corrupted by white noise at 0 and 5 dB S/N. The noisy spectra were shifted down for clarity.

The frequencies of the first three formant (F1–F3) peaks as well as their trajectory over time (i.e., the formant transitions) provide valuable cues to listeners for vowel [29], glide [30], and stop-consonant perception [31]. As the examples in Figures 4.7 and 4.8 demonstrate, the lowest two formant peaks are not affected in noise as much as the higher formant peaks. But to what extent is there reliable F1 and F2 information in noise?

The study in [26] showed that F1 is preserved to a certain degree in noise. Figure 4.9 plots the percent of frames for which F1 and F2 were reliably detected in babble as a function of the S/N ratio. These data were based on acoustic analysis of 11 vowels produced in the /hVd/ context by 23 different female speakers and 20 male speakers. Acoustic analysis indicated that F1 was detected more reliably in noise than F2. In multitalker babble at −5 dB S/N, for instance, F1 was identified 60% of the time whereas F2 was identified only 30% of the time (these values were obtained by summing the percentages of "F1 only" and "F1&F2" in Figure 4.9). The results from [26] suggest that in extremely noisy conditions, listeners are able to identify vowels based on a relatively accurate F1 representation and partial F2 representation.

In summary, noise may distort the shape of the spectrum, change its slope, and reduce the spectral dynamic range (see Figure 4.8), but the frequency locations of the lower formant peaks are preserved to some degree (see example in Figure 4.7).

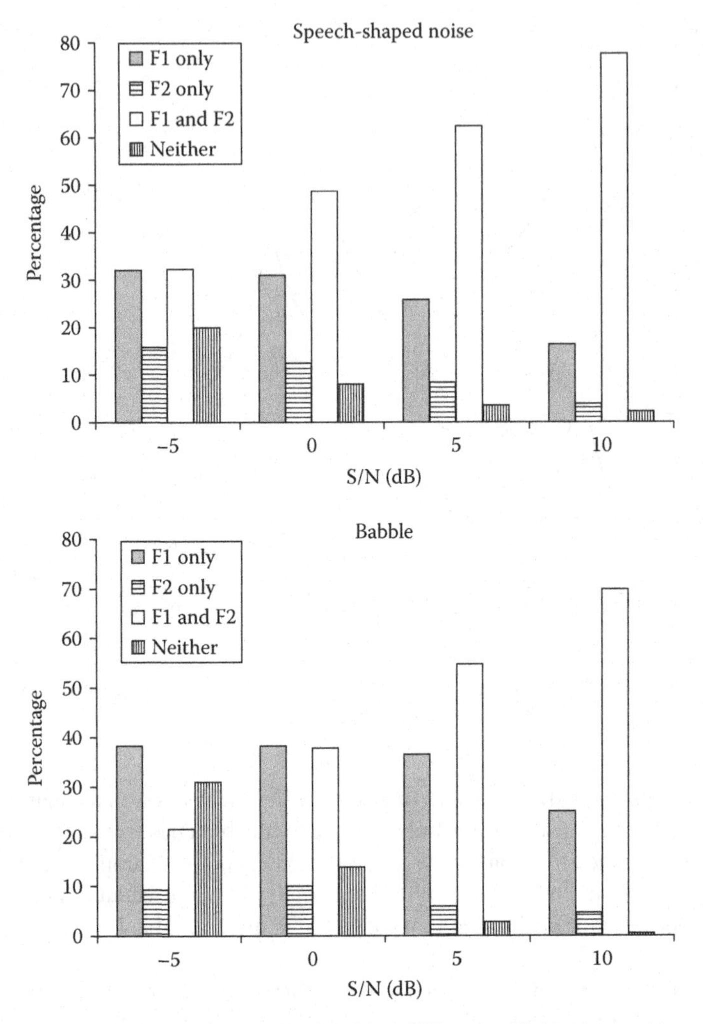

FIGURE 4.9 Percentage of frames for which F1 and F2 were reliably detected in multitalker babble and speech-shaped noise as a function of the S/N ratio. (From Parikh, G. and Loizou, P., *J. Acoust. Soc. Am.*, 118(6), 3874, 2005. With permission.)

4.2.3 Periodicity

As described in Chapter 3, the opening and closing of the vocal folds during voicing produces periodic waveforms (voiced segments of speech). The time duration of one cycle of the vocal folds' opening or closing is known as the fundamental period, and the reciprocal of the fundamental period is known as the vocal pitch or fundamental frequency (F0). The fundamental frequency F0 varies from a low frequency of around 80 Hz for male speakers to a high frequency of 280 Hz for children [29]. The presence or absence of periodicity signifies the distinction between voiced and

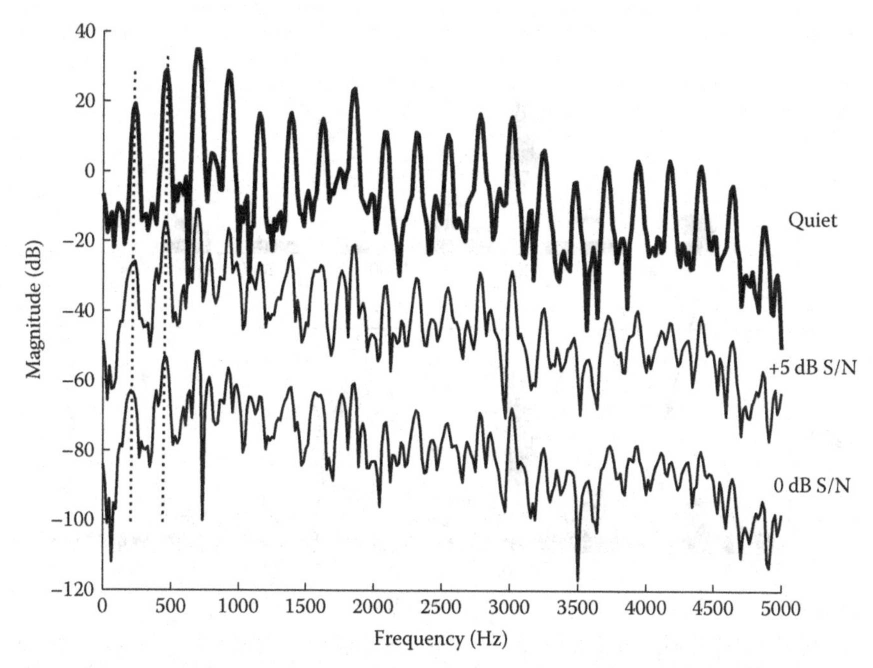

FIGURE 4.10 Example FFT-magnitude spectra of the vowel /eh/ corrupted by multitalker babble at 0 and 5 dB S/N. The noisy-magnitude spectra were shifted down for better clarity.

unvoiced sounds (e.g., between [d] and [t]). The F0 periodicity is also responsible for the perception of vocal pitch, intonation, prosody, and perception of lexical tone in tonal languages.

The voiced segments of speech (e.g., vowels) are quasi-periodic in the time domain and harmonic in the frequency domain. The periodicity of speech is broadly distributed across frequency and time and is robust in the presence of noise. Figure 4.10 shows the FFT spectra of the vowel /eh/ in quiet and in noise. It is clear that the lower harmonics are preserved in noise, at least up to 1 kHz. This suggests that listeners have access to relatively accurate F0 information in noise. Such information, as we will discuss later (Section 4.3.3), is important for understanding speech in situations where two or more people are speaking simultaneously [32].

4.2.4 Rapid Spectral Changes Signaling Consonants

Unlike vowels, consonants are short in duration and have low intensity. Consequently, they are more vulnerable to noise or distortion, compared to vowels. The duration of the /b/ burst, for instance, can be as brief as 5–10 ms. Vowels on the other hand can last as long as 300 ms [33].

Formant transitions associated with vowel or diphthong production are slow and gradual. In contrast, consonants (particularly stop consonants) are associated with rapid spectral changes and rapid formant transitions. In noise, these rapid spectral

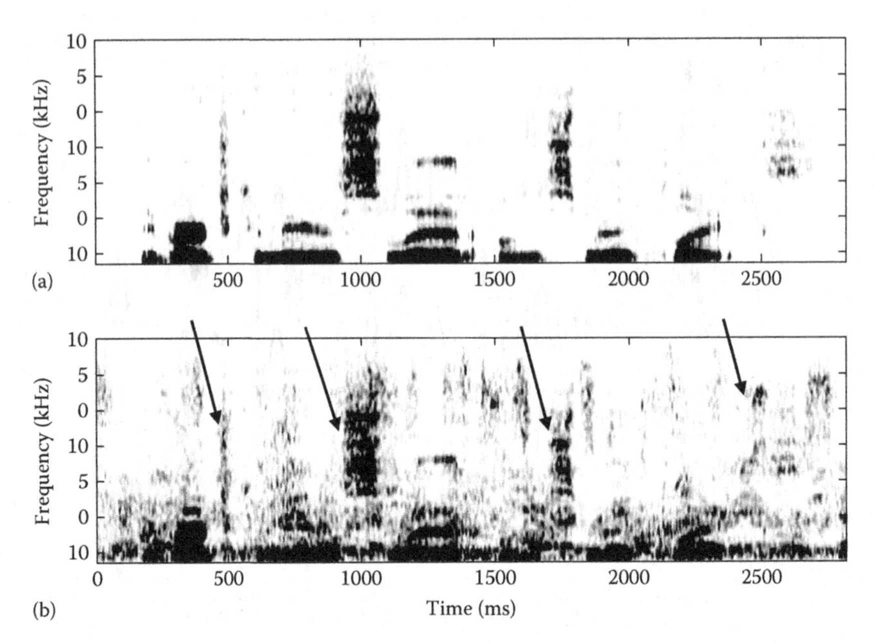

FIGURE 4.11 Spectrogram of the sentence "The birch canoe slid on the smooth planks" in quiet (a) and in +5dB babble (b). Arrows indicate the onsets of some of the high-frequency consonants.

changes are preserved to some degree and serve as landmarks signaling the presence of consonants. Figure 4.11 shows example spectrograms of a sentence embedded in +5dB babble noise. Note that the low-frequency (and intense) vowels alternate frequently with the high-frequency (and weak) consonants, resulting in sudden spectral changes. For instance, the low-frequency spectral dominance at near 500, 1000, and 1700ms is followed by a sudden dispersion of spectral energy across the spectrum. These sudden spectral changes coincide with the onsets of consonants. Although for the most part the high-frequency information is smeared and heavily masked by the noise, the onsets of most of the consonants are preserved (see arrows in Figure 4.11). There is evidence from neurophysiologic studies (e.g., [34]), suggesting that peripheral or central adaptation mechanisms exist that improve the prominence of spectral components with sudden onsets. The response of auditory nerve fibers to tone bursts is maximal at the onset of the stimulus, and gradually decays to its steady-state value.

4.3 PERCEPTUAL STRATEGIES FOR LISTENING IN NOISE

In a previous section (Section 4.1), we described how listeners are able to carry a conversation in the most adverse conditions, which might include highly reverberant rooms with multiple speakers in the background. But, how can the auditory system achieve such a feat? For one, the speech signal itself is shielded in many ways from external distortion (see Section 4.2). Furthermore, human listeners utilize several perceptual strategies that facilitate speech segregation. These listening strategies are discussed next.

4.3.1 Auditory Streaming

Consider a mixture of sounds consisting of speech and other sources, including, say, the sound of the wind blowing through the window, cars passing by, a telephone ringing, etc. Bregman [2] proposed that humans can analyze such an auditory scene and are able to segregate speech from the other sources by grouping together components of a sound mixture according to their sources. He referred to the components belonging to the same source as *auditory streams*.

Two different types of groupings were suggested as necessary to segregate speech by (1) linking events that follow one another in time (sequential grouping), and (2) integrating components that occur at the same time in different regions of the spectrum (simultaneous grouping). Sequential grouping can be done by tracking characteristics of the speech signal that vary slowly over time. For instance, listeners might exploit trajectories of formant peaks that vary slowly over time and frequency to track a voice in background noise. Simultaneous grouping can be done by exploiting differences in pitch (F0) between competing voices, differences in the shape of the spectrum envelope, and differences in the spatial location of the sources. In running speech, pitch (F0) is always changing, and two voices are not likely to follow exactly the same pitch contour at the same time. Segregation based on F0 can be done, for instance, by looking for one or more harmonics that can account for as many of the frequency components in the spectrum as possible, and then allocating all the components belonging to the same fundamental frequency (F0) to the same auditory stream. This suggests a *harmonic sieve* mechanism that excludes harmonic components whose frequencies do not correspond to integer multiples of a given fundamental frequency. Such a mechanism was proposed as a plausible model of pitch perception [35].

According to Bregman [2], the foregoing two grouping mechanisms are governed by primitive auditory constraints such as the constraint that most speech characteristics (e.g., F0, formants) tend to be continuous and change slowly over time. They are called primitive in that they probably exist from infancy, that is, they are innate, and do not rely on higher cognitive functions. Primitive auditory constraints utilize a bottom-up approach to auditory scene analysis. Bregman [2, Chapter 4] further proposed that auditory scene analysis is governed by learned constraints, which he called schema-based constraints. These constraints utilize a top-down approach to auditory scene analysis. The schema-driven segregation process is presumed to involve the activation of stored (learned) knowledge of familiar patterns in the acoustic environment (e.g., sounds of musical instruments, bells ringing, etc.), including learned knowledge of the language (e.g., language structure, semantics, grammar). Evidence of schema-based segregation is provided by studies of sine-wave speech [36]. When the formant trajectories of a sentence are replaced by sine waves following the formant frequencies, listeners can frequently recognize the words in the sentence, despite the fact that the synthesized sentence sounds unnatural, synthetic, and robotic. Listeners must be utilizing speech-specific knowledge about production to be able to fuse the perceived formant tracks into a single auditory stream. Such knowledge is acquired from extended exposure to the acoustic properties of speech.

4.3.2 Listening in the Gaps and Glimpsing

As mentioned earlier, there is evidence from several studies confirming that it is more difficult to identify words in the presence of steady-state noise than in the presence of a single competing speaker. The difference in SRT (50% intelligibility level) can be large, ranging from a low of 6 dB [5] to a high of 10 dB [4]. This difference is attributed to the fact that listeners are exploiting the silent gaps or waveform "valleys" in the competing signal to recognize the words in the target sentence. These gaps or amplitude valleys can potentially enable listeners to "glimpse" entire syllables or words of the target voice. During the gaps in the competing signal, the local (segmental) SNR is quite favorable. Clearly, the local SNR will be fluctuating over time, yet the listeners are able to exploit the local high-SNR segments of the noisy signal and extract (glimpse) useful information. Note that a similar situation occurs when the noise and speech signals are spatially separated. Listeners are able to utilize the "better" ear, that is, the ear with the highest SNR, to recognize the target voice. Humans possess a remarkable ability to exploit segments of noisy speech with highest SNR in both monaural and binaural listening situations.

The listening-in-the-gaps account of speech segregation falls apart, however, when there are large numbers (more than 4) of competing voices present because the masker waveform becomes nearly continuous, leaving no silent gaps in the waveform (see Figure 4.1). In such situations, different listening strategies are probably employed.

A different view of glimpsing was proposed by Cooke [37,38], extending and generalizing the aforementioned idea of listening in the gaps. This new view was based on a different definition of what constitutes a *glimpse*: "a time-frequency region that contains a reasonably undistorted 'view' of local signal properties" [38]. Useful signal properties may include signal energy or presence of reliable F0 and formant frequency information. Glimpses of speech in background noise may, for instance, comprise all time-frequency areas or slices having a local SNR exceeding a certain threshold value (e.g., 3 dB). The assumption is that the listeners are able to detect "useful" glimpses of speech, which are possibly occurring at different times and occupying different regions of the spectrum, and are able to integrate all these glimpses (as different pieces of the puzzle) to recognize the target speech. Computational models of glimpsing were developed for robust automatic speech recognition by modifying the recognition process to allow for the possibility of "missing data" [39,40]. Despite the attractive appeal of glimpsing as a means of speech separation, there still remain several issues to be resolved. Foremost among those issues is the question of what constitutes a "useful" glimpse and whether glimpses contain sufficient information to support identification of the target signal.

4.3.3 Use of F0 Differences

It is generally accepted that it is easier to recognize competing speech when the target and masker voices are of opposite sex. The difference in F0 between male and female voices could be as large as 100 Hz [29]. Several studies have demonstrated that the difference in fundamental frequencies of the masker and target voices is critically important for recognizing speech in competing voices. Brokx and Nooteboom [32] first demonstrated this by artificially modifying the speech of two talkers to have a monotonous (i.e., flat F0 contour) pitch and then synthesizing the monotonous sentences with an LPC vocoder. They varied the F0 difference between the target and masker voices from 0 to 12 semitones (1 octave). Results indicated that word identification accuracy was the lowest when the target and masker had the same F0 and gradually improved with increasing differences in F0 (see Figure 4.12). A mere difference of 3 semitones (F0 = 100 Hz vs. F0 = 120 Hz) was sufficient to produce a significant increase in the number of words identified from 40% correct to 60% correct. Identification accuracy was low when the pitch of the two voices was exactly 1 octave apart, which is the condition where every second harmonic of the higher-pitched voice coincides with a harmonic of the lower-pitched voice. These findings were replicated and extended by Bird and Darwin [41], who showed that identification accuracy continues to improve up to an F0 difference of 8 semitones (see Figure 4.12).

A similar outcome has emerged from studies examining the contribution of F0 in the perception of "double vowels" [42]—pairs of vowels played simultaneously on different fundamentals (F0). The listeners' task is to identify both vowels. Several studies demonstrated that performance is above the chance level even when the two vowels have the same F0 [42–44]. Identification improves significantly, however, as the F0 difference is increased from 0 to 2 semitones, but does not improve further beyond 2 semitones. Overall, the contribution of F0 is greater and more evident for "double sentences" [32,41] than for "double vowels" [43].

The separation of two voices on the basis of fundamental frequency is believed to be mediated by simultaneous grouping mechanisms. Harmonics corresponding to the same F0 are presumably grouped together to form a single auditory stream. Such a grouping, for example, can potentially aid the listeners to identify and track

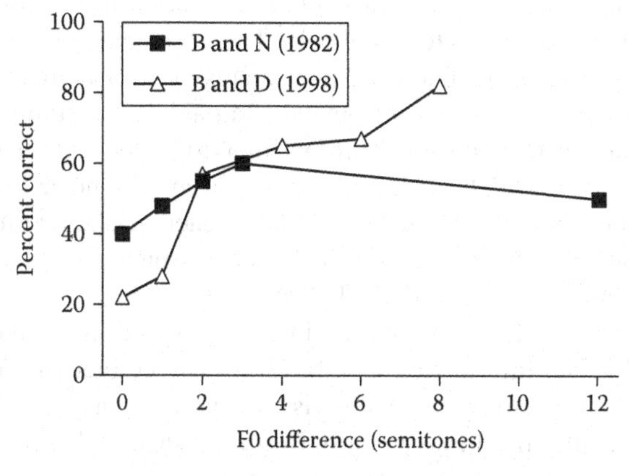

FIGURE 4.12 Results from two studies (B and N [32] and B and D [41]) on intelligibility of sentences corrupted by a single interfering talker as a function of the F0 difference of the target and interfering talkers. The F0 difference is expressed in semitones with 12 semitones equaling 1 octave.

(over time) formant peaks belonging to the target speaker. A number of algorithms have used this principle for automatic separation of two voices [45–47].

4.3.4 Use of Linguistic Knowledge

Intelligibility of speech in adverse conditions is greatly influenced by the ability of listeners to exploit linguistic knowledge, particularly when the cues contained in the acoustic signal are weak. The presence of semantic context, in particular, can lead to higher intelligibility of sentences as it restricts the range of plausible words [48].

Early experiments by Treisman [49] demonstrated that the linguistic content of the interfering message can greatly influence speech recognition. Competing speech in the same language and similar in content as the target speech was found to be the most disruptive. Least disruptive was competing speech spoken in an unfamiliar foreign language. Access to learned knowledge about the language provides linguistic constraints useful in a schema-based perceptual segregation process [2].

4.3.5 Use of Spatial and Visual Cues

In real-world environments (e.g., in a crowded restaurant), competing voices originate from different locations in space. The acoustic signals arriving at the two ears of the listener will have different intensities (ILDs) and different times of arrival (ITDs). The ILD and ITD cues are used by listeners in spatial segregation of voices. The ILD cues alone, by virtue of providing access to a "better ear," provide a large benefit in speech intelligibility, provided the noise sources are not symmetrically located around the listener [20]. The ITD cues alone are effective cues for tracking a particular sound over time, but are not effective for segregating the speech of a single talker from competing talkers [50]. In concert, the ILD and ITD cues provide a large binaural advantage in situations where the speech and noise sources are spatially separated [12].

In real-world environments, and particularly in face-to-face communication settings, listeners also have access to visual cues. The visual cues provide synchronization between the acoustic signal and the movements of the articulators (e.g., tongue, lip). Having access to such visual information can aid in discrimination of certain confusable consonants (e.g., /p/ vs. /t/, /m/ vs. /n/) differing in place of articulation. Discrimination of /t/ vs. /p/, for instance, can be difficult in noise in the absence of visual cues, but it becomes extremely easy if the listener watches the lips of the target speaker. It is relatively easy to identify the labial consonants (e.g., /p/, /b/) because these consonants are produced with the lips closed.

Several studies have demonstrated the intelligibility benefit gained by integrating acoustic and visual information [51]. In [51], sentence recognition in noise was assessed in both auditory-only and audio-visual conditions, using sentences ranging in lip reading difficulty from easy to hard. Results indicated that the overall benefit conferred by visual cues was equivalent to an effective improvement in the SNR of 11 dB. As expected, the better lip readers benefited more than the poor lip readers. Other studies also demonstrated a significant benefit in intelligibility even when limited amounts of acoustic information supplemented speech reading [52].

4.4 SUMMARY

The present chapter provided a brief overview of auditory scene analysis by human listeners. Human listeners (with normal hearing) are able to carry on a conversation in the most adverse conditions for two main reasons. First, the information in speech is shielded from distortion in several ways (see Section 4.2). More precisely, the speech signal possesses a number of properties (e.g., low-pass shape of speech spectrum, spectral peaks) that protect the information contained in the signal from external distortion and interference. In the context of noise reduction algorithms, this suggests that these properties (e.g., spectral peaks, F0 information) need to be preserved to avoid any degradation in speech intelligibility. Second, multiple listening strategies are used by listeners to accommodate various listening scenarios where not all cues might necessarily be present (Section 4.3). In the absence of visual and spatial cues (e.g., listening via the telephone), for instance, listeners must be using alternative listening strategies (e.g., F0 differences between the target speech and competing talkers, linguistic constraints, glimpsing, etc.) to communicate in noisy environments.

The area of auditory scene analysis is vast and remains an active topic of research not only for scientists interested in cognition but also for people interested in developing computational models for automatic speech separation. This chapter has barely scratched the surface of this topic. For more information on auditory scene analysis, the interested reader is referred to reviews [3,14,53–56] as well as books [2,57].

REFERENCES

1. Cherry, E. (1953), Some experiments on the recognition of speech with one and with two ears, *J. Acoust. Soc. Am.*, 25, 975–979.
2. Bregman, A. (1990), *Auditory Scene Analysis*, Cambridge, MA: MIT Press.
3. Assmann, P. and Summerfield, Q. (2004), The perception of speech under adverse conditions, in Greenberg, S., Ainsworth, W., Popper, A., and Fay, R. (Eds.), *Speech Processing in the Auditory System*, New York: Springer Verlag, pp. 231–308.
4. Miller, G. (1947), The masking of speech, *Psychol. Bull.*, 44(2), 105–129.
5. Festen, J. and Plomp, R. (1990), Effects of fluctuating noise and interfering speech on the speech-reception threshold for impaired and normal hearing, *J. Acoust. Soc. Am.*, 88, 1725–1736.
6. Levitt, H. and Rabiner, L. (1967), Binaural release from masking for speech and gain in intelligibility, *J. Acoust. Soc. Am.*, 42(3), 601–608.
7. Carhart, R., Tillman, T., and Greetis, E. (1969), Perceptual masking in multiple sound backgrounds, *J. Acoust. Soc. Am.*, 45(3), 694–703.
8. Duquesnoy, A. (1983), Effect of a single interfering noise or speech source upon the binaural sentence intelligibility of aged persons, *J. Acoust. Soc. Am.*, 74(3), 739–743.
9. Drullman, R. and Bronkhorst, A. (2000), Multichannel speech intelligibility and speaker recognition using monaural, binaural, and 3D auditory presentation, *J. Acoust. Soc. Am.*, 107(4), 2224–2235.
10. Brungart, D. (2001), Informational and energetic masking effects in the perception of two simultaneous talkers, *J. Acoust. Soc. Am.*, 109(3), 1101–1109.
11. Bronkhorst, A. and Plomp, R. (1992), Effect of multiple speechlike maskers on binaural speech recognition in normal and impaired hearing, *J. Acoust. Soc. Am.*, 92(6), 3132–3139.

12. Hawley, M., Litovsky, R., and Culling, J. (2004), The benefit of binaural hearing in a cocktail party: Effect of location and type of interferer, *J. Acoust. Soc. Am.*, 115(2), 833–843.
13. Peissig, J. and Kollmeier, B. (1997), Directivity of binaural noise reduction in spatial multiple noise-source arrangements for normal and impaired listeners, *J. Acoust. Soc. Am.*, 101(3), 1660–1670.
14. Bronkhorst, A. (2000), The cocktail party phenomenon: A review of research on speech intelligibility in multiple-talker conditions, *Acustica*, 86, 117–128.
15. Hawley, M., Litovsky, R., and Colburn, H. (1999), Intelligibility and localization of speech signals in a multi-source environment, *J. Acoust. Soc. Am.*, 105, 3436–3448.
16. Yost, W., Dye, R., and Sheft, S. (1996), A simulated "cocktail party" with up to three sound sources, *Percept. Psychophys.*, 58(7), 1026–1036.
17. Blauert, J., Brueggen, M., Bronkhorst, A., Drullman, R., Reynaud, G., Pellieux, L., Krebber, W., and Sottek, R. (1998), The AUDIS catalog of human HRTFs, *J. Acoust. Soc. Am.*, 103, 3082.
18. IEEE Subcommittee (1969), IEEE recommended practice for speech quality measurements, *IEEE Trans. Audio Electroacoust.*, AU-17(3), 225–246.
19. Noble, W. and Perrett, S. (2002), Hearing speech against spatially separate competing speech versus competing voice, *Percept. Psychophys.*, 64(8), 1325–1336.
20. Bronkhorst, A. and Plomp, R. (1988), The effect of head-induced interaural time and level differences on speech intelligibility in noise, *J. Acoust. Soc. Am.*, 83(4), 1508–1516.
21. Culling, J., Hawley, M., and Litovsky, R. (2004), The role of head-induced interaural time and level differences in the speech reception threshold for multiple interfering sound sources, *J. Acoust. Soc. Am.*, 116(2), 1057–1065.
22. Levitt, H. and Rabiner, L. (1967), Predicting binaural gain in intelligibility and release from masking for speech, *J. Acoust. Soc. Am.*, 42(4), 820–829.
23. Nabelek, A. and Robinson, P. (1982), Monaural and binaural speech perception in reverberation for listeners of various ages, *J. Acoust. Soc. Am.*, 71, 1242–1248.
24. Moncur, J. and Dirks, D. (1967), Binaural and monaural speech intelligibility in reverberation, *J. Speech Hear. Res.*, 10, 186–195.
25. Byrne, D., Dillon, H., Tran, K., Arlinger, S., Wilbraham, K., Cox, R., Hagerman et al. (1994), An international comparison of long-term average speech spectra, *J. Acoust. Soc. Am.*, 96, 2108–2120.
26. Parikh, G. and Loizou, P. (2005), The influence of noise on vowel and consonant cues, *J. Acoust. Soc. Am.*, 118(6), 3874–3888.
27. Young, E. and Sachs, M. (1979), Representation of steady-state vowels in the temporal aspects of the discharge patterns of populations of auditory nerve fibers, *J. Acoust. Soc. Am.*, 66(5), 1381–1403.
28. Patterson, R. and Moore, B. (1986), Auditory filters and excitation patterns as representations of auditory frequency selectivity, in Moore, B. (Ed.), *Frequency Selectivity in Hearing*, London, U.K.: Academic Press.
29. Peterson, G. and Barney, H. (1952), Control methods used in a study of the vowels, *J. Acoust. Soc. Am.*, 24(2), 175–184.
30. O'Connor, J., Gerstman, L., Liberman, A., Delattre, P., and Cooper, F. (1957), Acoustic cues for the perception of initial/w, j, r, l/in English, *Word*, 13, 24–43.
31. Delattre, P., Liberman, A., and Cooper, F. (1955), Acoustic loci and transitional cues for consonants, *J. Acoust. Soc. Am.*, 27, 769–774.
32. Brokx, J. and Nooteboom, S. (1982), Intonation and perception of simultaneous voices, *J. Phonetics*, 10, 23–26.
33. Hillenbrand, J., Getty, L., Clark, M., and Wheeler, K. (1995), Acoustic characteristics of American English vowels, *J. Acoust. Soc. Am.*, 97(5), 3099–3111.

34. Delgutte, B. (1980), Representation of speech-like sounds in the discharge patterns of auditory-nerve fibers, *J. Acoust. Soc. Am.*, 68(3), 843–857.
35. Duifhuis, H., Willems, L., and Sluyter, R. (1982), Measurement of pitch on speech: An implementation of Goldstein's theory of pitch perception, *J. Acoust. Soc. Am.*, 71, 1568–1580.
36. Remez, R., Rubin, P., Pisoni, D., and Carrell, T. (1981), Speech perception without traditional cues, *Science*, 212, 947–950.
37. Cooke, M. (2003), Glimpsing speech, *J. Phonetics*, 31, 579–584.
38. Cooke, M. (2005), Making sense of everyday speech: A glimpsing account, in Divenyi, P. (Ed.), *Speech Separation by Humans and Machines*, New York: Kluwer Academic Publishers, pp. 305–314.
39. Cooke, M., Green, P., and Crawford, M. (1994), Handling missing data in speech recognition, *Proceedings of International Conference on Spoken Language Processing*, Yokohama, Japan, pp. 1555–1558.
40. Cooke, M., Green, P., Josifovski, L., and Vizinho, A. (2001), Robust automatic speech recognition with missing and uncertain acoustic data, *Speech Commun.*, 34, 267–285.
41. Bird, J. and Darwin, C. (1998), Effects of a difference in fundamental frequency in separating two sentences, in Palmer, A., Rees, A., Summerfield, Q., and Meddis, R. (Eds.), *Psychophysical and Physiological Advances in Hearing*, London, U.K.: Whurr.
42. Scheffers, M. (1983), Sifting vowels: Auditory pitch analysis and sound segregation, PhD thesis, Rijksuniversiteit te Groningen, Groningen, the Netherlands.
43. Assmann, P. and Summerfield, Q. (1990), Modeling the perception of concurrent vowels: Vowels with different fundamental frequencies, *J. Acoust. Soc. Am.*, 88, 680–697.
44. Culling, J. and Darwin, C. (1993), Perceptual separation of simultaneous vowels: Within and across-formant grouping by F0, *J. Acoust. Soc. Am.*, 93, 3454–3467.
45. Parsons, T. (1976), Separation of speech from interfering speech by means of harmonic selection, *J. Acoust. Soc. Am.*, 60, 656–660.
46. Stubbs, R. and Summerfield, Q. (1988), Evaluation of two voice-separation algorithms using normal-hearing and hearing-impaired listeners, *J. Acoust. Soc. Am.*, 84(4), 1238–1249.
47. Denbigh, P. and Zhao, J. (1992), Pitch extraction and separation of overlapping speech, *Speech Commun.*, 11, 119–126.
48. Miller, G., Heise, G., and Lichten, W. (1951), The intelligibility of speech as a function of the context of the test materials, *J. Exp. Psychol.*, 41, 329–335.
49. Treisman, A. (1964), Verbal cues, language, and meaning in selective attention, *Am. J. Psychol.*, 77(2), 206–219.
50. Culling, J. and Summerfield, Q. (1995), Perceptual separation of concurrent speech sounds: Absence of across-frequency grouping by common interaural delay, *J. Acoust. Soc. Am.*, 98, 785–797.
51. MacLeod, A. and Summerfield, Q. (1987), Quantifying the contribution of vision to speech perception in noise, *Br. J. Audiol.*, 21, 131–141.
52. Breeuwer, M. and Plomp, R. (1984), Speechreading supplemented with frequency-selective sound pressure information, *J. Acoust. Soc. Am.*, 76(3), 686–691.
53. Cooke, M. and Ellis, D. (2001), The auditory organization of speech and other sources in listeners and computational models, *Speech Commun.*, 35, 141–177.
54. Darwin, C. and Carlyon, R. (1995), Auditory grouping, in Moore, B. (Ed.), *Hearing*, San Diego, CA: Academic Press, pp. 387–424.
55. Moore, B. and Gockel, H. (2002), Factors influencing sequential stream segregation, *Acustica*, 88, 320–332.
56. Darwin, C. (1997), Auditory grouping, *Trends Cogn. Sci.*, 1, 327–333.
57. Divenyi, P. (2005), *Speech Separation by Humans and Machines*, Norwell, MA: Kluwer Academic Publishers.

Part II

Algorithms

5 Spectral-Subtractive Algorithms

The spectral-subtractive algorithm is historically one of the first algorithms proposed for noise reduction. More papers have been written describing variations of this algorithm than any other algorithm. It is based on a simple principle. Assuming additive noise, one can obtain an estimate of the clean signal spectrum by subtracting an estimate of the noise spectrum from the noisy speech spectrum. The noise spectrum can be estimated and updated, during periods when the signal is absent. The assumption made is that noise is stationary or a slowly varying process and that the noise spectrum does not change significantly between the updating periods. The enhanced signal is obtained by computing the inverse discrete Fourier transform of the estimated signal spectrum using the phase of the noisy signal. The algorithm is computationally simple as it only involves a forward and an inverse Fourier transform.

The simple subtraction processing comes at a price. The subtraction process needs to be done carefully to avoid any speech distortion. If too much is subtracted, then some speech information might be removed, whereas if too little is subtracted, then much of the interfering noise remains. Many methods have been proposed to alleviate, and in some cases eliminate, most of the speech distortion introduced by the spectral subtraction process. This chapter introduces the basic spectral subtraction algorithm [1] and describes some of the variations of the algorithm aimed at reducing speech and noise distortion.

5.1 BASIC PRINCIPLES OF SPECTRAL SUBTRACTION

Assume that $y(n)$, the noise-corrupted input signal, is composed of the clean speech signal $x(n)$ and the additive noise signal, $d(n)$, that is,

$$y(n) = x(n) + d(n) \tag{5.1}$$

Taking the discrete-time Fourier transform of both sides gives

$$Y(\omega) = X(\omega) + D(\omega) \tag{5.2}$$

We can express $Y(\omega)$ in polar form as follows:

$$Y(\omega) = |Y(\omega)|\, e^{j\phi_y(\omega)} \tag{5.3}$$

where

$|Y(\omega)|$ is the magnitude spectrum

$\phi_y(\omega)$ is the phase (spectrum) of the corrupted noisy signal

The noise spectrum $D(\omega)$ can also be expressed in terms of its magnitude and phase spectra as $D(\omega) = |D(\omega)| e^{j\varphi_d(\omega)}$. The magnitude noise spectrum $|D(\omega)|$ is unknown, but can be replaced by its average value computed during nonspeech activity (e.g., during speech pauses). Similarly, the noise phase $\phi_d(\omega)$ can be replaced by the noisy speech phase $\phi_y(\omega)$ (more on this in Section 5.2). This is partly motivated by the fact that phase that does not affect speech intelligibility [2] may affect speech quality to some degree. After making these substitutions to Equation 5.2, we can obtain an estimate of the clean signal spectrum:

$$\hat{X}(\omega) = [|Y(\omega)| - |\hat{D}(\omega)|]e^{j\phi_y(\omega)} \tag{5.4}$$

where $|\hat{D}(\omega)|$ is the estimate of the magnitude noise spectrum made during nonspeech activity. We henceforth use the symbol "^" to indicate the *estimated* spectrum or *estimated* parameter of interest. The enhanced speech signal can be obtained by simply taking the inverse Fourier transform of $\hat{X}(\omega)$.

Equation 5.4 summarizes the underlying principle of spectral subtraction. Compute the magnitude spectrum of the noisy speech via the fast Fourier transform (FFT) and keep an estimate of the noise spectrum when speech is not present. Subtract the noise magnitude spectrum from the noisy speech magnitude spectrum (hence the name "spectral subtraction") and, finally, take the inverse Fourier transform of the difference spectra (using the noisy phase) to produce the enhanced speech signal.

Note that the magnitude spectrum of the enhanced signal, $|\hat{X}(\omega)| = (|Y(\omega)| - |\hat{D}(\omega)|)$, can be negative owing to inaccuracies in estimating the noise spectrum. The magnitude spectra, however, cannot be negative; hence, caution needs to be exercised when subtracting the two spectra to ensure that $|\hat{X}(\omega)|$ is always nonnegative. One solution to this is to half-wave-rectify the difference spectra, that is, set the negative spectral components to zero as follows:

$$|\hat{X}(\omega)| = \begin{cases} |Y(\omega)| - |\hat{D}(\omega)| & \text{if } |Y(\omega)| > |\hat{D}(\omega)| \\ 0 & \text{else} \end{cases} \tag{5.5}$$

The half-wave rectification process is only one of many ways of ensuring nonnegative $|\hat{X}(\omega)|$. Other methods can be used and will be described later on in the chapter.

The preceding derivation of the magnitude spectral subtraction algorithm can be easily extended to the power spectrum domain. In some cases, it might be best to work with power spectra rather than magnitude spectra. To obtain the short-term power spectrum of the noisy speech, we multiply $Y(\omega)$ in Equation 5.2 by its conjugate $Y^*(\omega)$. In doing so, Equation 5.2 becomes

$$\begin{aligned} |Y(\omega)|^2 &= |X(\omega)|^2 + |D(\omega)|^2 + X(\omega) \cdot D^*(\omega) + X^*(\omega)D(\omega) \\ &= |X(\omega)|^2 + |D(\omega)|^2 + 2\,\mathrm{Re}\{X(\omega)D^*(\omega)\} \end{aligned} \tag{5.6}$$

The terms $|D(\omega)|^2$, $X(\omega) \cdot D^*(\omega)$, and $X^*(\omega) \cdot D(\omega)$ cannot be obtained directly and are approximated as $E\{|D(\omega)|^2\}$, $E\{X^*(\omega) \cdot D(\omega)\}$, and $E\{X(\omega) \cdot D^*(\omega)\}$, where $E[\cdot]$ denotes the expectation operator. Typically, $E\{|D(\omega)|^2\}$ is estimated during nonspeech activity and is denoted by $|\hat{D}(\omega)|^2$. If we assume that $d(n)$ is zero mean and uncorrelated with the clean signal $x(n)$, then the terms $E\{X^*(\omega) \cdot D(\omega)\}$ and $E\{X(\omega) \cdot D^*(\omega)\}$ reduce to zero. Thus, after using the preceding assumptions, the estimate of the clean speech power spectrum can be obtained as follows:

$$|\hat{X}(\omega)|^2 = |Y(\omega)|^2 - |\hat{D}(\omega)|^2 \tag{5.7}$$

The preceding equation describes the *power spectrum subtraction algorithm*. As mentioned earlier, the estimated power spectrum $|\hat{X}(\omega)|^2$ in Equation 5.7 is not guaranteed to be positive, but can be half-wave-rectified as shown in Equation 5.5. The enhanced signal is finally obtained by computing the inverse Fourier transform of $|\hat{X}(\omega)|$ (obtained by taking the square root of $|\hat{X}(\omega)|^2$), using the phase of the noisy speech signal. Note that if we take the inverse Fourier transform of both sides in Equation 5.7, we get a similar equation in the autocorrelation domain, that is,

$$r_{\hat{x}\hat{x}}(m) = r_{yy}(m) - r_{\hat{d}\hat{d}}(m) \tag{5.8}$$

where $r_{\hat{x}\hat{x}}(m)$, $r_{yy}(m)$, and $r_{\hat{d}\hat{d}}(m)$ are the autocorrelation sequences of the estimated clean signal, the noisy speech signal, and the estimated noise signals, respectively. Hence, the subtraction could in principle be performed in the autocorrelation domain. Such a technique was proposed by Weiss et al. [3, 4, p. 561] and referred to as the INTEL technique. Weiss et al. [3] also proposed doing the subtraction in the cepstrum domain.

Equation 5.7 can also be written in the following form:

$$|\hat{X}(\omega)|^2 = H^2(\omega)|Y(\omega)|^2 \tag{5.9}$$

where

$$H(\omega) = \sqrt{1 - \frac{|\hat{D}(\omega)|^2}{|Y(\omega)|^2}} \tag{5.10}$$

In the context of linear system theory, $H(\omega)$ is known as the system's transfer function (Chapter 2). In speech enhancement, we refer to $H(\omega)$ as the *gain function* or *suppression function*. Note that $H(\omega)$ in Equation 5.10 is real and, in principle, is always positive, taking values in the range of $0 \le H(\omega) \le 1$. Negative values are sometimes obtained owing to inaccurate estimates of the noise spectrum. $H(\omega)$ is called the *suppression function* because it provides the amount of suppression (or attenuation, as $0 \le H(\omega) \le 1$) applied to the noisy power spectrum $|Y(\omega)|^2$ at a given frequency to obtain the enhanced power spectrum $|\hat{X}(\omega)|^2$. The shape of the suppression function is unique to a particular speech enhancement algorithm. For that reason, we often compare different algorithms by comparing their corresponding suppression functions. The fact that $H(\omega)$ is real-valued implies that $h(n)$, that is, its inverse Fourier transform, is evenly symmetric around zero and, therefore, noncausal. In the time domain, Equation 5.9 corresponds to a noncausal filtering operation. A method was proposed in [5] that modified the suppression function $H(\omega)$ so that Equation 5.9 corresponded to a causal filtering operation in the time domain and will be discussed later on in Section 5.9.

A more generalized version of the spectral subtraction algorithm is given by

$$|\hat{X}(\omega)|^p = |Y(\omega)|^p - |\hat{D}(\omega)|^p \tag{5.11}$$

where p is the power exponent, with $p = 1$ yielding the original magnitude spectral subtraction [1] and $p = 2$ yielding the power spectral subtraction algorithm. The general form of the spectral subtraction algorithm is shown in Figure 5.1.

It is important to note that Equations 5.7 and 5.11 are only approximations because of the presence of the cross terms. The cross terms in Equation 5.6 are zero only in the statistical sense, assuming that the expectations are carried out using sufficient data and assuming that the signals are stationary. Speech, however, is nonstationary. In most applications, the speech signal is processed on a frame-by-frame basis (using 20–30 ms windows), and the cross-expectation terms might not necessarily be zero. This was demonstrated in [6] and is shown in Figure 5.2. Speech was corrupted by multitalker babble at +5 dB S/N. Figure 5.2 plots the values of the noisy speech power spectrum $|Y(\omega)|^2$ along with the *cross terms* $2 \cdot \text{Re}[X(\omega) \cdot D^*(\omega)]$ computed using a 30 ms speech frame. As can be seen, the cross terms are not negligible, at least in the low frequencies, compared to the values of the power spectrum of the noisy speech signal. In the low frequencies, the values of the cross terms are comparable to the noisy speech magnitudes, but are small, and perhaps negligible, in the extremely high frequencies. Despite the fact that the cross terms might not be negligible across the whole spectrum (as shown in Figure 5.2), most spectral subtraction

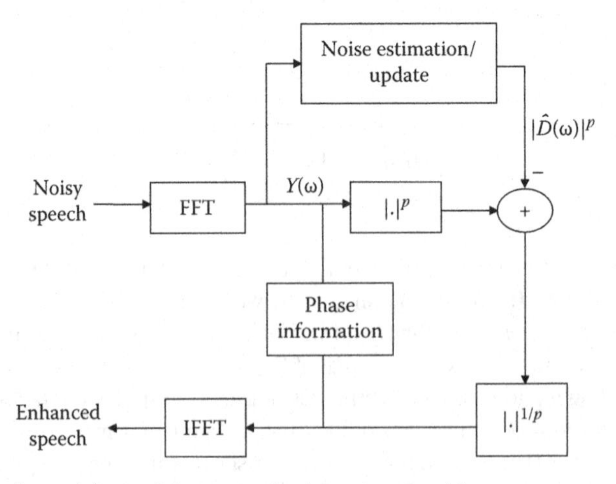

FIGURE 5.1 General form of the spectral subtraction algorithm.

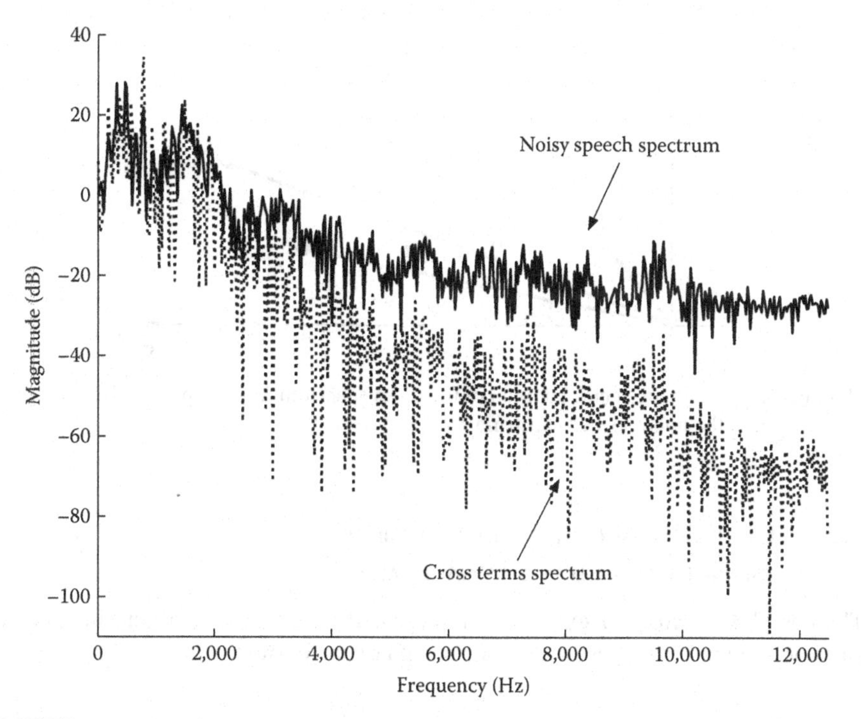

FIGURE 5.2 Plot of the cross terms' spectrum, that is, 2 Re{$X(\omega)D^*(\omega)$}, superimposed on the noisy speech spectrum for a signal embedded in +5 dB S/N multitalker babble noise.

algorithms assume for simplicity that these terms are zero. A method for estimating the cross terms was proposed in [7]. The implications of discarding the cross terms are discussed next using a geometric view of spectral subtraction.

5.2 GEOMETRIC VIEW OF SPECTRAL SUBTRACTION

From Equation 5.2, we note that the noisy spectrum $Y(\omega_k)$ at frequency ω_k is obtained by summing two complex-valued spectra at frequency ω_k. As such, $Y(\omega_k)$ can be represented geometrically in the complex plane as the sum of two complex numbers, $X(\omega_k)$ and $D(\omega_k)$. This is illustrated in Figure 5.3, which shows the representation of $Y(\omega_k)$ as a vector addition of $X(\omega_k)$ and $D(\omega_k)$ in the complex plane. Representing the noisy spectrum $Y(\omega_k)$ geometrically in the complex plane (see Figure 5.3) can provide valuable insights to the spectral subtraction approach that might otherwise not be obvious. For one, such a geometric viewpoint can provide upper bounds on the difference between the phases of the noisy and clean spectra [8]; that is, it will tell us, for instance, the conditions under which it is safe to make the assumption that the phase of the clean signal spectrum can be replaced by that of the noisy speech spectrum. It will also tell us whether it is theoretically possible to recover exactly the clean signal magnitude $|X(\omega)|$ given the noisy speech spectrum $Y(\omega_k)$ and under what conditions. Finally, it will tell us how discarding the cross terms in Equation 5.6 affects the prospects of obtaining accurate estimates of the magnitude spectrum.

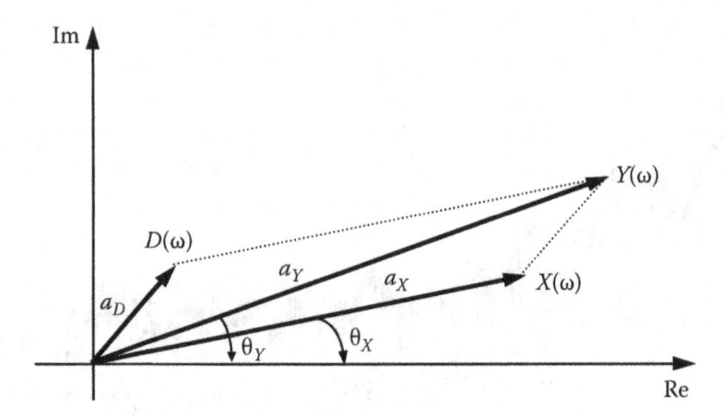

FIGURE 5.3 Complex vector addition of the clean spectrum $X(\omega)$ with the noise spectrum $D(\omega)$ to obtain the noisy speech spectrum $Y(\omega)$.

5.2.1 Upper Bounds on the Difference between the Noisy and Clean Signals' Phases

The complex spectrum $Y(\omega_k)$ can be represented by either its real and imaginary parts or in polar form by its magnitude and phase as follows:

$$Y(\omega_k) = a_Y e^{j\theta_Y} \tag{5.12}$$

where

a_Y denotes the magnitude spectrum (i.e., $a_Y \triangleq |Y(\omega_k)|$)
θ_Y denotes the phase spectrum

We drop for now the frequency variable ω_k for convenience. Similarly, we represent the clean signal and noise spectra in polar form as follows:

$$X(\omega_k) = a_X e^{j\theta_X}, \quad D(\omega_k) = a_D e^{j\theta_D} \tag{5.13}$$

We are interested in determining an upper bound of the difference between the noisy and clean phases, that is, $\theta_Y - \theta_X$. To do that, we consider the vector diagram shown in Figure 5.4. The phase difference $\theta_Y - \theta_X$ is given in general by the following equation [8]:

$$\tan(\theta_Y - \theta_X) = \frac{a_D \sin(\theta_D - \theta_X)}{a_X + a_D \cos(\theta_D - \theta_X)} \tag{5.14}$$

It is easy to see from Figure 5.4 that the phase difference reaches its maximum value when the noise and clean signal vectors are orthogonal to each other, that is, when

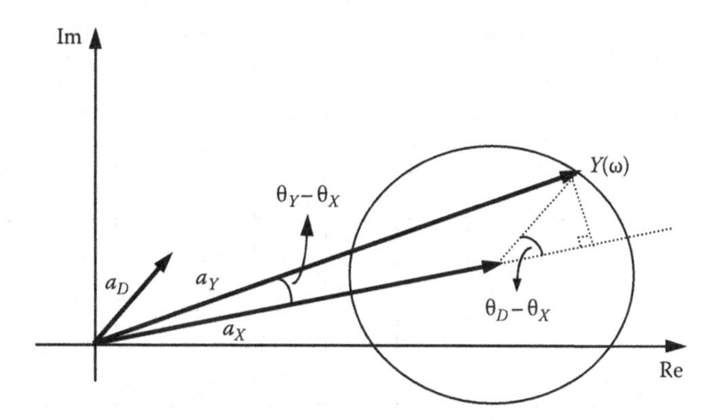

FIGURE 5.4 Diagram illustrating the trigonometric relationship of the phase difference between the noisy and clean signals.

$\theta_D - \theta_X = \pi/2$. Substituting $\pi/2$ for $\theta_D - \theta_X$ in Equation 5.14 and solving for the phase difference, we get the following upper bound:

$$(\theta_Y - \theta_X)\Big|_{\theta_D - \theta_X = \pi/2} \triangleq \theta_{\max} = \tan^{-1}\frac{a_D}{a_X} \tag{5.15}$$

Note that the preceding upper bound is valid for $|\theta_D - \theta_X| < \pi/2$ and the upper bound for $|\theta_D - \theta_X| > \pi/2$ is π. Defining

$$\xi = \frac{a_x^2}{a_d^2} \tag{5.16}$$

as the instantaneous spectral signal-to-noise ratio (SNR) at frequency bin ω_k, we can express Equation 5.15 as follows:

$$\theta_{\max} = \tan^{-1}\frac{1}{\sqrt{\xi}} \tag{5.17}$$

Figure 5.5 plots the upper bound of the difference between the noisy and clean phases as a function of the SNR defined in Equation 5.16. As expected, the larger the SNR, the smaller the difference between the noisy (θ_Y) and clean phases (θ_X). This suggests that it is safe to replace the phase of the clean signal spectrum at a specific frequency bin with the phase of the noisy spectrum, provided that the corresponding SNR in that bin is large. In the context of speech enhancement, we can adopt the following strategy: as long as the phase difference is not perceptible by the auditory system, we can use the noisy phase. Listening experiments conducted in [8] suggest that the smallest detectable phase difference is between $\pi/8$ and $\pi/4$. Therefore, provided that the spectral SNR is larger than approximately 8 dB (Figure 5.5) for all frequencies, we should not be able to perceive the noisy phase. Otherwise, mismatch in phase might be perceived as "roughness" in quality.

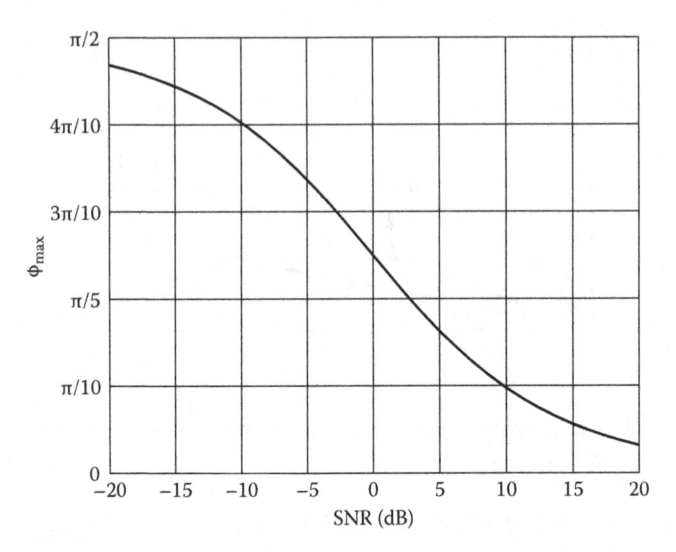

FIGURE 5.5 Upper bound of the phase difference of the noisy and clean signals as a function of SNR in dB.

5.2.2 Alternate Spectral-Subtractive Rules and Theoretical Limits

The preceding section demonstrated that the signal phase need not be recovered exactly as long as the spectral SNR is high enough. Turning now to the signal magnitude spectrum estimation problem, we seek to answer the question of whether it is possible to recover with high accuracy the magnitude spectrum of the clean signal if we have access to relatively accurate estimates of the noise magnitude. Of related interest is the answer to the question of whether access to phase information is critical for recovering the signal magnitude spectrum; that is, does accurate signal magnitude estimation require accurate phase estimation? To answer these questions, we next derive alternate spectral-subtractive rules to those given in Section 5.1 and examine the relationship between the signals' magnitudes and phases.

We start by setting the real and imaginary parts of the two sides of Equation 5.2 equal to each other, using the notation in Equations 5.12 and 5.13:

$$a_Y \cos(\theta_Y) = a_X \cos(\theta_X) + a_D \cos(\theta_D) \tag{5.18}$$

$$a_Y \sin(\theta_Y) = a_X \sin(\theta_X) + a_D \sin(\theta_D) \tag{5.19}$$

By squaring Equations 5.18 and 5.19 and adding them together, we get

$$a_Y^2 = a_X^2 + a_D^2 + 2a_X a_D \cos(\theta_X - \theta_D) \tag{5.20}$$

It is easy to see that the preceding equation is identical to Equation 5.6 since

$$\text{Re}\{X(\omega)D^*(\omega)\} = a_X a_D \cos(\theta_X - \theta_D) \tag{5.21}$$

Equation 5.20 is a quadratic function of a_X and has the following two solutions:

$$a_X = -a_D c_{XD} \pm \sqrt{a_D^2(c_{XD}^2 - 1) + a_Y^2} \tag{5.22}$$

where c_{XD} is defined as follows:

$$c_{XD} \triangleq \cos(\theta_X - \theta_D) \tag{5.23}$$

The fact that the cross terms in Equation 5.20 are a function of the clean signal magnitude and phase prohibits us from using it for enhancement. A different form of the equation can be derived, however, with cross terms that are functions of the noisy speech magnitude and phase:

$$a_X^2 = a_Y^2 + a_D^2 - 2a_Y a_D \cos(\theta_Y - \theta_D) \tag{5.24}$$

It is clear that if $\cos(\theta_Y - \theta_D) = 1$, the preceding equation reduces to the standard subtraction rule given in Equation 5.5. As we will see shortly, $\cos(\theta_Y - \theta_D) \approx 1$ when the SNR is low.

Different algebraic manipulations of Equations 5.18 and 5.19 result in different expressions for the clean signal magnitude. For instance, the clean signal magnitude a_X can also be obtained using the following equation:

$$a_X = a_Y c_{XY} \pm \sqrt{a_Y^2\left(c_{XY}^2 - 1\right) + a_D^2} \tag{5.25}$$

where c_{XY} is defined as follows:

$$c_{XY} \triangleq \cos(\theta_X - \theta_Y) \tag{5.26}$$

Equations 5.22 and 5.25 are two (of many) spectral-subtractive rules that can be used in lieu of the standard subtraction rule given in Equation 5.5. As we show next, the standard subtraction rule is a special case of the preceding two equations under certain conditions.

If, for instance, $c_{XD} = 0$ in Equation 5.22, then we get $a_X^2 = a_Y^2 - a_D^2$. Geometrically, $c_{XD} = 0$ if the signal and noise vectors are orthogonal to each other since $\cos(\pm\pi/2) = 0$. Statistically, if the clean signal and noise spectra are orthogonal (i.e., $E\{X(\omega_k)D(\omega_k)\} = 0$) and have zero mean, then they are uncorrelated. This is consistent with the common assumption that the clean signal and noise are uncorrelated. Hence, under the condition that the signal and noise vectors are orthogonal to each other, the standard power subtraction rule (Equation 5.5) is very accurate. Based on Equation 5.20, we infer that the power spectral subtraction rule (Equation 5.7) is also accurate under the same conditions. It is worth mentioning here that if the phase difference $(\theta_X - \theta_D)$ is assumed to be uniformly distributed in $[-\pi, \pi]$, then it can be shown that $E[c_{XD}] = 0$ [9, p. 135].

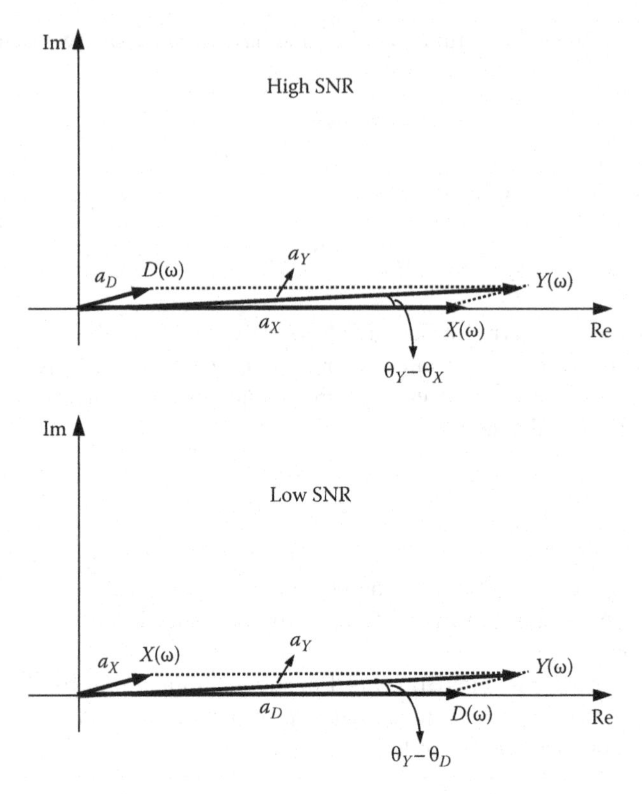

FIGURE 5.6 Geometric view of high- and low-SNR conditions.

If $c_{XY} = 1$ in Equation 5.25 and we take the negative sign, then we have $a_X = a_Y - a_D$. Geometrically, $c_{XY} = 1$ if the noisy and clean signal vectors are colinear, that is, point in the same direction. As shown in Figure 5.6, the noisy and clean signal vectors are approximately colinear when the SNR is high, that is, when $a_X \gg a_D$. Hence, under high-SNR conditions, the standard subtraction rule (Equation 5.5) is very accurate. It is interesting to note that the subtractive rule in Equation 5.25 bears a striking resemblance to the maximum-likelihood rule derived in [10] (see Chapter 7).

The subtractive rules given in Equations 5.22 and 5.25 are simple to use and more accurate than those given in Equations 5.5 and 5.7, as they make no statistical assumptions about the relationship between the clean signal and the noise, thus taking into account the presence of the cross terms. However, the subtractive rules (Equations 5.22 and 5.25) are ambiguous regarding the sign (±) in that we have no simple way of knowing which sign to use. Alternative subtractive rules can be derived with no sign ambiguity by algebraically manipulating Equations 5.18 and 5.19 to avoid the quadratic terms in a_X. A sample of those rules follows:

$$a_X = a_Y c_{YX} - a_D c_{XD} \tag{5.27}$$

$$a_X = \frac{a_Y c_{YD} - a_D}{c_{XD}} \tag{5.28}$$

$$a_X = \frac{a_Y - a_D c_{YD}}{c_{XY}} \tag{5.29}$$

$$a_X^2 = \left(a_Y - a_D c_{YD}\right)^2 + a_D^2\left(1 - c_{YD}^2\right) \tag{5.30}$$

$$a_X^2 = \left(a_D - a_Y c_{YD}\right)^2 + a_Y^2\left(1 - c_{YD}^2\right) \tag{5.31}$$

$$a_X^2 = \frac{a_D^2\left(1 - c_{YD}^2\right)}{\left(1 - c_{YX}^2\right)} \tag{5.32}$$

$$a_X^2 = \frac{a_Y^2\left(1 - c_{YD}^2\right)}{\left(1 - c_{XD}^2\right)} \tag{5.33}$$

We can make a few interesting observations about the preceding rules. Starting with Equation 5.30, if $c_{YD} = 1$, then we have $a_X = a_Y - a_D$. Geometrically, $c_{YD} = 1$ if the noisy and noise vectors are colinear, that is, point in the same direction. As shown in Figure 5.6, the noisy and noise vectors are approximately colinear when the SNR is low, that is, when $a_D \ll a_X$. Hence, under low-SNR conditions, Equation 5.30 reduces to the standard subtraction rule given in Equation 5.5.

If $c_{YX} \approx 1$, corresponding to a high-SNR (spectral) condition (see Figure 5.6), then we observe that Equation 5.27 resembles the oversubtraction rule proposed in [11], with the oversubtraction factor given explicitly by c_{XD} (more on this in Section 5.4). Unlike the approach in [11], where the oversubtraction factor was always larger than (or equal to) one, the value of c_{XD} is always smaller than (or equal to) one.

Equation 5.32 offers an explicit relationship for the instantaneous (spectral) SNR (as defined in Equation 5.16) in terms of the signal/noise phases alone:

$$\xi \triangleq \frac{a_X^2}{a_D^2} = \frac{1 - c_{YD}^2}{1 - c_{YX}^2} \tag{5.34}$$

The preceding equation is consistent with the geometric interpretation of high- and low-SNR conditions (see Figure 5.6). More specifically, if $c_{YX} \approx 1$, the denominator will be small, resulting in large values of ξ, that is, a high-SNR situation. Likewise, if $c_{YD} \approx 1$, the numerator will be small, resulting in small values of ξ, that is, a low-SNR situation.

Last, Equation 5.33 provides an explicit relationship of the suppression function $a_X - a_Y$ in terms of the phase differences between the noisy/clean and noise signals:

$$h \triangleq \frac{a_X}{a_Y} = \sqrt{\frac{1 - c_{YD}^2}{1 - c_{XD}^2}} \tag{5.35}$$

In principle, multiplication of the noisy magnitude a_Y by the preceding suppression function (also called *gain function*) should yield the clean signal amplitude a_X. It is noteworthy that this suppression function reduces to the suppression function of the power spectral subtraction method (i.e., Equation 5.10) if $c_{XD} = 0$, that is, if the signal and noise are orthogonal to each other or, equivalently, if they are statistically uncorrelated. To prove this, after solving for c_{YD} in Equation 5.28 with $c_{XD} = 0$, we get:

$$c_{YD} = \frac{a_D}{a_Y} \tag{5.36}$$

Substituting the preceding equation in Equation 5.35, we get Equation 5.10. In view of this analysis, we can say that the suppression rule given in Equation 5.35 is the true and exact suppression rule for spectral-subtractive algorithms if no assumptions are made about the statistical relationship between the signal and noise. In contrast, the suppression rule given in Equation 5.10 is merely an approximation as it assumes that $c_{XD} = 0$, that is, that the clean signal and noise are orthogonal to each other.

The aforementioned subtractive rules depend on the estimation of phase differences between the noisy (or clean) and noise signals, which by itself, however, is a difficult task, and no methods currently exist to determine these phases accurately. The preceding analysis, however, suggests a few avenues worth investigating for phase estimation. One possibility is to derive and make use of explicit relationships between the phases of noisy and noise signals as done in Equation 5.14 based on trigonometric principles. Another possibility is to use Equations 5.20 and 5.24 and solve explicitly for c_{YD} and c_{XD}, yielding

$$c_{YD} = \frac{a_Y^2 + a_D^2 - a_X^2}{2a_Y a_D} \tag{5.37}$$

$$c_{XD} = \frac{a_Y^2 - a_X^2 - a_D^2}{2a_X a_D} \tag{5.38}$$

Similarly, it is easy to show that c_{YX} can be obtained by the following equation:

$$c_{YX} = \frac{a_Y^2 + a_X^2 - a_D^2}{2a_X a_Y} \tag{5.39}$$

Clearly, the main obstacle in using the preceding equations to estimate the phase differences between the signal and noise signals is their dependency on the clean signal amplitude, which we do not have. One possible solution is to use previously estimated values of a_X, thereby making the implicit assumption that the magnitude spectra do not change drastically from frame to frame.

In summary, the preceding geometric analysis of spectral subtraction led us to the following conclusions:

1. It is safe to use the noisy phase in place of the clean signal phase, provided the spectral SNR is high enough. Based on the data provided in [8], the phase difference should not be perceivable if the spectral SNR is at least 8 dB.
2. Phase estimation is critically important for accurate signal magnitude estimation. In fact, it is not possible to recover the magnitude spectrum of the clean signal exactly even if we have access to the noise signal. Access to phase information is needed. The subtractive rule derived in Equation 5.33, for instance, demonstrates that if we somehow have access to the phase difference between the noisy (and clean) signals and the noise, then we can recover the signal magnitude exactly without needing explicit information about the noise magnitude. It is possible, however, that knowledge about the noise magnitude might be implicitly embedded in the phase differences between the noisy (or clean) signal and the noise signal (e.g., see Equation 5.37).

5.3 SHORTCOMINGS OF THE SPECTRAL SUBTRACTION METHOD

We now turn our attention to the spectral-subtractive rules discussed in Section 5.1, which have been studied the most. Although the spectral subtraction algorithm can be easily implemented to effectively reduce the noise present in the corrupted signal, it has a few shortcomings. As mentioned earlier, the modified speech spectrum obtained from Equation 5.7, as well as the spectra obtained using the subtractive rules given in the previous section, may contain some negative values owing to errors in estimating the noise spectrum. The simplest solution is to half-wave-rectify these values (i.e., set the negative values to zero) to ensure a nonnegative magnitude spectrum. This nonlinear processing of the negative values, however, creates small, isolated peaks in the spectrum occurring at random frequency locations in each frame. Converted in the time domain, these peaks sound similar to tones with frequencies that change randomly from frame to frame; that is, tones that are turned on and off at the analysis frame rate (every 20–30 ms). This type of "noise" introduced by the half-wave rectification process has been described as warbling with tonal quality and is commonly referred to in the literature [11] as *musical noise*. Musical noise is more prominent in the unvoiced segments of speech where the noise power is comparable to the speech power. In some cases, this musical noise can be more disturbing to the listener than the original distortions caused by the interfering noise. Figure 5.7 shows an example magnitude spectra of the enhanced signal after half-wave rectification. The isolated spectral peaks are clearly indicated in the figure.

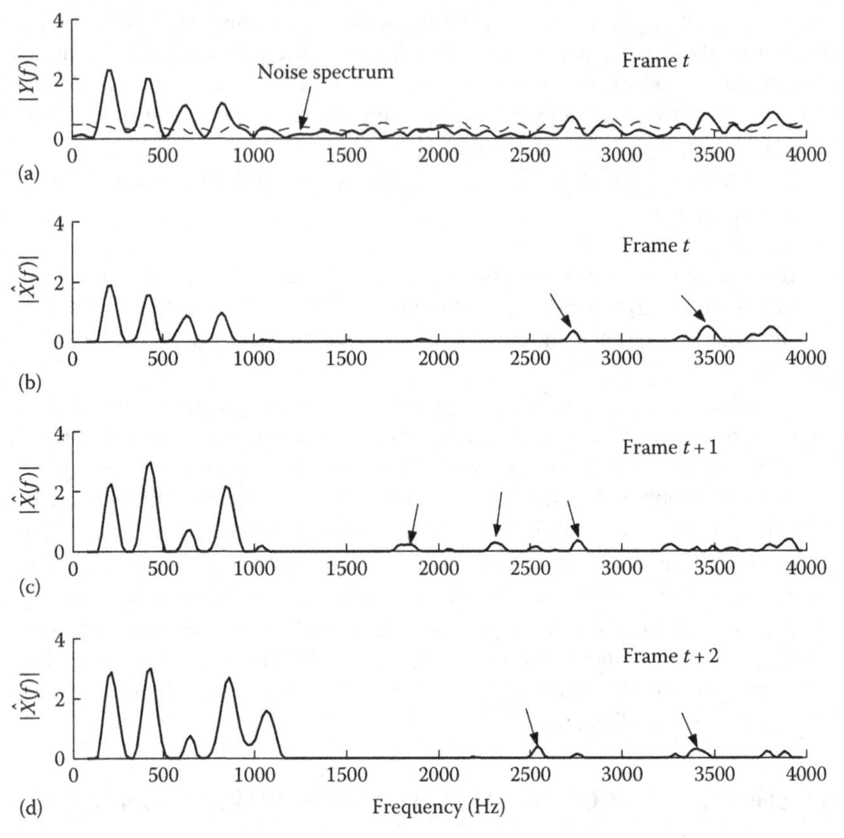

FIGURE 5.7 Example magnitude spectra of the enhanced signal following half-wave rectification in the subtraction process. Arrows show the isolated peaks responsible for musical noise. (a) Noisy speech spectrum along with the noise spectrum (dashed line); (b) enhanced signal spectrum at frame t; (c) enhanced signal spectrum at frame $t + 1$; and (d) enhanced signal spectrum at frame $t + 2$.

Another relatively minor shortcoming of the spectral subtraction approach is the use of noisy phase that produces a roughness in the quality of the synthesized speech. The phases of the noise-corrupted signal are not enhanced before being combined with the modified spectrum to regenerate the enhanced time signal. This is because the presence of noise in the phase information does not contribute much to the degradation of speech quality. Although this is especially true at high SNRs (>5 dB) and at low SNRs (<0 dB), the noisy phase can lead to a perceivable roughness in the speech signal, contributing to the reduction in speech quality. Experiments conducted [8,12] have corroborated this fact. Estimating the phase of the clean speech is a difficult task and greatly increases the complexity of the enhancement algorithm. The distortion due to noisy phase information is not very significant compared to that of the magnitude spectrum, especially for high SNRs. As mentioned in Section 5.2, the noisy phase is imperceptible, provided the spectral SNR is large. In brief, the use of the noisy phase information is considered to be an acceptable practice in the reconstruction of the enhanced speech signal.

Combating musical noise is much more critical than finding methods to preserve the original phase. For that reason, much effort has been focused on finding methods to reduce musical noise. Before discussing these methods, it is important to state some of the factors that contribute to musical noise:

1. Nonlinear processing of the negative subtracted spectral components.
2. Inaccurate estimate of the noise spectrum. As the noise spectrum cannot be directly obtained, we are forced to use an averaged estimate of the noise. Hence, there are some significant variations between the estimated noise spectrum and the actual noise content present in the instantaneous speech spectrum. The subtraction of these quantities results in the presence of isolated residual noise levels of large variance.
3. Large variance in the estimates of the noisy and noise signal spectra [13]. Most algorithms use periodogram-type spectral estimators, which are known to have a large variance even when long-duration windows are used [14].
4. Large variability in the suppression or gain function (Equation 5.10).

Much research has been done to find ways to combat the problem of musical noise [15–18]. It is extremely difficult to minimize musical noise without affecting the speech signal itself in some way, and, in general, there is a trade-off between the amount of noise reduction and speech distortion introduced. In the following sections, we describe some of the techniques that have been proposed to reduce musical noise and therefore improve the performance of the standard spectral subtraction algorithm.

5.4 SPECTRAL SUBTRACTION USING OVERSUBTRACTION

The approach taken by Boll [1] to reduce musical noise was to spectrally floor any negative subtracted spectral components rather than to set them to zero (Equation 5.5). The floor value was determined by taking the minimum spectral value from adjacent frames. More precisely, Equation 5.5 was modified to

$$|\hat{X}_i(\omega)| = \begin{cases} |Y_i(\omega)| - |\hat{D}(\omega)| & \text{if } |Y_i(\omega)| - |\hat{D}(\omega)| > \max|\hat{D}(\omega)| \\ \min\limits_{j=i-1,i,i+1} |\hat{X}_j(\omega)| & \text{else} \end{cases} \quad (5.40)$$

where $|\hat{X}_i(\omega)|$ denotes the enhanced spectrum estimated in frame i, and $|\hat{D}(\omega)|$ is the spectrum of the noise obtained during nonspeech activity. The underlying idea of Equation 5.40 is to retain the information if the current frame is a low-energy segment (e.g., unvoiced segment/s/) or use a better estimate of the noise if several consecutive frames do not contain speech. The main drawback of this approach, however, is that it requires access to future enhanced spectra, and such an approach may not be amenable to real-time implementation.

A different approach that does not require access to future information was proposed by Berouti et al. [11]. Their method consists of subtracting an overestimate of the noise power spectrum, while preventing the resultant spectral components from going below a preset minimum value (spectral floor). Their proposed technique had the following form:

$$|\hat{X}(\omega)|^2 = \begin{cases} |Y(\omega)|^2 - \alpha|\hat{D}(\omega)|^2 & \text{if } |Y(\omega)|^2 > (\alpha+\beta)|\hat{D}(\omega)|^2 \\ \beta|\hat{D}(\omega)|^2 & \text{else} \end{cases} \quad (5.41)$$

where

α is the oversubtraction factor ($\alpha \geq 1$)

β ($0 < \beta << 1$) is the spectral floor parameter

The main motivation of using the oversubtraction factor and the spectral flooring is as follows. When we subtract the estimate of the noise spectrum from the noisy speech spectrum, there remain peaks in the spectrum. Some of those peaks are broadband (encompassing a wide range of frequencies) whereas others are narrow band, appearing as spikes in the spectrum. By oversubtracting the noise spectrum, that is, by using $\alpha > 1$, we can reduce the amplitude of the broadband peaks and, in some cases, eliminate them altogether. This by itself, however, is not sufficient because the deep valleys surrounding the peaks still remain in the spectrum. For that reason, spectral flooring is used to "fill in" the spectral valleys and possibly mask the remaining peaks by the neighboring spectral components of comparable value. The valleys between peaks are no longer deep when $\beta > 0$ compared to when $\beta = 0$. Berouti et al. [11] found that speech processed by Equation 5.41 had less musical noise than that processed by Equation 5.5.

The two parameters α and β offer a great amount of flexibility to the spectral subtraction algorithm. The parameter β controls the amount of remaining residual noise and the amount of perceived musical noise. If the spectral floor parameter β is too large, then the residual noise will be audible but the musical noise will not be perceptible. Conversely, if β is too small, the musical noise will become annoying but the residual noise will be markedly reduced. Figure 5.8 shows the effect of varying the value of β on the spectrum for a fixed value of α.

The parameter α affects the amount of speech spectral distortion caused by the subtraction in Equation 5.41. If α is too large, then the resulting signal will be severely distorted to the point that intelligibility may suffer. Figure 5.9 shows the effect of varying the value of α on the spectrum for a fixed value of β. Experimental results showed that for best noise reduction with the least amount of musical noise, α should be small for high-SNR frames (i.e., when speech is present) and large for low-SNR frames (i.e., for low-energy segments or during pauses). Berouti et al. [11] suggested that the parameter α should vary from frame to frame according to

$$\alpha = \alpha_0 - \frac{3}{20}SNR \quad -5\text{ dB} \leq SNR \leq 20\text{ dB} \quad (5.42)$$

where

α_0 is the desired value of α at 0 dB SNR

SNR is the short-time SNR estimated in each frame

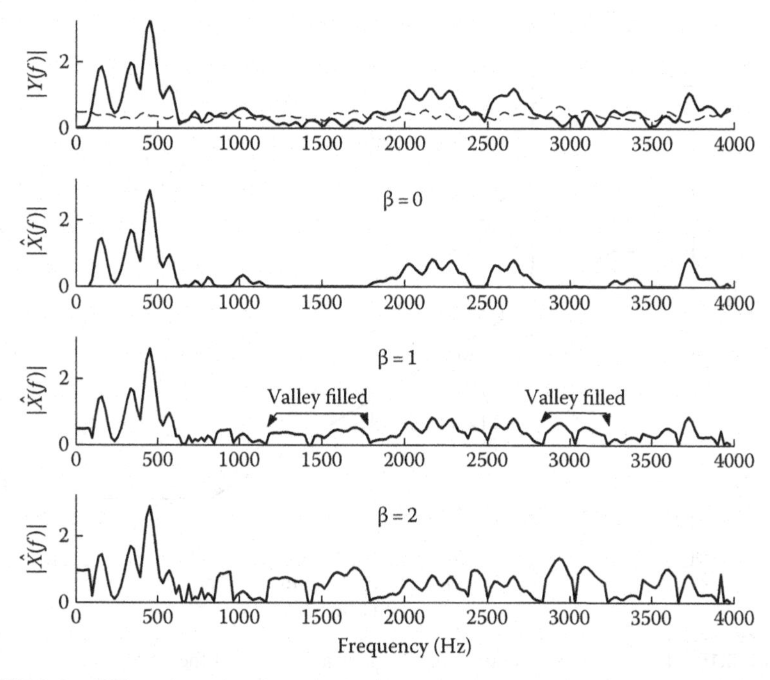

FIGURE 5.8 Effect of varying the value of spectral floor parameter β for a fixed value of α.

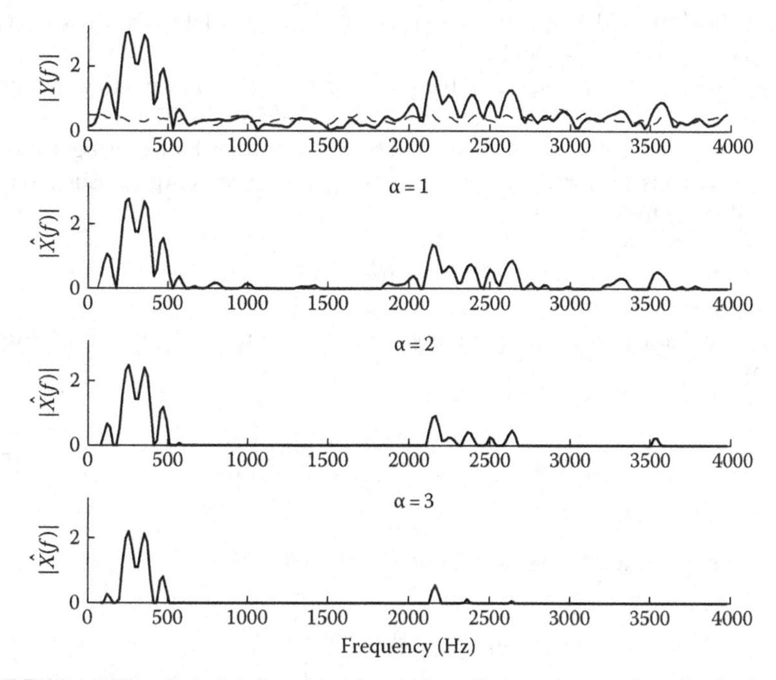

FIGURE 5.9 Effect of varying the value of oversubtraction parameter α for a fixed value of β.

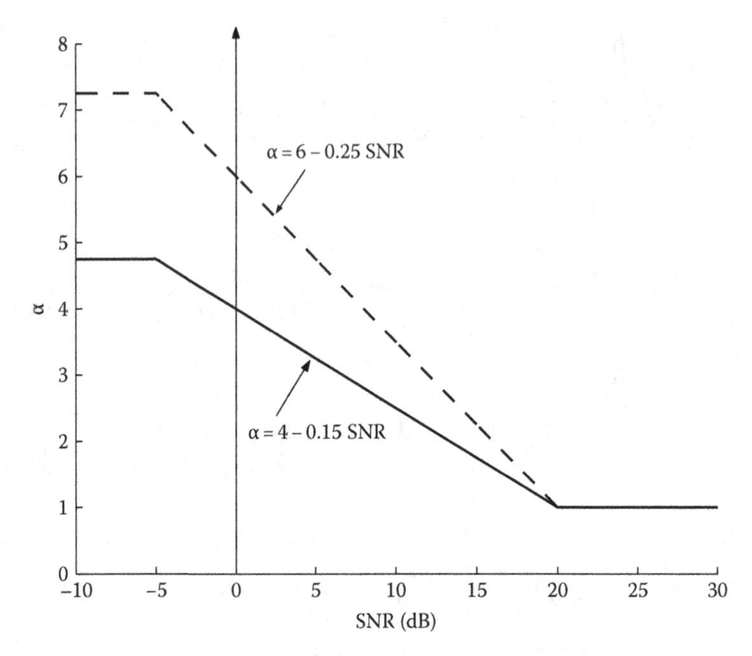

FIGURE 5.10 Plot of the oversubtraction factor as a function of the SNR.

Note that this is not the true SNR as we do not have access to the clean signal. It is an *a posteriori* estimate of the SNR computed based on the ratio of the noisy speech power to the estimated noise power. Figure 5.10 shows the plot of the value of α as a function of the *a posteriori* SNR.

The effect of the parameter α on the spectrum can be seen by plotting the attenuation curves as a function of the SNR for different values of α. These curves give us the amount of attenuation (in dB) incurred by the spectral subtraction algorithm. To obtain the suppression (or attenuation) curves, we first need to express Equation 5.41 in the following form:

$$|\hat{X}(\omega)| = H(\omega) \cdot |Y(\omega)| \tag{5.43}$$

where $H(\omega)$ can be viewed as a time-varying filter. From Equation 5.41, $H(\omega)$ is given by

$$H(\omega) = \left(\frac{|Y(\omega)|^2 - \alpha |\hat{D}(\omega)|^2}{|Y(\omega)|^2} \right)^{1/2} \tag{5.44}$$

The preceding equation can also be written as follows:

$$H(\omega) = \left(\frac{\gamma(\omega) - \alpha}{\gamma(\omega)} \right)^{1/2} \tag{5.45}$$

where $\gamma(\omega)$ is the *a posteriori* SNR at frequency ω and is defined as follows:

$$\gamma(\omega) = \frac{|Y(\omega)|^2}{|\hat{D}(\omega)|^2} \tag{5.46}$$

Figure 5.11 plots $H(\omega)$ (Equation 5.45) as a function of $\gamma(\omega)$ for different values of the parameter α. More attenuation is increasingly applied for larger values of α. So, for example, if the *a posteriori* SNR is 8 dB (i.e., $\gamma(\omega) = 8$ dB) at frequency ω, then the attenuation obtained with $\alpha = 1$ will be −0.74 dB, with $\alpha = 3$ it will be −2.8 dB, and with $\alpha = 5$ it will be −6.8 dB. Heavier attenuation is therefore obtained with larger values of α.

The attenuation curves of Figure 5.11 also tell us when flooring occurs. If $\alpha = 5$, for instance, spectral flooring occurs when the *a posteriori* SNR is smaller than 7 dB. If $\alpha = 3$, spectral flooring occurs when the *a posteriori* SNR is smaller than 5 dB, and if $\alpha = 1$, spectral flooring occurs when the *a posteriori* SNR is smaller than 0 dB. This then suggests that spectral flooring occurs more often when α is large compared to when α is small. This continuing spectral flooring of the enhanced spectra contributes to speech distortion. Another factor that contributes to the spectral distortion is the nonuniform distribution of $\gamma(\omega)$ values across the spectrum. It is possible, for instance, that in a given frame, the low-frequency components are, say, attenuated by as much as 7 dB, while

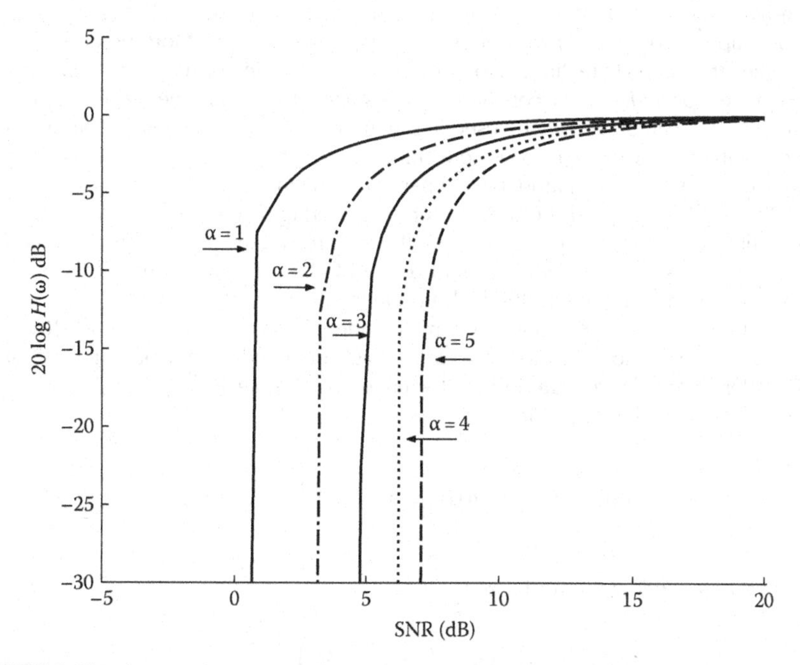

FIGURE 5.11 Attenuation curves of the spectral subtraction algorithm for different values of the oversubtraction factor α.

the high-frequency components are attenuated by 1 dB. The magnitude spectrum attenuation is clearly nonuniform across the spectrum and therefore may cause additional spectral distortion.

Extensive experiments were performed by Berouti et al. [11] to determine the optimum values of α and β. The function in Equation 5.42 shown in Figure 5.10 was found to work quite well for α with the best α_0 value set in the range of 3–6. The spectral flooring parameter β was found to be dependent on the value of the *a posteriori* SNR. For high noise levels (SNR = −5 dB), they suggested that β be in the range of 0.02–0.06, and for lower noise levels (SNR $\geq$ 0 dB), β in the range of 0.005–0.02. A 25–35 ms analysis window was recommended. Using an analysis frame shorter than 20 ms resulted in rough speech quality. The influence of α and the effect of the power exponent on performance were also investigated by others [13,19–21]. Vary and Martin [21, p. 407] recommended an oversubtraction factor between 1.3 and 2 for low-SNR conditions. For high-SNR conditions, a subtraction factor less than one was recommended. This was consistent with the findings reported by Kushner et al. [20], in the context of speech recognition and by the theoretical analysis presented in [13] as well the geometric analysis presented in Section 5.2. More specifically, when the SNR is high, $c_{YX} \approx 1$ in Equation 5.27, the exact subtraction factor is given by c_{XD} (Equation 5.23), which is always less than (or equal to) one.

Example 5.1

Design a spectral-subtractive rule of the form given in Equation 5.41 that provides more suppression in the high frequencies than the low ones. More precisely, we like the attenuation to be limited to 20 dB for $f > 2.5$ kHz and to 10 dB for $f < 2.5$ kHz when the *a posteriori* SNR (Equation 5.46) is smaller than 5 dB. The preceding suppression rule can potentially be used in situations where we know beforehand that most of the energy of the noise is concentrated in the high frequencies (>2.5 kHz in this example), with small amounts of energy leaking in the low frequencies.

To design the desired suppression rule, we need to determine the values of the oversubtraction factors that can achieve the required attenuation at the prescribed *a posteriori* SNR (5 dB). Two values of α need to be computed, one for the low-frequency band and one for the high-frequency band.

In the high-frequency band, we limit the attenuation to a maximum of −20 dB. We can use Equation 5.45 to solve for the high-frequency oversubtraction factor α_H. After setting the *a posteriori* SNR $\gamma(\omega)$ to $10^{5/10}$ (since $10\log_{10}(10^{5/10}) = 5$ dB), we get the following equation:

$$20\log_{10} H(\omega) = -20 \text{ dB} = 20\log_{10}\left(\frac{10^{5/10} - \alpha_H}{10^{5/10}}\right)^{1/2} \tag{5.47}$$

In the linear domain, we have

$$10^{-20/20} = \left(\frac{10^{5/10} - \alpha_H}{10^{5/10}}\right)^{1/2} \tag{5.48}$$

After solving for α_H in the preceding equation, we get $\alpha_H = 3.13$. Similarly, we can solve for the low-frequency factor α_L in the following equation:

$$-10\ \text{dB} = 20\log_{10}\left(\frac{10^{5/10} - \alpha_L}{10^{5/10}}\right)^{1/2} \tag{5.49}$$

After solving for α_L in the preceding equation, we get $\alpha_L = 2.84$. We are now ready to express the desired suppression rules for the low- and high-frequency bands.

For $f > 2.5$ kHz:

$$|\hat{X}(f)|^2 = \begin{cases} |Y(f)|^2 - 2.84|\hat{D}(f)|^2 & \text{if } |Y(f)|^2 > \sqrt{10}\,|\hat{D}(f)|^2 \\ 10^{-1}|Y(f)|^2 & \text{else} \end{cases} \tag{5.50}$$

For $f > 2.5$ kHz:

$$|\hat{X}(f)|^2 = \begin{cases} |Y(f)|^2 - 3.13|\hat{D}(f)|^2 & \text{if } |Y(f)|^2 > \sqrt{10}\,|\hat{D}(f)|^2 \\ 10^{-2}|Y(f)|^2 & \text{else} \end{cases} \tag{5.51}$$

Note that the spectral flooring ensures that the attenuation does not exceed −10 dB in the low frequencies and −20 dB at the high frequencies when the *a posteriori* SNR is less than 5 dB. In Equations 5.50 and 5.51, the spectrum was spectrally floored to the noisy speech. Alternatively, it could be floored to the noise spectrum.

As illustrated by the preceding example and foregoing discussion, the choice of the two parameters, α and β, clearly influences the performance of spectral subtraction algorithms. Different algorithms have been proposed in the literature depending on how these two parameters were chosen, and these algorithms are described next.

5.5 NONLINEAR SPECTRAL SUBTRACTION

In the implementation of the spectral subtraction algorithm proposed by Berouti et al. [11], it was assumed that noise affects all spectral components equally. Consequently, a single oversubtraction factor α is used to subtract an overestimate of the noise over the whole spectrum. That is not the case, however, with real-world noise (e.g., car noise and cafeteria noise). Certain types of interfering noise may affect the low-frequency region of the spectrum more than the high-frequency region (see Section 1.1.1). This suggests the use of a frequency-dependent subtraction factor to account for different types of noise.

The nonlinear spectral subtraction (NSS) proposed in [22] is basically a modification of the method proposed in [11] by making the oversubtraction factor frequency dependent and the subtraction process nonlinear. Larger values are subtracted at frequencies with low SNR levels, and smaller values are subtracted at frequencies with high SNR levels.

The subtraction rule used in the nonlinear subtraction algorithm has the following form:

$$|\hat{X}(\omega)| = \begin{cases} |\bar{Y}(\omega)| - a(\omega)N(\omega) & \text{if } |\bar{Y}(\omega)| > a(\omega)N(\omega) + \beta \cdot |\bar{D}(\omega)| \\ \beta |\bar{Y}(\omega)| & \text{else} \end{cases} \quad (5.52)$$

where
β is the spectral floor (set to 0.1 in [22])
$|\bar{Y}(\omega)|$ and $|\bar{D}(\omega)|$ are the smoothed estimates of noisy speech and noise, respectively
$\alpha(\omega)$ is a frequency-dependent subtraction factor
$N(\omega)$ is a nonlinear function of the noise spectrum

The smoothed estimates of the noisy speech (denoted as $|\bar{Y}(\omega)|$) and noise (denoted as $|\bar{D}(\omega)|$) are obtained as follows:

$$\begin{aligned} |\bar{Y}_i(\omega)| &= \mu_y |\bar{Y}_{i-1}(\omega)| + (1-\mu_y)|Y_i(\omega)| \\ |\bar{D}_i(\omega)| &= \mu_d |\bar{D}_{i-1}(\omega)| + (1-\mu_d)|\hat{D}_i(\omega)| \end{aligned} \quad (5.53)$$

where
$|Y_i(\omega)|$ is the magnitude spectrum of the noisy speech obtained in the ith frame
$|\hat{D}_i(\omega)|$ is the estimate of the magnitude spectrum of the noise for the ith frame
The constants μ_y, μ_d take values in the range $0.1 \le \mu_y \le 0.5$ and $0.5 \le \mu_d \le 0.9$

The $N(\omega)$ term is obtained by computing the maximum of the noise magnitude spectra, $|\hat{D}_i(\omega)|$, over the past 40 frames:

$$N(\omega) = \max_{i-40 \le j \le i} (|\hat{D}_j(\omega)|) \quad (5.54)$$

Note that in [11], $\alpha(\omega)$ is constant for all frequencies but varies from frame to frame depending on the *a posteriori* SNR. For the $\alpha(\omega)$ function in Equation 5.52, several nonlinear functions were suggested in [22], providing different types of weighting to the SNR. One of many functions considered [22] had the following form:

$$\alpha(\omega) = \frac{1}{1 + \gamma\rho(\omega)} \quad (5.55)$$

where γ is a scaling factor, and $\rho(\omega)$ is the square root of the *a posteriori* SNR estimate, that is,

$$\rho(\omega) = \frac{|\bar{Y}(\omega)|}{|\bar{D}(\omega)|} \quad (5.56)$$

Note that the function in Equation 5.55 is similar to the oversubtraction function proposed by Berouti et al. [11] (see Figure 5.10) in that it applies a small weight to frequencies with high *a posteriori* SNR [i.e., large values of $\rho(\omega)$] values and a large weight to frequencies with low-SNR [i.e., for small values of $\rho(\omega)$] values. In contrast to the oversubtraction algorithm, the weighting is applied to each individual frequency bin separately. The preceding nonlinear subtraction algorithm was successfully used in [22] as a preprocessor to enhance the performance of speech recognition systems in noise.

5.6 MULTIBAND SPECTRAL SUBTRACTION

A multiband approach to spectral subtraction was proposed in [23,24]. The motivation behind this approach is similar to that of NSS. It is based on the fact that, in general, noise will not affect the speech signal uniformly over the whole spectrum. Some frequencies will be affected more adversely than others depending on the spectral characteristics of the noise (see Chapter 1). This is best illustrated in Figure 5.12, which shows plots of the *a posteriori* SNR of four frequency bands estimated over time. As this example shows, the segmental SNR in the high-frequency bands (e.g., band 4) is in some instances significantly lower than the SNR of the low-frequency bands (e.g., band 2) by as much as 15 dB.

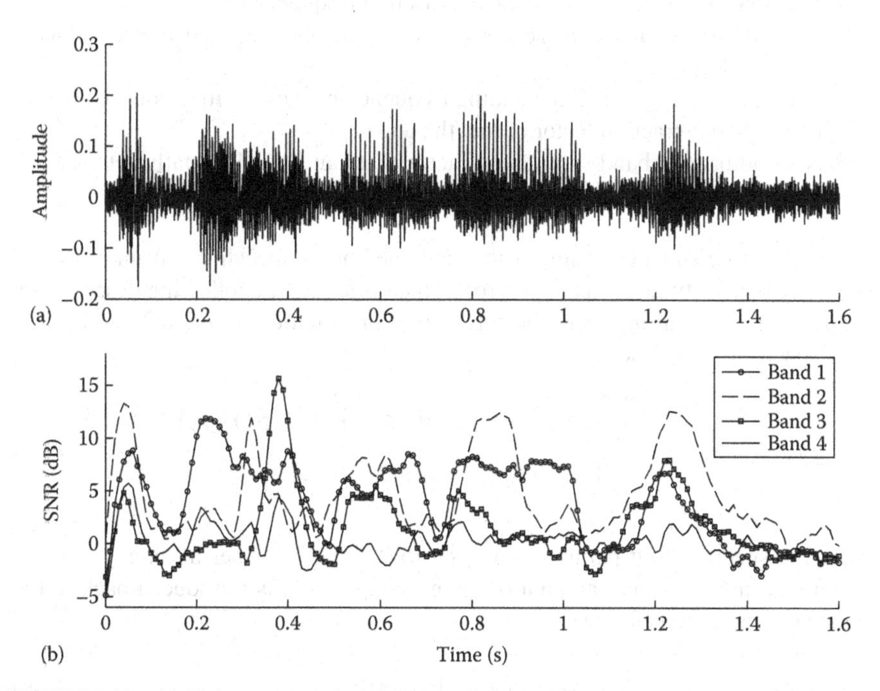

FIGURE 5.12 (a) Noisy sentence in +5 dB speech-shaped noise and (b) four-band SNR values plotted over time. These SNR values were obtained by dividing the spectrum into four linearly spaced bands and computing the *a posteriori* SNR of each band at each frame of speech.

The main difference between the multiband and the NSS algorithms is in the estimation of the oversubtraction factors. The MB approach estimates one subtraction factor for each frequency band, whereas the NSS algorithm estimates one subtraction factor for each frequency bin. One drawback of estimating one subtraction factor for each frequency bin is that the SNR of each frequency bin can change radically from frame to frame. These radical changes are partly responsible for the speech distortion (musical noise) encountered in spectral subtraction [25]. In contrast, as shown in Figure 5.12, the band SNRs do not change as radically. Consequently, the speech distortion is expected to be markedly reduced with the multiband approach.

In the multiband approach [23,24,26], the speech spectrum is divided into N nonoverlapping bands, and spectral subtraction is performed independently in each band. The process of splitting the speech signal into different bands can be performed either in the time domain by using band-pass filters or in the frequency domain by using appropriate windows. The latter method was adopted because it is computationally more economical to implement.

The estimate of the clean speech spectrum in the ith band is obtained by [24]

$$|\hat{X}_i(\omega_k)|^2 = |\bar{Y}_i(\omega_k)|^2 - \alpha_i \cdot \delta_i \cdot |\hat{D}_i(\omega_k)|^2 \quad b_i \le \omega_k \le e_i \tag{5.57}$$

where

$\omega_k = 2\pi k/N$ ($k = 0, 1, \ldots, N-1$) are the discrete frequencies

$|\hat{D}_i(\omega_k)|^2$ is the estimated noise power spectrum (obtained and updated during speech-absent segments)

b_i and e_i are the beginning and ending frequency bins of the ith frequency band

α_i is the oversubtraction factor of the ith band

δ_i is an additional band-subtraction factor that can be individually set for each frequency band to customize the noise removal process

In the preceding equation, $\bar{Y}_i(\omega_k)$ is the smoothed noisy speech spectrum of the ith frequency band estimated in the preprocessing stage (see the following description). Negative values resulting from the subtraction in Equation 5.57 are floored to the noisy spectrum as follows:

$$|\hat{X}_i(\omega_k)|^2 = \begin{cases} |\hat{X}_i(\omega_k)|^2 & \text{if } |\hat{X}_i(\omega_k)|^2 > \beta |\bar{Y}_i(\omega_k)|^2 \\ \beta |\bar{Y}_i(\omega_k)|^2 & \text{else} \end{cases} \tag{5.58}$$

where the spectral floor parameter β is set to 0.002. To further mask any remaining musical noise, a small amount of the noisy spectrum is introduced back to the enhanced spectrum as follows:

$$|\bar{\bar{X}}_i(\omega_k)|^2 = |\hat{X}_i(\omega_k)|^2 + 0.05 \cdot |\bar{Y}_i(\omega_k)|^2 \tag{5.59}$$

where $|\bar{\bar{X}}_i(\omega_k)|^2$ is the newly enhanced power spectrum.

The band-specific oversubtraction factor α_i is a function of the segmental SNR_i of the ith frequency band and is computed as follows:

$$\alpha_i = \begin{cases} 4.75 & SNR_i < -5 \\ 4 - \frac{3}{20}(SNR_i) & -5 \le SNR_i \le 20 \\ 1 & SNR_i > 20 \end{cases} \tag{5.60}$$

where the band SNR_i is given by

$$SNR_i\,(\text{dB}) = 10\log_{10}\left(\frac{\sum_{\omega_k=b_i}^{e_i} |\bar{Y}_i(\omega_k)|^2}{\sum_{\omega_k=b_i}^{e_i} |D_i(\omega_k)|^2}\right) \tag{5.61}$$

Although the use of the oversubtraction factor α_i provides a degree of control over the noise subtraction level in each band, the use of multiple frequency bands and the use of the δ_i weights provided an additional degree of control within each band. The values for δ_i in Equation 5.57 are empirically determined and set to

$$\delta_i = \begin{cases} 1 & f_i \le 1\ \textbf{kHz} \\ 2.5 & 1\ \textbf{kHz} < f_i \le \frac{Fs}{2} - 2\ \textbf{kHz} \\ 1.5 & f_i > \frac{Fs}{2} - 2\ \textbf{kHz} \end{cases} \tag{5.62}$$

where

f_i is the upper frequency of the ith band
Fs is the sampling frequency in Hz

The motivation for using smaller δ_i values for the low-frequency bands is to minimize speech distortion, as most of the speech energy is present in the lower frequencies. Relaxed subtraction is also used for the high-frequency bands. The preceding parameter can be customized for different types of noise encountered in various applications.

The block diagram of the multiband method proposed in [24,26] is shown in Figure 5.13. The signal is first windowed, and the magnitude spectrum is estimated using the FFT. The noisy speech spectrum is then preprocessed to produce a smoothed estimate of the spectrum (further details follow). Next, the noise and speech spectra are divided into N contiguous frequency bands, and the oversubtraction factors for each

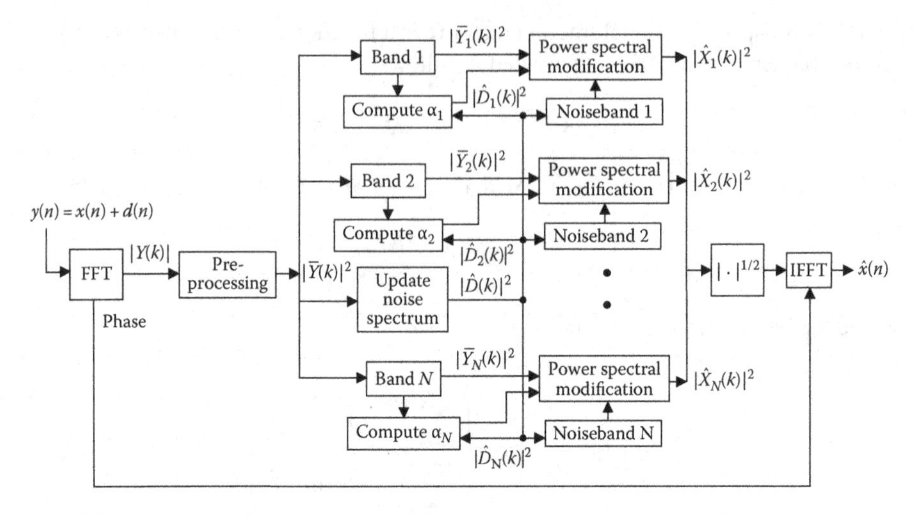

FIGURE 5.13 Block diagram of the multiband spectral subtraction algorithm.

band are calculated. The individual frequency bands of the estimated noise spectrum are subtracted from the corresponding bands of the noisy speech spectrum. Last, the modified frequency bands are recombined, and the enhanced signal is obtained by taking the IFFT of the enhanced spectrum using the noisy speech phase.

The motivation behind the preprocessing stage is to reduce the variance of the spectral estimate and consequently reduce the residual noise. The preprocessing serves to precondition the input data to surmount the distortion caused by errors in the subtraction process. Hence, instead of directly using the power spectrum of the signal, a smoothed version of the power spectrum is used. Smoothing of the magnitude spectrum as per [1] was found to reduce the variance of the speech spectrum and contribute to speech quality improvement. Smoothing of the estimated noise spectrum was not found to be helpful in reducing residual noise [26]. A weighted spectral average is taken over preceding and succeeding frames of speech as follows:

$$|\overline{Y_j}(\omega_k)| = \sum_{i=-M}^{M} W_i \, |Y_{j-i}(\omega_k)| \tag{5.63}$$

where

$|\overline{Y_j}(\omega_k)|$ is the preprocessed noisy magnitude spectrum of the jth frame

$|Y_i(\omega_k)|$ is the noisy magnitude spectrum

W_i $(0 < W < 1)$ are the weights assigned to each frame

The averaging is done over M preceding and M succeeding frames of speech. The number of frames M is limited to 2 to prevent smearing of spectral information. The weights W_i were empirically determined and set to W_i = [0.09, 0.25, 0.32, 0.25, 0.09]. Figure 5.14 shows the effect of smoothing and local averaging on

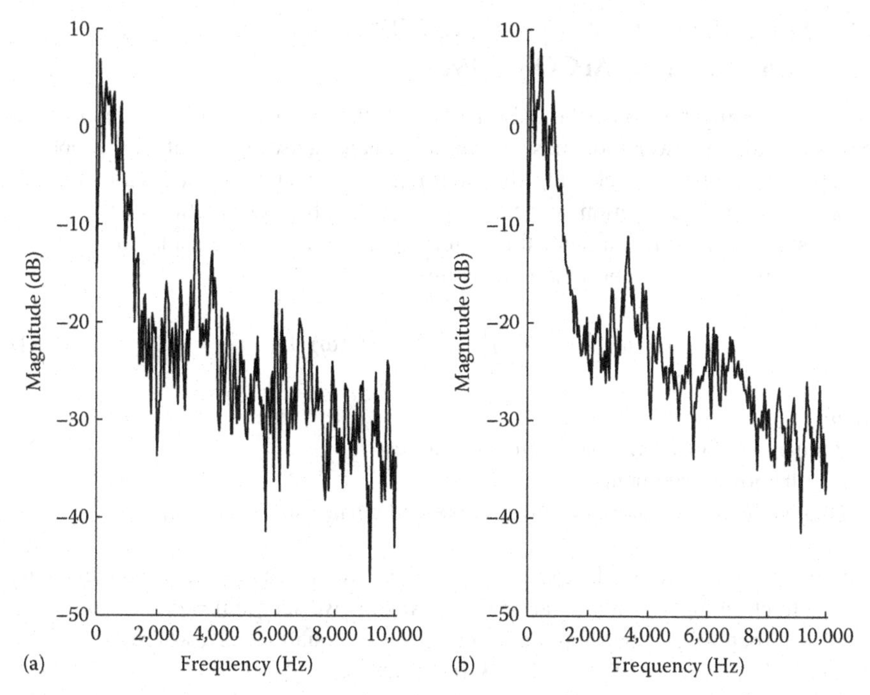

FIGURE 5.14 Effect of local averaging on the spectrum. (a) The original power spectrum of noisy speech obtained using the FFT. (b) The weighted spectral average taken over preceding and succeeding frames of speech using Equation 5.63.

the spectrum. Local or magnitude averaging was also shown by others [1,27] to improve the quality of processed speech.

Several experiments were conducted [24,26] to investigate the effect of varying the number of frequency bands and frequency spacing on performance. Performance was assessed using the Itakura–Saito (IS) spectral distance measure (see Chapter 11 for more details). The IS distance showed marked improvement (i.e., it decreased) when the number of bands increased from one to four. Considerably smaller improvements were noted when the number of bands increased beyond four. The improvement in speech quality was also evident. Three different types of frequency spacing were investigated: linear, logarithmic, and mel spacing. All three spacing methods exhibited comparable performance in terms of spectral distance values and speech quality, with the exception of logarithmic spacing, which caused some distortion in the lower frequency ranges.

The aforementioned multiband approach is similar to the algorithm proposed in [23], which was based on a critical-band partition of the spectrum. In [23], the spectrum was divided into a considerably larger number of bands (18 critical bands were used in [23], whereas 4–8 linearly spaced bands were used in [24]). The two methods also differed in the value of the oversubtraction factor in Equation 5.57. A fixed value for the oversubtraction factor was used in [23] for all bands, whereas a different value was used in the MB approach [24] for each band, depending on the corresponding segmental SNR of that band.

5.7 MINIMUM MEAN SQUARE ERROR SPECTRAL SUBTRACTION ALGORITHM

In the preceding methods, the subtractive parameters α and β were determined experimentally and were not chosen optimally in any sense. Sim et al. [28] proposed a method for optimally selecting the subtractive parameters in the mean-squared-error sense. Their derivation was based on a parametric formulation of the generalized spectral subtraction algorithm. More specifically, they considered a general version of the spectral subtraction algorithm:

$$|\hat{X}(\omega)|^p = \gamma_p(\omega)|Y(\omega)|^p - \alpha_p(\omega)|\hat{D}(\omega)|^p \tag{5.64}$$

where

$\gamma_p(\omega)$ and $\alpha_p(\omega)$ are the parameters of interest
p is the power exponent
$\hat{D}(\omega)$ is the average noise spectrum obtained during nonspeech activity

Note that if we set $\gamma_p(\omega) = 1$, $\alpha_p(\omega) = \alpha$, and $p = 2$, then Equation 5.64 reduces to the oversubtraction algorithm (Equation 5.41). Also, if we set $\gamma_p(\omega) = c_{YX}$, $\alpha_p(\omega) = c_{XD}$, and $p = 1$, then we get the subtractive rule given in Equation 5.27, where c_{YX} and c_{XD} are defined in Equations 5.26 and 5.23, respectively.

The parameters $\gamma_p(\omega)$ and $\alpha_p(\omega)$ can be determined optimally by minimizing the mean square of the error spectrum:

$$e_p(\omega) = |X_p(\omega)|^p - |\hat{X}(\omega)|^p \tag{5.65}$$

where $|X_p(\omega)|^p$ is the clean speech spectrum, assuming an "ideal" spectral subtraction model. It is assumed here that the noisy speech spectrum consists of the sum of two independent spectra, the $|X_p(\omega)|^p$ spectrum and the true noise spectrum. That is, it is assumed that the following equation holds for some constant p:

$$|Y(\omega)|^p = |X_p(\omega)|^p + |D(\omega)|^p \tag{5.66}$$

where $D(\omega)$ is the true noise spectrum. In theory, the preceding equation holds for $p = 1$ assuming that the phases of the clean signal spectrum are equal to the phases of the noise spectrum. By minimizing the mean-square error of the error spectrum $e_p(\omega)$, that is, $E[\{e_p(\omega)\}^2]$, with respect to $\gamma_p(\omega)$ and $\alpha_p(\omega)$, we get the following optimal subtractive parameters:

$$\alpha_p(\omega) = \frac{\xi^p(\omega)}{1+\xi^p(\omega)} \tag{5.67}$$

$$\gamma_p(\omega) = \frac{\xi^p(\omega)}{1+\xi^p(\omega)}\{1-\xi^{-p/2}(\omega)\} \tag{5.68}$$

where

$$\xi(\omega) = \frac{E[|X_p(\omega)|^2]}{E[|D(\omega)|^2]} \tag{5.69}$$

The preceding equations were derived after making the assumption that the individual spectral components of speech and noise are statistically independent and zero-mean complex-Gaussian random variables (see Chapter 7). This assumption was necessary to simplify the solution. Substituting Equations 5.67 and 5.68 into Equation 5.64 yields the optimal parametric estimator:

$$|\hat{X}(\omega)| = \left\{ \frac{\xi^p(\omega)}{1+\xi^p(\omega)} \left[|Y(\omega)|^p - (1-\xi^{-p/2}(\omega))\,|\hat{D}(\omega)|^p \right] \right\}^{1/p} \tag{5.70}$$

The preceding estimator was derived by making no assumptions about the relationship between the two parameters $\gamma_p(\omega)$ and $\alpha_p(\omega)$ and was therefore referred to as the unconstrained estimator. Sim et al. [28] also considered constraining the two parameters to be equal to each other, that is, $\gamma_p(\omega) = \alpha_p(\omega)$ and derived a different estimator. The derived optimal constrained estimator had the following form:

$$|\hat{X}(\omega)| = \left\{ \frac{\xi^p(\omega)}{\delta_p+\xi^p(\omega)} \left[|Y(\omega)|^p - |\hat{D}(\omega)|^p \right] \right\}^{1/p} \tag{5.71}$$

where δ_p is constant for a given power exponent p ($\delta_p = 0.2146$, 0.5, and 0.7055 for $p = 1$, 2, and 3, respectively). To limit overattenuation of low-energy speech segments, a lower spectral bound was further applied to Equation 5.71. The smoothed lower-bound spectrum was obtained by averaging an attenuated version of the noisy speech spectrum, $\mu Y(\omega)$ $(0 < \mu < 1)$, with the enhanced and smoothed spectrum estimated in the previous frame, that is,

$$\mu\,|\bar{Y}(\omega)| = 0.5(\mu\,|Y(\omega)| + |\bar{X}_{prev}(\omega)|) \tag{5.72}$$

where $\mu|\bar{Y}(\omega)|$ denotes the smoothed lower spectral bound. That is, if the enhanced spectral value in Equation 5.71 is found to be smaller than $\mu Y(\omega)$, it is set equal to $\mu|\bar{Y}(\omega)|$. The final constrained estimator had the following form:

$$|\bar{X}(\omega)| = \begin{cases} |\hat{X}(\omega)| & \text{if } |\hat{X}(\omega)| \geq \mu\,|Y(\omega)| \\ \mu\,|\bar{Y}(\omega)| & \text{else} \end{cases} \tag{5.73}$$

Note that the term $|\bar{X}_{prev}(\omega)|$ used in Equation 5.72 is based on the preceding equation and not on Equation 5.71. The preceding parameter μ (set in the range 0.05–0.2 in [28]) served as a spectral flooring constant, much like the parameter in β Equation 5.41.

The term $\xi(\omega)$ in Equation 5.69 corresponds to the ratio of the signal power to noise power and is often referred to as the *a priori* SNR. Unfortunately, this term cannot be computed exactly as we do not have access to the clean signal. Following the approach proposed in [29], Sim et al. [28] approximated the *a priori* SNR as follows:

$$\xi(\omega) \approx (1-\eta)\max\left(\frac{|Y(\omega)|^2}{|\hat{D}(\omega)|^2}-1,0\right)+\eta\frac{|\hat{X}_{prev}(\omega)|^2}{|\hat{D}(\omega)|^2} \tag{5.74}$$

where η is a smoothing constant (set to 0.96) and $|\hat{X}_{prev}(\omega)|$ is the enhanced spectrum computed in the previous frame. Equation 5.74 is basically a weighted average of the current instantaneous SNR (first term) and the old SNR (second term). Further details regarding the derivation of Equation 5.74 can be found in Chapter 7. The estimate of the noise spectrum was smoothed and updated in a similar way.

The preceding two estimators were evaluated [28] and compared against the standard spectral subtraction algorithm [11] using objective measures, namely, the SNR and log-likelihood measures. Significant improvements over the standard spectral subtraction algorithm (for the same value of p) were observed only for low SNR levels (≤ 5 dB). For the constrained estimator, $\mu = 0.1$ (Equation 5.73) was used. Performance obtained with $p = 1$ and 2 was nearly the same.

Analysis of the two estimators showed that the suppression function (computed as $|\hat{X}(\omega)|/|Y(\omega)|$) of the unconstrained estimator had a similar trend as that of the minimum mean square error (MMSE) estimator [29]. Comparison between the suppression functions of the two estimators revealed that the constrained estimator provided more noise attenuation than the unconstrained estimator, particularly for low-energy speech segments. Subjective listening tests confirmed that the constrained estimator resulted in lower levels of residual noise. In fact, when μ was set to 0.10, the residual noise levels were found to be perceptually comparable to the levels obtained using the MMSE estimator [29].

5.8 EXTENDED SPECTRAL SUBTRACTION

In most spectral subtraction algorithms, it is assumed that an estimate of the noise spectrum is available. Such an estimate can be obtained, for instance, using a voice activity detector (VAD) or a noise estimation algorithm (to be discussed in Chapter 9). An alternative and computationally simple approach that continually estimates the noise spectrum without requiring a VAD algorithm was proposed in [30,31]. The key feature of the proposed algorithm is the continuous update of the background noise spectrum even during speech activity.

The proposed method, termed extended spectral subtraction (ESS), is based on a combination of adaptive Wiener filtering (Chapter 6) and spectral subtraction principles. Wiener filtering is used to estimate the noise spectrum, which is then subtracted from the noisy speech signal. The block diagram of the ESS algorithm is given in Figure 5.15.

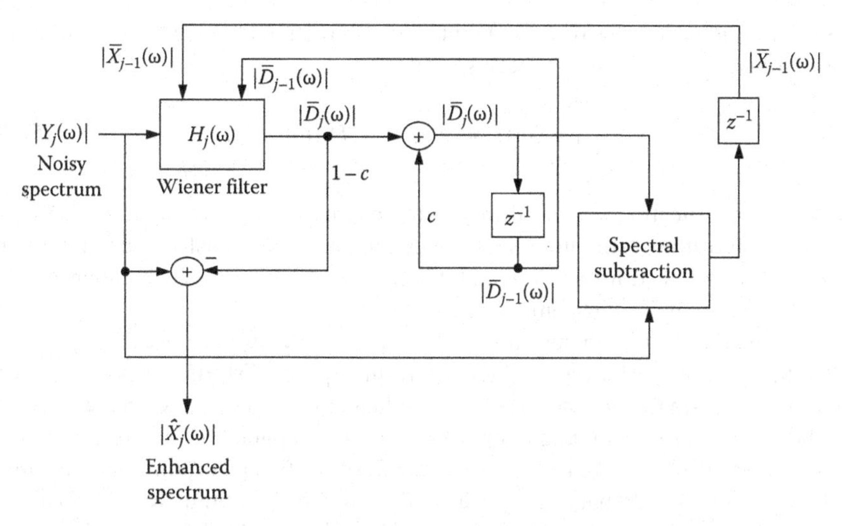

FIGURE 5.15 Block diagram of the extended spectral subtraction algorithm.

The Wiener filter approximation for frame j is based on preceding spectral estimates and is given by

$$H_j(\omega) = \left(\frac{|\bar{D}_{j-1}(\omega)|^2}{|\bar{X}_{j-1}(\omega)|^2 + |\bar{D}_{j-1}(\omega)|^2} \right)^{1/2} \tag{5.75}$$

where

$|\bar{D}_{j-1}(\omega)|^2$ is the smoothed estimate of the noise power spectrum
$|\bar{X}_{j-1}(\omega)|^2$ is the smoothed power spectrum of the enhanced signal at frame $j-1$

Note that the Wiener filter in Equation 5.75 estimates the noise spectrum of the previous frame because it is based on previous estimates of the enhanced signal. It is therefore based on the assumption that the spectral characteristics of the noise do not change drastically from the previous frame. The smoothed noise estimate is obtained according to

$$|\bar{D}_j(\omega)| = c\,|\bar{D}_{j-1}(\omega)| + (1-c)\,|\hat{D}_j(\omega)| \tag{5.76}$$

where c is a smoothing constant ($0 < c < 1$) and $|\hat{D}_j(\omega)|$ is the current estimate of the noise spectrum obtained by applying the Wiener filter (computed in the previous frame) to the input noisy speech spectrum, that is,

$$|\hat{D}_j(\omega)| = H_j(\omega)\,|Y_j(\omega)| \tag{5.77}$$

Finally, the enhanced spectrum is obtained by subtracting the preceding noise spectrum estimate from the noisy speech spectrum:

$$|\hat{X}_j(\omega)| = |Y_j(\omega)| - |\hat{D}_j(\omega)| \tag{5.78}$$

Half-wave rectification was used in [31] to ensure nonnegative values for $|\hat{X}_j(\omega)|$. The ESS algorithm estimates the noise spectrum continuously as per Equation 5.77 without the need for a VAD, and it therefore allows for speech enhancement in nonstationary noise environments.

Experimental results indicated that the smoothing constant c used in Equation 5.76 influenced the performance of the algorithm. Speech distortion was noted when the c value was small, but a more audible residual noise was noted when it was large. The best range for c was found to be $0.8 < c < 0.99$, and good results were obtained with $c = 0.95$. The performance of the extended subtraction algorithm was compared to the algorithm in [32] that employed a noise estimation algorithm. Results, in terms of SNR improvement, showed that the two algorithms yielded comparable performance. The design implementation details and the effect in performance of various parameters are described in greater detail in [31].

5.9 SPECTRAL SUBTRACTION USING ADAPTIVE GAIN AVERAGING

As mentioned earlier, two of the factors responsible for the musical noise in spectral-subtractive algorithms were the large variance in the spectral estimate and the variability in the gain function. To address the first issue, Gustafsson et al. [5] suggested dividing the current analysis frame into smaller subframes and obtaining a lower resolution spectrum. The individual spectra in each subframe were subsequently averaged to obtain a lower-variance spectrum. To address the second issue, Gustafsson et al. [5] proposed smoothing the gain function over time using adaptive exponential averaging. Furthermore, to circumvent the noncausal filtering due to the use of a zero-phase gain function, Gustafsson et al. suggested introducing a linear phase in the gain function. The proposed spectral subtraction algorithm reduced overall the processing delay to a fraction of the analysis frame duration.

Figure 5.16 shows the block diagram of the proposed spectral subtraction algorithm [5]. The input signal is divided into L-sample frames and further subdivided into subframes consisting of M ($M < L$) samples each. The computed spectra in each subframe are averaged to produce a low-variance *magnitude* spectrum estimate, denoted by $|\bar{Y}_i^{(M)}(\omega)|$, where the superscript indicates the number of spectral components (i.e., size of FFT), and the subscript i indicates the frame number. From $\bar{Y}_i^{(M)}(\omega)$, a lower-resolution gain function is formed as follows:

$$G_i^{(M)}(\omega) = 1 - k\frac{\left|\hat{D}_i^{(M)}(\omega)\right|}{\left|\bar{Y}_i^{(M)}(\omega)\right|} \tag{5.79}$$

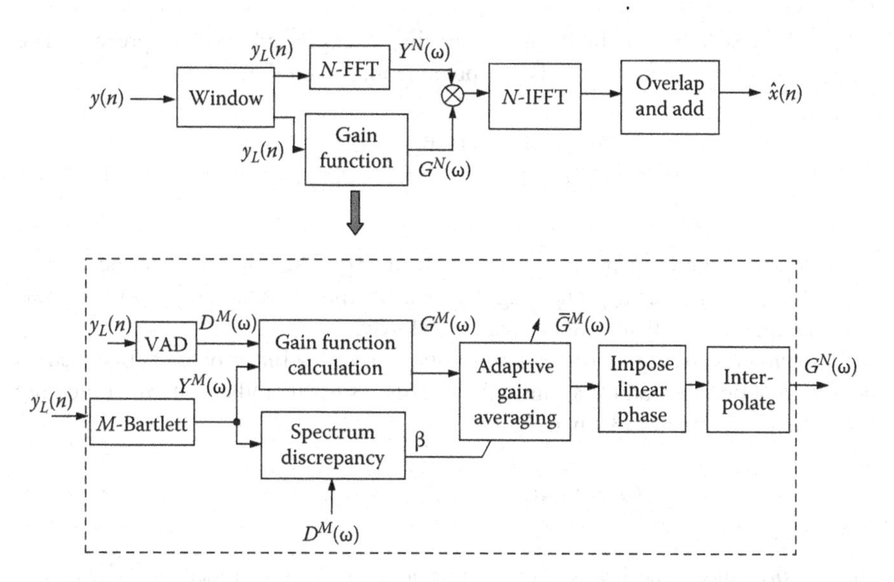

FIGURE 5.16 Block diagram of the spectral subtraction algorithm with adaptive gain averaging.

where

k is a subtraction factor (set to $k = 0.7$ in [5])

$|\hat{D}_i^{(M)}(\omega)|$ denotes the estimated magnitude spectrum of the noise updated during speech-absent segments of speech

To reduce the variability of the gain function, $G_i^{(M)}(\omega)$ is averaged over time according to

$$\bar{G}_i^{(M)}(\omega) = a_i \bar{G}_{i-1}^{(M)}(\omega) + (1 - a_i) G_i^{(M)}(\omega) \tag{5.80}$$

where $\bar{G}_i^{(M)}(\omega)$ denotes the smoothed gain function in frame i, and a_i is an adaptive smoothing parameter. The adaptive averaging parameter a_i is derived from a spectral discrepancy measure β_i defined as follows:

$$\beta_i = \min\left\{ \frac{\sum_{\omega_k=0}^{M-1} \left| |\bar{Y}_i^{(M)}(\omega_k)| - |\hat{D}_i^{(M)}(\omega_k)| \right|}{\sum_{\omega_k=0}^{M-1} |\hat{D}_i^{(M)}(\omega_k)|}, 1 \right\} \tag{5.81}$$

The preceding discrepancy measure assesses in a crude way spectral change relative to the background noise. A small discrepancy value would suggest a relatively stationary background noise situation, whereas a large discrepancy value would suggest situations in which speech or highly varying background noise is present. The adaptive averaging parameter a_i is computed from β_i as follows:

$$a_i = \begin{cases} \gamma a_{i-1} + (1-\gamma)(1-\beta_i) & \text{if } a_{i-1} < 1-\beta_i \\ 1-\beta_i & \text{Otherwise} \end{cases} \quad (5.82)$$

where γ is a smoothing parameter (γ = 0.8 in [5]). The adaptive parameter a_i is allowed to decrease rapidly, enabling the gain function to adapt quickly to the new input signal, but is only allowed to increase slowly.

Following the averaging operation in Equation 5.80, a linear phase is imposed on the gain function to produce a causal filter. This results in a filter with the following time-domain symmetry [33, p. 621]:

$$g_M(n) = \pm g_M(M-1-n) \quad n = 0, 1, \ldots, M-1 \quad (5.83)$$

where $g_M(n)$ denotes the inverse Fourier transform of the gain function $\bar{G}_i^{(M)}(\omega)$. The resulting filter has a delay of $(M-1)/2$, which is a fraction of the original frame length (L).

Finally, after imposing a linear phase on the gain function, $\bar{G}_i^{(M)}(\omega)$ is interpolated from the M-point function to form an N-point function, where N is the size of the FFT. Note that N is chosen so that $N > L + M$, thus avoiding circular convolution effects (see Chapter 2). The resulting output signal is obtained by computing the inverse FFT of

$$\hat{X}_i^{(N)}(\omega) = \bar{G}_i^{(N)}(\omega) \cdot Y_i^{(N)}(\omega) \quad (5.84)$$

where

$\hat{X}_i^{(N)}(\omega)$ is the enhanced complex spectrum
$\bar{G}_i^{(N)}(\omega)$ is the N-point interpolated gain function (which is now complex-valued)
$Y_i^{(N)}(\omega)$ is the complex spectrum of the noisy speech, obtained after zero padding the L-sample input signal

Note that the inverse FFT of $\hat{X}_i^{(N)}(\omega)$ in Equation 5.84 yields the linear convolution of the gain function $g_M(n)$ ($n = 0, 1, \ldots, M-1$) with the noisy signal $y(n)$, $n = 0, 1, \ldots, L-1$.

Figure 5.17 shows an example estimate of the gain function obtained with and without adaptive averaging for a fixed frequency bin. Figure 5.17b shows the gain function given in Equation 5.79 with no averaging, and Figure 5.17c shows the gain function given in Equation 5.80 obtained with adaptive averaging. The gain function shown in Figure 5.17b changes drastically, particularly during speech-absent segments of speech (see, for example, the segments at $t < 0.5$ s and $t > 2.5$ s). In contrast, the gain function in Figure 5.17c is relatively smoother. Figure 5.17d shows the adaptive averaging parameter a_i computed using Equation 5.82. Large values of a_i are obtained when the spectral discrepancy value is small, suggesting

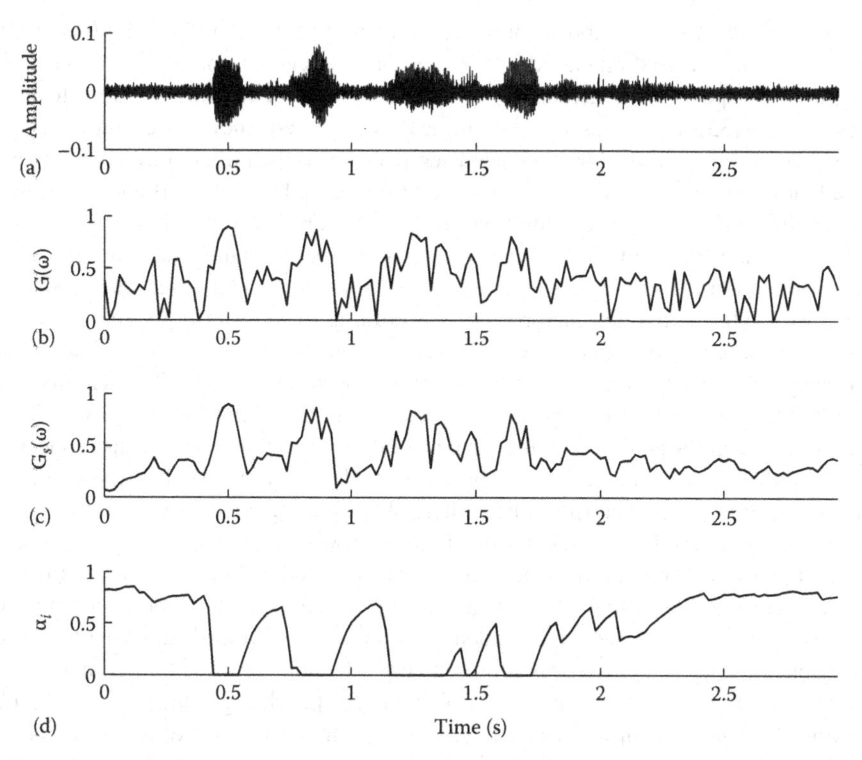

FIGURE 5.17 (a) A sample noisy sentence. Example gain functions (for a fixed frequency) obtained (b) without averaging, (c) with averaging (Equation 5.80). (d) The instantaneous values of the smoothing parameter a_i used in the gain averaging.

stationary background noise situations (see, for example, the segments at $t < 0.5$ s and $t > 2.5$ s). Small values of a_i are obtained when speech is present (see, for example, the segments near $t \approx 1.25$ s and $t \approx 0.8$ s).

The following parameters were found in [5] to work well for speech sampled at 8 kHz: $L = 160$, $M = 32$, and $N = 256$. Magnitude spectral subtraction was used in [5], as indicated in Equation 5.79, although, in practice, power spectral subtraction could have been used. Experimental results reported in [5] indicated significant improvement in performance over the conventional spectral subtraction algorithm.

5.10 SELECTIVE SPECTRAL SUBTRACTION

The aforementioned methods treated all speech segments equally, making no distinction between voiced and unvoiced segments. Motivated by the spectral differences between vowels and consonants (Chapter 3), several researchers have proposed algorithms that treated the voiced and unvoiced segments differently. The resulting spectral-subtractive algorithms were therefore selective for different classes of speech sounds.

A two-band spectral subtraction algorithm was proposed in [34]. The incoming speech frame was first classified into voiced or unvoiced by comparing the energy of the noisy speech to a threshold. For voiced frames, an algorithm similar to that described in [35] was first used to determine the cutoff frequency above which speech was considered to be stochastic. Voiced segments were then filtered into two bands, one below the determined cutoff frequency (low-passed speech) and one above the determined cutoff frequency (high-passed speech). Different algorithms were then used to enhance the low-passed and high-passed speech signals accordingly. The oversubtraction algorithm was used for the low-passed speech based on the short-term FFT. The subtraction factor was set according to short-term SNR as per [11]. For high-passed voiced speech as well as for unvoiced speech, the spectral subtraction algorithm was employed with a different spectral estimator. The Thomson's multiwindow spectral estimator [36] was used in place of the FFT estimator. The main motivation was to reduce the variance of the spectrum at the high-frequency regions of the spectrum, which can be more stochastic in nature than the low-frequency regions of the spectrum. The authors [34] reported that the musical noise was significantly reduced when the two-band approach was used.

A dual excitation speech model, similar to that used in low-rate speech coding [37], was proposed in [38] for speech enhancement. In the proposed approach, speech was decomposed into two independent components—a voiced and an unvoiced component. That is, speech was represented as the sum of these two components (note that this is not equivalent to classifying each speech segment into voiced and unvoiced). Voiced component analysis was performed first by extracting the fundamental frequency and the harmonic amplitudes. The noisy estimates of the harmonic amplitudes were adjusted according to some rule to account for any noise that might have leaked to the harmonics. Following that, the unvoiced component spectrum was computed by subtracting the voiced spectrum from the noisy speech spectrum. Then, a two-pass system, which included a modified Wiener filter, was used to enhance the unvoiced spectrum. Finally, the enhanced speech consisted of the sum of the enhanced voiced and unvoiced components.

A voiced–unvoiced spectral subtraction scheme was also proposed in [39]. Speech frames were first classified as being voiced or unvoiced based on energy and zero-crossing measurements. The unvoiced spectra were first spectrally sharpened by convolving the log of the noisy speech spectrum with a sharpening function of the following form:

$$H(\omega) = \begin{cases} -3c/2L & -L/2 \le \omega \le -L/6 \\ 3(1+c)/L & -L/6 \le \omega \le L/6 \\ -3c/2L & L/6 \le \omega \le L/2 \\ 0 & \text{Otherwise} \end{cases} \tag{5.85}$$

where $0 < c < 0.5$, and L is the width of the spectral sharpening function, set to 2.4% of the signal bandwidth, that is, $L = 0.024\pi$. If the convolved spectral output was found to be negative, it was set to the noisy speech spectrum. Note that a similar sharpening function was used in [40] for modeling lateral inhibition. The main motivation behind spectral sharpening was to increase the spectral contrast, that is, make the spectral peaks more pronounced while suppressing the spectral valleys. This was intended to mitigate the spectral flattening effect of noise. The spectrally sharpened spectrum was subsequently subtracted from the noisy speech spectrum using the oversubtraction rule [11]. The negative subtracted spectral components were set to a spectral minimal bound, which was computed using the LPC spectrum of the noise-subtracted signal (this signal was obtained by passing the noisy speech signal once through the spectral subtraction algorithm). The spectral minimum bound comprised the smoothed spectral envelope of speech and was therefore used to smooth out the spectral discontinuities produced by the spectral subtraction rule. The voiced and speech-absent noisy spectra were similarly subtracted from the noisy speech spectra using the oversubtraction rule. The negative subtracted spectral components were set to the masking threshold levels computed using the procedure described in [41]. Simulation results indicated that the proposed approach was better, in terms of input–output SNR, than the approach in [11] by about 0.98 dB in low-SNR (<0 dB) conditions.

In sum, treating voiced and unvoiced segments differently can bring about substantial improvements in performance. However, the major challenge with such algorithms is making accurate and reliable voiced/unvoiced decisions, particularly at low-SNR conditions.

5.11 SPECTRAL SUBTRACTION BASED ON PERCEPTUAL PROPERTIES

In the preceding methods, the subtractive parameters were either computed experimentally, based on the short-term SNR levels [11], or obtained optimally in a mean-square-error sense [28]. No perceptual properties of the auditory system have been exploited. In this section, we present an algorithm proposed by Virag [42] that incorporates psychoacoustically motivated constraints in the spectral subtraction process. The main objective of this algorithm is to render the residual noise perceptually inaudible and ultimately improve the intelligibility of enhanced speech by taking into account the properties of the human auditory system.

Virag [42] suggested adapting the spectral subtraction parameters α and β in Equation 5.41 based on masking threshold levels. The proposed method was based on the following idea. If the estimated masking threshold at a particular frequency is low, the residual noise level might be above the threshold and will therefore be audible. The subtraction parameters should therefore attain their maximal values at that frequency. Similarly, if the masking threshold level is high at a certain frequency, the residual noise will most likely be masked and consequently will be inaudible. The subtraction parameters should attain their minimal values at that frequency. The choice of the subtraction parameters was therefore guided by a nonlinear function of the auditory masking thresholds as follows:

$$\alpha(\omega) = F_a[\alpha_{\min}, \alpha_{\max}, T(\omega)] \tag{5.86}$$

$$\beta(\omega) = F_b[\beta_{\min}, \beta_{\max}, T(\omega)] \tag{5.87}$$

where $T(\omega)$ was the masking threshold, α_{min} and α_{max} were set to 1 and 6, respectively, and the spectral flooring constants β_{min} and β_{max} were set to 0 and 0.02, respectively. The $F_a(\omega)$ function had the following boundary conditions:

$$F_a(\omega) = \begin{cases} a_{max} & \text{if } T(\omega) = T(\omega)_{min} \\ a_{min} & \text{if } T(\omega) = T(\omega)_{max} \end{cases} \tag{5.88}$$

where $T(\omega)_{min}$ and $T(\omega)_{max}$ are the minimal and maximal values, respectively, of the masking thresholds estimated in each frame. The values of the function $F_a(\omega)$ between these two extreme values were interpolated based on the values of $T(\omega)$. Similarly, the function $F_b(\omega)$ was computed using β_{min} and β_{max} as the boundary conditions. As in NSS [22], the values of the subtractive parameters $\alpha(\omega)$ and $\beta(\omega)$ were frequency dependent in the sense that different values are used for different frequencies. The main advantage of Virag's approach lies in the use of noise-masking thresholds $T(\omega)$ rather than SNR levels for adjusting the parameters $\alpha(\omega)$ and $\beta(\omega)$. The masking thresholds $T(\omega)$ provide a smoother evolution from frame to frame than the SNR and are also better correlated with perception than the SNR.

The preceding algorithm requires accurate computation of the masking thresholds, which are typically derived from the clean speech signal. As only the noisy signal is available, the threshold calculation can be done by first obtaining a rough estimate of the clean signal with a simple power spectral subtraction scheme. In [42], adjustments were made in the threshold computation to account for the fact that the residual noise produced from the first pass of the spectral subtraction algorithm might alter the tonality of the signal and consequently shift the estimated threshold at high frequencies. Following the threshold calculation and the estimation of the subtractive parameters $\alpha(\omega)$ and $\beta(\omega)$, the noisy speech spectrum was subjected to the oversubtraction rule (Equation 5.41). The proposed algorithm was evaluated in [42] using objective measures and subjective tests and found to yield better quality than the NSS and standard spectral subtraction algorithms.

5.12 PERFORMANCE OF SPECTRAL SUBTRACTION ALGORITHMS

The spectral subtraction algorithm was evaluated extensively in many studies, primarily using objective measures such as SNR improvement and spectral distances (e.g., IS measure). These measures (see Chapter 11) assess how closely the enhanced signal matches the original signal in the time or frequency domain. As such, they are only partly correlated with speech intelligibility and speech quality. The intelligibility and speech quality measures reflect the true performance of speech enhancement algorithms in realistic scenarios. Ideally, the spectral subtraction algorithm should improve both intelligibility and quality of speech in noise. Results from the literature, however, suggest that this was not the case. Several have assessed the performance of spectral-subtractive algorithms in terms of intelligibility and quality using formal listening tests. In such tests, a group of normal-hearing listeners is invited to listen, either through headphones or speakers located in a sound-treated room, to processed sentences and asked to either identify the words spoken and/or rate the quality of processed speech. Intelligibility is typically assessed by counting the number of words identified correctly. Next, we present the results of subjective listening and intelligibility studies of noisy speech enhanced by spectral-subtractive algorithms.

Boll [1] performed intelligibility and quality measurements using the diagnostic rhyme test (DRT) (see Chapter 10), which consisted of 192 words produced by a single speaker. In his evaluation, speech from the DRT database was recorded in a helicopter environment and presented to normal-hearing listeners. Results indicated that spectral subtraction did not decrease speech intelligibility scores, but improved speech quality particularly in the areas of pleasantness and inconspicuousness of the background noise.

Lim [43] evaluated the intelligibility of nonsense sentences in white noise at −5, 0, and +5 dB S/N processed by a generalized spectral subtraction algorithm (Equation 5.11). Half-wave rectification was used in the subtraction (Equation 5.5). The intelligibility of processed speech was evaluated for various power exponents, p, ranging from $p = 0.25$ to $p = 2$ (power spectral subtraction). One hundred nonsense sentences were processed for each S/N condition and for each power exponent. Results indicated that the spectral subtraction algorithm did not degrade speech intelligibility except when $p = 0.25$. There was no significant difference between the intelligibility scores obtained with $p = 0.5$, 1, and 2 in all S/N conditions. Similar findings were also reported by others [19].

Kang and Fransen [44] evaluated the quality of noise processed by the spectral subtraction algorithm and then fed to a 2400 bps LPC vocoder. In their study, the spectral subtraction algorithm was used as a preprocessor to reduce the input noise level. The Diagnostic Acceptability Measure (DAM) test (see Chapter 10) was used to evaluate the speech quality of 10 sets of noisy speech sentences recorded at actual military platforms containing helicopter, tank, and jeep noise. Listeners listened to 12 phonetically balanced sentences processed by the spectral subtraction algorithm and LPC vocoder and rated the overall quality on 21 different dimensions that described the speech quality, the background (e.g., hissing, buzzing), and the voice signal (e.g., fluttering, muffled, crackling). Results indicated that the spectral subtraction algorithm improved the quality of speech. The average DAM scores improved consistently by six points for all types of noise tested. The largest improvements in speech quality were noted for relatively stationary noise sources.

Hu and Loizou [45] compared the performance of the spectral subtraction algorithm with gain averaging [5] (see Section 5.9) against the performance of the multiband spectral subtraction algorithm [24] (see Section 5.6) using formal subjective listening tests conducted according to ITU-T P.835 [46]. The ITU-T P.835 methodology is designed to evaluate the speech quality along three dimensions: signal distortion, noise distortion, and overall quality (see Chapter 11 for more details). Results indicated that the multiband spectral subtraction algorithm performed the best consistently across all noise conditions, in terms of overall quality. In terms of noise distortion, the multiband and gain averaging algorithms performed equally well, except in 5 dB train and 10 dB street conditions, in which the multiband algorithm performed significantly better (i.e., it yielded lower noise distortion). In terms of speech distortion, the multiband and gain averaging algorithms performed equally well in most conditions except in 5 dB car noise and in 10 dB street noise, in which the multiband algorithm performed significantly better (i.e., it yielded lower speech distortion). In brief, the multiband algorithm generally performed better than the gain averaging algorithm in overall quality, signal, and noise distortion. Further details about the subjective comparison of spectral-subtractive algorithms as well as other algorithms can be found in Chapter 12.

Overall, most studies confirmed that the spectral subtraction algorithm improves speech quality but not speech intelligibility. In fact, in some cases, depending on the subtractive parameters chosen, speech intelligibility may decrease [43]. Intuitively, one would expect that by improving speech quality, speech intelligibility should improve, but that is not the case. In subjective listening tests, listeners seem to prefer the quality of speech that has minimal noise present without paying much attention to the fact that there might be missing speech information caused by the spectral subtraction process. Speech that is "less noisy" seems to be preferred in general by most listeners. The spectral subtraction algorithm does an excellent job in removing noise but at the expense of eliminating occasionally low-energy speech information, which explains the lack of improvement in speech intelligibility. The low-energy segments of speech are the first to be lost in the subtraction process (see Figure 5.9), particularly when oversubtraction is used. Intelligibility does not degrade, however, even after removing low-energy, but perceptually important, segments of speech owing to the inherent redundancy of information present in the speech signal. This redundancy, along with the use of high-level linguistic knowledge (e.g., context), enables listeners to "fill in" missing information.

Last, it should be noted that most intelligibility tests were conducted using implementations that subtracted noise spectra estimated from speech-absent segments of speech. Recently, better techniques were proposed that estimate and update the noise spectra continuously (see Chapter 9 for more details). It remains to be seen whether spectral subtraction algorithms incorporating sophisticated noise-estimation algorithms will produce improvements in speech intelligibility.

5.13 SUMMARY

This chapter described various spectral-subtractive algorithms proposed for speech enhancement. These algorithms are computationally simple to implement as they only involve a forward and an inverse Fourier transform. However, the simple subtraction processing involved comes at a price. The subtraction of the noise spectra from the noisy spectra introduces a distortion in the signal known as *musical noise*. We presented different techniques that mitigated the musical noise distortion to some degree. The techniques proposed in [5,24], in particular, produced minimal, if any, musical noise distortion. Different variations of spectral subtraction were developed over the years. The most common variation involved the use of an oversubtraction factor that controlled to some degree the amount of speech spectral distortion caused by the subtraction process and the use of a spectral floor that prevented the resultant spectral components from going below a preset minimum value. The spectral floor value controlled the amount of remaining residual noise and the amount of perceived musical noise. Different methods were proposed for computing the oversubtraction factor based on different criteria that included linear [11] and nonlinear functions [22] of the spectral SNR of individual frequency bins or bands [24] and psychoacoustic masking thresholds [42]. Evaluation of the spectral-subtractive algorithms revealed that these algorithms improve speech quality when used at the front end of speech coders.

REFERENCES

1. Boll, S. F. (1979), Suppression of acoustic noise in speech using spectral subtraction, *IEEE Trans. Acoust. Speech Signal Process.*, 27(2), 113–120.
2. Paliwal, K. and Alsteris, L. (2005), On the usefulness of STFT phase spectrum in human listening tests, *Speech Commun.*, 45(2), 153–170.
3. Weiss, M., Aschkenasy, E., and Parsons, T. (1974), Study and the development of the INTEL technique for improving speech intelligibility, Technical Report NSC-FR/4023, Nicolet Scientific Corporation, Northvale, NJ.
4. Deller, J., Hansen, J. H. L., and Proakis, J. (2000), *Discrete-Time Processing of Speech Signals*, New York: IEEE Press.
5. Gustafsson, H., Nordholm, S., and Claesson, I. (2001), Spectral subtraction using reduced delay convolution and adaptive averaging, *IEEE Trans. Speech Audio Process.*, 9(8), 799–807.
6. Bhatnagar, M. (2002), A modified spectral subtraction method combined with perceptual weighting for speech enhancement, Master's thesis, Department of Electrical Engineering, University of Texas-Dallas, Richardson, TX.
7. Hu, Y., Bhatnagar, M., and Loizou, P. (2001), A cross-correlation technique for enhancing speech corrupted with correlated noise, *Proceedings of IEEE International Conference on Acoustic Speech Signal Processing*, Vol. 1, Salt Lake City, UT, pp. 673–676.
8. Vary, P. (1985), Noise suppression by spectral magnitude estimation: Mechanism and theoretical limits, *Signal Process.*, 8, 387–400.
9. Papoulis, A. and Pillai, S. (2002), *Probability, Random Variables and Stochastic Processes*, 4th ed., New York: McGraw-Hill.
10. McAulay, R. J. and Malpass, M. L. (1980), Speech enhancement using a soft-decision noise suppression filter, *IEEE Trans. Acoust. Speech Signal Process.*, 28, 137–145.
11. Berouti, M., Schwartz, M., and Makhoul, J. (1979), Enhancement of speech corrupted by acoustic noise, *Proceedings of IEEE International Conference on Acoustic Speech Signal Processing*, Washington, DC, pp. 208–211.
12. Schroeder, M. (1975), Models of hearing, *Proc. IEEE*, 63(9), 1332–1350.
13. Handel, P. (1995), Low-distortion spectral subtraction for speech enhancement, *Proceeding of the Eurospeech*, Madrid, Spain, pp. 1549–1552.
14. Stoica, P. and Moses, R. (1997), *Introduction to Spectral Analysis*, Upper Saddle River, NJ: Prentice Hall.
15. Goh, Z., Tan, K., and Tan, B. (1998), Postprocessing method for suppressing musical noise generated by spectral subtraction, *IEEE Trans. Speech Audio Process.*, 6(3), 287–292.
16. Crozier, P., Cheetham, B., Holdt, C., and Munday, E. (1993), Speech enhancement employing spectral subtraction and linear predictive analysis, *Electron. Lett.*, 29(12), 1094–1095.
17. Seok, J. and Bae, K. (1999), Reduction of musical noise in spectral subtraction method using subframe phase randomisation, *Electron. Lett.*, 35(2), 123–125.
18. Beh, J. and Ko, H. (2003), A novel spectral subtraction scheme for robust speech recognition: Spectral subtraction using spectral harmonics of speech, *Proceedings of IEEE International Conference on Acoustic Speech Signal Processing*, Vol. 1, Hong Kong, Hong Kong, pp. 648–651.

19. Niederjohn, R., Lee, P., and Josse, F. (1987), Factors related to spectral subtraction for speech in noise enhancement, *Proc. SPIE*, Cambridge, MA, pp. 985–996.
20. Kushner, W., Goncharoff, V., Wu, C., Nguyen, V., and Damoulakis, J. (1989), The effects of subtractive-type speech enhancement/noise reduction algorithms on parameter estimation for improved recognition and coding in high noise environments, *Proceedings of IEEE International Conference on Acoustic Speech Signal Processing*, Vol. 1, Glasgow, Scotland, pp. 211–214.
21. Vary, P. and Martin, R. (2006), *Digital Speech Transmission: Enhancement, Coding and Error Concealment*, Chichester, England: John Wiley & Sons.
22. Lockwood, P. and Boudy, J. (1992), Experiments with a Non-linear Spectral Subtractor (NSS), Hidden Markov Models and the projections, for robust recognition in cars, *Speech Commun.*, 11(2–3), 215–228.
23. Singh, L. and Sridharan, S. (1998), Speech enhancement using critical band spectral subtraction, *Proceedings of International Conference on Spoken Language Processing*, Sydney, NSW, Australia, pp. 2827–2830.
24. Kamath, S. and Loizou, P. (2002), A multi-band spectral subtraction method for enhancing speech corrupted by colored noise, *Proceedings of IEEE International Conference on Acoustic Speech Signal Processing,* Orlando, FL.
25. Cappe, O. (1994), Elimination of the musical noise phenomenon with the Ephraim and Malah noise suppressor, *IEEE Trans. Speech Audio Process.*, 2(2), 346–349.
26. Kamath, S. (2001), A multi-band spectral subtraction method for speech enhancement, Master's thesis, Department of Electrical Engineering, University of Texas-Dallas, Richardson, TX.
27. Arslan, L., McCree, A., and Viswanathan, V. (1995), New methods for adaptive noise suppression, *Proceedings of IEEE International Conference on Acoustic Speech Signal Processing*, Detroit, MI, pp. 812–815.
28. Sim, B., Tong, Y., Chang, J., and Tan, C. (1998), A parametric formulation of the generalized spectral subtraction method, *IEEE Trans. Speech Audio Process.*, 6(4), 328–337.
29. Ephraim, Y. and Malah, D. (1984), Speech enhancement using a minimum mean-square error short-time spectral amplitude estimator, *IEEE Trans. Acoust. Speech Signal Process.*, 32(6), 1109–1121.
30. Sovka, P. (1995), Extended spectral substraction: Description and preliminary results, Technical Report R95-2, Prague, CTU, Faculty of Electrical Engineering, Prague, Czech Republic.
31. Sovka, P., Pollack, P., and Kybic, J. (1996), Extended spectral subtraction, *Proceedings of European Conference on Signal Processing Communication*, Trieste, Italy, pp. 963–966.
32. Martin, R. (1994), Spectral subtraction based on minimum statistics, *Proceedings of European Signal Processing*, Edinburgh, Scotland, pp. 1182–1185.
33. Proakis, J. and Manolakis, D. (1996), *Digital Signal Processing*, 3rd ed., Upper Saddle River, NJ: Prentice Hall.
34. He, C. and Zweig, G. (1999), Adaptive two-band spectral subtraction with multi-window spectral estimation, *Proceedings of IEEE International Conference on Acoustic Speech Signal Processing*, Vol. 2, Phoenix, AZ, pp. 793–796.
35. Makhoul, J., Viswanathan, R., Schwartz, R., and Huggins, A. (1978), A mixed source model for speech compression and synthesis, *J. Acoust. Soc. Am.*, 64(6), 1577–1581.
36. Thomson, D. (1982), Spectrum estimation and harmonic analysis, *Proc. IEEE*, 70(9), 1055–1096.
37. Hardwick, J. and Lim, J. (1988), A 4.8kbps multi-band excitation speech coder, *Proceedings of IEEE International Conference on Acoustic Speech Signal Processing*, Vol. 1, New York, NY, pp. 374–377.

38. Hardwick, J., Yoo, C., and Lim, J. (1993), Speech enhancement using the dual excitation speech model, *Proceedings of IEEE International Conference on Acoustic Speech Signal Processing*, Vol. 2, Minneapolis, MN, pp. 367–370.
39. Kim, W., Kang, S., and Ko, H. (2000), Spectral subtraction based on phonetic dependency and masking effects, *IEE Proc.—Vision Image Signal Process.*, 147(5), 423–427.
40. Cheng, Y. and O'Shaughnessy, D. (1991), Speech enhancement based conceptually on auditory evidence, *IEEE Trans. Acoust. Speech Signal Process.*, 39(9), 1943–1954.
41. Johnston, J. (1988), Transform coding of audio signals using perceptual noise criteria, *IEEE J. Select. Areas Commun.*, 6, 314–323.
42. Virag, N. (1999), Single channel speech enhancement based on masking properties of the human auditory system, *IEEE Trans. Speech Audio Process.*, 7(3), 126–137.
43. Lim, J. (1978), Evaluation of a correlation subtraction method for enhancing speech degraded by additive noise, *IEEE Trans. Acoust. Speech Signal Process.*, 37(6), 471–472.
44. Kang, G. S. and Fransen, J. (1989), Quality improvement of LPC processed noisy speech by spectral subtraction, *IEEE Trans. Acoust. Speech Signal Process.*, 37, 939–942.
45. Hu, Y. and Loizou, P. (2006), Subjective comparison of speech enhancement algorithms, *Proceedings of IEEE International Conference on Acoustic Speech Signal Processing*, Vol. I, pp. 153–156.
46. ITU-T (2003), Subjective test methodology for evaluating speech communication systems that include noise suppression algorithm, ITU-T Recommendation P.835.

6 Wiener Filtering

The spectral-subtractive algorithms described in Chapter 5 were based largely on intuitive and heuristically based principles. More specifically, these algorithms exploited the fact that noise is additive, and one can obtain an estimate of the clean signal spectrum simply by subtracting the noise spectrum from the noisy speech spectrum. The enhanced signal spectrum was not derived in an optimal way. We now turn our attention to Wiener filtering approach that derives the enhanced signal by optimizing a mathematically tractable error criterion, the mean-square error.

6.1 INTRODUCTION TO WIENER FILTER THEORY

Consider the statistical filtering problem given in Figure 6.1. The input signal goes through a linear and time-invariant system to produce an output signal $y(n)$. We are to design the system in such a way that the output signal, $\hat{d}(n)$, is as close (in some sense) to the desired signal, $d(n)$, as possible. This can be done by computing the estimation error, $e(n)$, and making it as small as possible. The optimal filter that minimizes the estimation error is called the *Wiener filter*, named after the mathematician Norbert Wiener [1], who first formulated and solved this filtering problem in the continuous domain.

It should be noted that one of the constraints placed on the filter is that it is linear, thus making the analysis easy to handle. In principle, the filter could be finite impulse response (FIR) or infinite impulse response (IIR), but often FIR filters are used because (1) they are inherently stable and (2) the resulting solution is linear and computationally easy to evaluate. Assuming an FIR system (see Figure 6.2), we have

$$\hat{d}(n) = \sum_{k=0}^{M-1} h_k y(n-k) \quad n = 0,1,2,\ldots \tag{6.1}$$

where

$\{h_k\}$ are the FIR filter coefficients
M is the number of coefficients

Next, we need to compute the filter coefficients $\{h_k\}$ so that the estimation error, that is, $d(n) - \hat{d}(n)$, is minimized. The mean square of the estimation error is commonly used as a criterion for minimization, and the optimal filter coefficients can be derived in the time or frequency domain.

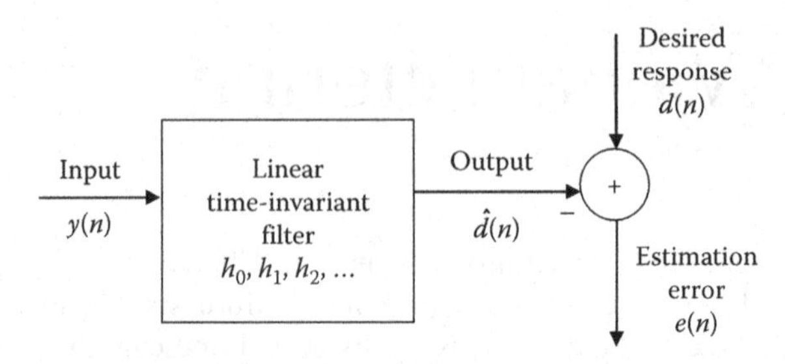

FIGURE 6.1 Block diagram of the statistical filtering problem.

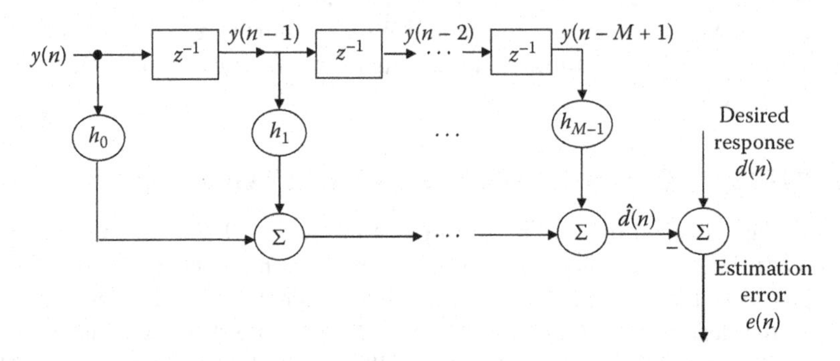

FIGURE 6.2 Block diagram of the optimum filtering problem using an M-tap FIR filter.

6.2 WIENER FILTERS IN THE TIME DOMAIN

We henceforth assume that the input signal $y(n)$ and the desired signal $d(n)$ are realizations of jointly wide-sense stochastic processes. We first compute the estimation error $e(n)$ as

$$\begin{aligned} e(n) &= d(n) - \hat{d}(n) \\ &= d(n) - \mathbf{h}^T\mathbf{y} \end{aligned} \tag{6.2}$$

where

$\mathbf{h}^T = [h_0, h_1, h_2, \ldots, h_{M-1}]$ is the filter coefficient vector

$\mathbf{y}^T = [y(n), y(n-1), y(n-2), \ldots, y(n-M+1)]$ is the input vector containing the past M samples of the input

To find the optimal filter coefficients, we minimize the mean-square value of $e(n)$, that is, $E[e^2(n)]$, where $E[\cdot]$ is the expectation operator. The mean-squared error is given by

$$\begin{aligned} J = E[e^2(n)] &= E(d(n) - \mathbf{h}^T\mathbf{y})^2 \\ &= E[d^2(n)] - 2\mathbf{h}^T E[\mathbf{y}d(n)] + \mathbf{h}^T E[\mathbf{y}\mathbf{y}^T]\mathbf{h} \\ &= E[d^2(n)] - 2\mathbf{h}^T\mathbf{r}_{yd} + \mathbf{h}^T\mathbf{R}_{yy}\mathbf{h} \end{aligned} \tag{6.3}$$

where

$\mathbf{r}_{yd}^{-} \triangleq E[\mathbf{y}d(n)] = E[(y(n)y(n-1)\ldots y(n-M+1))d(n)]$ is the cross-correlation vector ($M \times 1$) between the input and desired signals

$\mathbf{R}_{yy} = E[\mathbf{y}\mathbf{y}^T]$ is the autocorrelation matrix ($M \times M$) of the input signal

The superscript in $\mathbf{r}_{yd}^{-}$ is used to indicate that the mth element of the cross-correlation vector is in fact $r_{yd}(-m)$. From Equation 6.3, we deduce that the mean-square error J is a quadratic function of the coefficients $\mathbf{h}$ and therefore has a single (global) minimum. If, for example, the filter has only two coefficients, $\mathbf{h} = [h_0, h_1]$, then the error surface will have the shape of a bowl with a single minimum.

For the cost function J to attain its smallest value, we require all the elements of the gradient vector to be zero, that is,

$$\frac{\partial J}{\partial h_k} = 0 = 2E\left[e(n)\frac{\partial e(n)}{\partial h_k}\right], \quad k = 0, 1, \ldots, M-1 \tag{6.4}$$

From Equation 6.2, $\frac{\partial e(n)}{\partial h_k} = -y(n-k)$, and the previous equation simplifies to

$$\frac{\partial J}{\partial h_k} = -2E[e(n)y(n-k)] = 0, \quad k = 0, 1, \ldots, M-1 \tag{6.5}$$

The preceding equation gives the necessary and sufficient condition for the cost function J to attain its minimum. The estimation error $e(n)$ needs to be orthogonal to the input signal $y(n)$ [two random variables x and z are orthogonal if $E(x \cdot z) = 0$]. This statement constitutes the well-known *orthogonality principle* of optimum linear filtering.

Next, we continue with the derivation of the optimal filter coefficients. Using matrix and vector derivatives properties, we evaluate the derivative of J with respect to the vector $\mathbf{h}$ as

$$\frac{\partial J}{\partial \mathbf{h}} = -2\mathbf{r}_{yd}^{-} + 2\mathbf{h}^T\mathbf{R}_{yy} = 0 \tag{6.6}$$

Solving for $\mathbf{h}$ in Equation 6.6, we get the optimal filter coefficients $\mathbf{h}^*$:

$$\mathbf{R}_{yy}\mathbf{h}^* = \mathbf{r}_{yd}^{-} \tag{6.7}$$

We can express the preceding equation as

$$\sum_{k=0}^{M-1} h_k r_{yy}(m-k) = r_{yd}(-m), \quad m = 0, 1, \ldots, M-1 \tag{6.8}$$

which clearly shows that the filter coefficients, h_k, can be obtained by solving M systems of equations with M unknowns, $\{h_k\}$. Solving for $\mathbf{h}^*$ in Equation 6.7, we get

$$\mathbf{h}^* = \mathbf{R}_{yy}^{-1}\mathbf{r}_{yd}^{-} \tag{6.9}$$

The preceding solution in Equation 6.9 is known as the *Wiener–Hopf* solution [2] and can also be expressed in matrix form as

$$\begin{bmatrix} h_0 \\ h_1 \\ h_2 \\ \vdots \\ h_{M-1} \end{bmatrix} = \begin{bmatrix} r_{yy}(0) & r_{yy}(1) & r_{yy}(2) & \cdots & r_{yy}(M-1) \\ r_{yy}(1) & r_{yy}(0) & r_{yy}(1) & \cdots & r_{yy}(M-2) \\ r_{yy}(2) & r_{yy}(1) & r_{yy}(0) & \cdots & r_{yy}(M-3) \\ \vdots & \vdots & \vdots & \ddots & \vdots \\ r_{yy}(M-1) & r_{yy}(M-2) & \cdots & r_{yy}(1) & r_{yy}(0) \end{bmatrix}^{-1} \begin{bmatrix} r_{yd}(0) \\ r_{yd}(-1) \\ r_{yd}(-2) \\ \vdots \\ r_{yd}(-M+1) \end{bmatrix} \tag{6.10}$$

Because the input signal is assumed to be wide-sense stationary, the autocorrelation matrix $\mathbf{R}_{yy}$ is symmetric and Toeplitz (values along each diagonal are the same). Efficient numerical techniques exist, such as the Levinson–Durbin algorithm, for inverting the matrix $\mathbf{R}_{yy}$ [3].

To find the minimum of the mean-squared error J, we substitute the optimal filter vector (Equation 6.9) in Equation 6.3 to get

$$\begin{aligned} J_{\min} &= E[d^2(n)] - 2\left(\mathbf{R}_{yy}^{-1}\mathbf{r}_{yd}^{-}\right)^T \mathbf{r}_{yd}^{-} + \left(\mathbf{R}_{yy}^{-1}\mathbf{r}_{yd}^{-}\right)^T \mathbf{R}_{yy}\mathbf{R}_{yy}^{-1}\mathbf{r}_{yd}^{-} \\ &= E[d^2(n)] - 2\left(\mathbf{r}_{yd}^{-}\right)^T \mathbf{R}_{yy}^{-T}\mathbf{r}_{yd}^{-} + \left(\mathbf{r}_{yd}^{-}\right)^T \mathbf{R}_{yy}^{-T}\mathbf{r}_{yd}^{-} \\ &= E[d^2(n)] - \left(\mathbf{r}_{yd}^{-}\right)^T \mathbf{R}_{yy}^{-T}\mathbf{r}_{yd}^{-} \\ &= E[d^2(n)] - \left(\mathbf{r}_{yd}^{-}\right)^T \mathbf{h}^* \end{aligned} \tag{6.11}$$

In the preceding derivation, we made use of the fact that $\mathbf{R}_{yy}$ is symmetric and therefore $\mathbf{R}_{yy}^{-T} = \mathbf{R}_{yy}^{-1}$.

6.3 WIENER FILTERS IN THE FREQUENCY DOMAIN

In the previous section, we considered a finite duration impulse response. Now, we consider a two-sided, infinite duration filter of the form

$$\hat{d}(n) = \sum_{k=-\infty}^{\infty} h_k y(n-k) \quad -\infty < n < \infty \tag{6.12}$$

Unlike the scenario in Equation 6.1, suppose now that we are allowed to use past as well as future data to estimate $d(n)$ at time index n. The preceding filter is termed the *Wiener smoother filter.* It is easy to show that the Wiener–Hopf equations for the smoothing filter are similar to those in Equation 6.8:

$$\sum_{k=-\infty}^{\infty} h_k r_{yy}(m-k) = r_{yd}(-m), \quad -\infty < m < \infty \tag{6.13}$$

Unlike Equation 6.8, the preceding equations are valid for all m.

Note that from Equation 6.12, the output signal $\hat{d}(n)$ can be obtained by convolving the system's impulse response $\{h_k\}$ with the input signal $y(n)$, that is,

$$\hat{d}(n) = h(n) * y(n) \tag{6.14}$$

where * denotes convolution. Therefore, in the frequency domain, we have

$$\hat{D}(\omega) = H(\omega)Y(\omega) \tag{6.15}$$

where $H(\omega)$ and $Y(\omega)$ are the discrete-time Fourier transforms of $h(n)$ and $y(n)$, respectively. We can define the estimation error at frequency ω_k as

$$\begin{aligned} E(\omega_k) &= D(\omega_k) - \hat{D}(\omega_k) \\ &= D(\omega_k) - H(\omega_k)Y(\omega_k) \end{aligned} \tag{6.16}$$

Next, we need to compute $H(\omega)$ that minimizes the mean-square error, that is, $E[|E(\omega_k)|^2]$, in the frequency domain (note that $E(\omega_k)$ is complex valued). The mean-square error is given by

$$\begin{aligned} E\left[|E(\omega_k)|^2\right] &= E\{[D(\omega_k) - H(\omega_k)Y(\omega_k)]^*[D(\omega_k) - H(\omega_k)Y(\omega_k)]\} \\ &= E\left[|D(\omega_k)|^2\right] - H(\omega_k)E\left[D^*(\omega_k)Y(\omega_k)\right] - H^*(\omega_k)E[Y^*(\omega_k)D(\omega_k)] \\ &\quad + |H(\omega_k)|^2 E\left[|Y(\omega_k)|^2\right] \end{aligned} \tag{6.17}$$

Noting that $P_{yy}(\omega_k) = E|Y(\omega_k)|^2$ is the power spectrum of $y(n)$, and $P_{yd}(\omega_k) = E[Y(\omega_k)D^*(\omega_k)]$ is the cross-power spectrum of $y(n)$ and $d(n)$, we can express the mean-square error as

$$\begin{aligned} J_2 = E[|E(\omega_k)|^2] &= E[|D(\omega_k)|^2] - H(\omega_k)P_{yd}(\omega_k) - H^*(\omega_k)P_{dy}(\omega_k) \\ &\quad + |H(\omega_k)|^2 P_{yy}(\omega_k) \end{aligned} \tag{6.18}$$

To find the optimal filter $H(\omega_k)$, we take the complex derivative of the mean-square error J_2 with respect to $H(\omega_k)$ and set it equal to zero to get

$$\frac{\partial J_2}{\partial H(\omega_k)} = H^*(\omega_k)P_{yy}(\omega_k) - P_{yd}(\omega_k)$$

$$= [H(\omega_k)P_{yy}(\omega_k) - P_{dy}(\omega_k)]^* = 0 \quad (6.19)$$

after using the fact that $P_{yd}(\omega_k) = P_{dy}^*(\omega_k)$. Solving for $H(\omega_k)$, we get the general form of the Wiener filter in the frequency domain:

$$H(\omega_k) = \frac{P_{dy}(\omega_k)}{P_{yy}(\omega_k)} \quad (6.20)$$

Note that $H(\omega_k)$ is complex valued because the cross-power spectrum $P_{dy}(\omega_k)$ is generally complex.

The preceding equation can alternatively be derived by taking the Fourier transform of both sides in Equation 6.13. The left side is the convolution of $r_{yy}(k)$ with h_k, which in the frequency domain becomes the product of the Fourier transforms of $r_{yy}(k)$ and h_k, that is, it is $H(\omega)P_{yy}(\omega)$. The Fourier transform of $r_{yd}(-m)$ is equal to $P_{yd}^*(\omega)$, or, equivalently, $P_{dy}(\omega)$. Therefore, we have $H(\omega)P_{yy}(\omega) = P_{dy}(\omega)$, in agreement with Equation 6.20.

Equations 6.7 and 6.20 comprise the general equations of the Wiener filters in the time and frequency domain, respectively, and can be used in any system configuration (see [4,5] for more applications of the Wiener filter). Depending on the application at hand, however, the desired signal, $d(n)$, will be different and, consequently, different, and sometimes simplified forms of the Wiener filter can be derived.

6.4 WIENER FILTERS AND LINEAR PREDICTION

If the desired signal in Figure 6.1 is set equal to the input signal, that is, $d(n) = y(n)$, then the Wiener filter becomes a linear prediction filter. That is, the Wiener filter attempts to predict the present input value $y(n)$ based on M past input values $[y(n-1), y(n-2), \ldots, y(n-M)]$. The estimated signal $\hat{d}(n)$ shown in Figure 6.2 filter takes now the following form:

$$\hat{d}(n) = \sum_{k=1}^{M} h_k y(n-k) \quad n = 0, 1, 2, \ldots \quad (6.21)$$

Note that we no longer use the coefficient h_0. The error between the predicted value $\hat{d}(n)$ and the true value, $d(n) = y(n)$, is given by

$$e(n) = d(n) - \hat{d}(n)$$

$$= y(n) - \sum_{k=1}^{M} h_k \, y(n-k) \quad (6.22)$$

Minimization of the preceding error (in the mean-square sense) with respect to the coefficients $[h_1, h_2,\ldots,h_M]$ leads to the same form of solution given in Equation 6.7. According to Equation 6.7, to find the optimal filter coefficients, we will need to compute the new (because the input is shifted) autocorrelation matrix $\mathbf{R}_{yy}$ and the new cross-correlation vector $\mathbf{r}_{\bar{y}d}$.

Let $\bar{\mathbf{y}}^T = [y(n-1), y(n-2),\ldots, y(n-M)]$ be the new input vector containing M past values. The autocorrelation matrix of the input signal vector $\bar{\mathbf{y}}^T$ is given by

$$\bar{\mathbf{R}}_{yy} = E[\bar{\mathbf{y}}\cdot\bar{\mathbf{y}}^T] = \begin{bmatrix} r_{yy}(0) & r_{yy}(1) & r_{yy}(2) & \cdots & r_{yy}(M-1) \\ r_{yy}(1) & r_{yy}(0) & r_{yy}(1) & \cdots & r_{yy}(M-2) \\ r_{yy}(2) & r_{yy}(1) & r_{yy}(0) & \cdots & r_{yy}(M-3) \\ \vdots & \vdots & \vdots & \ddots & \vdots \\ r_{yy}(M-1) & r_{yy}(M-2) & \cdots & r_{yy}(1) & r_{yy}(0) \end{bmatrix} \tag{6.23}$$

which is identical to the matrix derived earlier, because $y(n)$ being a wide-sense stationary process is invariant to a time shift. The cross-correlation vector between the input vector and the desired response is

$$\begin{aligned} \mathbf{r}_{\bar{y}d} &\triangleq E[\bar{\mathbf{y}}d(n)] = E[\bar{\mathbf{y}}y(n)] = E[(y(n-1)\cdots y(n-M))y(n)] \\ &= [r_{yy}(1), r_{yy}(2),\ldots, r_{yy}(M)] \end{aligned} \tag{6.24}$$

Hence, according to Equation 6.7, the optimal filter coefficients that minimize the mean-square error (Equation 6.22) between the predicted and the true values can be computed by solving the following system of equations:

$$\begin{bmatrix} r_{yy}(0) & r_{yy}(1) & r_{yy}(2) & \cdots & r_{yy}(M-1) \\ r_{yy}(1) & r_{yy}(0) & r_{yy}(1) & \cdots & r_{yy}(M-2) \\ r_{yy}(2) & r_{yy}(1) & r_{yy}(0) & \cdots & r_{yy}(M-3) \\ \vdots & \vdots & \vdots & \ddots & \vdots \\ r_{yy}(M-1) & r_{yy}(M-2) & \cdots & r_{yy}(1) & r_{yy}(0) \end{bmatrix} \begin{bmatrix} h_1 \\ h_2 \\ h_3 \\ \vdots \\ h_M \end{bmatrix} = \begin{bmatrix} r_{yy}(1) \\ r_{yy}(2) \\ r_{yy}(3) \\ \vdots \\ r_{yy}(M) \end{bmatrix} \tag{6.25}$$

These are the Wiener–Hopf equations for the one-step linear predictor based on past M samples. These equations are identical to the Yule–Walker equations used to solve for the auto regressive (AR) parameters of an AR process [3]. The values of $[-h(1),-h(2),\ldots,-h(M)]$ are also known as the *linear prediction coefficients*. Various computationally efficient methods can be used to solve the preceding system of equations, avoiding matrix inversion. Specifically, because the autocorrelation matrix $\bar{\mathbf{R}}_{yy}$ is symmetric and Toeplitz, the Levinson–Durbin recursive algorithm is often used to solve the preceding system of equations [3].

The minimum prediction error is given according to Equation 6.11 by

$$
\begin{aligned}
J_{\min} &= E[y^2(n)] - \mathbf{r}_y{}^T\mathbf{h}^* \\
&= r_{yy}(0) - \sum_{k=1}^{M} r_{yy}(k)h(k)
\end{aligned}
\tag{6.26}
$$

As will be seen later, the minimum prediction error is also equal to the gain of an all-pole speech production model.

In the preceding linear prediction problem, we set the desired signal equal to the input signal. If, now, the input signal contains additive noise, that is, $y(n) = x(n) + n(n)$, and the desired signal is set equal to the clean signal, that is, $d(n) = x(n)$, then the Wiener filter will attempt to estimate the clean signal. In other words, it will try to "filter" the noise out. The Wiener filter in this system configuration can be used for noise reduction. Next, we derive the Wiener filters for noise reduction applications.

6.5 WIENER FILTERS FOR NOISE REDUCTION

In speech enhancement applications, the input signal $y(n)$ in Figure 6.2 is the noisy speech signal:

$$
y(n) = x(n) + n(n) \tag{6.27}
$$

where

$x(n)$ is the clean speech signal
$n(n)$ is the noise signal

The desired signal $d(n)$ in Figure 6.2 is the clean (noise-free) signal $x(n)$, that is, $d(n) = x(n)$. The objective of the Wiener filter is therefore to produce an estimate of the clean signal $x(n)$.

We can derive the corresponding Wiener filters in the time or frequency domain, using Equations 6.7 and 6.20. To evaluate the time-domain Wiener filter, we need first to compute $\mathbf{R}_{yy}$. Expressing Equation 6.27 in vector notation, we have by definition

$$
\begin{aligned}
\mathbf{R}_{yy} &= E[\mathbf{y}\mathbf{y}^T] = E[(\mathbf{x}+\mathbf{n})(\mathbf{x}+\mathbf{n})^T] \\
&= E[\mathbf{x}\mathbf{x}^T] + E[\mathbf{n}\mathbf{n}^T] + E[\mathbf{x}\mathbf{n}^T] + E[\mathbf{n}\mathbf{x}^T] \\
&= \mathbf{R}_{xx} + \mathbf{R}_{nn}
\end{aligned}
\tag{6.28}
$$

The last two expectations in the preceding equation are zero, because the signal and noise are assumed to be uncorrelated and zero mean. The cross-correlation vector

$\mathbf{r}_{\bar{y}d}$ in Equation 6.7 is equal to $\mathbf{r}_{xx}$ because the signal and noise signals are assumed to be uncorrelated. Therefore, the resulting Wiener filter in the time domain has the form

$$\mathbf{h}^* = (\mathbf{R}_{xx} + \mathbf{R}_{nn})^{-1}\mathbf{r}_{xx} \tag{6.29}$$

As shown here, the Wiener filter $\mathbf{h}^*$ is a function of the autocorrelation of the clean signal $x(n)$ (which we do not have access to), and therefore it is not realizable. Interesting asymptotic relationships about the values of the optimal Wiener filter $\mathbf{h}^*$ can be derived by rewriting Equation 6.29 as follows [6]:

$$\mathbf{h}^* = \left[\frac{\mathbf{I}}{\text{SNR}} + \hat{\mathbf{R}}_{nn}^{-1}\hat{\mathbf{R}}_{xx}\right]^{-1}\hat{\mathbf{R}}_{nn}^{-1}\hat{\mathbf{R}}_{xx}\mathbf{u}_1 \tag{6.30}$$

where

$$\text{SNR} = \frac{E\{x^2(n)\}}{E\{n^2(n)\}} = \frac{\sigma_x^2}{\sigma_n^2} \tag{6.31}$$

is the signal-to-noise ratio (SNR), $\mathbf{I}$ is the identity matrix ($M \times M$), $\mathbf{u}_1^T = [1, 0, \ldots, 0]$ ($1 \times M$), and $\hat{\mathbf{R}}_{xx} \triangleq \mathbf{R}_{xx}/\sigma_x^2$, $\hat{\mathbf{R}}_{nn} \triangleq \mathbf{R}_{nn}/\sigma_n^2$. From Equation 6.30, we can write the following asymptotic relationships about the Wiener filter for large and small SNR values:

$$\begin{aligned} \lim_{\text{SNR}\to\infty} \mathbf{h}^* &= \mathbf{u}_1 \\ \lim_{\text{SNR}\to 0} \mathbf{h}^* &= \mathbf{0} \end{aligned} \tag{6.32}$$

The first relationship shows that when the SNR is extremely large, the Wiener filter does not provide noise reduction because $\mathbf{u}_1^T\mathbf{y} = y(n)$, that is, the observed noisy signal passes unaltered. Consequently, no speech distortion is imparted to the speech signal by the Wiener filter when the SNR is large. In contrast, the second relationship in Equation 6.32 suggests that when the SNR is extremely low, the output of the Wiener filter is heavily attenuated. This attenuation produces undesirable distortion in the speech signal. We will revisit the trade-off between speech and noise distortion in Section 6.9.1.

Next, we derive the Wiener filter in the frequency domain. Taking the Fourier transform of the signals in Equation 6.27, we get

$$Y(\omega_k) = X(\omega_k) + N(\omega_k) \tag{6.33}$$

According to Equation 6.20, we need to compute $P_{dy}(\omega_k)$ and $P_{yy}(\omega_k)$. Given that $D(\omega_k) = X(\omega_k)$, and after using Equation 6.33, we get

$$\begin{aligned} P_{dy}(\omega_k) &= E\left[X(\omega_k)\{X(\omega_k)+N(\omega_k)\}^*\right] \\ &= E\left[X(\omega_k)X^*(\omega_k)\right]+E\left[X(\omega_k)N^*(\omega_k)\right] \\ &= P_{xx}(\omega_k) \end{aligned} \tag{6.34}$$

Similarly,

$$\begin{aligned} P_{yy}(\omega_k) &= E\left[\{X(\omega_k)+N(\omega_k)\}\{X(\omega_k)+N(\omega_k)\}^*\right] \\ &= E\left[X(\omega_k)X^*(\omega_k)\right]+E\left[N(\omega_k)N^*(\omega_k)\right]+E\left[X(\omega_k)N^*(\omega_k)\right] \\ &\quad +E\left[N(\omega_k)X^*(\omega_k)\right]=P_{xx}(\omega_k)+P_{nn}(\omega_k) \end{aligned} \tag{6.35}$$

Finally, after substituting Equations 6.34 and 6.35 in Equation 6.20, we get the Wiener filter in the frequency domain:

$$H(\omega_k)=\frac{P_{xx}(\omega_k)}{P_{xx}(\omega_k)+P_{nn}(\omega_k)} \tag{6.36}$$

Note that $H(\omega_k)$ is real, nonnegative, and even, because (a) both $P_{nn}(\omega_k) \geq 0$ and $P_{xx}(\omega_k) \geq 0$ and (b) the power spectra $P_{nn}(\omega_k)$ and $P_{xx}(\omega_k)$ have even symmetry. The fact that $H(\omega_k)$ is even and real suggests that the impulse response, h_k, must be even as well. This in turn suggests that h_k is not causal; therefore, the Wiener filter is not realizable.

By defining ξ_k

$$\xi_k \triangleq \frac{P_{xx}(\omega_k)}{P_{nn}(\omega_k)} \tag{6.37}$$

as the *a priori* SNR at frequency ω_k, we can also express the Wiener filter in Equation 6.36 as

$$H(\omega_k)=\frac{\xi_k}{\xi_k+1} \tag{6.38}$$

Note that $0 \leq H(\omega_k) \leq 1$, and $H(\omega_k) \approx 0$ when $\xi_k \to 0$ (i.e., at extremely low-SNR regions) and $H(\omega_k) \approx 1$ when $\xi_k \to \infty$ (i.e., at extremely high-SNR regions). These asymptotic relationships in the frequency domain are in line with the asymptotic relationships in the time domain given in Equation 6.32. So, according to Equation 6.38, the Wiener filter emphasizes portions of the spectrum where the SNR is high and attenuates portions of the spectrum where the SNR is low. This is illustrated in

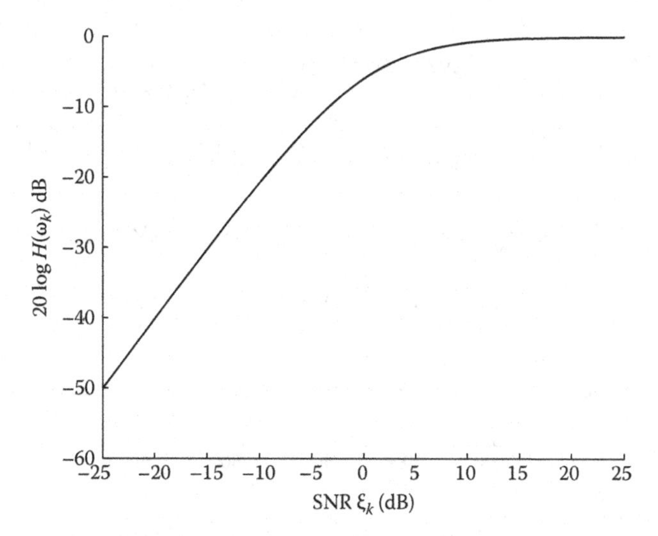

FIGURE 6.3 Attenuation curve of the Wiener filter as a function of the *a priori* SNR.

Figure 6.3, which plots $H(\omega_k)$ as a function of ξ_k in dB. Note that for $\xi_k > 10$ dB, no attenuation is performed since $H(\omega_k) \approx 1$. Thus, the Wiener filter attenuates each frequency component in proportion to the estimated SNR (ξ_k) of that frequency.

Figure 6.4 shows an example of the estimated Wiener filter for a voiced segment of speech embedded in white noise. The true values of the *a priori* SNR ξ_k are shown in panel d. The ξ_k values follow for the most part the input noisy spectrum, at least when the additive noise is white. The Wiener filter response (in dB) is plotted in panel e. It is clear that no attenuation is applied to the noisy speech spectrum when ξ_k is large (see for example the 2000–4000 Hz frequency region). Large attenuation of about −30 to −40 dB is applied when ξ_k is small (see, for example, the 4000–8000 Hz frequency region). Therefore, the amount of attenuation applied by the Wiener filter is proportional to the SNR of each frequency component (i.e., ξ_k).

Example 6.1

Consider the following sine wave embedded in noise:

$$\begin{aligned} y(n) &= x(n) + w(n) \\ &= \sin(2\pi f n + \theta) + w(n) \end{aligned} \tag{6.39}$$

where

f is the normalized frequency ($-1/2 < f < 1/2$)
θ is the phase of the sine wave assumed to be uniformly distributed in $[0, 2\pi]$
$w(n)$ is white Gaussian noise with zero mean and variance σ^2

Derive the time- and frequency-domain Wiener filters assuming an M-tap FIR filter. Assume that $M = 2$, $\sigma^2 = 2$, and $f = 0.2$.

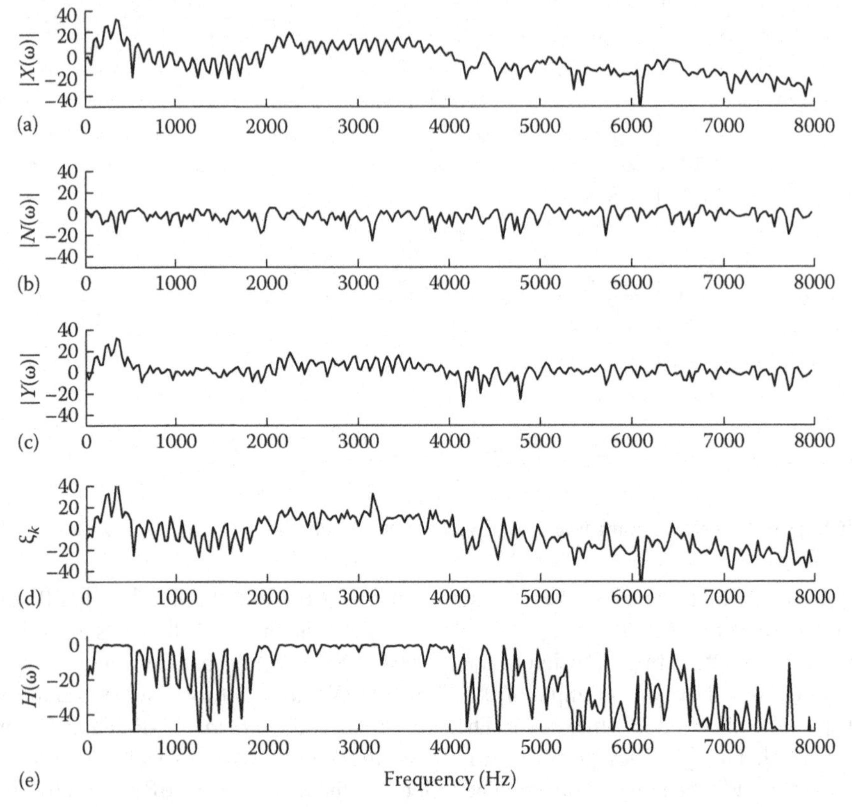

FIGURE 6.4 Wiener filter response for a voiced speech segment embedded in white noise. The clean noise and noisy speech spectra (in dB) are shown in panels (a) through (c), respectively. Panel (d) shows the true *a priori* SNR values (in dB), and panel (e) shows the Wiener filter response (in dB).

We know that $x(n)$ is a zero-mean, wide-sense stationary process and has the following autocorrelation:

$$r_{xx}(m) = \frac{1}{2}\cos(2\pi f m) \tag{6.40}$$

To obtain the mean-square error or performance function J, we first need to estimate the autocorrelation matrix and cross-correlation vector given in Equation 6.3. For the signal in Equation 6.39, we know that $\mathbf{R}_{yy} = \mathbf{R}_{xx} + \mathbf{R}_{nn}$ (Equation 6.28) and $\mathbf{r}_{yd} = \mathbf{r}_{xx}$, because $d(n) = x(n)$. The mean-square error can then be written as

$$\begin{aligned} J &= E[d^2(n)] - 2\mathbf{h}^T\mathbf{r}_{yd} + \mathbf{h}^T\mathbf{R}_{yy}\mathbf{h} \\ &= E[x^2(n)] - 2\mathbf{h}^T\mathbf{r}_{xx} + \mathbf{h}^T(\mathbf{R}_{xx} + \mathbf{R}_{nn})\mathbf{h} \\ &= r_{xx}(0) - 2\mathbf{h}^T\mathbf{r}_{xx} + \mathbf{h}^T\left(\mathbf{R}_{xx} + \sigma_w^2\mathbf{I}\right)\mathbf{h} \end{aligned} \tag{6.41}$$

where **I** denotes the identity matrix ($M \times M$). From Equation 6.40, the input correlation matrix is given by

$$\mathbf{R}_{xx} = \begin{bmatrix} r_{xx}(0) & r_{xx}(1) \\ r_{xx}(1) & r_{xx}(0) \end{bmatrix} = \begin{bmatrix} 0.5 & 0.5\cos(2\pi 0.2) \\ 0.5\cos(2\pi 0.2) & 0.5 \end{bmatrix}$$

$$= \begin{bmatrix} 0.5 & 0.154 \\ 0.154 & 0.5 \end{bmatrix} \tag{6.42}$$

and $\mathbf{r}_{xx} = [0.5 \quad 0.154]^T$. The mean-square error can be expressed as

$$J = r_{xx}(0) - 2\mathbf{h}^T\mathbf{r}_{xx} + \mathbf{h}^T\left(\mathbf{R}_{xx} + \sigma_w^2\mathbf{I}\right)\mathbf{h}$$

$$= 0.5 - 2[h_0\ h_1]\begin{bmatrix} 0.5 \\ 0.154 \end{bmatrix} + [h_0\ h_1]\begin{bmatrix} 0.5+2 & 0.154 \\ 0.154 & 0.5+2 \end{bmatrix}\begin{bmatrix} h_0 \\ h_1 \end{bmatrix}$$

$$= 0.5 - h_0 - 0.308h_1 + 0.308h_0h_1 + 2.5\left(h_0^2 + h_1^2\right) \tag{6.43}$$

The plot of the performance surface J is given in Figure 6.5. The minimum of J is attained at $\mathbf{h}^T = [0.197 \quad 0.049]$. We can also obtain the optimal Wiener filter using Equation 6.29:

$$\mathbf{h} = (\mathbf{R}_{xx} + \mathbf{R}_{nn})^{-1}\mathbf{r}_{xx}$$

$$= (\mathbf{R}_{xx} + 2\mathbf{I})^{-1}\mathbf{r}_{xx}$$

$$= \begin{bmatrix} 2.5 & 0.154 \\ 0.154 & 2.5 \end{bmatrix}^{-1}\begin{bmatrix} 0.5 \\ 0.154 \end{bmatrix}$$

$$= \begin{bmatrix} 0.197 \\ 0.0496 \end{bmatrix} \tag{6.44}$$

in agreement with the minimum of the performance surface given in Equation 6.43.

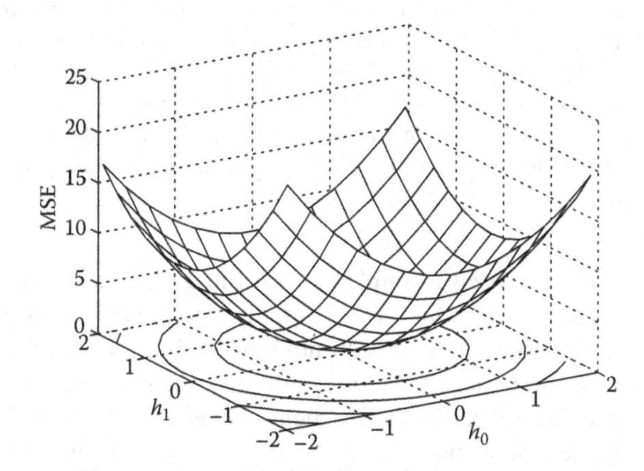

FIGURE 6.5 Quadratic performance surface for Example 6.1. The mean-squared error is plotted vertically, and the filter coefficients h_0 and h_1 are plotted horizontally. The optimum filter coefficient vector is $h^* = [0.197\ 0.049]$.

Next, we compute the Wiener filter in the frequency domain for an arbitrary number, M, of FIR taps. First, we need to compute $P_{xx}(\omega_k)$, which by definition is the Fourier transform of $r_{xx}(m)$ given in Equation 6.40:

$$P_{xx}(\omega) = \sum_{m=-M}^{M} r_{xx}(m)\exp(-j\omega m)$$

$$= \sum_{m=-M}^{M} 0.5\cos(2\pi fm)\exp(-j\omega m) \tag{6.45}$$

Realizing that $P_{xx}(\omega)$ is the Fourier transform of a windowed cosine signal (see Section 2.4), we get

$$P_{xx}(\omega) = \frac{1}{4}\left[\frac{\sin\left(\left(M+\frac{1}{2}\right)(\omega - w_0)\right)}{\sin\left((\omega - w_0)/2\right)} + \frac{\sin\left(\left(M+\frac{1}{2}\right)(\omega + w_0)\right)}{\sin\left((\omega + w_0)/2\right)}\right] \tag{6.46}$$

where $\omega_0 = 2\pi f_0$ and $f_0 = 0.2$ in this example. The Wiener filter at frequency ω_k is then given by

$$H(\omega_k) = \frac{P_{xx}(\omega_k)}{P_{xx}(\omega_k) + P_{nn}(\omega_k)}$$

$$= \frac{P_{xx}(\omega_k)}{P_{xx}(\omega_k) + 2} \tag{6.47}$$

with $P_{xx}(\omega_k)$ given by Equation 6.46. Figure 6.6 plots $H(\omega_k)$ for different number of FIR tap coefficients, M. For small M, we note a hump centered around ω_0. As M gets larger, the filter becomes more localized around the input signal frequency, ω_0. Thus, the Wiener filter passes only frequencies in the neighborhood of ω_0, which is the frequency region of interest. Asymptotically, as $M \to \infty$, $P_{xx}(\omega_k)$ becomes a delta function, and the Wiener filter becomes an "ideal" noise reduction filter in that it attenuates all frequencies but the input signal frequency, ω_0.

Note that in the preceding example, we assumed that the autocorrelation of the desired signal is known, which is admittedly a nonrealistic assumption. The example was intended to provide insight into the capability of the Wiener filter to remove or reduce noise under idealistic conditions, in which the autocorrelation or, more generally, the second-order moments of the desired signal are known. Numerous techniques were proposed for estimating the Wiener filter from the noisy speech signal and will be discussed later. Next, we examine some variations of the Wiener filter.

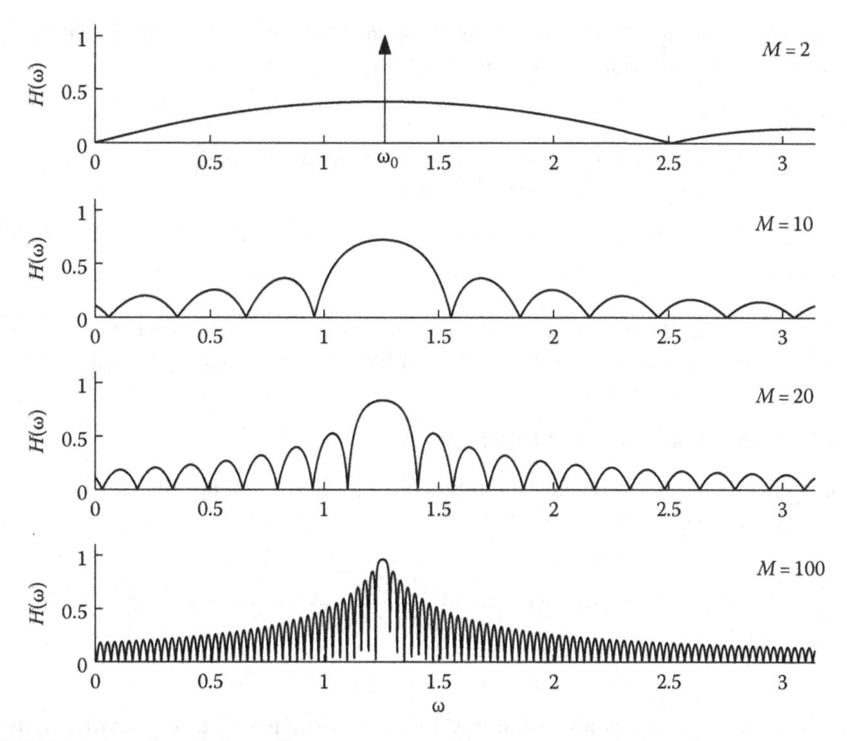

FIGURE 6.6 Plot of Wiener filter response as a function of the number of FIR taps, M. The signal frequency, ω_0, of the input sinusoid is indicated in the top panel.

6.5.1 Square-Root Wiener Filter

Suppose that we use the square root of the Wiener filter. Then the output of the Wiener filter in the frequency domain will be

$$\hat{X}(\omega_k) = \sqrt{H(\omega_k)}Y(\omega_k) \tag{6.48}$$

Let us now estimate the power spectrum of the estimated signal, $\hat{x}(n)$. After using Equation 6.48, we get

$$\begin{aligned} E|\hat{X}(\omega_k)|^2 &= \left(\sqrt{H(\omega_k)}\right)^2 E|Y(\omega_k)|^2 \\ P_{\hat{x}\hat{x}}(\omega_k) &= H(\omega_k)\,P_{yy}(\omega_k) \\ P_{\hat{x}\hat{x}}(\omega_k) &= \frac{P_{xx}(\omega_k)}{P_{xx}(\omega_k)+P_{nn}(\omega_k)}P_{yy}(\omega_k) \end{aligned} \tag{6.49}$$

Because the signal and noise are assumed to be uncorrelated, we have $P_{yy}(\omega_k) = P_{xx}(\omega_k) + P_{nn}(\omega_k)$, and Equation 6.49 simplifies to

$$P_{\hat{x}\hat{x}}(\omega_k) = \frac{P_{xx}(\omega_k)}{P_{xx}(\omega_k) + P_{nn}(\omega_k)}\left[P_{xx}(\omega_k) + P_{nn}(\omega_k)\right]$$
$$= P_{xx}(\omega_k) \quad (6.50)$$

Thus, in noise, the power spectrum of the output of the square-root Wiener filter $[\hat{P}_{xx}(\omega_k)]$ is identical to the power spectrum of the noise-free signal $[P_{xx}(\omega_k)]$.

6.5.2 Parametric Wiener Filters

More generally, we can consider the following parametric Wiener filters [7]:

$$H(\omega_k) = \left(\frac{P_{xx}(\omega_k)}{P_{xx}(\omega_k) + \alpha P_{nn}(\omega_k)}\right)^{\beta} \quad (6.51)$$

for some parameters α and β. The traditional and square-root Wiener filters discussed so far are special cases of Equation 6.51. If $\alpha = \beta = 1$, then we get the traditional Wiener filter; and if $\alpha = 1$, $\beta = 1/2$, we get the square-root Wiener filter. By varying the parameters α and β, we can obtain various types of Wiener filters with different attenuation characteristics. To examine the effect of these two parameters on attenuation, we first express Equation 6.51 in terms of ξ_k:

$$H(\omega_k) = \left(\frac{\xi_k}{\alpha + \xi_k}\right)^{\beta} \quad (6.52)$$

Figure 6.7 plots the filter attenuation as a function of ξ_k for a fixed value of α ($\alpha = 1$) and for different values of β. As can be seen, the parameter β affects the attenuation at extremely low SNR levels. Heavier attenuation is applied when β is large and $\xi_k = 0$ dB. For instance, when $\xi_k = -20$ dB and $\beta = 1$, we get about -40 dB attenuation, and when $\beta = 2$, we get -80 dB attenuation. The parameter β therefore provides a mechanism that can be used to artificially increase the signal attenuation. Increasing the signal attenuation, however, comes at a price. Although the residual noise might be reduced considerably by increasing β, speech distortion will most likely be introduced as a consequence.

Figure 6.8 plots attenuation as a function of ξ_k for a fixed value of β ($\beta = 1$) and for different values of α. As can be seen, the parameter shifts the attenuation curves down with increasing values of α. As a result, it influences attenuation at both high

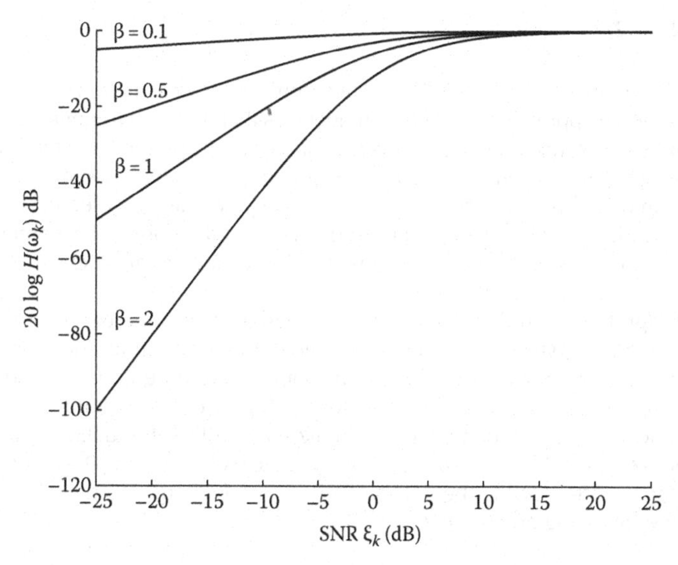

FIGURE 6.7 Attenuation curves for the parametric Wiener filter obtained using different values of β and for a fixed value of α ($\alpha = 1$).

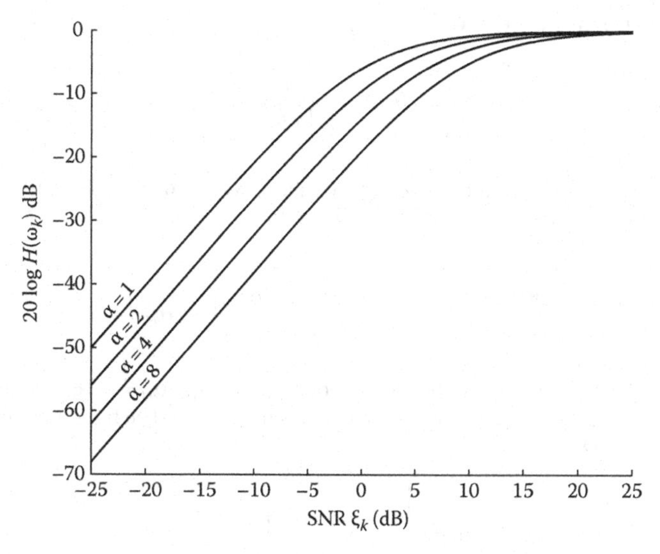

FIGURE 6.8 Attenuation curves for the parametric Wiener filter obtained using different values of α and for a fixed value of β ($\beta = 1$).

and low SNR levels. The attenuation caused by large values of α in extremely low SNR levels is not as large as that caused by increasing the parameter β (Figure 6.7). Compared to the parameter β, parameter α offers more flexibility as it can influence attenuation at both low and high SNR levels. A method for adjusting the parameter α will be given in Sections 6.10 and 6.11.

Example 6.2

Design a parametric Wiener filter of the form given in Equation 6.52, which provides more suppression in the low frequencies than the high frequencies. More precisely, we like the attenuation to be limited to −20 dB for $f < 1$ kHz and to −10 dB for $f > 1$ kHz when the *a priori* SNR ξ_k (in dB) is negative. Assume that $\beta = 1$ in Equation 6.52. The preceding Wiener filter can potentially be used in situations in which we know beforehand that most of energy of the noise is concentrated in the low frequencies (<1 kHz in this example) with small amounts of energy leaking in the high frequencies.

To design the desired Wiener filter, we need to determine the values of the parameter α in Equation 6.52 that can achieve the required attenuation at the prescribed *a priori* SNR (0 dB). Two values of α need to be computed, one for the low-frequency band and the other for the high-frequency band.

In the low-frequency band, we would like to limit the attenuation to a maximum of −20 dB. We can use Equation 6.52 to solve for the low-frequency parameter α_L. After setting the *a priori* SNR ξ_k to 1 [because $10 \log_{10}(1) = 0$ dB], we get the following equation:

$$20\log_{10} H(\omega) = -20 \text{ dB} = 20\log_{10}\left(\frac{1}{1+\alpha_L}\right) \tag{6.53}$$

In the linear domain, we have

$$10^{-20/20} = \frac{1}{1+\alpha_L} \tag{6.54}$$

After solving for α_L in the preceding equation, we get $\alpha_L = 9$. Similarly, we can solve the high-frequency parameter α_H in the following equation:

$$20\log_{10} H(\omega) = -10 \text{ dB} = 20\log_{10}\left(\frac{1}{1+\alpha_H}\right) \tag{6.55}$$

After solving for α_H in the preceding equation, we get $\alpha_H = 2.16$. We are now ready to express the desired suppression rules for the low- and high-frequency bands.

For $f < 1$ kHz:

$$\hat{X}(f) = \begin{cases} \dfrac{\hat{\xi}_k}{\hat{\xi}_k + 9} Y(f) & \text{if } \hat{\xi}_k > 1 \\ 10^{-1} Y(f) & \text{else} \end{cases} \tag{6.56}$$

For $f > 1$ kHz:

$$\hat{X}(f) = \begin{cases} \dfrac{\hat{\xi}_k}{\hat{\xi}_k + 2.16} Y(f) & \text{if } \hat{\xi}_k > 1 \\ 10^{-1/2} Y(f) & \text{else} \end{cases} \tag{6.57}$$

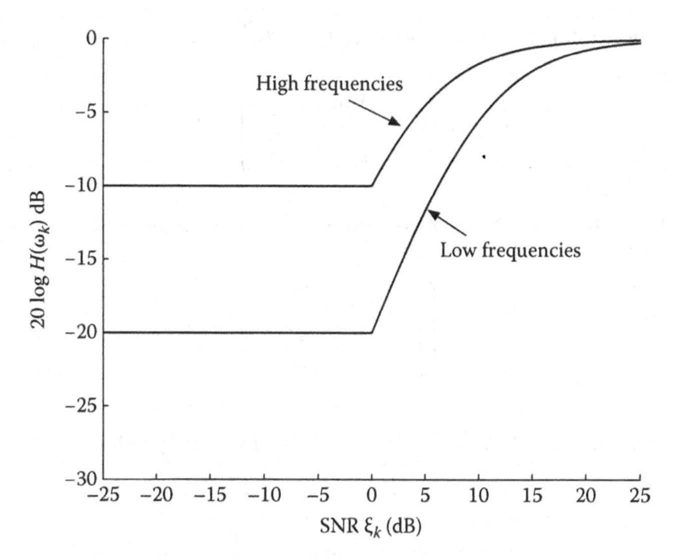

FIGURE 6.9 Wiener filter suppression curves for Example 6.2.

where $\hat{\xi}_k$ denotes the estimated *a priori* SNR. The preceding suppression curves [(i.e., $20\ \log_{10}(|\hat{X}(f)|/|Y(f)|)$] are plotted in Figure 6.9 as a function of the *a priori* SNR. Note that the spectral flooring ensures that the attenuation does not exceed −10 dB in the high frequencies and −20 dB at the low frequencies when the estimated *a priori* SNR is negative. The preceding implementations of the Wiener filter require estimates of the *a priori* SNR $\hat{\xi}_k$. Methods for estimating $\hat{\xi}_k$ will be discussed later (see Section 6.10) and in Chapter 7.

The parameters α and β in Equation 6.51 are typically fixed beforehand and then used throughout to enhance the noisy speech spectrum in each frame. Alternatively, the parameters can be varied in some way in each frame to control the trade-off between speech and noise distortion. Some of the techniques proposed for adapting the parameter α for every speech frame will be discussed later in Sections 6.10 and 6.11.

Next, we show that some of the common speech enhancement algorithms are special cases of the parametric Wiener filters (Equation 6.51) [7]. To do that, we first make the following approximation:

$$P_{xx}(\omega_k) \approx \left|\hat{X}(\omega_k)\right|^2 \tag{6.58}$$

that is, we approximate the true power spectral density of $x(n)$ by the estimated short-term magnitude spectrum squared. We know that the output of the Wiener filter in the frequency domain is given by

$$\hat{X}(\omega_k) = H(\omega_k)\,Y(\omega_k) \tag{6.59}$$

and after substituting Equation 6.58 in Equation 6.51, we get

$$\hat{X}(\omega_k) = \left(\frac{\left|\hat{X}(\omega_k)\right|^2}{\left|\hat{X}(\omega_k)\right|^2 + aP_{nn}(\omega_k)} \right)^{\beta} Y(\omega_k) \tag{6.60}$$

After taking the magnitudes of both sides, we get the following implicit equation:

$$\left|\hat{X}(\omega_k)\right| = \left(\frac{\left|\hat{X}(\omega_k)\right|^2}{\left|\hat{X}(\omega_k)\right|^2 + aP_{nn}(\omega_k)} \right)^{\beta} \left|Y(\omega_k)\right| \tag{6.61}$$

Let us consider first the case when $\beta = 1/2$. After squaring both sides of Equation 6.61, we get

$$\left|\hat{X}(\omega_k)\right|^2 = \left(\frac{\left|\hat{X}(\omega_k)\right|^2}{\left|\hat{X}(\omega_k)\right|^2 + aP_{nn}(\omega_k)} \right) \left|Y(\omega_k)\right|^2 \tag{6.62}$$

from which we can solve for $|\hat{X}(\omega_k)|$:

$$\left|\hat{X}(\omega_k)\right| = \left[\left|Y(\omega_k)\right|^2 - aP_{nn}(\omega_k) \right]^{1/2} \tag{6.63}$$

This is, of course, the spectral (over) subtraction method proposed by Berouti et al. [8], where a is the oversubtraction factor.

Now, if we set $\beta = 1$ in Equation 6.61, we get the following quadratic equation in $|\hat{X}(\omega_k)|$:

$$\left|\hat{X}(\omega_k)\right|^2 - \left|\hat{X}(\omega_k)\right| \left|Y(\omega_k)\right| + aP_{nn}(\omega_k) = 0 \tag{6.64}$$

One of the solutions of the preceding quadratic equation is given by

$$\left|\hat{X}(\omega_k)\right| = \frac{1}{2}\left|Y(\omega_k)\right| + \frac{1}{2}\sqrt{\left|Y(\omega_k)\right| - 4aP_{nn}(\omega_k)} \tag{6.65}$$

which, for $a = 1/4$, is identical to the maximum-likelihood method proposed in [9] and described in Chapter 7.

6.6 ITERATIVE WIENER FILTERING

As mentioned earlier, the Wiener filter is noncausal and, therefore, not realizable. For one thing, it requires knowledge about the power spectrum of the clean signal, which we do not have. In this section, we present a method for estimating the Wiener filter in an iterative fashion. In particular, we consider an iterative procedure, where in the $(i+1)$ iteration, the enhanced signal spectrum is estimated by

$$\hat{X}_{i+1}(\omega_k) = H_i(\omega_k)\, Y(\omega_k) \tag{6.66}$$

where $H_i(\omega_k)$ denotes the Wiener filter obtained in the ith iteration. We can consider the following two-step procedure at iteration i to estimate $H_i(\omega_k)$:

Step 1: Obtain an estimate of the Wiener filter $H_i(\omega_k)$ based on the enhanced signal $\hat{x}_i(n)$. In the first iteration, initialize $\hat{x}_i(n)$ with the noisy speech signal $y(n)$.

Step 2: Filter the noisy signal $y(n)$ through the newly obtained Wiener filter $H_i(\omega_k)$ according to Equation 6.66, to get the new enhanced signal, $\hat{x}_{i+1}(n)$. Use $\hat{x}_{i+1}(n)$ in place of $\hat{x}_i(n)$ in Step 1 and repeat the foregoing procedure.

As with all iterative algorithms, there is the issue of convergence. We would like the iterative algorithm to improve, in some sense, the enhanced signal at each iteration. Such an algorithm was proposed by Lim and Oppenheim [10] in the context of estimating all-pole AR model parameters from noisy speech. In their approach, speech was assumed to have been generated by an AR process, and the task was to estimate the clean AR parameters. Hence, with this approach, the problem of speech enhancement was reduced to the estimation of AR parameters assumed to have been used to generate the clean signal. The speech enhancement problem was consequently converted to a parameter estimation problem.

6.6.1 Mathematical Speech Production Model

As described in Section 3.3, speech can be thought to be the response of a linear time-invariant system, the vocal tract, to a periodic excitation for voiced speech and randomlike excitation for unvoiced speech. The vocal tract system has the following all-pole form in the z-domain:

$$V(z) = \frac{g}{A(z)} = \frac{g}{1 - \sum_{k=1}^{p} a_k z^{-k}} \tag{6.67}$$

where

g is the gain of the system

$\{a_k\}$ are the all-pole coefficients, which can be obtained using Equation 6.25

p is the number of all-pole coefficients

In the time domain, the speech signal $x(n)$ is described by the following difference equation:

$$x(n) = \sum_{k=1}^{p} a_k x(n-k) + g \cdot w(n), \quad n = 0, 1, \ldots, N-1 \tag{6.68}$$

where $w(n)$ is the input excitation to the system. We assume that $w(n)$ is white Gaussian noise with zero mean and unit variance. We can express the preceding equation more compactly as

$$x(n) = \mathbf{a}^T \mathbf{x}_p + g \cdot w(n) \tag{6.69}$$

where $\mathbf{a}^T = [a_1, a_2, \ldots, a_p]$ and $\mathbf{x}_p^T = [x(n-1), x(n-2), \ldots, x(n-p)]$. Note that Equation 6.68 requires initial conditions for $n < p$, and we denote the initial condition vector by $\mathbf{x}_I$, where $\mathbf{x}_I^T = [x(-1), x(-2), \ldots, x(-p)]$.

Now, in noise, we have

$$\begin{aligned} y(n) &= x(n) + d(n) \\ &= \mathbf{a}^T \mathbf{x}_p + g \cdot w(n) + d(n) \end{aligned} \tag{6.70}$$

where $d(n)$ is the noise signal assumed to be Gaussian with zero mean and variance σ_d^2. From Equation 6.68, it is clear that the input (clean) signal $x(n)$ depends on a total of $2p + 1$ parameters: the p values of the coefficient vector $\mathbf{a}$, the p initial values $\mathbf{x}_I$, and the gain term, g. The preceding speech production model offers an alternative to the speech enhancement problem. Rather than trying to estimate the clean signal $x(n)$ itself, we can instead estimate the parameters assumed to have been used to generate the signal according to Equation 6.70. As we will see shortly, the gain term g can easily be obtained using Parseval's theorem, and the p initial values $\mathbf{x}_I$ do not affect the estimation of $\mathbf{a}$, at least in noise. We are then left with the problem of estimating the all-pole model parameters a from the noisy speech signal. One can use linear prediction techniques to estimate a (according to Equation 6.25) in noise, but, generally, the estimated coefficients will not be accurate. Hence, alternative methods are needed for estimating the coefficients $\mathbf{a}$ of the clean signal from the noisy signal.

6.6.2 Statistical Parameter Estimation of the All-Pole Model in Noise

Statistical estimation techniques were used by Oppenheim and Lim [10] to estimate the all-pole parameters a in noise. In particular, maximum *a posteriori* (MAP) techniques were used. In the initial approach, Oppenheim and Lim [10] considered maximizing the probability of observing $\mathbf{a}$, given the noisy speech signal, $p(\mathbf{a} \mid \mathbf{y})$, that is, they sought solution to the problem:

$$\mathbf{a}_{MAP} = \max_{a} p(\mathbf{a} \mid \mathbf{y}) \tag{6.71}$$

where $\mathbf{y}^T = [y(0), y(1), \ldots, y(N-1)]$ is the noisy speech vector. Maximization of $p(\mathbf{a} \mid \mathbf{y})$ resulted, however, in a nonlinear problem, which could not be solved easily.

Instead, a suboptimal iterative procedure was considered, which was computationally tractable. They considered the MAP estimation of $x(n)$, given the noisy observations $y(n)$ and the coefficients $\mathbf{a}$, that is, they considered maximization of the conditional density $p(\mathbf{x} \mid \mathbf{a}, \mathbf{y})$. The gain term g and the initial conditions $\mathbf{x}_I$ were assumed to be known. The following iterative procedure was suggested:

Step 1: Based on an initial estimate of $\mathbf{a}$, which we denote by $\mathbf{a}_0$, estimate $\mathbf{x}$ by maximizing $p(\mathbf{x} \mid \mathbf{a}_0, \mathbf{y})$. Denote this first estimate of $\mathbf{x}$ by $\mathbf{x}_1$.

Step 2: Use $\mathbf{x}_1$ to form a new estimate of $\mathbf{a}$, which we denote by $\mathbf{a}_1$. The coefficients $\mathbf{a}$ can be obtained using linear prediction techniques. Go to Step 1 and use $\mathbf{a}_1$ in place of $\mathbf{a}_0$.

The preceding procedure is repeated iteratively to obtain a better (in some statistical sense) estimate of the coefficients $\mathbf{a}$. In fact, it was proved [10] that the preceding iterative procedure is guaranteed to converge to a local maximum of the joint probability density $p(\mathbf{a}, \mathbf{x} \mid \mathbf{y})$.

To implement Step 1 in the preceding iterative algorithm, we need to maximize $p(\mathbf{x} \mid \mathbf{a}_i, \mathbf{y})$ over all $x(n)$. From Bayes' rule, $p(\mathbf{x} \mid \mathbf{a}_i, \mathbf{y})$ can be written as

$$p(\mathbf{x} \mid \mathbf{a}_i, \mathbf{y}) = \frac{p(\mathbf{y} \mid \mathbf{a}_i, \mathbf{x})\, p(\mathbf{x} \mid \mathbf{a}_i)}{p(\mathbf{y} \mid \mathbf{a}_i)} \tag{6.72}$$

where $\mathbf{a}_i$ are the coefficients obtained at the ith iteration. The denominator is not a function of $x(n)$ and can therefore be ignored in the maximization. We assume that the gain term g and initial vector $\mathbf{x}_I$ are known in all the probability density terms in Equation 6.72. The MAP estimate of $\mathbf{x}$ needed in Step 1 is therefore given by

$$\mathbf{x}_{MAP} = \max_x p(\mathbf{x} \mid \mathbf{a}_i, \mathbf{y}) = \max_x p(\mathbf{y} \mid \mathbf{a}_i, \mathbf{x})\, p(\mathbf{x} \mid \mathbf{a}_i) \tag{6.73}$$

The conditional density $p(\mathbf{y} \mid \mathbf{a}_i, \mathbf{x})$ is Gaussian with mean $x(n)$ and variance σ_d^2 (same variance as the noise $d(n)$) and therefore has the following form:

$$p(\mathbf{y} \mid \mathbf{a}_i, \mathbf{x}) = \frac{1}{\left(2\pi\sigma_d^2\right)^{N/2}} \exp\left[-\frac{1}{2\sigma_d^2}\sum_{n=0}^{N-1}\left(y(n) - x(n)\right)^2\right] \tag{6.74}$$

The conditional density $p(\mathbf{x} \mid \mathbf{a}_i)$ is also Gaussian with mean $\mathbf{a}^T\mathbf{x}_p$ and variance g^2 and is given by

$$p(\mathbf{x} \mid \mathbf{a}_i) = \frac{1}{\left(2\pi g^2\right)^{N/2}} \exp\left[-\frac{1}{2g^2}\sum_{n=0}^{N-1}\left(x(n) - \mathbf{a}^T\mathbf{x}_p\right)^2\right] \tag{6.75}$$

Substituting Equations 6.74 and 6.75 in Equation 6.72, we get an expression for $p(\mathbf{x} \mid \mathbf{a}_i, \mathbf{y})$:

$$p(\mathbf{x} \mid \mathbf{a}_i, \mathbf{y}) = C\frac{1}{\left(4\pi^2 g^2\sigma_d^2\right)^{N/2}} \exp\left[-\frac{1}{2}\Delta_p\right] \tag{6.76}$$

where C is a constant, and Δ_p is given by

$$\Delta_p = \frac{1}{g^2}\sum_{n=0}^{N-1}\left(x(n) - \mathbf{a}^T\mathbf{x}_p\right)^2 + \frac{1}{\sigma_d^2}\sum_{n=0}^{N-1}(y(n) - s(n))^2 \tag{6.77}$$

Maximization of $p(\mathbf{x} \mid \mathbf{a}_i, \mathbf{y})$ with respect to $x(n)$ is equivalent to minimization of the Δ_p term, because the exponent in Equation 6.76 is negative. The estimation of $x(n)$ (in Step 1) can therefore be done by minimizing Δ_p or equivalently by choosing $\mathbf{x}$, such that

$$\frac{\partial \Delta_p}{\partial x(n)} = 0, \quad n = 0, 1, \ldots, N-1 \tag{6.78}$$

The preceding equation yields a linear system of N equations with N unknowns. The number N of samples used in analysis, however, could be large, and therefore, the solution could be computationally expensive.

Fortunately, the solution to Equation 6.78 can be simplified by observing that Δ_p can be expressed in the form $(\mathbf{x} - \mathbf{m}_i)^T\Sigma^{-1}(\mathbf{x} - \mathbf{m}_i)$, for some vector $\mathbf{m}_i$ and matrix Σ^{-1}. We could therefore express the conditional density $p(\mathbf{x} \mid \mathbf{a}_i, \mathbf{y})$ as

$$p(\mathbf{x} \mid \mathbf{a}_i, \mathbf{y}) = C\frac{1}{\left(4\pi^2 g^2 \sigma_d^2\right)^{N/2}}\exp\left[-\frac{1}{2}\left(\mathbf{x} - \mathbf{m}_i\right)^T \sum_i^{-1}\left(\mathbf{x} - \mathbf{m}_i\right)\right] \tag{6.79}$$

where

Σ_i is a covariance matrix

$\mathbf{m}_i$ is a mean vector (closed-form expressions for Σ_i and $\mathbf{m}_i$ can be found in [11, eq. 6.19]). According to the preceding equation, the conditional density $p(\mathbf{x} \mid \mathbf{a}_i, \mathbf{y})$ is jointly Gaussian, and, therefore, the MAP estimate of $\mathbf{x}$ is equivalent to the minimum mean-square error (MMSE) estimate of $\mathbf{x}$ [12]. This is because the MMSE estimate of $\mathbf{x}$ is also the mean of the *a posteriori* density $p(\mathbf{x} \mid \mathbf{a}_i, \mathbf{y})$. Since the conditional density $p(\mathbf{x} \mid \mathbf{a}_i, \mathbf{y})$ is jointly Gaussian, the maximum and the mean of $p(\mathbf{x} \mid \mathbf{a}_i, \mathbf{y})$ are identical. Furthermore, for large values of N (i.e., long-duration frames), we do not need to evaluate the mean of $p(\mathbf{x} \mid \mathbf{a}_i, \mathbf{y})$, but can use the noncausal Wiener filter to obtain the MMSE estimate of $\mathbf{x}$.

In summary, the MAP estimate of $\mathbf{x}$ (Equation 6.73, or, equivalently, the solution to Equation 6.78) can be simply obtained by filtering the noisy signal $y(n)$ through the Wiener filter:

$$H(\omega) = \frac{P_{xx}(\omega)}{P_{xx}(\omega) + \sigma_d^2} \tag{6.80}$$

where $P_{xx}(\omega)$ is the power spectrum of $x(n)$, given $\mathbf{a}_i$ and g, that is,

$$P_{xx}(\omega) = \frac{g^2}{\left|1 - \sum_{k=1}^{p} a_k e^{-jk\omega}\right|^2} \tag{6.81}$$

where the coefficients a_k in the preceding equation correspond to $\mathbf{a}_i$. Therefore, Step 1 can alternatively be implemented using Wiener filters.

The gain term g in Equation 6.81 can be estimated by requiring that the variance of the noisy speech signal, $y(n)$, be equal to the sum of the variances of the clean signal and the noise (because $x(n)$ and $d(n)$ are uncorrelated and zero mean):

$$\sigma_y^2 = \sigma_x^2 + \sigma_d^2 \tag{6.82}$$

where σ_y^2 is the variance (which is also the energy) of $y(n)$ and σ_x^2 is the variance of the estimated signal $x(n)$. We can compute the signal variance σ_x^2 of the estimated signal in the frequency domain using Parseval's theorem:

$$\begin{aligned}\sigma_x^2 &= \sum_{n=0}^{N-1} x^2(n) = \frac{1}{2\pi}\int_{-\pi}^{\pi} P_{xx}(\omega)d\omega \\ &= \frac{1}{2\pi}\int_{-\pi}^{\pi} \frac{g^2}{\left|1-\sum_{k=1}^{p} a_k e^{-jk\omega}\right|^2} d\omega\end{aligned} \tag{6.83}$$

Therefore, substituting Equation 6.83 in Equation 6.82, we get the following equation for g:

$$\frac{1}{2\pi}\int_{-\pi}^{\pi} \frac{g^2}{\left|1-\sum_{k=1}^{p} a_k e^{-jk\omega}\right|^2} d\omega = \frac{1}{N}\sum_{n=0}^{N-1} y^2(n) - \sigma_d^2 \tag{6.84}$$

from which we can solve for g^2:

$$g^2 = \frac{\frac{2\pi}{N}\sum_{n=0}^{N-1} y^2(n) - 2\pi\sigma_d^2}{\int_{-\pi}^{\pi} \frac{1}{\left|1-\sum_{k=1}^{p} a_k e^{-jk\omega}\right|^2} d\omega} \tag{6.85}$$

Note that the denominator in the integral can be evaluated by computing the Fourier transform of the all-pole coefficients (zero padded to N). Next, we outline the iterative Wiener filter algorithm proposed in [10].

Iterative Wiener Filtering Algorithm:

Initialization: Initialize the initial signal estimate, $\mathbf{x}_0$, to the noisy signal, that is, set $\mathbf{x}_0 = \mathbf{y}$

For iterations $i = 0, 1, 2, \ldots$, do the following:

Step 1: Given the estimated signal $\mathbf{x}_i$ at iteration i, compute the all-pole coefficients $\mathbf{a}_i$ using linear prediction techniques.

Step 2: Using $\mathbf{a}_i$, estimate the gain term g^2 according to Equation 6.85.

Step 3: Compute the short-term power spectrum of the signal $\mathbf{x}_i$:

$$P_{x_i x_i}(\omega) = \frac{g^2}{\left|1 - \sum_{k=1}^{p} a_i(k) e^{-jk\omega}\right|^2} \tag{6.86}$$

where $\{a_i(k)\}$ are the coefficients estimated in Step 1.

Step 4: Compute the Wiener filter:

$$H_i(\omega) = \frac{P_{x_i x_i}(\omega)}{P_{x_i x_i}(\omega) + \sigma_d^2} \tag{6.87}$$

Step 5: Estimate the spectrum of the enhanced signal:

$$X_{i+1}(\omega) = H_i(\omega) Y(\omega)$$

where $Y(\omega)$ is the spectrum of the noisy speech signal, $y(n)$. Compute the inverse Fourier transform of $X_{i+1}(\omega)$ to get the enhanced signal $\mathbf{x}_{i+1}$ in the time domain.

Step 6: Go to Step 1 using $\mathbf{x}_{i+1}$ for the estimated signal and repeat until a convergence criterion is met or repeat for a specified number of iterations.

In the preceding algorithm, we assumed that the additive noise is white Gaussian with zero mean and variance σ_d^2. For colored noise, Equation 6.87 takes the form

$$H_i(\omega) = \frac{P_{x_i x_i}(\omega)}{P_{x_i x_i}(\omega) + \hat{P}_{dd}(\omega)} \tag{6.88}$$

where $\hat{P}_{dd}(\omega)$ is the estimate of the noise power spectrum obtained during speech-absent frames. The noise variance σ_d^2 needed for the computation of the gain term in Equation 6.85 can alternatively be computed in the frequency domain as

$$\sigma_d^2 = \frac{1}{2\pi} \int_{-\pi}^{\pi} \hat{P}_{dd}(\omega) d\omega \tag{6.89}$$

In principle, the preceding iterative algorithm is run until a convergence criterion is met. In practice, however, the preceding algorithm is run for a fixed number of iterations.

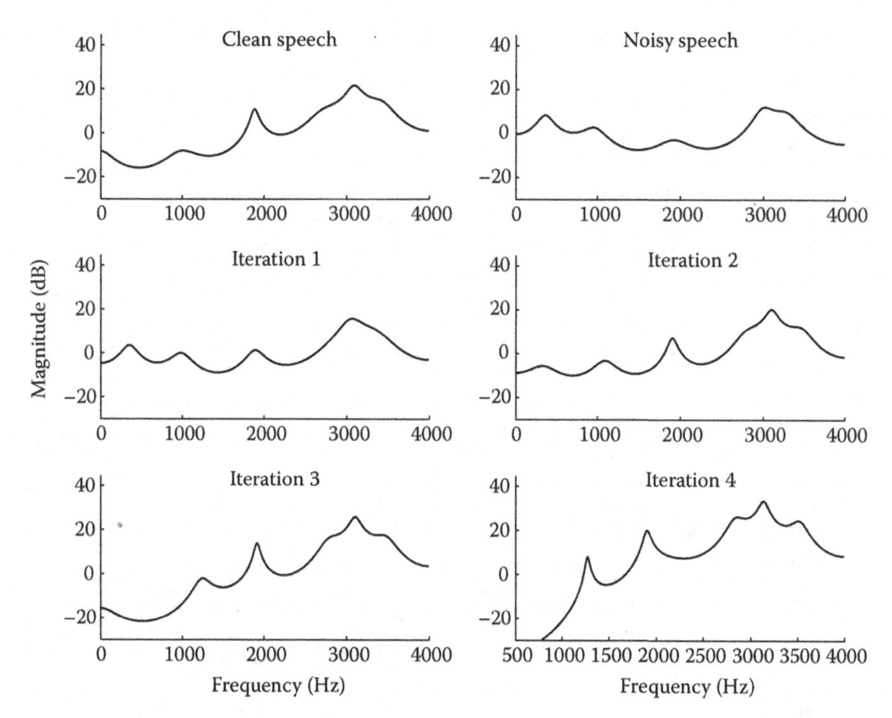

FIGURE 6.10 LPC spectra obtained at each iteration of the iterative Wiener filtering algorithm for an unvoiced speech segment.

Three to seven iterations have been found to be sufficient most of the time [11,13]. Figure 6.10 shows the estimated spectra as a function of iteration number for an unvoiced speech segment. For this example, three iterations seemed to be sufficient. Figure 6.11 shows the estimated spectra as a function of iteration number for a voiced speech segment. For this example, the algorithm was run for eight iterations. As is evident from Figure 6.11, allowing more iterations is not necessarily beneficial. Compare, for instance, the spectrum obtained at iteration 8 with that obtained at iteration 3. The formant bandwidths of the spectrum at iteration 8 are considerably smaller than those of the clean speech signal and those at iterations 3 and 4. Also, the spectral peak at $f = 3000\,\text{Hz}$ is much sharper at the eighth iteration compared to the same peak at the third or fourth iterations. This suggests that the pole magnitudes of the AR model must be moving toward the unit circle. Also, the lower two formant peaks are split into two additional peaks. The presence of spurious peaks suggests that the pole locations of the AR model must be moving as well.

The preceding examples illustrated some of the issues associated with iterative Wiener filtering:

1. It is not clear what convergence criterion to use or when to terminate the iterative algorithm. Knowing when to terminate the algorithm is critical for best performance.

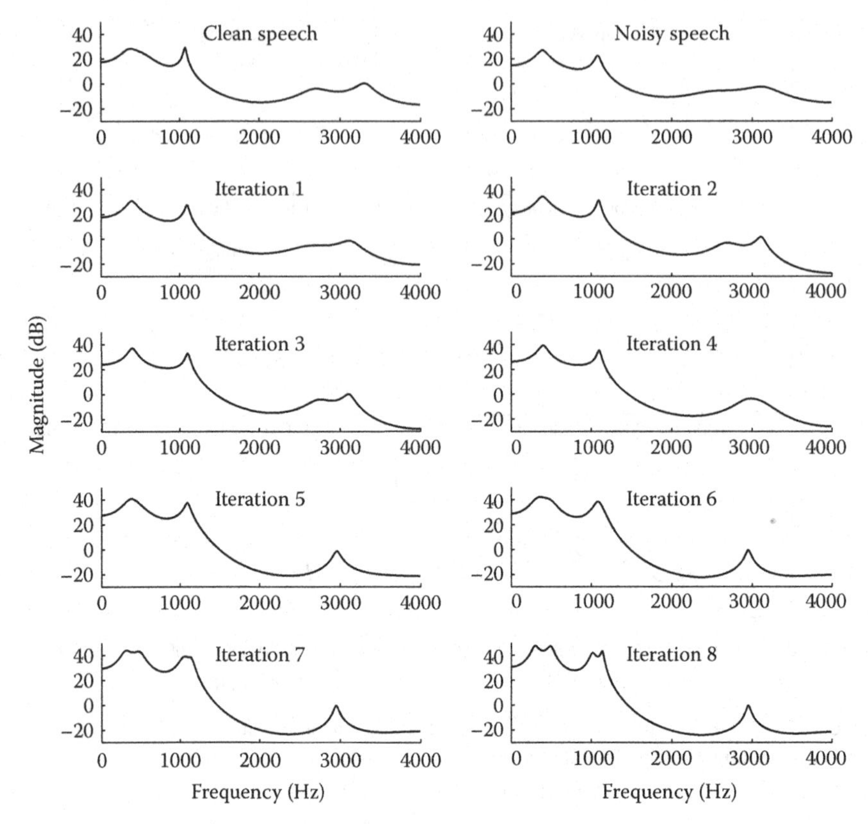

FIGURE 6.11 LPC spectra obtained at each iteration of the iterative Wiener filtering algorithm for a voiced speech segment.

2. The all-pole spectrum might have unnaturally sharp peaks, which in turn can affect the quality of speech.
3. Spurious spectral peaks might be generated if the algorithm is run for too many iterations.

No good and reliable solution has been found to address the first issue regarding the "optimal" number of iterations. Even worse, the optimal number of iterations seems to be different for different types of sounds. In [11], the authors noted that vowels needed on average three iterations for best overall speech quality, whereas the glides needed two iterations, and the nasals, liquids, and affricates needed five to six iterations.

Several solutions have been proposed to address the second and third issues [13–16]. These two issues can be dealt with by imposing spectral constraints on the characteristics of the all-pole spectrum. For one, we can impose spectral continuity constraints to ensure that the spectra obtained at a given frame are not too different from those obtained at previous or future frames. This is motivated by the fact that the vocal tract characteristics do not change drastically from frame to frame. Second, we can impose constraints at the iteration level to ensure that only valid all-pole spectra are generated.

6.7 IMPOSING CONSTRAINTS ON ITERATIVE WIENER FILTERING

Spectral constraints can therefore be imposed across time (interframe) and across iterations (intraframe) to improve the performance of the iterative Wiener filtering algorithm. Next, we describe some of the proposed spectral constraints [11,13,14].

6.7.1 Across-Time Spectral Constraints

Perhaps, the simplest approach of imposing across-time constraints is to apply temporal smoothing on the estimated spectrum of the form

$$P_{xx}^{(k)}(\omega) = \tau P_{xx}^{(k-1)}(\omega) + (1-\tau)P_{xx}^{(k)}(\omega) \tag{6.90}$$

where

$P_{xx}^{(k)}(\omega)$ denotes the spectrum estimate at frame k
τ is a smoothing constant ($0 \le \tau \le 1$)

Better yet, rather than using a fixed value for τ, we can make τ time varying. When the spectrum is changing rapidly, as in voiced-to-unvoiced transitions, for instance, we can apply little temporal smoothing. On the other hand, we can increase the smoothing when the spectrum is relatively stationary, as during a vowel segment. We can therefore change the smoothing constant τ according to some measure of stationarity of the signal spectrum. Such an approach was described in [17,18], where τ was estimated by mapping the spectral derivative of the signal spectrum (based on the computation of the first-order difference between the present and immediate past spectrum) to a time-varying constant taking values between 0 and 1. The resulting smoothed spectrum was obtained according to

$$P_{xx}^{(k)}(\omega) = \tau(k)P_{xx}^{(k-1)}(\omega) + (1-\tau(k))P_{xx}^{(k)}(\omega) \tag{6.91}$$

where $\tau(k)$ is now the time-varying smoothing constant ($0 \le \tau(k) \le 1$).

Alternatively, we can impose constraints directly on the all-pole parameters $\mathbf{a}^{(k)}$, because the poles of the linear prediction polynomial $A(z)$ affect the shape of the spectrum. Spectral constraints on the all-pole parameters estimated at frame k, $\mathbf{a}^{(k)}$, can be imposed using the all-pole parameters estimated in neighboring past (i.e., $\mathbf{a}^{(k-1)}$, $\mathbf{a}^{(k-2)}$,…) and future frames (i.e., $\mathbf{a}^{(k+1)}$, $\mathbf{a}^{(k+2)}$,…).

As mentioned earlier, the all-pole spectra might have unnaturally sharp peaks. Such peaks can be generated when the magnitudes of the poles of the $A(z)$ polynomial (see Equation 6.67) move too close to the unit circle. A simple approach can be adopted to constrain the magnitude of the poles by evaluating the all-pole polynomial in Equation 6.86 at a circle of radius r, that is, evaluate $A(re^{j\omega})$, where r is a parameter that controls the formant bandwidth. We can thus replace the denominator in Equation 6.86 with

$$\left|A\left(re^{j\omega}\right)\right|^2 = \left|1 - \sum_{k=1}^{M} a_i(k) r^k e^{-k\omega}\right|^2 \tag{6.92}$$

For $r < 1$, the preceding evaluation moves the poles toward the interior of the unit circle and increases the formant bandwidth, that is, it broadens the formant peaks (see example in Figure 6.12). Similarly, we can impose angular constraints on the poles to limit the movement of the pole locations within a prescribed angular window or equivalently constrain the movement of the formant peaks within a small region. To do that, we will need a root-solving algorithm to obtain the M poles of the $A(z)$ polynomial. Because root solving is computationally expensive and numerically inaccurate, a more robust procedure was sought in [13] to implement the preceding constraints.

The line spectral frequency (LSF) representation of the all-pole coefficients was considered in [13]. The LSF representation expresses the forward and backward linear predictive coding (LPC) polynomials in terms of two polynomials, $P(z)$ and $Q(z)$ [19, p. 116]. The angles of the roots of these two polynomials are called the *line spectrum frequencies*, which we denote by l_i (i = 1, 2, …, M). The odd-indexed LSP frequencies are termed the *position parameters* and correspond roughly to the

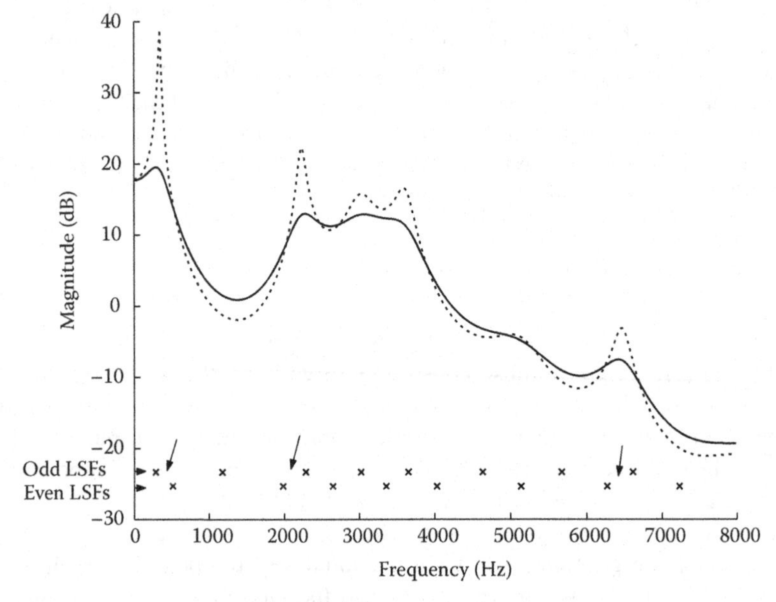

FIGURE 6.12 LPC spectrum $(1/|A(e^{(jw)})|^2$ of a 30 ms segment of the vowel/i/ is shown in solid lines, and the modified LPC spectrum, $1/|A(re^{(jw)})|^2$, using $r = 0.94$, is shown in dashed lines.

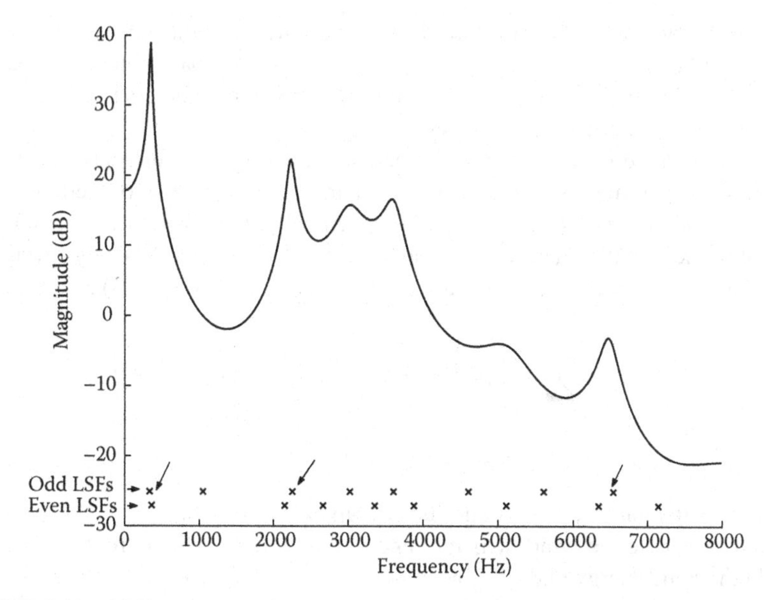

FIGURE 6.13 LPC spectrum of a 30 ms segment of the vowel/i/. The odd and even line spectral frequencies (LSFs) are plotted at the bottom.

formant frequency locations: $p_i = l_{2i-1}$ for $i = 1, 2, \ldots, M/2$. The distance between the roots of the $P(z)$ polynomial from the closest roots of the $Q(z)$ polynomial provides the *difference parameters*, which are indicative of the formant frequency bandwidth (see example in Figure 6.13). This corresponds roughly to the distance between the odd-indexed and even-indexed LSFs. The smaller the distance, the smaller the bandwidth of the formant. The difference parameters, d_i, are given by

$$|d_i| = \min_{j=-1,1} \left| l_{2i+j} - l_{2i} \right|, \quad i = 1,2,\ldots,M/2 \tag{6.93}$$

Figure 6.13 plots the LPC spectrum of the vowel/i/along with the corresponding LSFs, which are shown at the bottom. Note that the odd- and even-indexed LSFs pointed by the arrows are close to each other, suggesting that the corresponding difference parameters are small. More precisely, the estimated difference parameters for this example are $|d_i|$ = {28.05, 689.33, 101.23, 335.34, 250.34, 501.04, 498.22, 196.39} Hz. Small values of difference parameters are indeed associated with narrow formant bandwidths. Note, for example, the narrow bandwidth of the first formant located at about 400 Hz. The corresponding difference parameter is 28.05 Hz. In contrast, the bandwidth of the first formant shown in Figure 6.12 is wide, and the corresponding difference parameters are considerably larger. The estimated difference parameters for the spectrum shown in Figure 6.12 with broadened formants are $|d_i|$ = {231.17, 649.60, 301.84, 333.90, 296.58, 505.07, 533.03, 344.68} Hz. Hence, the values of the difference parameters are indicative of the formant bandwidth.

The LSFs provide us with a way of constraining both the formant frequency locations and formant bandwidths. We can use the position parameters to constrain movement of the formant frequencies and the difference parameters to constrain the bandwidths of the formant frequencies.

To reduce frame-to-frame formant frequency drifting, we can apply constraints to the position parameters [13]. The position parameters, p_i, are smoothed over time using past and future values of p_i. More specifically, the position parameter estimated at frame k on the ith iteration, denoted as $\hat{p}_j^{(i)}(k)$, is smoothed using a weighted triangular window with a variable base of support (one to five frames) as follows:

$$\hat{p}_j^{(i)}(k) = \sum_{m=-L}^{L} R \cdot \left[1 - \frac{|m|}{W}\right] p_j^{(i)}(k+m), \quad j = 1, 2, \ldots, M/2 \tag{6.94}$$

where

L denotes the number of past and future frames

R and W denote the window height and width, both of which are dependent on both frame energy and LSF index j

The height and width (R and W) of the triangular window varies, depending on whether the frame is classified as voiced or unvoiced (including background noise). The voiced or unvoiced classification is done by comparing the frame energy against a preset threshold. If a frame is classified as unvoiced (or noise), the lower formant frequencies are smoothed over a narrower triangle width compared to the higher formant frequencies.

No smoothing is performed on the difference parameters. However, if a difference parameter falls below a small value, $d_{\min}$, it is floored to that value. This is done to avoid obtaining spectra with unnaturally small formant bandwidths that could potentially degrade speech quality. Values in the range $0.015 \leq d_{\min} \leq 0.031$ rads were found to yield good quality.

Following the smoothing and limiting of the preceding parameters, the position and difference parameters are combined to form the new, constrained all-pole coefficients needed in the Wiener filter (Equation 6.86).

6.7.2 Across-Iterations Constraints

In addition to across-time constraints, across-iterations constraints can also be imposed [11,13,14]. The constraints are not applied to the all-pole coefficients directly but are applied to the autocorrelation coefficients, which are used to derive the all-pole coefficients. More specifically, the kth autocorrelation lag estimated in the ith iteration, denoted as $r_{xx}^{(i)}(k)$, is computed as a weighted combination of the kth lags from previous iterations:

$$r_{xx}^{(i)}(k) = \sum_{m=0}^{i-1} \psi_m r_{xx}^{(i-m)}(k) \tag{6.95}$$

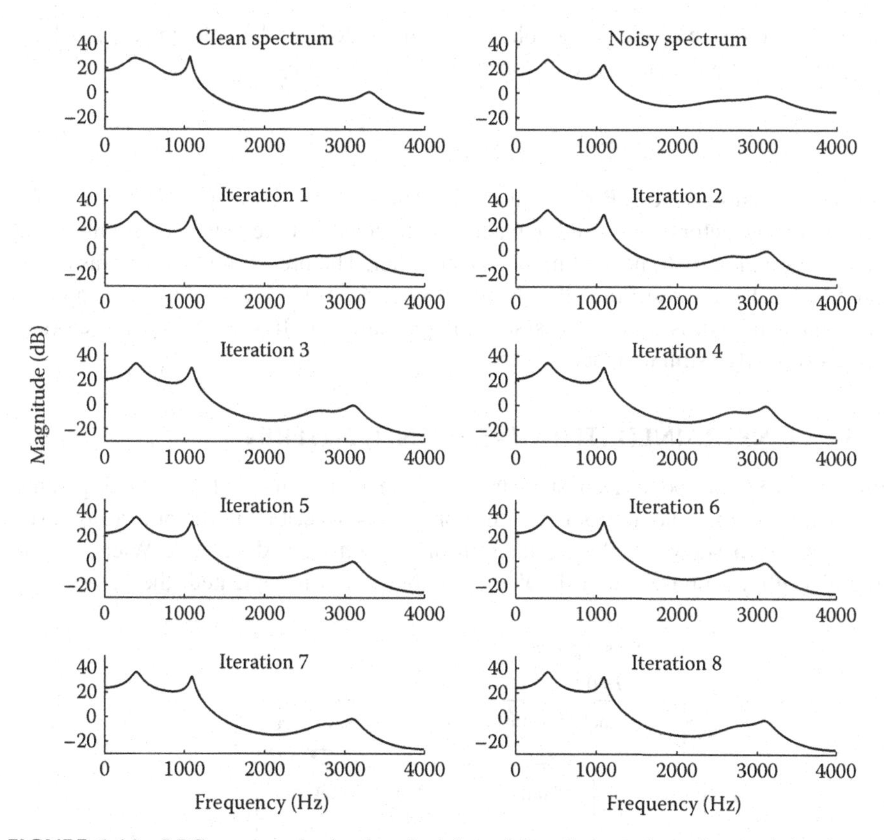

FIGURE 6.14 LPC spectra obtained as function of iteration number after applying inter-frame constraints on the autocorrelation function.

where ψ_m denote the weights satisfying the condition: $\Sigma_m \psi_m = 1$. Figure 6.14 shows the effect on the spectra after applying the preceding autocorrelation constraint on the same frame of speech used in Figure 6.11. For this example, a triangular type of weighting of the form $\psi_m = R \cdot \left(1 - \frac{m}{i}\right)$ (for $0 \leq m \leq i - 1$, where R is chosen so that $\Sigma_m \psi_m = 1$) is applied to the autocorrelation lags, placing more emphasis on recent autocorrelation lags and less emphasis on lags obtained in previous iterations. As can be seen by comparing the spectra obtained at the eighth iteration in Figures 6.11 and 6.14, the formant bandwidths no longer become smaller, and the formants no longer move with increasing iteration.

A codebook-based method was proposed in [14] for applying across-iterations constraints. A codebook of all-pole coefficients was first trained using a large database of clean speech. Then, rather than using the estimated all-pole coefficients $\mathbf{a}_i$ at iteration i, the codebook vector $\mathbf{c}_j$, closest to $\mathbf{a}_i$ was chosen satisfying the following condition:

$$d(\mathbf{a}_i, \mathbf{c}_j) \leq d(\mathbf{a}_i, \mathbf{c}_k), \quad k = 1, 2, \ldots, L \tag{6.96}$$

where L is the size of the codebook ($L = 1024$ yielded good results in [14]), and $d(\cdot)$ denotes the Mahalanobis-type distortion measure given by

$$d(\mathbf{a}_i, \mathbf{c}_j) = (\mathbf{a}_i - \mathbf{c}_j)^T \hat{R}_{xx} (\mathbf{a}_i - \mathbf{c}_j) \tag{6.97}$$

where $\hat{R}_{xx}$ denotes the estimated autocorrelation matrix corresponding to $\mathbf{a}_i$. The selected codevector $\mathbf{c}_j$ was used in place of $\mathbf{a}_i$ to construct the power spectrum of the signal (Equation 6.86) needed in the Wiener filter. The preceding method was based on the idea that the resulting all-pole power spectra based on $\mathbf{c}_j$ ought to have normal formant bandwidths and possess speechlike characteristics, as the codevectors $\mathbf{c}_j$ were originally estimated from clean speech.

6.8 CONSTRAINED ITERATIVE WIENER FILTERING

Various types of spectral constraints were investigated in [11,13], including some of the across-time and across-iterations constraints described in the preceding text.

Figure 6.15 shows the block diagram of the constrained iterative Wiener filtering algorithm proposed in [13]. Of all the constraints investigated, the across-time

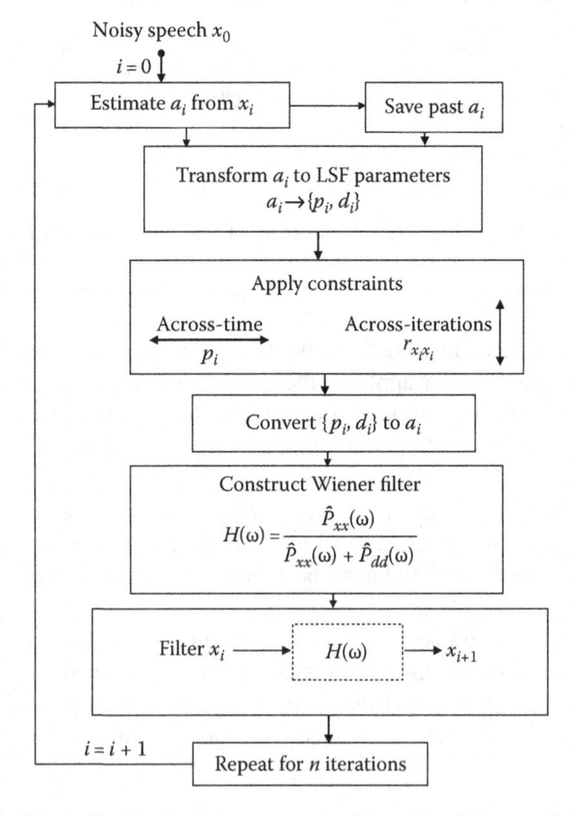

FIGURE 6.15 Block diagram of the constrained iterative Wiener filtering algorithm proposed in [13].

constraints on the position parameters given by Equation 6.94 and the across-iterations constraints on the autocorrelation lags as specified by Equation 6.95 were found to yield the highest performance in terms of the Itakura–Saito (IS) objective measure. Larger improvements in performance were obtained by the constrained approach when compared to the unconstrained Wiener filtering approach [10] and the spectral subtraction approach. Detailed evaluation of individual sound classes (e.g., nasals, stops, glides, and fricatives) indicated that the constrained approach consistently improved the performance for all sound classes. Furthermore, unlike the unconstrained approach, the constrained approach reached the best overall speech quality at the same iteration, independent of SNR and sound class. The optimum terminating iteration (determined by observing the smallest, across all iterations, IS measure between the estimated all-pole spectra and the clean spectra) in the constrained approach was found consistently to be the seventh iteration.

The constrained approach proposed in [13] was evaluated primarily using sentences corrupted with additive white Gaussian noise. Large improvements in performance were noted with white Gaussian noise, and relatively smaller ones were noted with colored noise sources. This was not surprising because no special considerations were given for colored noise. Colored noise, such as automobile highway noise, does not affect the spectrum uniformly, but rather affects only a small portion of the spectrum. Consequently, for low-frequency noise degradations of the spectrum, it might not be desirable to apply spectral constraints to the high-frequency regions of the spectrum. Ideally, the spectral constraints should be applied selectively to the regions of the spectrum that have been corrupted the most by noise. In the case of car noise, for instance, the constraints should be applied primarily to the low-frequency portion of the spectrum and not the high-frequency portion.

Such an approach was proposed in [20], by decomposing the signal into a set of Q linearly spaced frequency bands. The amount of spectral smoothing imposed on each band was controlled by limiting the number of iterations allowed in each band according to the degree of spectral degradation in that band. The idea was to reduce the terminating iteration in spectral regions of high SNR and to increase the terminating iteration in spectral regions of low SNR; that way, spectral smoothing constraints are imposed primarily on spectral regions that were affected the most by the colored noise.

The terminating iteration for subband k, denoted as $TI(k)$, was a linear function of the subband SNR and was determined using the following equation:

$$TI(k) = \left\lceil \left(IT_{\max} - IT_{\min}\right) \frac{\text{SNR}_{\max} - \text{SNR}(k)}{\text{SNR}_{\max} - \text{SNR}_{\min}} \right\rceil + IT_{\min}, \quad 1 \le k \le Q \tag{6.98}$$

where $\lceil \cdot \rceil$ denotes the nearest integer, $\text{SNR}_{\max} = 25\,\text{dB}$, $\text{SNR}_{\min} = -5\,\text{dB}$, $IT_{\min} = 1$ was the minimum terminating iteration allowed, $IT_{\max} = 4$ was the maximum terminating iteration allowed, and SNR(k) is the (*a posteriori*) SNR estimate of the SNR in subband k:

$$\text{SNR}(k) = 10 \log_{10} \left(\frac{E_x(k)}{E_n(k)} - 1 \right) \tag{6.99}$$

where

$E_x(k)$ is the energy of the noisy speech signal in subband k
$E_n(k)$ is the energy of the noise in subband k estimated during speech-absent frames.

The algorithm proposed in [20] was implemented using the following steps:

Step 1: Obtain enhanced speech $\mathbf{x}_i$ at the ith iteration as in [13] by applying the autocorrelation and position parameters constraints (Equations 6.94 and 6.95).

Step 2: Decompose $\mathbf{x}_i$ into Q subbands and evaluate the terminating iterations for each subband as per Equation 6.98. If the current iteration is equal to $TI(k)$ (i.e., if $TI(k) = i$), then retain the kth subband signal as the final estimate of the current subband.

Step 3: Repeat Step 1 until terminating iteration $IT_{\max}$ is reached.

Step 4: Sum up the Q subband signals to recover the enhanced signal.

In their simulations, eight linearly spaced frequency bands (i.e., $Q = 8$) were used, and the algorithm was evaluated using a variety of colored and nonstationary noise sources including fan, aircraft cockpit, and street noise. The proposed algorithm performed consistently better than the algorithm in [13] for all noises and SNRs examined.

6.9 CONSTRAINED WIENER FILTERING

So far, we have focused our attention on iterative Wiener filtering techniques for speech enhancement, which imposed within-frame and across-frame constraints on the all-pole spectra. Imposing across-time spectral constraints proved to be beneficial in improving speech quality. However, the main limitation of that approach is that it is not amenable to real-time implementation, as it would require access to future frames. Also, the spectral constraints were applied heuristically to Wiener filtering and were primarily motivated by knowledge of speech production and perception principles. Alternatively, we can impose constraints on the Wiener filter in an optimal fashion by including the constraints in the derivation of the Wiener filter; that is, we can consider finding an optimal filter that minimizes a mean-square error criterion subject to certain constraints. Next, we derive a Wiener filter that considers the speech and noise distortions as constraints. The derived Wiener filter does no longer need to be implemented iteratively.

6.9.1 Mathematical Definitions of Speech and Noise Distortions

Before deriving the optimally constrained Wiener filters, we first need to formalize the mathematical definition of speech and noise distortion* [6,21], at least in the context of linear estimators (e.g., Wiener estimator).

As mentioned earlier, we consider the linear estimator $\hat{X}(\omega) = H(\omega) \cdot Y(\omega)$ of the signal spectrum, where $Y(\omega)$ is the spectrum of the noisy signal and $H(\omega)$ is

* Caution needs to be exercised about the mathematical definitions of speech and noise distortion. It is unclear, and undetermined, whether these mathematical definitions correlate well with the human listener's subjective ratings of speech and noise distortion (more on this in Chapters 10 and 11).

the unknown filter, also called *estimator.* We can decompose the estimation error into two components, $\varepsilon_x(\omega)$ and $\varepsilon_d(\omega)$, as follows:

$$\begin{aligned}\varepsilon(\omega) &= \hat{X}(\omega) - X(\omega)\\ &= H(\omega)\cdot Y(\omega) - X(\omega) = H(\omega)\cdot(X(\omega)+D(\omega)) - X(\omega)\\ &= (H(\omega)-1)\cdot X(\omega) + H(\omega)\cdot D(\omega)\\ &= \varepsilon_x(\omega) + \varepsilon_d(\omega)\end{aligned} \tag{6.100}$$

where $D(\omega)$ is the spectrum of the noise signal. The power spectra of $\varepsilon_x(\omega)$ and $\varepsilon_d(\omega)$ are given by

$$\begin{aligned}E\left[\varepsilon_x^2(\omega)\right] &= (H(\omega)-1)^2 P_{xx}(\omega)\\ E\left[\varepsilon_d^2(\omega)\right] &= (H(\omega))^2 P_{dd}(\omega)\end{aligned} \tag{6.101}$$

The overall mean-square estimation error, $E[\varepsilon(\omega)]^2$, can be expressed as the sum of these two components, that is,

$$\begin{aligned}E[\varepsilon(\omega)]^2 &= E[\varepsilon_x(\omega)]^2 + E[\varepsilon_d(\omega)]^2\\ d_T(\omega) &= d_X(\omega) + d_D(\omega)\end{aligned} \tag{6.102}$$

The first term, $(H(\omega) - 1)^2 \cdot P_{XX}(\omega)$, represents the effect of the filter $H(\omega)$ on the signal power spectrum and quantifies in some way the speech distortion introduced by the estimator $H(\omega)$. This is to be expected because the estimator $H(\omega)$ will not eliminate the noise completely and will therefore affect both the signal and the additive noise. Similarly, the second term, $(H(\omega))^2 \cdot P_{dd}(\omega)$, quantifies the noise distortion introduced by the estimator $H(\omega)$.

From Equation 6.101, we see that both distortion components are quadratic functions of $H(\omega)$ and are plotted in Figure 6.16. The steepness of the parabolas depends on the signal and noise power spectra, and for the example shown in Figure 6.16, we assume that $P_{xx}(\omega) = P_{dd}(\omega)$ (i.e., $\xi_k = 1$). If we choose $H(\omega) = 1$, then we minimize the speech distortion (i.e., $d_X(\omega) = 0$). However, the noise distortion will be large. At the other extreme, if we choose $H(\omega) = 0$, then we minimize the noise distortion (i.e., $d_D(\omega) = 0$), but the speech distortion will be large. Hence, it is clear from Figure 6.16 that there is a trade-off between speech and noise distortion. For this example, the optimal Wiener gain is $H_W(\omega) = 1/2$, and the noise distortion is equal to the speech distortion.

We know that the Wiener filter minimizes the total mean-square error $E[\varepsilon(\omega)]^2$, and according to Figure 6.16, the Wiener filter is obtained as the minimum of the $d_T(\omega)$ parabola. Consider now two possible scenarios for the estimated Wiener filter. If the signal is strong and the noise weak [i.e., $P_{xx}(\omega) >> P_{dd}(\omega)$], then the Wiener filter yields a large noise distortion but a small speech distortion. This can be seen in Figure 6.17b. At the other extreme, if the signal is weak and the noise strong [i.e., $P_{xx}(\omega) << P_{dd}(\omega)$], then the speech distortion will be large

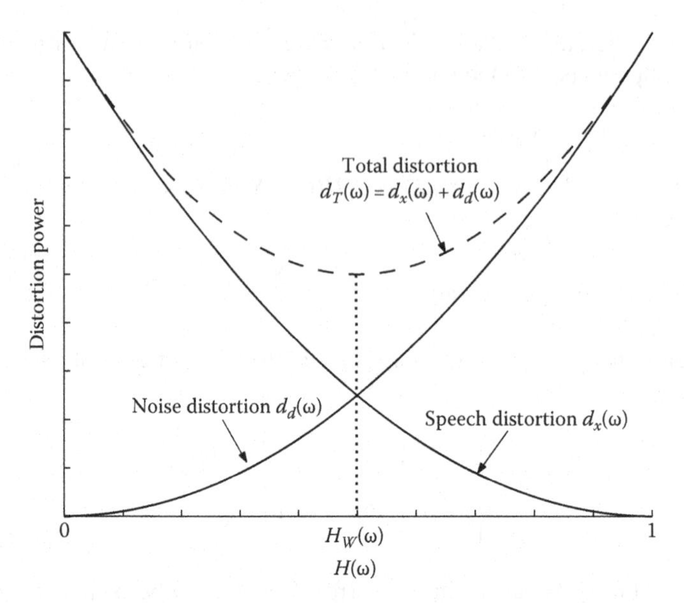

FIGURE 6.16 Plot of speech and noise distortion power as a function of the estimator function $H(\omega)$, where $0 \leq H(\omega) \leq 1$. For this example, it is assumed that $P_{xx}(\omega) = P_{dd}(\omega)$. The Wiener estimator, indicated as $H_W(\omega)$, is obtained as the spectral weighting value, $H(\omega)$, corresponding to the minimum of the total-distortion parabola.

(see Figure 6.17a), whereas the noise distortion will be small. Therefore, depending on the power of the signal and the noise (or equivalently, the ratio of the signal to noise power, i.e., the *a priori* SNR), the speech and noise distortion will vary over time. Hence, the traditional Wiener filter offers no way of controlling individually the noise and speech distortion. In addition, it is not possible to always choose $H(\omega)$ so that the estimation error falls below a certain threshold level, say, a masking threshold.

If we place equal weight on the noise and speech distortions, we can consider choosing $H(\omega)$ so that the two distortions are at least equal to each other. This avoids the possibility of one of the two distortions being disproportionately larger than the other. This can be done by setting $d_X(\omega) = d_D(\omega)$ in Equation 6.101 and solving for $H(\omega)$. In doing so, we get a quadratic function in $H(\omega)$ with the following solution*:

$$H_E(\omega_k) = \frac{1}{1 + \sqrt{\dfrac{P_{dd}(\omega_k)}{P_{xx}(\omega_k)}}}$$

$$= \frac{\sqrt{\xi_k}}{\sqrt{\xi_k} + 1} \tag{6.103}$$

* The second solution of the quadratic equation does not always satisfy the constraint: $0 \leq H(\omega) \leq 1$.

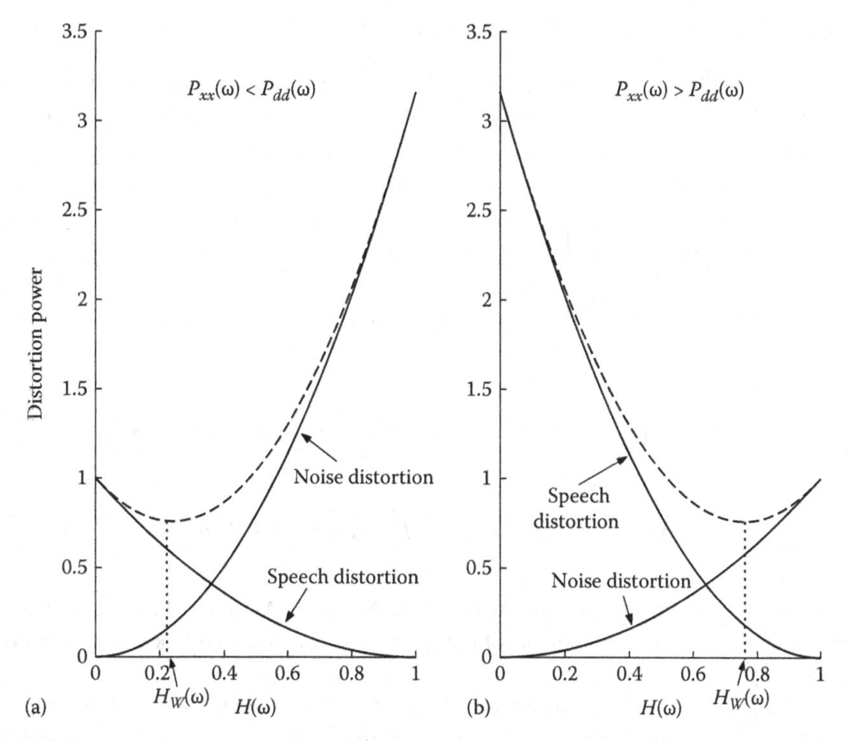

FIGURE 6.17 Wiener estimator in two scenarios. (a) Plot of speech and noise distortion power as a function of the estimator $H(\omega)$ for $P_{xx}(\omega) < P_{dd}(\omega)$. For this example, $P_{dd}(\omega) = 3.16 \cdot P_{xx}(\omega)$ corresponding to −5 dB *a priori* SNR. (b) Plot of speech and noise distortion power as a function of the estimator function $H(\omega)$ for $P_{xx}(\omega) > P_{dd}(\omega)$. For this example, $P_{xx}(\omega) = 3.16 \cdot P_{dd}(\omega)$ corresponding to 5 dB *a priori* SNR. The Wiener estimator is indicated as $H_W(\omega)$ in both scenarios and is equal to $H_W(\omega) = 0.24$ for scenario (a) and $H_W(\omega) = 0.76$ for scenario (b).

Comparing the preceding filter $H_E(\omega)$ to the Wiener filter in Figure 6.17a, we see that the $H_E(\omega)$ filter yields smaller speech distortion but larger noise distortion. This holds in general provided that $P_{xx}(\omega_k) < P_{dd}(\omega_k)$ or $\xi_k < 1$. In contrast, for the example given in Figure 6.17b, the $H_E(\omega)$ filter yields smaller noise distortion but larger speech distortion, and this is true in general when $P_{xx}(\omega) > P_{dd}(\omega)$. So, if we want to minimize the speech distortion while allowing for a variable noise distortion, we can choose the $H_E(\omega)$ filter if the estimated *a priori* SNR is $\xi_k < 1$ and the Wiener filter otherwise. Although a viable approach, it has two drawbacks: First, much like the Wiener filter, we cannot choose $H(\omega)$ so that both speech and noise distortions always fall below a certain threshold. Second, the speech and noise distortions will vary over time.

An alternative option is to try to limit the noise distortion while allowing for a variable speech distortion. It is clear from Figure 6.16 that we can always find $H(\omega)$ so that the noise (or speech) distortion always falls below a preset threshold level. We can therefore consider minimizing the speech distortion while constraining the noise distortion to fall below a preset threshold level. The optimal filter can thus be derived by solving a constrained minimization problem. Such an approach was proposed in [22,23] and is described next.

6.9.2 Limiting the Noise Distortion Level

Let $\mathbf{y} = \mathbf{x} + \mathbf{d}$ denote the noisy speech vector consisting of the clean signal vector $\mathbf{x}$ and additive noise $\mathbf{d}$. Let F denote the N-point discrete Fourier transform matrix given by

$$F = \frac{1}{\sqrt{N}} \begin{bmatrix} 1 & 1 & \cdots & 1 \\ 1 & e^{j\omega_0} & \cdots & e^{j(N-1)\omega_0} \\ \vdots & \vdots & \ddots & \vdots \\ 1 & e^{j(N-1)\omega_0} & \cdots & e^{j(N-1)(N-1)\omega_0} \end{bmatrix} \tag{6.104}$$

where $\omega_0 = 2\pi/N$. The Fourier transform of the noisy speech vector $\mathbf{y}$ can then be written as

$$\mathbf{Y}(\omega) = F^H \cdot \mathbf{y} = F^H \cdot \mathbf{x} + F^H \cdot \mathbf{d} = \mathbf{X}(\omega) + \mathbf{D}(\omega) \tag{6.105}$$

where H indicates the Hermitian operator and $\mathbf{X}(\omega)$ and $N(\omega)$ are the $N \times 1$ vectors containing the spectral components of the clean speech vector $\mathbf{x}$ and the noise vector $\mathbf{d}$, respectively.

Let $\hat{\mathbf{X}}(\omega) = G \cdot \mathbf{Y}(\omega)$ be the linear estimator of $\mathbf{X}(\omega)$, where G is now an $N \times N$ matrix. As we will show shortly, the derivation of the optimal estimator discussed in the previous section is a special case if we assume that G is a diagonal matrix. For now, we assume that the matrix G is a full $N \times N$ matrix. The estimation error in the frequency domain is given by

$$\begin{aligned} \varepsilon(\omega) &= \hat{\mathbf{X}}(\omega) - \mathbf{X}(\omega) \\ &= G \cdot \mathbf{Y}(\omega) - \mathbf{X}(\omega) = G \cdot (\mathbf{X}(\omega) + \mathbf{D}(\omega)) - \mathbf{X}(\omega) \\ &= (G - \mathbf{I}) \cdot \mathbf{X}(\omega) + G \cdot \mathbf{D}(\omega) \\ &= \varepsilon_x(\omega) + \varepsilon_d(\omega) \end{aligned} \tag{6.106}$$

where $\mathbf{I}$ is the identity matrix ($N \times N$) and $\{\varepsilon_x(\omega), \varepsilon_d(\omega)\}$ are the distortion terms. Using Equation 6.106, we can express the energy of the speech distortion as follows:

$$\begin{aligned} \varepsilon_{\mathbf{x}}^2 &= E\left(\varepsilon_{\mathbf{x}}^H(\omega) \cdot \varepsilon_{\mathbf{x}}(\omega)\right) = \text{tr}\left(E\left(\varepsilon_{\mathbf{x}}(\omega) \cdot \varepsilon_{\mathbf{x}}^H(\omega)\right)\right) \\ &= \text{tr}\left((G - \mathbf{I}) \cdot F^H \cdot E[\mathbf{x} \cdot \mathbf{x}^T] \cdot F \cdot (G - \mathbf{I})^H\right) \\ &= \text{tr}\left((G - \mathbf{I}) \cdot F^H \cdot R_{xx} \cdot F \cdot (G - \mathbf{I})^H\right) \end{aligned} \tag{6.107}$$

where R_{xx} is the $N \times N$ autocorrelation matrix of $\mathbf{x}$. Similarly, the energy of the noise distortion is given by

$$\begin{aligned} \varepsilon_d^2 &= E\left(\varepsilon_d^H(\omega) \cdot \varepsilon_d(\omega)\right) = \mathrm{tr}\left(E\left(\varepsilon_d(\omega) \cdot \varepsilon_d^H(\omega)\right)\right) \\ &= \mathrm{tr}\left(G \cdot F^H \cdot R_{dd} \cdot F \cdot G^H\right) \end{aligned} \tag{6.108}$$

To enhance speech with no noticeable distortion, we need to minimize the speech distortion (over all estimators G) while keeping the noise distortion below a threshold. We can therefore obtain the optimal linear estimator by solving the following constrained optimization problem:

$$\begin{aligned} &\min_G \varepsilon_{\mathbf{x}}^2 \\ &\text{subject to: } \frac{1}{N}\varepsilon_d^2 \le \delta \end{aligned} \tag{6.109}$$

where δ is a positive number corresponding to a preset threshold. The estimator derived in this way minimizes the energy of the speech distortion in the frequency domain while maintaining the energy of the residual noise (in the frequency domain) below the preset threshold δ. We can use the Lagrange method to solve the preceding problem. It can be shown that G satisfies the following equation:

$$G \cdot \left(F^H \cdot R_{xx} \cdot F + \mu \cdot F^H \cdot R_{dd} \cdot F\right) = F^H \cdot R_{xx} \cdot F \tag{6.110}$$

The preceding equation can be further simplified if we assume that G is a diagonal matrix. Furthermore, it can be shown that the matrices $F^H \cdot R_{\mathbf{xx}} \cdot F$ and $F^H \cdot R_{dd} \cdot F$ are asymptotically ($N \to \infty$) diagonal, assuming that the autocorrelation matrices R_{xx} and R_{dd} are Toeplitz. The diagonal elements of $F^H \cdot R_{\mathbf{xx}} \cdot F$ and $F^H \cdot R_{dd} \cdot F$ are the power spectrum components $P_{xx}(\omega_k)$ and $P_{dd}(\omega_k)$ of the clean speech vector $\mathbf{x}$ and noise vector $\mathbf{d}$, respectively, that is,

$$\begin{aligned} F^H \cdot R_{xx} \cdot F &= \mathrm{diag}(P_{xx}(0), P_{xx}(\omega_1), \ldots, P_{xx}(\omega_{N-1})) \\ F^H \cdot R_{dd} \cdot F &= \mathrm{diag}(P_{dd}(0), P_{dd}(\omega_1), \ldots, P_{dd}(\omega_{N-1})) \end{aligned} \tag{6.111}$$

Denoting the kth diagonal element of G by $g(k)$, we can simplify Equation 6.110 to

$$g(k) \cdot (P_{xx}(\omega_k) + \mu \cdot P_{dd}(\omega_k)) = P_{xx}(\omega_k) \tag{6.112}$$

The gain function $g(k)$ for the frequency component ω_k is therefore given by

$$g(k) = \frac{P_{xx}(\omega_k)}{P_{xx}(\omega_k) + \mu \cdot P_{dd}(\omega_k)} \tag{6.113}$$

which can also be expressed in terms of the *a priori* SNR ξ_k:

$$g(k) = \frac{\xi_k}{\xi_k + \mu} \tag{6.114}$$

The preceding equation is identical to the parametric Wiener filter given in Equation 6.52 (with $\beta = 1$), with the Lagrangian multiplier μ being the adjustable parameter.

It is worth noting that if we use the spectral subtraction algorithm to estimate $P_{xx}(\omega_k)$ in Equation 6.113, then the preceding gain function becomes identical to the spectral subtraction gain function. Specifically, let

$$\hat{P}_{xx}(\omega_k) = P_{yy}(\omega_k) - \mu \cdot P_{dd}(\omega_k) \tag{6.115}$$

be the estimate of $P_{xx}(\omega_k)$ in Equation 6.113. Then, after substituting Equation 6.115 in Equation 6.113, we get

$$g_{SS}(k) = 1 - \mu \frac{P_{dd}(\omega_k)}{P_{yy}(\omega_k)} \tag{6.116}$$

which is the gain function of the oversubtraction algorithm (Chapter 5). The oversubtraction factor used in [8] plays the same role as the Lagrangian multiplier μ.

Computing μ for a given threshold value δ is not straightforward, because of the nonlinear relationship between μ and δ. The equation relating μ to the threshold δ can be obtained by substituting Equation 6.114 in Equation 6.108 and making the assumption that $F^H \cdot R_{dd} \cdot F$ is asymptotically ($N \to \infty$) diagonal (see Equation 6.111):

$$\varepsilon_d^2 = \sum_{k=0}^{N-1} g^2(k) P_{dd}(\omega_k) = \sum_{k=0}^{N-1} \left(\frac{\xi_k}{\xi_k + \mu} \right)^2 P_{dd}(\omega_k) \leq \delta \tag{6.117}$$

The preceding equation provides the relationship between μ and the noise distortion and can therefore be used to assess the effect of μ on noise distortion. Similarly, we can obtain the relationship between the speech distortion ε_x^2 and μ:

$$\varepsilon_x^2 = \sum_{k=0}^{N-1} (1 - g(k))^2 P_{xx}(\omega_k) = \sum_{k=0}^{N-1} \left(\frac{\mu}{\xi_k + \mu} \right)^2 P_{xx}(\omega_k) \tag{6.118}$$

From Equations 6.117 and 6.118, we can see that the Lagrangian multiplier μ ($\mu \geq 0$) controls the trade-off between speech and noise distortions. A large μ, for instance, would produce more speech distortion but less residual noise. Conversely, a small μ would produce a smaller amount of speech distortion but more residual noise. Ideally, we would like to minimize the speech distortion in speech-dominated frames because the speech signal will mask the noise in those frames. Similarly, we would like to reduce the residual noise in noise-dominated frames. To accomplish that, we can make the value of μ dependent on the estimated segmental SNR. We can therefore choose the following equation for estimating μ:

$$\mu = \mu_0 - \left(\text{SNR}_{dB}\right)/s \tag{6.119}$$

where
μ_0 and s are constants chosen experimentally
SNR_{dB} is the segmental SNR

A different, and better, method for choosing μ based on psychoacoustically motivated constraints will be given in Section 6.11.

6.10 ESTIMATING THE WIENER GAIN FUNCTION

A noniterative approach was used in [22,24] for estimating the Wiener gain function (Equation 6.114). The focus was on getting a good (low-variance) estimate of the *a priori* SNR ξ_k needed in the Wiener gain function (Equation 6.114), because it is known [25] that a low-variance estimate of ξ_k can eliminate musical noise.

In [24], the *a priori* SNR ξ_k was estimated using the decision-directed method proposed in [26]. More specifically, ξ_k was estimated as a weighted combination of the past and present estimates of ξ_k (see Chapter 7 for more details). At frame m, $\hat{\xi}_k(m)$ was estimated as

$$\hat{\xi}_k(m) = \alpha \frac{|\hat{X}_k(m-1)|^2}{|D_k(m-1)|^2} + (1-\alpha)\max\left(\frac{|Y_k(m)|^2}{|D_k(m)|^2} - 1, 0\right) \tag{6.120}$$

where
α is a smoothing constant ($\alpha = 0.98$ in [24])
$\hat{X}_k(m-1)$ denotes the enhanced signal spectrum obtained at frame $m-1$
$Y_k(m)$, $D_k(m)$ denote the noisy speech and noise spectra, respectively

For $\alpha \approx 1$, $\hat{\xi}_k(m)$ in the preceding text can be viewed as a weighted combination of the past estimate of ξ_k and the current frame estimate, that is, $\hat{\xi}_k(m)$ can be approximated as $\hat{\xi}_k(m) \approx \alpha\hat{\xi}_k(m-1) + (1-\alpha)\tilde{\xi}(m)$, where $\tilde{\xi}_k(m)$ denotes the current frame estimate of ξ_k. This recursive relationship provides smoothness in the estimate of ξ_k and consequently can eliminate the musical noise [25]. Good performance was reported in [27] (see also Chapter 12) with the preceding algorithm. Speech enhanced by the preceding algorithm had little speech distortion but had notable residual noise.

A different approach was taken in [22] for estimating ξ_k based on the assumption that the variance of the ξ_k estimate is affected by the variance of the spectrum estimator, because, after all, ξ_k is computed as the ratio of two power spectra. This motivated the use of the low-variance spectrum estimators in [22] in place of the traditional periodogram-type spectrum estimators, which are computed as the square of the magnitude FFT spectra. More specifically, the multitaper method proposed in [28] was considered for estimating the power spectrum of the signal. The multitaper spectrum estimator of the signal $x(n)$ is given by

$$P_{xx}^{mt}(\omega) = \frac{1}{L}\sum_{k=0}^{L-1} P_k(\omega) \tag{6.121}$$

where L is the number of tapers used and

$$P_k(\omega) = \left|\sum_{n=0}^{N-1} t_k(n)x(n)e^{-j\omega n}\right|^2 \tag{6.122}$$

where $t_k(n)$ is the kth data taper (window) used for the kth spectral estimate. These tapers are chosen to be orthonormal, that is, $\Sigma_m t_k(m)t_j(m) = 0$ if $j \neq k$ and equal to 1 if $j = k$. The sine tapers [29] were used for $t_k(n)$:

$$t_k(n) = \sqrt{\frac{2}{N+1}}\sin\left(\frac{\pi k(n+1)}{N+1}\right) \quad n = 0,1,\ldots,N-1 \tag{6.123}$$

Wavelet-thresholding techniques can be used to further refine the spectral estimate and produce a smooth estimate of the logarithm of the spectrum [30].

Two different methods for estimating ξ_k were considered in [22], both based on wavelet thresholding the multitaper spectra of the noisy signal. Following multitaper spectral estimation, the *a priori* SNR ξ_k was approximated as $\hat{\xi}_k = \hat{P}_{xx}(\omega_k)/\hat{P}_{dd}(\omega_k)$, where

$$\hat{P}_{xx}(\omega) = P_{yy}(\omega) - \hat{P}_{dd}(\omega) \tag{6.124}$$

and $\hat{P}_{dd}(\omega)$ denotes the estimate of the noise spectrum obtained during speech-absent frames.

In the first method, the ratio of the multitaper spectra $\hat{P}_{xx}^{mt}(\omega)/\hat{P}_{dd}^{mt}(\omega)$ was formed, and the log of this ratio was wavelet-thresholded to get an estimate of ξ_k. It was shown in [22] that the log *a priori* SNR estimate, based on multitaper spectra denoted as ξ_k^{mt}, can be modeled as the true log *a priori* SNR, ξ_k, plus a Gaussian distributed noise $\zeta(k)$, that is,

$$\log\xi^{mt}(k) = \log\xi_k + \zeta(k) \tag{6.125}$$

where $\zeta(k)$ is approximately Gaussian distributed with zero mean and known variance. Because of the nature of $\zeta(k)$, wavelet denoising techniques [31,32] can be used to eliminate $\zeta(k)$ and therefore obtain a good estimate of ξ_k.

The second method is based on the assumption that a good estimate of the *a priori* SNR can be obtained using low-variance spectral estimates of $\hat{P}_{xx}(\omega)$ and $\hat{P}_{dd}(\omega)$. Specifically, the multitaper spectral estimates of $P_{yy}(\omega)$ and $\hat{P}_{dd}(\omega)$ are obtained first, and then the log of those estimates is wavelet-thresholded individually to obtain the refined spectrum of $\hat{P}_{xx}(\omega)$, denoted as $P_{xx}^{wmt}(\omega)$. The spectrum $P_{xx}^{wmt}(\omega)$ along with the wavelet-thresholded estimate of $\hat{P}_{dd}(\omega)$, denoted as $\hat{P}_{dd}^{wmt}(\omega)$, is then used to obtain an estimate of the *a priori* SNR, that is, $\hat{\xi}_k = \hat{P}_{xx}^{wmt}(\omega_k)/\hat{P}_{dd}^{wmt}(\omega_k)$.

The second method [22] was implemented in four steps. For each speech frame, do the following:

Step 1: Compute the multitaper power spectrum $P_{yy}^{mt}(\omega)$ of the noisy speech y using Equation 6.121, and estimate the multitaper power spectrum $P_{xx}^{mt}(\omega)$ of the clean speech signal by: $P_{xx}^{mt}(\omega) = P_{yy}^{mt}(\omega) - P_{dd}^{mt}(\omega)$, where $P_{dd}^{mt}(\omega)$ is the multitaper power spectrum of the noise obtained using noise samples collected during speech-absent frames. The number of tapers, L, was set to five. Any negative elements of $P_{xx}^{mt}(\omega)$ are floored as follows:

$$P_{xx}^{mt}(\omega) = \begin{cases} P_{yy}^{mt}(\omega) - P_{dd}^{mt}(\omega), & \text{if} \quad P_{yy}^{mt}(\omega) > (\beta+1)P_{dd}^{mt}(\omega) \\ \beta P_{dd}^{mt}(\omega), & \text{else} \end{cases}$$

where β is the spectral floor set to $\beta = 0.002$.

Step 2: Compute $Z(\omega) = \log P_{yy}^{mt}(\omega) + c$ [c is a constant determined as $c = -\phi(L) + \log L$, where $\phi(\cdot)$ is the digamma function] and then apply the discrete wavelet transform (DWT) to $Z(\omega)$ out to level q_0 to obtain the empirical DWT coefficients $z_{j,k}$ for each level j (q_0 was set to five in [22], based on listening tests). Eighth-order Daubechie's wavelets with least asymmetry and highest number of vanishing moments, for a given support, were used. Threshold the wavelet coefficients $z_{j,k}$ and apply the inverse DWT to the thresholded wavelet coefficients to obtain the refined log spectrum, $\log P_{yy}^{wmt}(\omega)$, of the noisy speech signal. Repeat this procedure to obtain the refined log spectrum, $\log P_{dd}^{wmt}(\omega)$, of the noise signal. The *a priori* SNR estimate $\hat{\xi}_k$ for frequency ω_k is finally computed as $\hat{\xi}_k = \hat{P}_{xx}^{wmt}(\omega_k)/\hat{P}_{dd}^{wmt}(\omega_k)$.

Step 3: Compute the μ value needed in Equation 6.114, according to the segmental SNR:

$$\mu = \begin{cases} \mu_0 - (\text{SNR}_{dB})/s & -5 < \text{SNR}_{dB} < 20 \\ 1 & \text{SNR}_{dB} \geq 20 \\ \mu_{\max} & \text{SNR}_{dB} \leq -5 \end{cases}$$

where μ_{max} is the maximum allowable value of μ (set to 10), $\mu_0 = (1 + 4\mu_{max})/5$, $s = 25/(\mu_{max} - 1)$, $SNR_{dB} = 10 \log_{10} SNR$, and the SNR is computed as

$$SNR = \frac{\sum_{k=0}^{N-1} P_{xx}^{wmt}(\omega_k)}{\sum_{k=0}^{N-1} P_{dd}^{wmt}(\omega_k)}$$

Step 4: Estimate the gain function $g(k)$ for frequency component ω_k using Equation 6.114. Obtain the enhanced spectrum $\hat{X}(\omega_k)$ by $\hat{X}(\omega_k) = g(k) \cdot Y(\omega_k)$. Apply the inverse FFT of $\hat{X}(\omega_k)$ to obtain the enhanced speech signal.

Two different wavelet-thresholding techniques were considered in Step 2, one based on universal level-dependent soft thresholding, and the other based on the heuristic Stein's unbiased risk estimator (SURE) method [31]. Objective and subjective listening tests showed that the heuristic SURE thresholding technique offered a slight advantage in performance. Listening tests showed no significant differences between the two methods discussed previously for estimating the *a priori* SNR ξ_k. The method described in Step 2 for estimating ξ_k was performed as well as the method based on wavelet-thresholding the ratio of $\hat{P}_{xx}^{mt}(\omega)/\hat{P}_{dd}^{mt}(\omega)$.

The proposed Wiener estimator based on wavelet-thresholding the multitaper spectra was compared against the subspace [33] and MMSE-LSA algorithms [34] using sentences corrupted at 0 and 5 dB SNR with speech-shaped and Volvo car noise. Formal listening tests indicated that the speech quality of the constrained Wiener method was found to be superior to the quality of the signal subspace method for both noise types. The speech quality of the constrained Wiener method was also found to be markedly better than the quality of the MMSE-LSA method for speech corrupted by car noise.

Listening tests in [22] showed that speech enhanced using multitaper spectra alone had some musical noise. The musical noise, however, was eliminated when the multitaper spectra were wavelet-thresholded. The authors postulated that the mechanisms responsible for that were similar to those in the MMSE method [26] and discussed in [25] (see also Chapter 7). More specifically, it was attributed to the better estimate of the *a priori* SNR ξ_k. Figure 6.18 shows example plots of the *a priori* SNR estimation for a single frequency component (312.5 Hz). As can be seen, the estimate of ξ_k obtained by wavelet-thresholding the multitaper spectra was smooth. In contrast, the estimate of ξ_k obtained with no wavelet-thresholding was more erratic. As pointed out in [25] and [35], it is this erratic behavior that produces the musical noise. Hence, the method that wavelet-thresholds the multitaper spectra eliminated the musical noise not by smoothing ξ_k directly as done by Equation 6.120, but by obtaining better (lower-variance) spectral estimates.

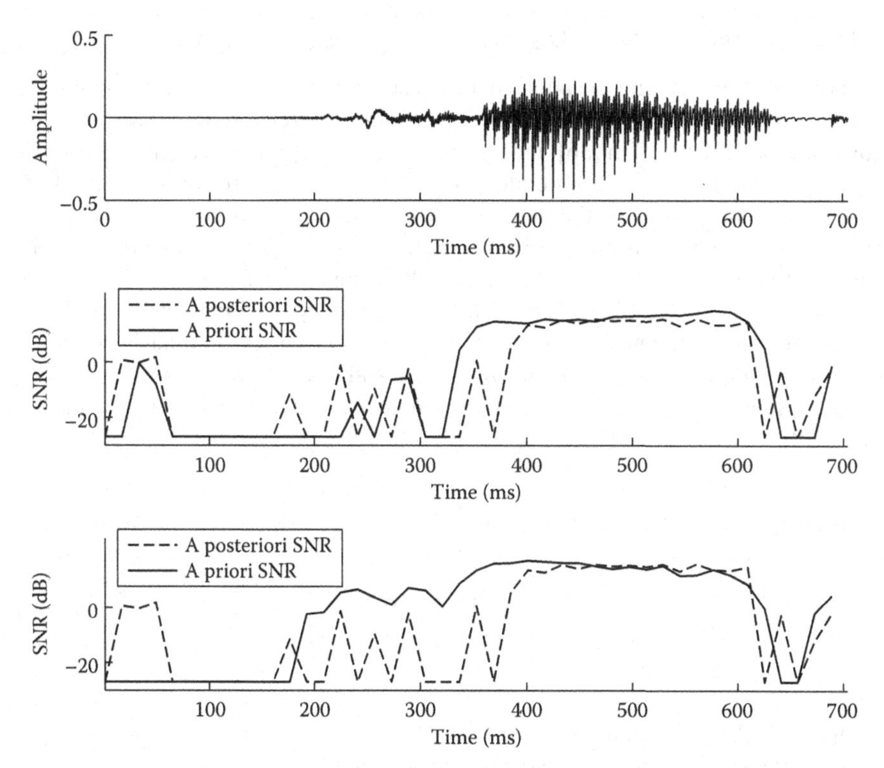

FIGURE 6.18 Estimation of the *a priori* SNR at frequency 312.5 Hz for the word *hayed* corrupted by speech-shaped noise at 15 dB. The top panel shows the clean speech file. The middle panel shows the *a priori* SNR ξ_k obtained by the multitaper method using sine tapers, and the bottom panel shows ξ_k obtained by wavelet-thresholding the multitaper spectra. The *a posteriori* SNR, defined as the ratio of the squared magnitude spectrum of the noisy speech to the noise spectrum, is shown in dashed lines for comparison. (Reprinted from Hu, Y. and Loizou, P., *IEEE Trans. Speech Audio Process.*, 12(1), 59, 2004. With permission.)

6.11 INCORPORATING PSYCHOACOUSTIC CONSTRAINTS IN WIENER FILTERING

In the preceding section, we described a method for minimizing the speech distortion while constraining the noise distortion to fall below a constant threshold value. Choosing and setting the appropriate threshold value, however, proved to be difficult owing to the resulting nonlinear relationship between the Lagrangian multiplier μ and the threshold value (see Equation 6.117). The nonlinear equation given in Equation 6.117 made it difficult to compute the μ value that would ensure that the noise distortion would fall below a given threshold. Also, there was no guarantee that the noise distortion would be rendered inaudible. Two psychoacoustically motivated methods were proposed in [21,36,37] to address these issues. The first approach proposes a method that shapes the noise distortion so as to render it inaudible, and the second approach uses the masking thresholds as constraints.

6.11.1 Shaping the Noise Distortion in the Frequency Domain

Rather than constraining the noise distortion to fall below a certain threshold, we can spectrally shape the noise distortion so that it is rendered audible. Such an approach was proposed in [36], motivated by the perceptually weighted error criterion used in low-rate speech coders (e.g., CELP). This error criterion exploits the masking properties of the auditory system and is based on the fact that the auditory system has a limited ability to detect quantization noise near the high-energy regions of the spectrum (e.g., near the formant peaks), as it is masked by the formant peaks and is therefore inaudible. Auditory masking can be exploited by shaping the frequency spectrum of the error so that less emphasis is placed near the formant peaks and more on the spectral valleys, where any amount of noise present will be audible. The error is shaped using the following perceptual filter [38]:

$$T(z) = \frac{A(z)}{A(z/\gamma)} = \frac{1 - \Sigma_{k=1}^{p} a_k z^{-k}}{1 - \Sigma_{k=1}^{p} a_k \gamma^k z^{-k}} \tag{6.126}$$

where

$A(z)$ is the LPC polynomial
a_k are the short-term linear prediction coefficients
γ is a parameter ($0 \leq \gamma \leq 1$) that controls the energy of the error in the formant regions
p is the prediction order.

Figure 6.19 shows an example of the spectrum of the perceptual filter for a speech segment extracted from the vowel/iy/in "heed." As can be seen, the perceptual filter places more emphasis on the spectral valleys and less emphasis near the formant peaks.

The preceding perceptual weighting filter was incorporated into the constrained Wiener filter to shape the noise distortion so as to make it inaudible. This was done by considering a perceptually weighted error criterion in place of the squared error criterion used in Equation 6.108. The perceptually weighted noise distortion $\varepsilon_{wd}(\omega)$ was obtained as follows:

$$\varepsilon_{wd}(\omega) = W_f \cdot \varepsilon_d(\omega) \tag{6.127}$$

where W_f is an N-dimensional diagonal perceptual weighting matrix given by

$$W_f = \begin{bmatrix} T(0) & 0 & \cdots & 0 \\ 0 & T(\omega_0) & \cdots & 0 \\ \vdots & \vdots & \ddots & \vdots \\ 0 & 0 & \cdots & T((N-1)\omega_0) \end{bmatrix} \tag{6.128}$$

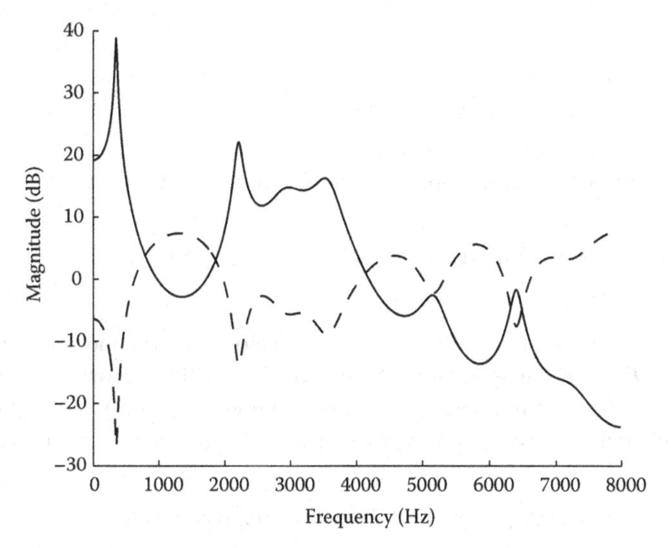

FIGURE 6.19 Example perceptual weighting filter (dashed lines) computed according to Equation 6.126 using $\gamma = 0.8$. The LPC spectrum (solid lines) is also shown for comparison.

where

$\omega_0 = 2\pi/N$

$T(\omega)$ is the frequency response of the perceptual filter given in Equation 6.126, that is, $T(\omega) = T(z)|_{z=\exp(j\omega)}$

We define the energy of the perceptually weighted noise distortion as

$$\begin{aligned}\varepsilon_{\mathbf{w}d}^2 &= E\left[\boldsymbol{\varepsilon}_{\mathbf{w}d}^H(\omega)\boldsymbol{\varepsilon}_{\mathbf{w}d}(\omega)\right] = \text{tr}\left(E\left[\boldsymbol{\varepsilon}_{\mathbf{w}d}(\omega)\boldsymbol{\varepsilon}_{\mathbf{w}d}^H(\omega)\right]\right)\\ &= \text{tr}\left(W_f E\left[\boldsymbol{\varepsilon}_d(\omega)\boldsymbol{\varepsilon}_d^H(\omega)\right]W_f^H\right)\end{aligned} \tag{6.129}$$

The new optimal linear estimator can be obtained by solving the following constrained optimization problem:

$$\begin{gathered}\min_G \varepsilon_{\mathbf{x}}^2\\ \text{subject to: } \frac{1}{N}\varepsilon_{\mathbf{w}d}^2 \le \delta\end{gathered} \tag{6.130}$$

The solution to the preceding problem can be found using similar techniques as mentioned earlier. Specifically, G is a stationary feasible point if it satisfies the gradient equation of the objective function:

$$J(G,\mu) = \varepsilon_{\mathbf{x}}^2 + \mu\left(\varepsilon_{\mathbf{w}d}^2 - N\delta\right) \tag{6.131}$$

and

$$\mu\left(\varepsilon_{wd}^2 - N\delta\right) = 0 \quad \text{for } \mu \geq 0 \tag{6.132}$$

where μ is the Lagrangian multiplier. From $\nabla_G J(G, \mu) = 0$, we have

$$\mu \cdot \left(W_f^H W_f\right) G \cdot F^H R_{dd} F + G \cdot F^H R_{xx} F = F^H R_{xx} F \tag{6.133}$$

Assuming, as mentioned earlier, that G is a diagonal matrix and that the matrices $F^H R_{xx} F$ and $F^H R_{dd} F$ are asymptotically diagonal, with the diagonal elements of $F^H R_{\mathbf{x}} F$ and $F^H R_{\mathbf{n}} F$ being the power spectrum components $P_{xx}(\omega_k)$ and $P_{dd}(\omega_k)$ of the clean speech and noise, respectively, we can simplify the preceding equation to

$$g(k) \cdot \left(P_{xx}(\omega_k) + \mu \left|T(\omega_k)\right|^2 P_{dd}(\omega_k)\right) = P_{xx}(\omega_k) \tag{6.134}$$

where $T(\omega_k)$ is the frequency response of the perceptual filter given in Equation 6.126. After solving for the gain function $g(k)$ for frequency component ω_k, we get

$$g(k) = \frac{P_{xx}(\omega_k)}{P_{xx}(\omega_k) + \mu \left|T(\omega_k)\right|^2 P_{dd}(\omega_k)} \tag{6.135}$$

Note that if $T(\omega_k) = 1$ for all frequencies, then the preceding equation reduces to Equation 6.113.

The preceding equation requires estimation of the perceptual filter $T(z)$ from the noisy signal. One possibility is to first enhance the signal (say, with spectral subtraction) and estimate $T(z)$ using the preenhanced signal. The major drawback of this approach, however, is that any distortion introduced in enhancing the signal in the first stage may lead to inaccurate estimates of $T(z)$ in the second stage. Alternatively, we can obtain $T(z)$ directly from the noisy speech. The second approach was taken in [36].

6.11.2 Using Masking Thresholds as Constraints

In Section 6.9, we derived the linear estimator that minimized the speech distortion while constraining the noise distortion to fall below a constant threshold level. The average (calculated across all frequencies) noise distortion was considered. If we now want to use the masking thresholds as constraints, we need to express the noise distortion at frequency ω_k. To do that, we first denote the kth spectral component of the noise distortion as

$$\varepsilon_{d,k} = \mathbf{e}_k^T \cdot \varepsilon_d(\omega) \tag{6.136}$$

where

$\varepsilon_d(\omega)$ is the noise distortion vector (Equation 6.106)

$\mathbf{e}_k^T$ is a selector that picks the kth component of ε_d, that is,

$$\mathbf{e}_k^T = [\underbrace{0\ldots0\ldots1}_{k}\ldots0\ldots0] \tag{6.137}$$

Having done that, we can now seek for an optimal estimator that minimizes the speech distortion, while requiring that the spectral energy of $\varepsilon_{d,k}$ be smaller than or equal to some preset threshold α_k ($\alpha_k \geq 0$, for $k = 1, 2, \ldots, N$) at frequency ω_k. These thresholds can be set to the masking threshold levels at the corresponding frequency.

Hence, we can obtain the optimal estimator by solving the following constrained optimization problem [37]:

$$\begin{gathered} \min_G \varepsilon_x^2 \\ \text{subject to: } \varepsilon_{d,k}^2 \leq \alpha_k \quad k = 1, 2, \ldots, N \end{gathered} \tag{6.138}$$

where $\varepsilon_{d,k}$ is given by Equation 6.136 and $\varepsilon_{d,k}^2 = E\left\{\left|\varepsilon_{d,k}\right|^2\right\}$. The solution to the preceding problem can be found using the method of Lagrangian multipliers. Specifically, G is a stationary feasible point if it satisfies the gradient equation of the objective function

$$J(G, \mu_1, \mu_2, \ldots, \mu_N) = \varepsilon_x^2 + \sum_{k=1}^{N} \mu_k \left(\varepsilon_{d,k}^2 - \alpha_k\right) \tag{6.139}$$

and

$$\mu_k \left(\varepsilon_{d,k}^2 - \alpha_k\right) = 0, \quad \text{for} \quad k = 1, 2, \ldots, N \tag{6.140}$$

where $\mu_k \geq 0$ is the kth Lagrangian multiplier of the constraint on the kth component of ε_d. After taking the derivative of the objective function in Equation 6.139 and setting it equal to zero, we get

$$\begin{gathered} \nabla_G J(G, \mu_1, \mu_2, \ldots, \mu_N) = 0 \\ GF^H R_{xx} F + \left(\sum_{k=1}^{N} \mu_k e_k e_k^T\right) G F^H R_{dd} F = F^H R_{xx} F \end{gathered} \tag{6.141}$$

Let Λ_μ be a diagonal matrix defined as $\Lambda_\mu = \Sigma_k \mu_k e_k e_k^T$, then the preceding equation can be rewritten as

$$GF^H R_{xx} F + \Lambda_\mu G F^H R_{dd} F_x = F^H R_{xx} F \tag{6.142}$$

To simplify matters, we assume that G is a diagonal matrix, that is, we assume that the gain is applied to each frequency component individually. As mentioned earlier, the matrices $F^H R_{xx}F$ and $F^H R_{dd}F$ are asymptotically diagonal, assuming that R_{xx} and R_{dd} are Toeplitz. The diagonal elements of $F^H R_{xx}F$ and $F^H R_{dd}F$ are the power spectrum components $P_{xx}(\omega)$ and $P_{dd}(\omega)$ of the clean speech and noise signals, respectively. Denoting the kth diagonal element of G by $g(k)$, we can rewrite Equation 6.142 as

$$g(k)\cdot\left(P_{xx}(\omega_k)+\mu_k P_{dd}(\omega_k)\right)=P_{xx}(\omega_k),\quad k=1,2,\ldots,N \tag{6.143}$$

Solving for the Wiener gain function, $g(k)$, of the kth frequency component, we get

$$\begin{aligned} g(k) &= \frac{P_{xx}(\omega_k)}{P_{xx}(\omega_k)+\mu_k P_{dd}(\omega_k)} \\ &= \frac{\xi_k}{\xi_k+\mu_k} \end{aligned} \tag{6.144}$$

where $\xi_k \triangleq P_{xx}(\omega_k)/P_{dd}(\omega_k)$. Note that the main difference between the preceding equation and Equation 6.114 is that the Lagrangian multipliers μ_k are now frequency specific. We can therefore use the μ_k values to set the constraints to the masking thresholds at frequency ω_k.

If we constrain the kth spectral component of the noise distortion to be lower than the masking threshold, denoted as T_k, in frequency bin k, then we can compute the μ_k values such that they meet this constraint. Assuming that the constraints α_k are set equal to the masking thresholds T_k and the equality in Equation 6.138 is satisfied, then $\varepsilon_{d,k}^2=\alpha_k$ implies that

$$g^2(k)P_{dd}(\omega_k)=T_k \tag{6.145}$$

Substituting Equation 6.144 in the preceding equation, with the condition that $\mu_k \geq 0$, we can obtain μ_k as

$$\mu_k=\max\left(\sqrt{\frac{P_{dd}(\omega_k)}{T_k}}-1,0\right)\frac{P_{xx}(\omega_k)}{P_{dd}(\omega_k)} \tag{6.146}$$

In terms of the *a priori* SNR ξ_k, μ_k can be expressed as

$$\mu_k=\max\left(\sqrt{\frac{P_{xx}(\omega_k)}{T_k\xi_k}}-1,0\right)\xi_k \tag{6.147}$$

Finally, plugging the preceding equation into Equation 6.144, we get an expression for $g(k)$:

$$g(k) = \frac{1}{1 + \max\left(\sqrt{\frac{P_{dd}(\omega_k)}{T_k}} - 1, 0\right)} \tag{6.148}$$

It is clear from the preceding equation that if the kth spectral component of the noise falls below the masking threshold (i.e., $P_{dd}(\omega_k) < T_k$), the gain $g(k)$ is set to 1, that is, no attenuation is applied because the kth noise spectral component is masked. Attenuation is applied only when the noise is above the masking threshold (i.e., $P_{dd}(\omega_k) > T_k$) and is therefore perceptible.

A similar gain function was derived in [21] using a simplified constrained minimization approach. Wanting to preserve background noise characteristics, the authors chose as the desired signal spectrum: $X_{DR}(\omega) = X(\omega) + \varsigma D(\omega)$, where ς defines the noise floor level. The error spectrum between the estimated spectrum obtained using a filter $H(\omega)$ and the desired spectrum $X_{DR}(\omega)$ can be expressed as

$$\begin{aligned}
\varepsilon(\omega) &= H(\omega)Y(\omega) - X_{DR}(\omega) \\
&= H(\omega)(X(\omega) + D(\omega)) - (X(\omega) + \varsigma D(\omega)) \\
&= (H(\omega) - 1)X(\omega) + (H(\omega) - \varsigma)D(\omega) \\
&= \varepsilon_x(\omega) + \varepsilon_d(\omega)
\end{aligned} \tag{6.149}$$

The second term defines the spectrum of the noise distortion. The energy of the noise distortion is computed as before as $E[\varepsilon_d^2(\omega)]$:

$$E[\varepsilon_d^2(\omega)] = (H(\omega) - \varsigma)^2 P_{dd}(\omega) \tag{6.150}$$

Note that this is the same distortion defined earlier, except that now the parabola is shifted to the right by ς, where $0 \leq \varsigma \leq 1$. The parameter ς provides an additional degree of freedom for controlling the noise distortion.

If we now want to mask the noise distortion, while allowing for a variable speech distortion, we can look for a linear estimator $H(\omega)$ that would keep the noise distortion at (or below) the masking threshold level. To do that, we set the noise distortion equal to the masking threshold:

$$\left(H(\omega_k) - \varsigma\right)^2 P_{dd}(\omega_k) = T_k \tag{6.151}$$

where T_k is the masking threshold level at frequency ω_k. Solving for $H(\omega)$ with the constraint $\varsigma \leq H(\omega_k) \leq 1$ leads to the following optimal estimator:

$$H(\omega_k) = \min\left(\sqrt{\frac{T_k}{P_{dd}(\omega_k)}} + \varsigma, 1\right) \tag{6.152}$$

Note from Equation 6.152 that if no speech is present, the masking threshold will be zero and $H(\omega_k) = \varsigma$. That is, the processed signal will be identical to the noise signal up to the attenuation factor ς, thus preserving the background noise characteristics. The noise floor factor ς was set to 0.1 in [21].

6.12 CODEBOOK-DRIVEN WIENER FILTERING

Next, we discuss an approach that uses codebooks of autoregressive spectra of the speech and noise signals to derive the Wiener filter gain function. This approach is motivated by the fact that many existing speech coders make use of codebooks of AR parameters for linear prediction synthesis. It seems reasonable, then, to want to take advantage of this and develop a speech enhancement algorithm that would integrate well with existing speech coders.

In this approach [39–41], the noisy speech spectrum is modeled as the sum of two AR spectra corresponding to the signal and noise signal spectra as follows:

$$\begin{aligned}\hat{P}_{yy}(\omega) &= \hat{P}_{xx}(\omega) + \hat{P}_{dd}(\omega) \\ &= \frac{\sigma_x^2}{|A_x(\omega)|^2} + \frac{\sigma_d^2}{|A_d(\omega)|^2}\end{aligned} \tag{6.153}$$

where σ_x^2 and σ_d^2 are the linear prediction gains of the signal and noise, respectively, and

$$A_x(\omega) = \sum_{k=0}^{p} \mathbf{a}_x(k)e^{j\omega k}, \quad A_d(\omega) = \sum_{k=0}^{q} \mathbf{a}_d(k)e^{j\omega k}, \tag{6.154}$$

where $\mathbf{a}_x = [a_x(0), a_x(1), \ldots, a_x(p)]$ and $\mathbf{a}_d = [a_d(0), a_d(1), \ldots, a_d(q)]$ are the AR coefficients of the clean and noise signals, respectively, with p and q being the respective AR-model orders. According to Equation 6.153, the following set of parameters is needed to completely represent the noisy speech spectrum $\hat{P}_{yy}(\omega)$: $\{\sigma_x^2, \sigma_d^2, \mathbf{a}_x, \mathbf{a}_d\}$. A total of $p + q + 2$ parameters are therefore needed to be estimated. The speech enhancement problem is thus reduced from that of needing to estimate the clean speech signal, to that of estimating the parameters $\{\sigma_x^2, \sigma_d^2, \mathbf{a}_x, \mathbf{a}_d\}$ assumed to have been used to generate the noisy speech signal.

We can solve the preceding parameter estimation problem by finding the best spectral fit between the observed noisy speech spectrum $P_{yy}(\omega)$ and the modeled noisy spectrum $\hat{P}_{yy}(\omega)$ with respect to a particular distortion measure; that is, we can estimate the unknown parameters by solving the following minimization problem:

$$\sigma_x^{*2}, \sigma_d^{*2}, \mathbf{a}_x^*, \mathbf{a}_d^* = \arg \min_{\sigma_x^2, \sigma_d^2, \mathbf{a}_x, \mathbf{a}_d} d\left(P_y(\omega), \hat{P}_y(\omega) \right) \tag{6.155}$$

where
 * is used to denote the optimal parameters
 $d(x,y)$ denotes the distortion measure between x and y

The distortion measure assesses how closely the modeled spectrum $\hat{P}_{yy}(\omega)$ fits the observed noisy speech spectrum $P_{yy}(\omega)$. The preceding minimization problem is difficult to solve, and the search space is vast. It can be simplified, however, if we restrict the search space by using codebooks of stored speech and noise AR spectra. We can store representative AR spectral shapes of the speech and noise signals in codebooks previously trained using a large database of speech. In doing so, we simplify the preceding minimization problem to the following:

$$\sigma_x^{*2}, \sigma_d^{*2} = \arg \min_{\mathbf{a}_x, \mathbf{a}_d} d\left(P_y(\omega), \hat{P}_y(\omega)\right) \tag{6.156}$$

where the search over all $\{\mathbf{a}_x, \mathbf{a}_d\}$ is now restricted over all pairs of $\{\mathbf{a}_x, \mathbf{a}_d\}$ contained in the speech and noise codebooks. So, for each combination of $\{\mathbf{a}_x, \mathbf{a}_d\}$, we can find the prediction gains $\left\{\sigma_x^2, \sigma_d^2\right\}$ that minimize a given spectral distortion measure. This simplifies the problem from that of needing to estimate $p + q + 2$ parameters to that of needing to estimate only two parameters, σ_x^2 and σ_d^2.

Several spectral distortion measures can potentially be used in Equation 6.156 to evaluate $d(P_y(\omega), \hat{P}_y(\omega))$. In [39], they considered the log-spectral distortion and the log-likelihood distortion measures. The log-spectral distortion measure between $P_{yy}(\omega)$ and $\hat{P}_{yy}(\omega)$ is given by

$$\begin{aligned} d\left(\hat{P}_{yy}(\omega), P_{yy}(\omega)\right) &= \frac{1}{2\pi} \int_0^{2\pi} \left| \ln \hat{P}_{yy}(\omega) - \ln P_{yy}(\omega) \right|^2 d\omega \\ &= \frac{1}{2\pi} \int_0^{2\pi} \left| \ln \left(\frac{\sigma_x^2}{|A_x(\omega)|^2} + \frac{\sigma_d^2}{|A_d(\omega)|^2} \right) - \ln P_{yy}(\omega) \right|^2 d\omega \end{aligned} \tag{6.157}$$

The preceding equation can be simplified to

$$d\left(\hat{P}_{yy}(\omega), P_{yy}(\omega)\right) = \frac{1}{2\pi}\int_0^{2\pi}\left|\ln\left(\frac{\sigma_x^2/|A_x(\omega)|^2 + \sigma_d^2/|A_d(\omega)|^2}{P_{yy}(\omega)}\right)\right|^2 d\omega$$

$$= \frac{1}{2\pi}\int_0^{2\pi}\left|\ln\left(\frac{\sigma_x^2/|A_x(\omega)|^2 + \sigma_d^2/|A_d(\omega)|^2}{P_{yy}(\omega)} - \frac{P_{yy}(\omega)}{P_{yy}(\omega)} + 1\right)\right|^2 d\omega$$

$$\approx \frac{1}{2\pi}\int_0^{2\pi}\left|\frac{\sigma_x^2/|A_x(\omega)|^2 + \sigma_d^2/|A_d(\omega)|^2 - P_{yy}(\omega)}{P_{yy}(\omega)}\right|^2 d\omega \tag{6.158}$$

after using the approximation $\ln(x + 1) \approx x$, for small x, that is, for small modeling errors. After partial differentiation of the preceding distortion measure with respect to σ_x^2 and σ_d^2, we get the following linear system of equations:

$$\begin{bmatrix} \left\|\frac{1}{P_{yy}^2(\omega)|A_x(\omega)|^4}\right\| & \left\|\frac{1}{P_{yy}^2(\omega)|A_x(\omega)|^2|A_d(\omega)|^2}\right\| \\ \left\|\frac{1}{P_{yy}^2(\omega)|A_x(\omega)|^2|A_d(\omega)|^2}\right\| & \left\|\frac{1}{P_{yy}^2(\omega)|A_d(\omega)|^4}\right\| \end{bmatrix}\begin{bmatrix}\sigma_x^2 \\ \sigma_d^2\end{bmatrix} = \begin{bmatrix} \left\|\frac{1}{P_{yy}(\omega)|A_x(\omega)|^2}\right\| \\ \left\|\frac{1}{P_{yy}(\omega)|A_d(\omega)|^2}\right\| \end{bmatrix} \tag{6.159}$$

where $\|f(\omega)\| \triangleq \int |f(\omega)| d\omega$. A similar system of equations can be derived using the log-likelihood distortion measure [39]. So, given the $\{A_x(\omega), A_d(\omega)\}$ terms, which can be retrieved from the speech and noise codebooks, respectively, and the observed power spectrum $P_{yy}(\omega)$, we can compute the optimal linear prediction gains σ_x^2 and σ_d^2 using the preceding equation.

To get a better spectral fit between the modeled and the observed spectra, it is necessary to use the AR spectrum of the observed noisy speech rather than the power spectrum estimated using the FFT. Thus, $P_{yy}(\omega)$ in the preceding equation is obtained as

$$P_{yy}(\omega) = \frac{\sigma_y^2}{|A_y(\omega)|^2}, \quad A_y(\omega) = \sum_{k=0}^{r} a_y(k)e^{-j\omega k} \tag{6.160}$$

where $a_y(k)$ are the AR coefficients of the noisy speech signal obtained using linear prediction analysis, and σ_y^2 is the linear prediction gain computed according to Equation 6.26 as

$$\sigma_y^2 = r_{yy}(0) - \sum_{k=1}^{r} a_y(k)r_{yy}(k) \tag{6.161}$$

where $r_{yy}(k)$ is the autocorrelation sequence of the noisy speech signal.

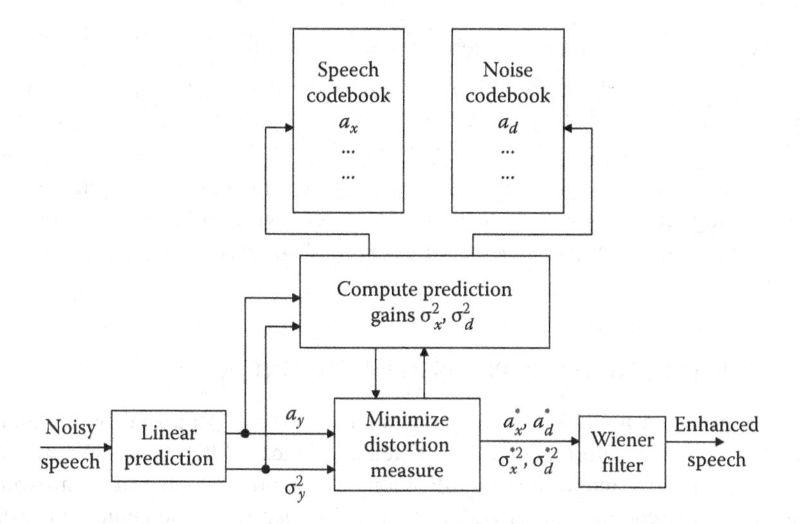

FIGURE 6.20 Block diagram of the codebook-driven Wiener filtering approach proposed in [39].

The codebook-driven Wiener filtering algorithm can be summarized as follows (see also block diagram in Figure 6.20). For each pair of speech and noise AR spectra from the respective codebooks, calculate first the prediction gains according to Equation 6.159 and then evaluate the distortion measure given in Equation 6.157. The speech and noise AR spectra that minimize the distortion measure over all pairs of $\{\mathbf{a}_x, \mathbf{a}_d\}$ stored in the codebooks are then used as the estimates of the clean and noise spectra in the Wiener filter:

$$H(\omega) = \frac{\dfrac{\sigma_x^{2*}}{|A_x^*(\omega)|^2}}{\dfrac{\sigma_x^{2*}}{|A_x^*(\omega)|^2} + \dfrac{\sigma_d^{2*}}{|A_d^*(\omega)|^2}} \tag{6.162}$$

where the asterisk (*) is used to indicate the optimal parameter values (and not complex conjugation).

An attractive feature of the preceding algorithm is the potential to perform well in the presence of nonstationary noise, because the use of noise codebooks eliminates the need for noise-estimation algorithms. The main drawback, however, is the complexity involved in the codebook search. The complexity is determined by the size of the two codebooks as well as the order of the AR models of speech and noise, p and q. The search, for instance, for a 1,024-level speech codebook and a 64-level noise codebook (as used in [39]) would involve a total of 65,536 (=1,024 × 64) distortion measure evaluations per frame. An iterative technique was proposed in [39] to reduce the codebook search complexity. Rather than performing a joint search of the best pair of all-pole coefficients $\{\mathbf{a}_x, \mathbf{a}_d\}$, a sequential search was conducted of the two codebooks. The speech codebook was searched first for the best $\{\mathbf{a}_x, \sigma_x^2, \sigma_d^2\}$ using an initial estimate of the AR spectrum of noise, $\mathbf{a}_d$, obtained using a noise-estimation algorithm. Then, the noise codebook was searched with $\mathbf{a}_x$ to obtain the best $\{\mathbf{a}_d, \sigma_x^2, \sigma_d^2\}$. The preceding two steps were repeated until there was no change in the distortion measure. Two to three iterations were found to be sufficient in [39]. The preceding algorithm was extended in [41] to account for different types of noise. A classified noise codebook scheme was proposed that used different noise codebooks for different noise types.

6.13 AUDIBLE NOISE SUPPRESSION ALGORITHM

Last, we discuss a novel speech enhancement algorithm proposed by Tsoukalas et al. [42,43], which, although not formulated as a Wiener filter, uses a Wiener-type function for spectral magnitude modification. The approach is based on a psychoacoustically derived quantity termed *audible noise spectrum*. The authors identified and derived, in a rigorous fashion, the residual noise that is audible and proposed a technique to suppress it.

Let $P_{xx}(\omega_k)$ and $P_{dd}(\omega_k)$ be the power spectra of the clean and noise signals, respectively, and $P_{dd}(\omega_k)$ be the power spectrum of the noisy speech signal. Based on the masking threshold levels, one can derive mathematically the audible spectral components. Generally, the audible spectral components are the ones lying above the masking threshold and can therefore be derived mathematically by taking the maximum between the power spectrum of speech and the corresponding masking threshold per frequency component. With this, let us define the audible spectrum of the noisy speech and the audible spectrum of the clean speech as $A_y(\omega_k)$ and $A_x(\omega_k)$:

$$A_y(\omega_k) = \max\{P_{yy}(\omega_k), T(\omega_k)\}$$
$$= \begin{cases} P_{yy}(\omega_k) & \text{if } P_{yy}(\omega_k) \geq T(\omega_k) \\ T(\omega_k) & \text{if } P_{yy}(\omega_k) < T(\omega_k) \end{cases} \tag{6.163}$$

$$A_x(\omega_k) = \max\{P_{xx}(\omega_k), T(\omega_k)\}$$
$$= \begin{cases} P_{xx}(\omega_k) & \text{if } P_{xx}(\omega_k) \geq T(\omega_k) \\ T(\omega_k) & \text{if } P_{xx}(\omega_k) < T(\omega_k) \end{cases} \tag{6.164}$$

where $T(\omega_k)$ is the masking threshold of frequency bin k. The spectral components that are perceived as noise, henceforth referred to as the *audible spectrum of additive noise*, can be expressed as the difference between the audible spectra of the noisy and clean speech; that is, the audible spectrum of the noise, denoted as $A_d(\omega_k)$, is expressed as

$$A_d(\omega_k) = A_y(\omega_k) - A_x(\omega_k) \tag{6.165}$$

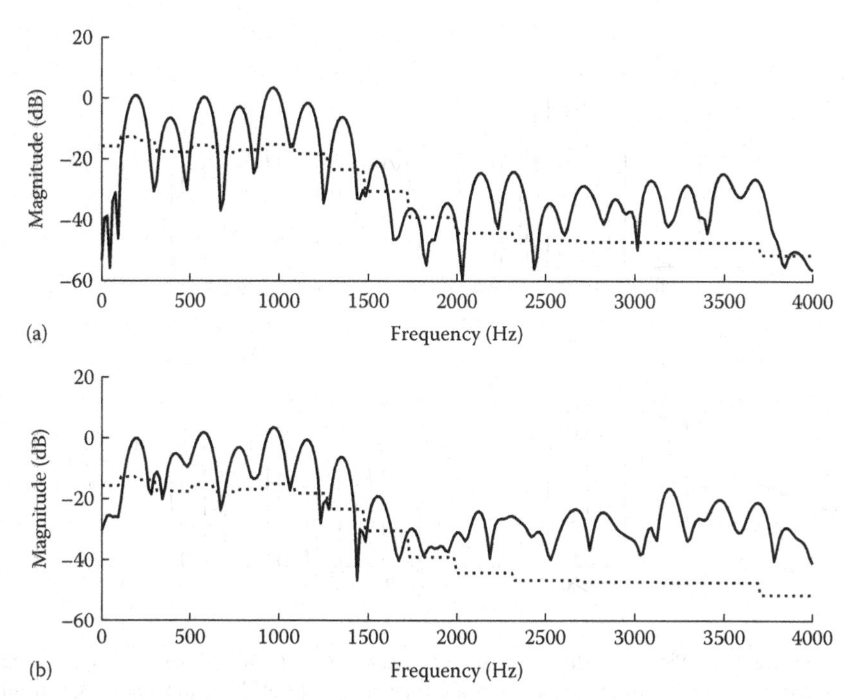

FIGURE 6.21 (a) Plot of clean speech spectrum (solid lines) along with the corresponding masking thresholds shown in dashed lines. (b) Plot of the noisy speech spectrum (solid lines) along with the corresponding masking thresholds. Masking thresholds were obtained using the clean signal.

Figure 6.21 shows power spectra of the clean and noisy signals, along with the masking threshold levels obtained using the clean signal. Figure 6.22a plots the difference spectra between the noisy and clean power spectra, that is, $P_{yy}(\omega_k) - P_{xx}(\omega_k)$, along with the masking thresholds. In principle, the difference spectrum corresponds to the noise spectrum (if we neglect the cross-power spectra terms). The audible noise spectrum, computed according to Equation 6.165, is also shown in Figure 6.22b and consists for the most part of noise spectral components lying above the masking threshold level (see Figure 6.22a). These components will be audible, as they lie above the masking threshold and will therefore need to be eliminated or reduced. The algorithm by Tsoukalas et al. [42] was designed to achieve just that.

A more detailed expression for $A_d(\omega_k)$ can be derived by substituting Equations 6.163 and 6.164 into Equation 6.165, yielding

$$A_d\left(\omega_k\right) = \begin{cases} P_{yy}(\omega_k) - P_{xx}(\omega_k) & \text{if } P_{yy}(\omega_k) \geq T(\omega_k) \text{ and } P_{xx}(\omega_k) \geq T(\omega_k) \quad \text{(I)} \\ P_{yy}(\omega_k) - T(\omega_k) & \text{if } P_{yy}(\omega_k) \geq T(\omega_k) \text{ and } P_{xx}(\omega_k) < T(\omega_k) \quad \text{(II)} \\ T(\omega_k) - P_{xx}(\omega_k) & \text{if } P_{yy}(\omega_k) < T(\omega_k) \text{ and } P_{xx}(\omega_k) \geq T(\omega_k) \quad \text{(III)} \\ 0 & \text{if } P_{yy}(\omega_k) < T(\omega_k) \text{ and } P_{xx}(\omega_k) < T(\omega_k) \quad \text{(IV)} \end{cases} \tag{6.166}$$

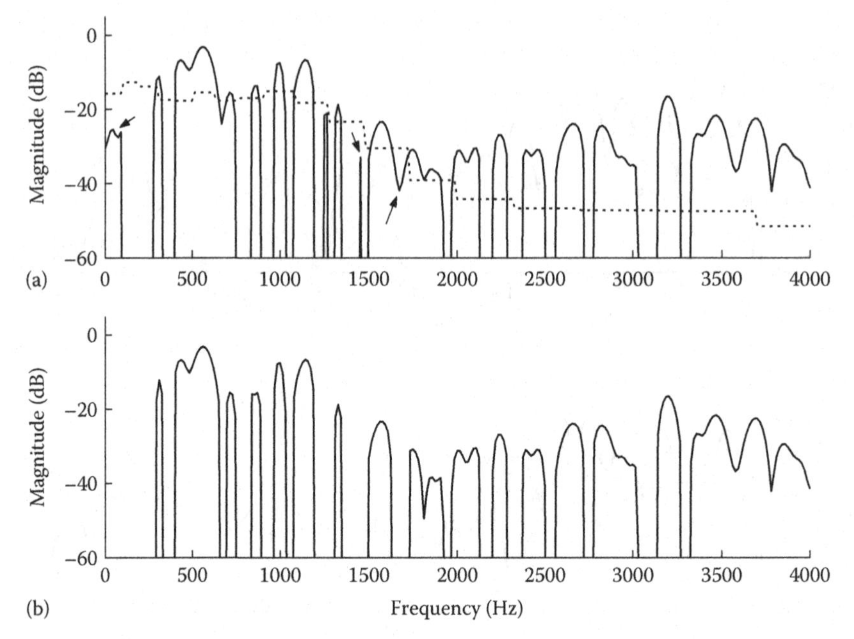

FIGURE 6.22 (a) Plot of the difference spectra, i.e., $P_{yy}(\omega_k) - P_{xx}(\omega_k)$, along with the masking threshold levels. Only positive differences are shown. (b) Plot of the audible noise spectrum $A_d(\omega_k)$. Only positive values of $A_d(\omega_k)$ are shown.

Examination of the preceding equation shows that the audible noise spectrum could either be negative or zero for cases III and IV. In these two cases, there is no audible noise present because $P_{yy}(\omega_k) < T(\omega_k)$; therefore, no modification needs to be made to the noisy speech power spectrum $P_{yy}(\omega_k)$. Case II, on the other hand, is always positive or zero (if $T(\omega_k) = P_{yy}(\omega_k)$), and clearly the audible noise needs to be removed or attenuated. Case I may be either positive, zero, or negative, depending on the values of $P_{yy}(\omega_k)$ and $P_{xx}(\omega_k)$. Of the four cases in Equation 6.166, only cases I and II need to be dealt with to render the noise inaudible. Therefore, the main objective of the proposed audible noise suppression algorithm is to modify the noisy speech spectrum $P_{yy}(\omega_k)$ in a way that would make the audible noise spectrum, $A_d(\omega_k)$, negative or zero. In doing so, the residual noise (produced after the spectral modification) will be made inaudible.

Suppose now that the noisy power spectrum $P_{yy}(\omega_k)$ is spectrally modified to yield the enhanced speech spectrum, denoted by $\hat{P}_{xx}(\omega_k)$. Then the modified audible noise spectrum, denoted by $\hat{A}_d(\omega_k)$, must satisfy the following condition:

$$\hat{A}_d(\omega_k) \leq 0 \quad 0 \leq k \leq N-1 \tag{6.167}$$

where N is the size of the FFT. Note that branches III and IV in Equation 6.166 will not be affected by the spectral modification, as they do not contribute to the audible noise components. For spectral modification of the noisy speech spectrum, Tsoukalas et al. [42] chose a parametric, Wiener-type function of the form

$$\hat{P}_{xx}(\omega_k) = \frac{P_{yy}^{\nu(k)}(\omega_k)}{\alpha^{\nu(k)}(\omega_k) + P_{yy}^{\nu(k)}(\omega_k)} P_{yy}(\omega_k) \tag{6.168}$$

where $\alpha(\omega_k)$ and $\nu(k)$ are time-frequency varying parameters, which are assumed to be positive. The preceding Wiener-type function was chosen because it allows for a flexible suppression of individual spectral components by appropriately manipulating the parameters $\alpha(\omega_k)$ and $\nu(k)$. As shown in [42], the main difference between the preceding suppression rule and the Wiener rule is that it provides relatively constant attenuation at low-input SNRs. In contrast, both spectral subtraction and Wiener filtering algorithms provide progressively heavy attenuation at very low SNRs (see Figure 6.3).

The optimal spectral modification of the noisy speech spectrum can be achieved by adjusting the parameters $\alpha(\omega_k)$ and $\nu(k)$ in Equation 6.168 to meet constraints I and II given in Equation 6.166 (constraints III and IV are not to be affected by the spectral modification)—that is, after substituting Equation 6.168 for $P_{yy}(\omega_k)$ in Equation 6.166, we can compute the parameters $\alpha(\omega_k)$ and $\nu(k)$ that satisfy constraints I and II:

$$\begin{aligned} &\frac{P_{yy}^{\nu(k)}(\omega_k)}{\alpha^{\nu(k)}(\omega_k) + P_{yy}^{\nu(k)}(\omega_k)} P_{yy}(\omega_k) - P_{xx}(\omega_k) \le 0, \quad \text{if } P_{xx}(\omega_k) \ge T(\omega_k) \quad \text{(I)} \\ &\frac{P_{yy}^{\nu(k)}(\omega_k)}{\alpha^{\nu(k)}(\omega_k) + P_{yy}^{\nu(k)}(\omega_k)} P_{yy}(\omega_k) - T(\omega_k) \le 0, \quad \text{if } P_{xx}(\omega_k) < T(\omega_k) \quad \text{(II)} \end{aligned} \tag{6.169}$$

To simplify matters, Tsoukalas et al. [42] chose to adapt $\alpha(\omega_k)$ for a fixed value of $\nu(k)$. The derived solution for the optimal $\alpha(\omega_k)$ had the disadvantage of relying on a good estimate of the whole clean speech spectrum; hence, they opted to estimate the critical-band spectrum of the clean speech signal instead. This reduced the dimensionality of the problem from that of needing to estimate N frequency components to that of estimating B critical-band components ($B = 22$ for a 16 kHz sampling frequency and $B = 18$ for telephone speech).

Two solutions were proposed for the estimation of the parameter $\alpha(\omega_k)$, one that relied on an estimate of the spectral minima within each critical band and the other that relied on an estimate of the auditory masking thresholds. The spectral minima solution had the form

$$\alpha_M(i) = \left(D_b(i) + X_{\min}(i)\right)\left[\frac{D_b(i)}{X_{\min}(i)}\right]^{1/\nu(i)}, \quad 1 \le i \le B \tag{6.170}$$

and the threshold solution had the form

$$\alpha_T(i) = (D_b(i) + T(i))\left[\frac{D_b(i)}{T(i)}\right]^{1/\nu(i)}, \quad 1 \le i \le B \tag{6.171}$$

where

B is the number of critical bands
$D_b(i)$ is the estimate of the noise spectrum in the ith critical band
$X_{\min}(i)$ is the minimum of the clean speech spectrum within the ith band
$T(i)$ is the estimated masking threshold of the ith band

Note that the parameters $\alpha_M(i)$ and $\nu(i)$ are now a function of the critical band and not the discrete frequency index ω_k and are assumed to be constant within each band. The preceding solutions (Equations 6.170 and 6.171) satisfy the constraint in Equation 6.167 when substituted in Equation 6.168, thereby suppressing any audible noise components present [42]. Because the clean speech spectrum is typically not available, a statistical estimator was derived for $X_{\min}(i)$ in Equation 6.170, based on the assumption that the probability distribution of the minimum spectral component had a Rayleigh form.

An iterative procedure can be used to get a good estimate of the auditory threshold values $T(i)$ in Equation 6.171, using an approach that resembled the iterative Wiener filtering algorithm [10] described earlier. Specifically, the procedure consisted of passing the noisy speech signal through the suppression function given in Equation 6.168 with $\nu(i) = 1$ several times. A better estimate of the clean speech signal is obtained at each iteration, and consequently, a more accurate estimate of the auditory masking thresholds $T(i)$ is expected to be derived. The jth iteration of the iterative procedure is given by

$$\hat{P}_{xx}^{(j)}(i) = \frac{\hat{P}_{xx}^{(j-1)}(i)}{\alpha^{(j)}(i) + \hat{P}_{xx}^{(j-1)}(i)} \hat{P}_{xx}^{(j-1)}(i) \tag{6.172}$$

where $\alpha^{(j)}(i)$ is given by:

$$\alpha^{(j)}(i) = D^{(j-1)}(i) + \frac{(D^{(j-1)}(i))^2}{T^{(j)}(i)} \tag{6.173}$$

where $D^{(j)}(i)$ indicates the estimate of the noise power in the ith band at iteration j. The preceding iterative algorithm was initialized with the noisy speech power spectrum, that is, $\hat{P}_{xx}^{(0)}(i) = P_{yy}(i)$. The initial approximation of the masking threshold in Equation 6.173, that is, $T^{(1)}(i)$, was based on an estimate of the clean spectrum obtained after passing the noisy speech signal through power spectrum subtraction.

The audible noise suppression algorithm based on the masking threshold method (Equation 6.171) is outlined in the following text. For each speech frame, do the following:

Step 1: Obtain the power spectrum $P_{yy}(\omega_k)$ of the noisy speech signal using the FFT. Save the phase of the noisy speech spectrum.

Step 2: Perform power spectrum subtraction to obtain an estimate of the clean power spectrum, $\hat{P}_{xx}(\omega_k)$.

Step 3: Estimate the masking thresholds using the spectrum obtained in Step 2, and use these masking thresholds as the initial $T^{(1)}(i)$ in Equation 6.173. Run the iterative algorithm given in Equations 6.172 and 6.173 to obtain a better estimate of the masking thresholds $T(i)$ (three iterations were found to be sufficient in [42]).

Step 4: Modify the noisy power spectrum $P_{yy}(\omega_k)$ according to Equations 6.168 and 6.171, using the masking threshold values obtained in Step 3. Set $\nu(i) = 1$ in Equation 6.168.

Step 5: Compute the inverse FFT of the magnitude spectrum estimated in Step 4 using the noisy speech phase spectrum.

Simulation results [42], based on objective measurements, showed that the algorithm was not too sensitive to the choice of $\nu(i)$, with $\nu(i) = 1$ (for all i) giving the best results. In addition to the objective measurement tests, several intelligibility tests were conducted using the diagnostic intelligibility rhyme test administered in both English and Greek. Results indicated that both estimators (based on spectral minima and threshold parameters) yielded large improvements in intelligibility at −5 dB SNR. For the English DRT test, both methods yielded about 30% improvement in intelligibility scores, and for the Greek DRT test, the minima estimator yielded a 20% improvement whereas the threshold estimator yielded a 13% improvement in intelligibility. The intelligibility of speech processed by the audible noise suppression algorithm was also evaluated in [44] with normal and hearing-impaired listeners. Small, but statistically significant, improvements in intelligibility were observed in some but not all of the tested noise conditions.

6.14 SUMMARY

This chapter described several variations of the Wiener filtering algorithm for speech enhancement applications. The Wiener filtering algorithm can be implemented either iteratively or noniteratively. The iterative algorithm generally assumed a model of the clean spectrum and attempted to estimate the parameters of the model iteratively. The AR speech production model (Equation 6.68) was used successfully in [10] for estimating the Wiener filter. The main drawback of the iterative Wiener filtering approach was that as additional iterations were performed, the speech formants shifted in location and decreased in formant bandwidth [13]. We described several methods [13,20] that imposed spectral constraints, both across frames and within each frame, to ensure that the AR spectra did not have unnaturally narrow formant bandwidths, and the formant peaks did not move erratically from frame to frame. The imposed constraints significantly improved the performance of the iterative Wiener filtering approach.

In Equation 6.38, we expressed the Wiener filter as a function of the ratio of the clean signal power spectrum to the noise power spectrum, that is, the *a priori* SNR. Several have attempted to estimate the *a priori* SNR, rather than the clean signal power spectrum [22,24,37]. Several noniterative Wiener filtering algorithms were proposed that focused on getting good estimates of the *a priori* SNR with the use of low-variance spectral estimators (multitaper based). We presented several psychoacoustically motivated Wiener filters [21,36,37] that were derived by solving a constrained minimization problem. More specifically, the Wiener filters were derived by minimizing the speech distortion subject to the noise distortion falling below a given threshold level (e.g., masking threshold).

The Wiener filters are derived under the assumption that the signals analyzed are stationary. The Wiener filters can also be extended to handle nonstationary signals and noise with the use of *Kalman filters*. Kalman filters can be viewed as sequential mean-square estimators of a signal embedded in noise [4, Chapter 10; 12, Chapter 13]. Kalman filters characterize the signal by a dynamical or state model; as such, the enhanced signal is obtained on a sample-by-sample basis rather than on a frame-by-frame basis, as done with the Wiener filters. Several speech enhancement methods based on Kalman filtering were proposed, and the interested reader can consult [45–49], and the references therein, for more details.

The Wiener filters are considered to be linear estimators of the clean signal spectrum, and they are optimal in the mean-square sense. These filters, however, are constrained to be linear; that is, the enhanced time-domain signal is obtained by convolving the noisy speech signal with a linear (Wiener) filter. Equivalently, in the frequency domain, the enhanced spectrum is obtained by multiplying the input (noisy) spectrum by the Wiener filter. The linear estimators, however, are not necessarily the best estimators of the clean signal spectrum. Nonlinear estimators of the clean signal spectrum could potentially yield better performance, and these estimators are discussed next.

REFERENCES

1. Wiener, N. (1949), *Extrapolation, Interpolation and Smoothing of Stationary Time Series with Engineering Applications*, Cambridge, MA: MIT Press.
2. Wiener, N. and Hopf, E. (1931), On a class of singular integral equations, *Proc. Russ. Acad. Math. Phys.*, pp. 696–706.
3. Marple, L. (1987), *Digital Spectral Analysis with Applications*, Englewood Cliffs, NJ: Prentice Hall.
4. Haykin, S. (2002), *Adaptive Filter Theory*, 4th ed., Englewood Cliffs, NJ: Prentice Hall.
5. Widrow, B. and Stearns, S. (1985), *Adaptive Signal Processing*, Englewood Cliffs, NJ: Prentice Hall.
6. Chen, J., Benesty, J., Huang, Y., and Doclo, S. (2006), New insights into the noise reduction Wiener filter, *IEEE Trans. Speech Audio Process.*, 14(4), 1218–1234.
7. Lim, J. and Oppenheim, A.V. (1979), Enhancement and bandwidth compression of noisy speech, *Proc. IEEE*, 67(12), 1586–1604.
8. Berouti, M., Schwartz, M., and Makhoul, J. (1979), Enhancement of speech corrupted by acoustic noise, *Proceedings of IEEE International Conference on Acoustics, Speech, Signal Processing*, Washington, DC, pp. 208–211.
9. McAulay, R.J. and Malpass, M.L. (1980), Speech enhancement using a soft-decision noise suppression filter, *IEEE Trans. Acoust. Speech Signal Process.*, 28, 137–145.
10. Lim, J. and Oppenheim, A.V. (1978), All-pole modeling of degraded speech, *IEEE Trans. Acoust. Speech Signal Process.*, 26(3), 197–210.
11. Hansen, J. (1988), Analysis and compensation of stressed and noisy speech with application to robust automatic recognition, PhD, dissertation Georgia Institute of Technology, Atlanta, GA.
12. Kay, S. (1993), *Fundamentals of Statistical Signal Processing: Estimation Theory,* Upper Saddle River, NJ: Prentice Hall.

13. Hansen, J. and Clements, M. (1991), Constrained iterative speech enhancement with application to speech recognition, *IEEE Trans. Signal Process.*, 39(4), 795–805.
14. Sreenivas, T. and Kirnapure, P. (1996), Codebook constrained Wiener filtering for speech enhancement, *IEEE Trans. Acoust. Speech Signal Process.*, 4(5), 383–389.
15. Hansen, J.H.L. and Clements, M. (1987), Iterative speech enhancement with spectral constraints, *Proceedings of IEEE International Conference on Acoustics, Speech, Signal Processing*, Dallas, TX, Vol. 12, pp. 189–192.
16. Hansen, J.H.L. and Clements, M. (1988), Constrained iterative speech enhancement with application to speech recognition, *Proceedings of IEEE International Conference on Acoustics, Speech, Signal Processing*, New York, Vol. 1, pp. 561–564.
17. Quatieri, T. and Dunn, R. (2002), Speech enhancement based on auditory spectral change, *Proceedings of IEEE International Conference on Acoustics, Speech, Signal Processing*, Vol. I, pp. 257–260.
18. Quatieri, T. and Baxter, R. (1997), Noise reduction based on spectral change, *IEEE Workshop on Applications of Signal Processing to Audio and Acoustics*, New Paltz, NY, pp. 8.2.1–8.2.4.
19. Furui, S. (2001), *Digital Speech Processing, Synthesis and Recognition*, 2nd ed., New York: Marcel Dekker.
20. Pellom, B. and Hansen, J. (1998), An improved (Auto:I, LSP:T) constrained iterative speech enhancement for colored noise environments, *IEEE Trans. Speech Audio Process.*, 6(6), 573–579.
21. Gustafsson, S., Jax, P., and Vary, P. (1998), A novel psychoacoustically motivated audio enhancement algorithm preserving background noise characteristics, *Proceedings of IEEE International Conference on Acoustics, Speech, Signal Processing*, Seattle, WA, pp. 397–400.
22. Hu, Y. and Loizou, P. (2004), Speech enhancement based on wavelet thresholding the multitaper spectrum, *IEEE Trans. Speech Audio Process.*, 12(1), 59–67.
23. Hu, Y. (2003), Subspace and multitaper methods for speech enhancement, PhD dissertation, University of Texas-Dallas, Richardson, TX.
24. Scalart, P. and Filho, J. (1996), Speech enhancement based on *a priori* signal to noise estimation, *Proceedings of IEEE International Conference on Acoustics, Speech, Signal Processing*, Atlanta, GA, pp. 629–632.
25. Cappe, O. (1994), Elimination of the musical noise phenomenon with the Ephraim and Malah noise suppressor, *IEEE Trans. Speech Audio Process.*, 2(2), 346–349.
26. Ephraim, Y. and Malah, D. (1984), Speech enhancement using a minimum mean-square error short-time spectral amplitude estimator, *IEEE Trans. Acoust. Speech Signal Process.*, 32(6), 1109–1121.
27. Hu, Y. and Loizou, P. (2006), Subjective comparison of speech enhancement algorithms, *Proceedings of IEEE International Conference on Acoustics, Speech, Signal Processing*, Toulouse, France, Vol. I, pp. 153–156.
28. Thomson, D. (1982), Spectrum estimation and harmonic analysis, *Proc. IEEE*, 70(9), 1055–1096.
29. Riedel, K. and Sidorenko, A. (1995), Minimum bias multiple taper spectral estimation, *IEEE Trans. Signal Process.*, 43, 188–195.
30. Walden, A., Percival, B., and McCoy, E. (1998), Spectrum estimation by wavelet thresholding of multitaper estimators, *IEEE Trans. Signal Process.*, 46, 3153–3165.
31. Donoho, D. (1995), De-noising by soft-thresholding, *IEEE Trans. Inform. Theory*, 41, 613–627.
32. Johnstone, I.M. and Silverman, B.W. (1997), Wavelet threshold estimators for data with correlated noise, *J. R. Stat. Soc. B*, 59, 319–351.
33. Hu, Y. and Loizou, P. (2003), A generalized subspace approach for enhancing speech corrupted by colored noise, *IEEE Trans. Speech Audio Process.*, 11, 334–341.

34. Ephraim, Y. and Malah, D. (1985), Speech enhancement using a minimum mean-square error log-spectral amplitude estimator, *IEEE Trans. Acoust. Speech Signal Process.*, 23(2), 443–445.
35. Vary, P. (1985), Noise suppression by spectral magnitude estimation: Mechanism and theoretical limits, *Signal Process.*, 8, 387–400.
36. Hu, Y. and Loizou, P. (2003), A perceptually motivated approach for speech enhancement, *IEEE Trans. Speech Audio Process.*, 11(5), 457–465.
37. Hu, Y. and Loizou, P. (2004), Incorporating a psychoacoustical model in frequency domain speech enhancement, *IEEE Signal Process. Lett.*, 11(2), 270–273.
38. Kroon, P. and Atal, B. (1992), Predictive coding of speech using analysis-by-synthesis techniques, in Furui, S. and Sondhi, M. (Eds.), *Advances in Speech Signal Processing*, New York: Marcel Dekker, pp. 141–164.
39. Srinivasan, S., Samuelsson, J., and Kleijn, B. (2003), Speech enhancement using a-priori information, *Proc. Eurospeech*, 2, 1405–1408.
40. Kuropatwinski, M. and Kleijn, B. (2001), Estimation of the excitation variances of speech and noise AR models for enhanced speech coding, *Proceedings of IEEE International Conference on Acoustics, Speech, Signal Processing*, Salt Lake City, UT, pp. 669–672.
41. Srinivasan, S., Samuelsson, J., and Kleijn, B. (2006), Codebook driven short-term predictor parameter estimation for speech enhancement, *IEEE Trans. Speech Audio Process.*, 14(1), 163–176.
42. Tsoukalas, D.E., Mourjopoulos, J.N., and Kokkinakis, G. (1997), Speech enhancement based on audible noise suppression, *IEEE Trans. Speech Audio Process.*, 5(6), 497–514.
43. Tsoukalas, D.E., Paraskevas, M., and Mourjopoulos, J.N. (1993), Speech enhancement using psychoacoustic criteria, *Proceedings of IEEE International Conference on Acoustics, Speech, Signal Processing*, Minneapolis, MN, pp. 359–362.
44. Arehart, K., Hansen, J., Gallant, S., and Kalstein, L. (2003), Evaluation of an auditory masked threshold noise suppression algorithm in normal-hearing and hearing-impaired listeners, *Speech Commun.*, 40, 575–592.
45. Paliwal, K. and Basu, A. (1987), A speech enhancement method based on Kalman filtering, *Proceedings of IEEE International Conference on Acoustics, Speech, Signal Processing*, Dallas, TX, Vol. 6, pp. 177–180.
46. Gibson, J., Koo, B., and Gray, S. (1991), Filtering of colored noise for speech enhancement and coding, *IEEE Trans. Signal Process.*, 39(8), 1732–1742.
47. Goh, Z., Tan, K., and Tan, B. (1999), Kalman-filtering speech enhancement method based on a voiced-unvoiced speech model, *IEEE Trans. Speech Audio Process.*, 7(5), 510–524.
48. Gabrea, M., Grivel, E., and Najim, M. (1999), A single microphone Kalman filter-based noise canceller, *IEEE Signal Process. Lett.*, 6(3), 55–57.
49. Gannot, S. (2005), Speech enhancement: Application of the Kalman filter in the Estimate-Maximize (EM) framework, in Benesty, J., Makino, S., and Chen, J. (Eds.), *Speech Enhancement*, Berlin, Germany: Springer, pp. 161–198.

7 Statistical-Model-Based Methods

In the previous chapter, we described the Wiener filter approach to speech enhancement. This approach derives in the mean-square sense the optimal complex discrete Fourier transform (DFT) coefficients of the clean signal. The Wiener filter approach yields a linear estimator of the complex spectrum of the signal and is optimal in the minimum mean-square-error (MMSE) sense when both the (complex) noise and speech DFT coefficients are assumed to be independent Gaussian random variables. In this chapter, we focus on nonlinear estimators of the magnitude (i.e., the modulus of the DFT coefficients) rather than the complex spectrum of the signal (as done by the Wiener filter), using various statistical models and optimization criteria. These nonlinear estimators take the probability density function (pdf) of the noise and the speech DFT coefficients explicitly into account and use, in some cases, non-Gaussian prior distributions. These estimators are often combined with soft-decision gain modifications that take the probability of speech presence into account.

The speech enhancement problem is posed in a statistical estimation framework [1]. Given a set of measurements that depend on an unknown parameter, we wish to find a nonlinear estimator of the parameter of interest. In our application, the measurements correspond to the set of DFT coefficients of the noisy signal (i.e., the noisy spectrum) and the parameters of interest are the set of DFT coefficients of the clean signal (i.e., the clean signal spectrum). Various techniques exist in the estimation theory literature [1] for deriving these nonlinear estimators and include the maximum-likelihood (ML) estimators and the Bayesian estimators (e.g., MMSE and maximum *a posteriori* estimators). These estimators differ primarily in the assumptions made about the parameter of interest (e.g., deterministic but unknown, random) and the form of optimization criteria used.

7.1 MAXIMUM-LIKELIHOOD ESTIMATORS

The ML approach [1, Chapter 7] is perhaps the most popular approach in statistical estimation theory for deriving practical estimators and is often used even for the most complicated estimation problems. It was first applied to speech enhancement by McAulay and Malpass [2].

Suppose that we are given an N-point data set $\mathbf{y} = \{y(0), y(1), \ldots, y(N-1)\}$ that depends on an unknown parameter θ. In speech enhancement, $\mathbf{y}$ (the observed data set) might be the noisy speech magnitude spectrum, and the parameter of interest, θ, might be the clean speech magnitude spectrum. Furthermore, suppose that we know the pdf of $\mathbf{y}$, which we denote by $p(\mathbf{y}; \theta)$. The pdf of $\mathbf{y}$ is parameterized by the unknown parameter θ, and we denote that by the semicolon. As the parameter θ affects the probability of **y**, we should be able to infer the values of θ from the observed values of **y**; that is, we can ask the question, *what value of* θ *most likely produced the observed data* **y**? Mathematically, we can look for the value of θ that maximizes $p(\mathbf{y}; \theta)$, that is,

$$\hat{\theta}_{ML} = \arg\max_{\theta} p(\mathbf{y};\theta) \tag{7.1}$$

The preceding estimate, $\hat{\theta}_{ML}$, is called the ML estimate of θ. The pdf $p(\mathbf{y}; \theta)$ is called the *likelihood function* as it can be viewed as a function of an unknown parameter (with **y** fixed). To find $\hat{\theta}_{ML}$, we differentiate $p(\mathbf{y}; \theta)$ with respect to θ, set the derivative equal to zero, and solve for θ. In some cases, it is more convenient to find $\hat{\theta}_{ML}$ by differentiating instead the log of $p(\mathbf{y}; \theta)$, which is called the log-likelihood function.

It is important to note that the parameter θ is assumed to be unknown but *deterministic*. This assumption differentiates the maximum likelihood estimate (MLE) approach from the Bayesian one (to be discussed in the next section), in which θ is assumed to be random. Before discussing the MLE approach to speech enhancement, we first introduce the notation that we will use throughout this chapter.

Let $y(n) = x(n) + d(n)$ be the sampled noisy speech signal consisting of the clean signal $x(n)$ and the noise signal $d(n)$. In the frequency domain, we have

$$Y(\omega_k) = X(\omega_k) + D(\omega_k) \tag{7.2}$$

for $\omega_k = 2\pi k/N$ and $k = 0, 1, 2, \ldots, N-1$, where N is the frame length in samples. The preceding equation can also be expressed in polar form as

$$Y_k e^{j\theta_y(k)} = X_k e^{j\theta_x(k)} + D_k e^{j\theta_d(k)} \tag{7.3}$$

where $\{Y_k, X_k, D_k\}$ denote the magnitudes and $\{\theta_y(k), \theta_x(k), \theta_d(k)\}$ denote the phases at frequency bin k of the noisy speech, clean speech, and noise, respectively.

In the ML approach, proposed by McAulay and Malpass [2], the magnitude and phase spectra of the clean signal, that is, X_k and $\theta_x(k)$, are assumed to be unknown but *deterministic*. The pdf of the noise Fourier transform coefficients $D(\omega_k)$ is assumed to be zero-mean, complex Gaussian. The real and imaginary parts of $D(\omega_k)$ are assumed to have variances $\lambda_d(k)/2$. Based on these two assumptions, we can form the probability density of the observed noisy speech DFT coefficients, $Y(\omega_k)$. The probability density of $Y(\omega_k)$ is also Gaussian with variance $\lambda_d(k)$ and mean $X_k e^{j\theta_x(k)}$:

$$\begin{aligned} p(Y(\omega_k)\,;\,X_k, \theta_x(k)) &= \frac{1}{\pi\lambda_d(k)} \exp\left[-\frac{|Y(\omega_k) - X_k e^{j\theta_x(k)}|^2}{\lambda_d(k)}\right] \\ &= \frac{1}{\pi\lambda_d(k)} \exp\left[-\frac{Y_k^2 - 2X_k \operatorname{Re}\left\{e^{-j\theta_x(k)} Y(\omega_k)\right\} + X_k^2}{\lambda_d(k)}\right] \end{aligned} \tag{7.4}$$

To obtain the ML estimate of X_k, we need to compute the maximum of $p(Y(\omega_k);$ $X_k, \theta_x(k))$ with respect to X_k. This is not straightforward, however, because $p(Y(\omega_k);$

X_k, $\theta_x(k)$) is a function of two unknown parameters: the magnitude and the phase. The phase parameter is considered to be a nuisance parameter (i.e., an undesired parameter), which can be easily eliminated by "integrating it out." More specifically, we can eliminate the phase parameter by maximizing instead the following average likelihood function:

$$p_L(Y(\omega_k);X_k)=\int_0^{2\pi}p(Y(\omega_k);X_k,\theta_x)\,p(\theta_x)\,d\theta_x \tag{7.5}$$

Note that for simplicity we drop the index k from the phase. Assuming a uniform distribution on $(0,2\pi)$ for the phase θ_x, that is, assuming that $p(\theta_x)=\frac{1}{2\pi}$ for $\theta_x\in[0,2\pi]$, the likelihood function becomes

$$p_L(Y(\omega_k);X_k)=\frac{1}{\pi\lambda_d(k)}\exp\left[-\frac{Y_k^2+X_k^2}{\lambda_d(k)}\right]\frac{1}{2\pi}\int_0^{2\pi}\exp\left[\frac{2X_k\,\mathrm{Re}\left(e^{-j\theta_x}Y(\omega_k)\right)}{\lambda_d(k)}\right]d\theta_x \tag{7.6}$$

The integral in the preceding equation is known as the modified Bessel function of the first kind (see Appendix A) and is given by

$$I_0(|x|)=\frac{1}{2\pi}\int_0^{2\pi}\exp[\mathrm{Re}(xe^{-j\theta_x})]\,d\theta_x \tag{7.7}$$

where $x=2X_kY(\omega_k)/\lambda_d(k)$. As shown in Figure 7.1, for values of $|x|>0.258$, the preceding Bessel function can be approximated as

$$I_0(|x|)\approx\frac{1}{\sqrt{2\pi|x|}}\exp(|x|) \tag{7.8}$$

and the likelihood function in Equation 7.6 simplifies to

$$p_L(Y(\omega_k);X_k)=\frac{1}{\pi\lambda_d(k)}\frac{1}{\sqrt{2\pi\frac{2X_kY_k}{\lambda_d(k)}}}\exp\left[-\frac{Y_k^2+X_k^2-2Y_kX_k}{\lambda_d(k)}\right] \tag{7.9}$$

After differentiating the log-likelihood function $\log p_L(Y(\omega_k);X_k)$ with respect to the unknown (parameter) X_k and setting the derivative to zero, we get the ML estimate of the magnitude spectrum:

$$\hat{X}_k=\frac{1}{2}\left[Y_k+\sqrt{Y_k^2-\lambda_d(k)}\right] \tag{7.10}$$

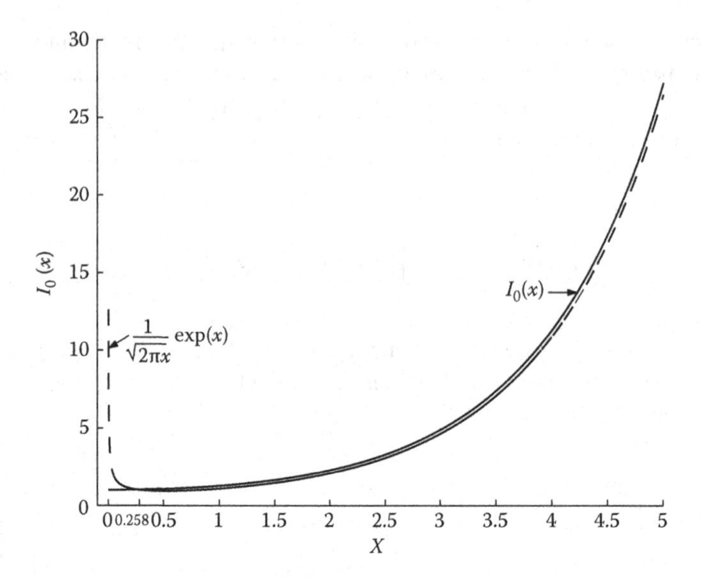

FIGURE 7.1 Plot of $I_0(x)$ and its approximation.

Using the noisy phase θ_y in place of θ_x, we can express the estimate of the clean signal (complex) spectrum as

$$\hat{X}(\omega_k) = \hat{X}_k e^{j\theta_y} = \hat{X}_k \frac{Y(\omega_k)}{Y_k}$$

$$= \left[\frac{1}{2} + \frac{1}{2}\sqrt{\frac{Y_k^2 - \lambda_d(k)}{Y_k^2}}\right] Y(\omega_k) \tag{7.11}$$

Letting $\gamma_k \triangleq Y_k^2 / \lambda_d(k)$ denote the *a posteriori* or measured signal-to-noise ratio (SNR) based on the observed data, the preceding equation can also written as

$$\hat{X}(\omega_k) = \left[\frac{1}{2} + \frac{1}{2}\sqrt{\frac{\gamma_k - 1}{\gamma_k}}\right] Y(\omega_k)$$

$$= G_{ML}(\gamma_k)\, Y(\omega_k) \tag{7.12}$$

where $G_{ML}(\gamma_k)$ denotes the gain function of the ML estimator.

Figure 7.2 plots the gain function $G_{ML}(\gamma_k)$ as a function of the *a posteriori* SNR γ_k. The gain functions of the power spectrum subtraction and Wiener filters are also plotted for comparison. As can be seen, the ML suppression rule provides considerably smaller attenuation compared to the power subtraction and Wiener suppression rules.

In the preceding derivation, we assumed that the signal magnitude and phase (X_k and θ_x) were unknown but deterministic. If we now assume that both signal and

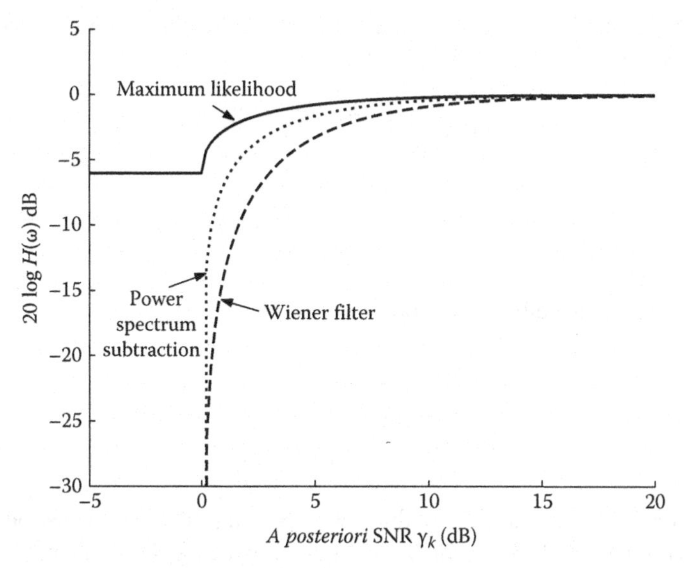

FIGURE 7.2 Suppression curve for the maximum-likelihood estimator.

speech DFT coefficients are modeled as independent, zero-mean Gaussian random processes, but it is the signal variance, $\lambda_x(k)$, that is unknown and deterministic, we get a different likelihood function. As the signal and noise are assumed to be independent, the variance of $Y(\omega_k)$, denoted as $\lambda_y(k)$, is given by $\lambda_y(k) = \lambda_x(k) + \lambda_d(k)$. Hence, the probability density of $Y(\omega_k)$ is given by

$$p(Y(\omega_k)\,;\lambda_x(k)) = \frac{1}{\pi[\lambda_x(k)+\lambda_d(k)]}\exp\left[-\frac{Y_k^2}{\lambda_x(k)+\lambda_d(k)}\right] \tag{7.13}$$

Maximizing the likelihood function $p(Y(\omega_k); \lambda_x(k))$ with respect to $\lambda_x(k)$, we get

$$\hat{\lambda}_x(k) = Y_k^2 - \lambda_d(k) \tag{7.14}$$

Assuming that $X_k^2 \approx \lambda_x(k)$ and $D_k^2 \approx \lambda_d(k)$ (and $Y_k^2 - \lambda_d(k) > 0$), we get an estimate of the signal magnitude spectrum:

$$\hat{X}_k = \sqrt{Y_k^2 - D_k^2} \tag{7.15}$$

Note that this estimator of X_k is nothing but the power spectrum subtraction estimator. Hence, the original power spectrum subtraction approach can be derived using ML principles by assuming that the signal and noise Fourier transform coefficients are modeled as independent Gaussian random processes and the signal variance, $\lambda_x(k)$, is unknown but deterministic.

As in Equation 7.12, we can compute the estimate of the clean signal spectrum obtained by power spectrum subtraction as

$$\hat{X}(\omega_k) = \hat{X}_k e^{j\theta_y} = \hat{X}_k \frac{Y(\omega_k)}{Y_k}$$

$$= \sqrt{\frac{Y_k^2 - \lambda_d(k)}{Y_k^2}}\, Y(\omega_k) \tag{7.16}$$

In terms of γ_k, the preceding equation can be written as

$$\hat{X}(\omega_k) = \sqrt{\frac{\gamma_k - 1}{\gamma_k}}\, Y(\omega_k)$$

$$= G_{PS}(\gamma_k)\, Y(\omega_k) \tag{7.17}$$

where $G_{PS}(\gamma_k)$ is the gain function of the power spectrum subtraction method. Finally, it is worth noting that if we substitute the ML estimate of $\lambda_x(k)$ (Equation 7.14) in the Wiener filter equation

$$\hat{X}(\omega_k) = \frac{\lambda_x(k)}{\lambda_x(k) + \lambda_d(k)} Y(\omega_k) \tag{7.18}$$

we get

$$\hat{X}(\omega_k) = \frac{Y_k^2 - \lambda_d(k)}{Y_k^2} Y(\omega_k)$$

$$= \frac{\gamma_k - 1}{\gamma_k}\, Y(\omega_k)$$

$$= G_{PS}^2(\gamma_k)\, Y(\omega_k) \tag{7.19}$$

Comparing Equation 7.17 with Equation 7.19, we see that the Wiener estimator is the square of the power spectrum subtraction estimator. Consequently, the Wiener estimator provides more spectral attenuation than the power spectrum subtraction estimator, for a fixed value of γ_k. This is also seen in Figure 7.2.

Finally, it should be pointed out that the ML suppression rule is never used by itself, because it does not provide enough attenuation (Figure 7.2). In [2] it was used in conjunction with a two-state model of speech that incorporated signal presence uncertainty. This model will be discussed later in more detail.

7.2 BAYESIAN ESTIMATORS

In the previous section, we discussed the ML approach for parameter estimation, in which we assumed that the parameter of interest, θ, was deterministic but unknown. Now, we assume that θ is a random variable, and we therefore need to estimate the realization of that random variable. This approach is called the *Bayesian* approach because its implementation is based on Bayes' theorem. The main motivation behind the Bayesian approach is the fact that if we have available *a priori* knowledge about θ, that is, if we know $p(\theta)$, we should incorporate that knowledge in the estimator to improve estimation accuracy. The Bayesian estimators typically perform better than the MLE estimators, as they make use of prior knowledge. Next, we describe methods that minimize the mean-square error (in the Bayesian sense) between the true and estimated magnitude spectra.

7.3 MMSE ESTIMATOR

We saw in the previous chapter that the Wiener estimator can be derived by minimizing the error between a linear model of the clean spectrum and the true spectrum. The Wiener estimator is considered to be the optimal (in the mean-square-error sense) complex spectral estimator, but is not the optimal spectral magnitude estimator. Acknowledging the importance of the short-time spectral amplitude (STSA) on speech intelligibility and quality, several authors have proposed optimal methods for obtaining the spectral amplitudes from noisy observations. In particular, optimal estimators were sought that minimized the mean-square error between the estimated and true magnitudes:

$$e = E\left\{\left(\hat{X}_k - X_k\right)^2\right\} \tag{7.20}$$

where

$\hat{X}_k$ is the estimate spectral magnitude at frequency ω_k
X_k is the true magnitude of the clean signal

The minimization of Equation 7.20 can be done in two ways, depending on how we perform the expectation. In the classical MSE approach, the expectation is done with respect to $p(\mathbf{Y}; X_k)$, where $\mathbf{Y}$ denotes the observed noisy speech spectrum, $\mathbf{Y} = [Y(\omega_0)\ Y(\omega_1) \cdots Y(\omega_{N-1})]$. In the Bayesian MSE approach, the expectation is done with respect to the joint pdf $p(\mathbf{Y}, X_k)$, and the Bayesian MSE is given by

$$BMSE(\hat{X}_k) = \iint (X_k - \hat{X}_k)^2\ p(\mathbf{Y}, X_k)\ d\mathbf{Y}dX_k \tag{7.21}$$

Minimization of the Bayesian MSE with respect to $\hat{X}_k$ leads to the optimal MMSE estimator given by [1]

$$\begin{aligned}\hat{X}_k &= \int X_k p(X_k \mid \mathbf{Y})\, dX_k \\ &= E[X_k \mid \mathbf{Y}] \\ &= E[X_k \mid Y(\omega_0)Y(\omega_1)\ldots Y(\omega_{N-1})]\end{aligned} \tag{7.22}$$

which is the mean of the *a posteriori* pdf of X_k. The posterior pdf of the clean spectral amplitudes, that is, $p(X_k \mid \mathbf{Y})$, is the pdf of the amplitudes after all the data (i.e., the complex noisy speech spectra, **Y**, in our case) are observed. In contrast, the *a priori* pdf of X_k, that is, $p(X_k)$, refers to the pdf of the clean amplitudes before the data are observed.

Note that there are two fundamental differences between the Wiener estimator and the MMSE estimator given in Equation 7.22. First, in the Wiener filter derivation, we assumed that $\hat{X}(\omega_k) = H_k Y(\omega_k)$ for some unknown filter H_k; that is, we assumed that there is a linear relationship between $Y(\omega_k)$ (the observed data) and $\hat{X}(\omega_k)$. Second, the Wiener filter is obtained by evaluating the mean of the posterior pdf of $X(\omega_k)$ rather than X_k; that is, it is given by $E[X(\omega_k) \mid Y(\omega_k)]$. The Wiener filter is therefore the optimal (in the MMSE sense) *complex spectrum* estimator and not the optimal *magnitude spectrum* estimator under the assumed model.

The MMSE estimator given in Equation 7.22, unlike the Wiener estimator, does not assume the existence of a linear relationship between the observed data and the estimator, but it does require knowledge about the probability distributions of the speech and noise DFT coefficients. Assuming that we do have prior knowledge about the distributions of the speech and noise DFT coefficients, we can evaluate the mean of the posterior pdf of X_k, that is, the mean of $p(X_k \mid \mathbf{Y})$.

Measuring the true probability distributions of the speech Fourier transform coefficients, however, has been difficult, largely because the speech (and sometimes the noise) signal is neither a stationary nor an ergodic process. Several have attempted to measure the probability distributions by examining the long-time behavior of the processes [3–5]. As argued in [6], however, it is questionable whether histograms of the Fourier coefficients, obtained using a large amount of data, measure the relative frequency of the Fourier transform coefficients rather than the true probability density of the Fourier transform coefficients.

To circumvent these problems, Ephraim and Malah [6] proposed a statistical model that utilizes the asymptotic statistical properties of the Fourier transform coefficients [7]. This model makes two assumptions:

1. The Fourier transform coefficients (real and imaginary parts) have a Gaussian probability distribution. The mean of the coefficients is zero, and the variances of the coefficients are time-varying owing to the nonstationarity of speech.
2. The Fourier transform coefficients are statistically independent and, hence, uncorrelated.

The Gaussian assumption is motivated by the central limit theorem, as the Fourier transform coefficients are computed as a sum of N random variables. Consider, for instance, the computation of the noisy speech Fourier transform coefficients, $Y(\omega_k)$:

$$Y(\omega_k) = \sum_{n=0}^{N-1} y(n)e^{-j\omega_k n} = y(0) + a_1 y(1) + a_2 y(2) + \cdots + a_{N-1} y(N-1) \tag{7.23}$$

where

$a_m = \exp(-j\omega_k m)$ are constants

$y(n)$ are the time-domain samples of the noisy speech signal

According to the central limit theorem [8], if the random variables $\{y(n)\}_{n=0}^{N-1}$ are statistically independent, the density of $Y(\omega_k)$ will be Gaussian. The central limit theorem also holds when sufficiently separated samples are weakly dependent [7], as is the case with the speech signal.

The uncorrelated assumption is motivated by the fact that the correlation between different Fourier coefficients approaches zero as the analysis frame length N approaches infinity [7,9]. The independence assumption is a direct consequence of the uncorrelated assumption, as it is known that if the Fourier coefficients are both uncorrelated and Gaussian, then they are also independent [8]. In speech applications, however, we are constrained by the nonstationarity of the speech signal to use analysis frame lengths on the order of 20–40ms. This may cause the Fourier transform coefficients to be correlated to some degree [10]. Despite that, overlapping analysis windows are typically used in practice. Although such "window overlap" clearly violates the assumption of uncorrelatedness, the resultant models have proved simple, tractable, and useful in practice. Models that take this correlation into account have also been proposed (see [11]).

7.3.1 MMSE Magnitude Estimator

To determine the MMSE estimator we first need to compute the posterior pdf of X_k, that is, $p(X_k \mid Y(\omega_k))$. We can use Bayes' rule to determine it as

$$\begin{aligned} p(X_k \mid Y(\omega_k)) &= \frac{p(Y(\omega_k) \mid X_k)\, p(X_k)}{p(Y(\omega_k))} \\ &= \frac{p(Y(\omega_k) \mid X_k)\, p(X_k)}{\int_0^{\infty} p(Y(\omega_k) \mid x_k)\, p(x_k)\, dx_k} \end{aligned} \tag{7.24}$$

where x_k is a realization of the random variable X_k. Note that $p(Y(\omega_k))$ is a normalization factor required to ensure that $p(X_k \mid Y(\omega_k))$ integrates to 1. Assuming statistical independence between the Fourier transform coefficients, that is,

$$E[X_k \mid Y(\omega_0)\, Y(\omega_1)\, Y(\omega_2) \cdots Y(\omega_{N-1})] = E[X_k \mid Y(\omega_k)] \tag{7.25}$$

and using the preceding expression for $p(x_k \mid Y(\omega_k))$, the estimator in Equation 7.22 simplifies to

$$\begin{aligned} \hat{X}_k &= E[X_k \mid Y(\omega_k)] \\ &= \int_0^{\infty} x_k p(x_k \mid Y(\omega_k))\, dx_k \\ &= \frac{\int_0^{\infty} x_k p(Y(\omega_k) \mid x_k)\, p(x_k)\, dx_k}{\int_0^{\infty} p(Y(\omega_k) \mid x_k)\, p(x_k)\, dx_k} \end{aligned} \tag{7.26}$$

Since

$$p(Y(\omega_k) \mid X_k)p(X_k) = \int_0^{2\pi} p(Y(\omega_k) \mid x_k, \theta_x)p(x_k, \theta_x)d\theta_x \tag{7.27}$$

where θ_x is the realization of the phase random variable of $X(\omega_k)$ (for clarity we henceforth drop the index k in θ_x), we get

$$\hat{X}_k = \frac{\int_0^\infty \int_0^{2\pi} x_k p(Y(\omega_k) \mid x_k, \theta_x)p(x_k, \theta_x)d\theta_x dx_k}{\int_0^\infty \int_0^{2\pi} p(Y(\omega_k) \mid x_k, \theta_x)p(x_k, \theta_x)d\theta_x dx_k} \tag{7.28}$$

Next, we need to estimate $p(Y(\omega_k) \mid x_k, \theta_x)$ and $p(x_k, \theta_x)$. From the assumed statistical model, we know that $Y(\omega_k)$ is the sum of two zero-mean complex Gaussian random variables. Therefore, the conditional pdf $p(Y(\omega_k) \mid x_k, \theta_x)$ will also be Gaussian:

$$p(Y(\omega_k) \mid x_k, \theta_x) = p_D(Y(\omega_k) - X(\omega_k)) \tag{7.29}$$

where $p_D(\cdot)$ is the pdf of the noise Fourier transform coefficients, $D(\omega_k)$. The preceding equation then becomes

$$p(Y(\omega_k) \mid x_k, \theta_x) = \frac{1}{\pi\lambda_d(k)} \exp\left\{-\frac{1}{\lambda_d(k)} \left|Y(\omega_k) - X(\omega_k)\right|^2\right\} \tag{7.30}$$

where $\lambda_D(k) = E\{|D(\omega_k)|^2\}$ is the variance of the kth spectral component of the noise. For complex Gaussian random variables, we know that the magnitude (X_k) and phase ($\theta_x(k)$) random variables of $X(\omega_k)$ are independent [12, p. 203] and can therefore evaluate the joint pdf $p(x_k, \theta_x)$ as the product of the individual pdfs, that is, $p(x_k, \theta_x) = p(x_k)\, p(\theta_x)$. The pdf of X_k is Rayleigh since $X_k = \sqrt{r(k)^2 + i(k)^2}$, where $r(k) = \text{Re}\{X(\omega_k)\}$ and $i(k) = \text{Im}\{X(\omega_k)\}$ are Gaussian random variables [12, p. 190]. The pdf of $\theta_x(k)$ is uniform in $(-\pi, \pi)$ (see proof in [12, p. 203]), and therefore the joint probability $p(x_k, \theta_x)$ is given by

$$p(x_k, \theta_x) = \frac{x_k}{\pi\, \lambda_x(k)} \exp\left\{-\frac{x_k^2}{\lambda_x(k)}\right\} \tag{7.31}$$

where $\lambda_x(k) = E\{|X(\omega_k)|^2\}$ is the variance of the kth spectral component of the clean signal. Substituting Equations 7.30 and 7.31 into Equation 7.26, we finally get the optimal MMSE magnitude estimator (see derivation in Appendix B):

$$\hat{X}_k = \sqrt{\lambda_k}\; \Gamma(1.5)\, \Phi(-0.5, 1; -v_k) \tag{7.32}$$

where $\Gamma(\cdot)$ denotes the gamma function, $\Phi(a, b; c)$ denotes the confluent hypergeometric function (Appendix A), λ_k is given by

$$\lambda_k = \frac{\lambda_x(k)\lambda_d(k)}{\lambda_x(k)+\lambda_d(k)} = \frac{\lambda_x(k)}{1+\xi_k} \tag{7.33}$$

and v_k is defined by

$$v_k = \frac{\xi_k}{1+\xi_k}\gamma_k \tag{7.34}$$

where γ_k and ξ_k are defined by

$$\gamma_k = \frac{Y_k^2}{\lambda_d(k)} \tag{7.35}$$

$$\xi_k = \frac{\lambda_x(k)}{\lambda_d(k)} \tag{7.36}$$

The terms ξ_k and γ_k are referred to as the *a priori* and *a posteriori* SNRs, respectively [6]. The *a priori* SNR ξ_k can be viewed as the true SNR of the kth spectral component, whereas the *a posteriori* SNR γ_k can be considered the observed or measured SNR of the kth spectral component after noise is added.

Equation 7.32 can also be written as

$$\hat{X}_k = \frac{\sqrt{v_k}}{\gamma_k}\,\Gamma(1.5)\,\Phi(-0.5, 1; -v_k)\,Y_k \tag{7.37}$$

since $\sqrt{\lambda_k}$ can be simplified using Equations 7.34 through 7.36 to

$$\begin{aligned}\sqrt{\lambda_k} &= \sqrt{\frac{\lambda_x(k)}{1+\xi_k}}\\ &= \sqrt{\frac{\xi_k\lambda_d(k)}{1+\xi_k}}\\ &= \sqrt{\frac{\xi_k Y_k^2}{(1+\xi_k)\gamma_k}\frac{\gamma_k}{\gamma_k}}\\ &= \sqrt{\frac{\xi_k\gamma_k}{(1+\xi_k)}\frac{1}{(\gamma_k)^2}}\,Y_k\\ &= \frac{\sqrt{v_k}}{\gamma_k}Y_k \end{aligned} \tag{7.38}$$

Finally, the confluent hypergeometric function in Equation 7.37 can be written in terms of Bessel functions using Equation A.14, and the MMSE estimator can be expressed as

$$\hat{X}_k = \frac{\sqrt{\pi}}{2}\frac{\sqrt{v_k}}{\gamma_k}\exp\left(-\frac{v_k}{2}\right)\left[(1+v_k)I_o\left(\frac{v_k}{2}\right)+v_kI_1\left(\frac{v_k}{2}\right)\right]Y_k \tag{7.39}$$

where $I_0(\cdot)$ and $I_1(\cdot)$ denote the modified Bessel functions of zero and first order, respectively (Appendix A).

Equation 7.39 or Equation 7.37 is preferred over the original equation (Equation 7.32), as we can express the estimated magnitude in terms of a gain function, that is, $\hat{X}_k = G(\xi_k, \gamma_k)Y_k$. The spectral gain function $G(\xi_k, \gamma_k)$

$$G(\xi_k,\gamma_k) = \frac{\hat{X}_k}{Y_k} = \frac{\sqrt{\pi}}{2}\frac{\sqrt{v_k}}{\gamma_k}\exp\left(-\frac{v_k}{2}\right)\left[(1+v_k)I_o\left(\frac{v_k}{2}\right)+v_kI_1\left(\frac{v_k}{2}\right)\right] \tag{7.40}$$

is a function of two parameters: the *a priori* SNR ξ_k and the *a posteriori* SNR value γ_k. To examine the dependency of ξ_k and γ_k on the gain function, we can plot $G(\xi_k, \gamma_k)$ as a function of the *a priori* SNR for fixed *a posteriori* SNR values. Figure 7.3 plots $G(\xi_k, \gamma_k)$ as a function of ξ_k for fixed values of $(\gamma_k - 1)$, referred to as the instantaneous SNR [6]. Note that for large values (~20dB) of the instantaneous SNR, the MMSE gain function is similar to the Wiener gain function, which is given by

$$G_W(\xi_k) = \frac{\xi_k}{\xi_k + 1} \tag{7.41}$$

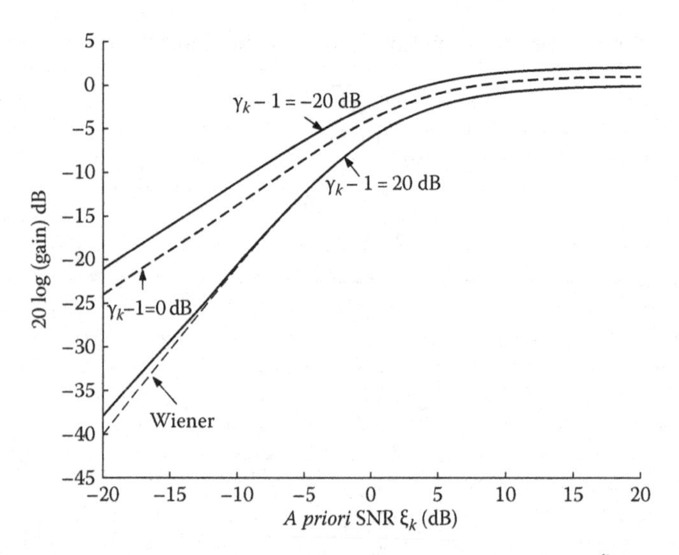

FIGURE 7.3 Attenuation curve of the MMSE estimator as a function of ξ_k.

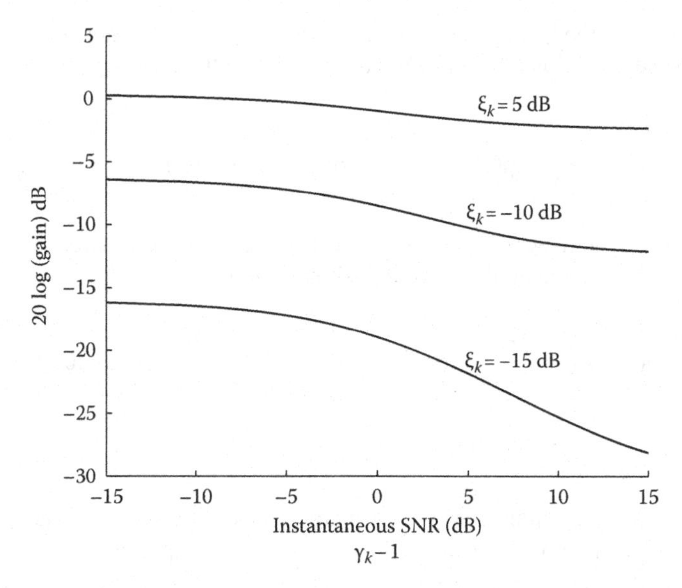

FIGURE 7.4 Attenuation curve of the MMSE estimator as a function of $\gamma_k - 1$.

In other words, the MMSE estimator behaves likes the Wiener estimator when ξ_k is large. Note that unlike the MMSE gain function, the Wiener gain function does not depend on the *a posteriori* SNR γ_k. The fact that $G(\xi_k, \gamma_k)$ depends on both ξ_k and γ_k will prove to be important for reducing the musical noise, and we will discuss this in Section 7.6.

The spectral gain function can alternatively be plotted as a function of the *a posteriori* SNR ($\gamma_k - 1$) and is shown in Figure 7.4 for fixed values of ξ_k. The fact that the suppression curve is relatively flat for a wide range of values of γ_k when $\xi_k \geq -10$ dB suggests that the *a posteriori* SNR γ_k has a small effect on suppression. This suggests that the *a priori* SNR ξ_k is the main parameter influencing suppression. The effect of γ_k on suppression is only evident for extremely low values of ξ_k (i.e., $\xi_k = -15$ dB). The behavior of γ_k is counterintuitive in that more suppression is applied when γ_k is high than when γ_k is low. This behavior will be explained in Section 7.6.

7.3.2 MMSE Complex Exponential Estimator

In the previous section, we derived the optimal spectral magnitude $\hat{X}_k$ given the noisy observations $Y(\omega_k)$. Having $\hat{X}_k$ alone, however, is not sufficient for constructing the enhanced signal spectrum. The phase is also needed to form $\hat{X}(\omega_k) = \hat{X}_k \exp(j\hat{\theta}_x(k))$. This raises the following question: Can the phase or the complex exponential be derived similarly in an optimal fashion using the same statistical model? If we could derive the optimal—in the MMSE sense—phase, then we could combine the phase estimator with the STSA estimator to construct the enhanced spectrum. Two methods were proposed in [6] for estimating the phases.

In the first method, the complex exponential MMSE estimator was derived by evaluating the conditional mean of the *a posteriori* pdf of the complex exponential of $X(\omega_k)$, that is,

$$\exp(j\hat{\theta}_x(k)) = E\{\exp(j\theta_x(k)) \mid Y(\omega_k)\} \tag{7.42}$$

using the same statistical model assumed for the STSA estimator. The derived MMSE complex exponential estimator had the form [6]

$$\exp(j\hat{\theta}_x(k)) = \frac{\sqrt{\pi}}{2}\sqrt{v_k}\exp\left(\frac{-v_k}{2}\right)\left[I_o\left(\frac{v_k}{2}\right) + I_1\left(\frac{v_k}{2}\right)\right]\exp(j\theta_y(k))$$

$$\triangleq B_k \exp(j\theta_y(k)) \tag{7.43}$$

Combining the preceding MMSE estimator $\exp(j\hat{\theta}_x(k))$ with the independently derived STSA estimator $\hat{X}_k$ results in the enhanced signal spectrum:

$$\hat{X}(\omega_k) = \hat{X}_k B_k \exp(j\theta_y(k)) \tag{7.44}$$

Note, however, that the new magnitude of $\hat{X}(\omega_k)$ (i.e., $\hat{X}_k B_k$) will not be optimal if $\hat{X}_k$ is already optimal. Thus, the fact that $|B_k|$ is not equal to 1 adversely affects the amplitude estimation, and for that reason, the preceding phase estimator was abandoned.

In the second method, a phase MMSE estimator was derived subject to the constraint that the modulus of the resulting estimator was 1. More specifically, the following constrained minimization problem was considered:

$$\min_{\exp(j\hat{\theta}_x)} E\{|\exp(j\theta_x) - \exp(j\hat{\theta}_x)|^2\}$$

$$\text{subject to: } |\exp(j\hat{\theta}_x)| = 1 \tag{7.45}$$

Using the method of Lagrange multipliers, the optimal solution can be shown to be

$$\exp(j\hat{\theta}_x) = \exp(j\theta_y) \tag{7.46}$$

That is, the noisy phase (θ_y) is the optimal—in the MMSE sense—phase. Note that this phase estimate does not affect the amplitude estimation, as it has a modulus of 1. For that reason, the noisy phase is commonly used for synthesizing the enhanced signal. Use of the noisy phase is often justified by the radial symmetry of the complex spectral prior in the complex plane. If the noise is assumed Gaussian (and hence is also radially symmetric), then the optimal phase estimate will be the noisy phase (as is the case with the Wiener estimator).

7.3.3 Estimating the *A Priori* SNR

The MMSE amplitude estimator (Equation 7.37) was derived under the assumption that the *a priori* SNR ξ_k and the noise variance ($\lambda_d(k)$) are known. In practice, however, we only have access to the noisy speech signal. The noise variance can be estimated easily assuming noise stationarity, and can in principle be computed during nonspeech activity with the aid of a voice activity detector or a noise estimation algorithm (Chapter 9). Estimating ξ_k, however, is considerably more difficult.

Ephraim and Malah [6] first examined the sensitivity of the amplitude estimator to inaccuracies of the *a priori* SNR ξ_k. They found the MMSE estimator to be relatively insensitive to small perturbations of the ξ_k value. More interesting was the finding that the MMSE estimator was more sensitive to underestimates rather than overestimates of the *a priori* SNR ξ_k.

Several methods were proposed [6,10,13–15] for estimating the *a priori* SNR ξ_k, and these methods are described next. The majority of these methods were extensions and improvements to the methods proposed in [6].

7.3.3.1 Maximum-Likelihood Method

An ML approach [6] can be used to estimate the *a priori* SNR ξ_k by first determining the unknown (and assumed to be deterministic) parameter $\lambda_x(k)$. Given $\lambda_x(k)$ and assuming that $\lambda_d(k)$ is estimated during nonspeech activity, we can obtain ξ_k using Equation 7.36. The estimation is based on L past consecutive observations of the noisy speech magnitudes $\mathbf{Y}_k(m) \triangleq \{Y_k(m), Y_k(m-1), \ldots, Y_k(m-L+1)\}$ obtained at the mth analysis frame for frequency bin k. Assuming statistical independence between the L observations and using the Gaussian statistical model, we can form the following likelihood function:

$$p(\mathbf{Y}_k(m); \lambda_x(k), \lambda_d(k)) = \prod_{j=0}^{L-1} \frac{1}{\pi(\lambda_x(k)+\lambda_d(k))} \exp\left(-\frac{Y_k^2(m-j)}{\lambda_x(k)+\lambda_d(k)}\right) \tag{7.47}$$

Maximizing the preceding likelihood function with respect to $\lambda_x(k)$, we get the estimate of $\lambda_x(k)$ for frame m:

$$\hat{\lambda}_x(k,m) = \begin{cases} \dfrac{1}{L}\displaystyle\sum_{j=0}^{L-1} Y_k^2(m-j) - \lambda_d(k,m) & \text{if nonnegative} \\ 0 & \text{else} \end{cases}$$

$$= \max\left(\frac{1}{L}\sum_{j=0}^{L-1} Y_k^2(m-j) - \lambda_d(k,m), 0\right) \tag{7.48}$$

After dividing both sides by $\lambda_d(k, m)$, we get

$$\hat{\xi}_k(m) = \max\left(\frac{1}{L}\sum_{j=0}^{L-1} \gamma_k(m-j) - 1, 0\right) \tag{7.49}$$

where $\gamma_k(m) \triangleq Y_k^2(m)/\lambda_d(k,m)$ denotes the *a posteriori* SNR of frame m, and the max(.) operator is used to ensure that $\hat{\xi}_k(m)$ is always nonnegative.

In practice, the running average in Equation 7.49 can be replaced by a recursive averaging operation:

$$\bar{\gamma}_k(m) = a\,\bar{\gamma}_k(m-1) + (1-a)\frac{\gamma_k(m)}{\beta} \tag{7.50}$$

where $0 \leq a < 1$ is a smoothing constant, and $\beta \geq 1$ is a correction factor. The final ML estimator of ξ_k has the form

$$\hat{\xi}_k(m) = \max(\bar{\gamma}_k(m) - 1, 0) \tag{7.51}$$

It is interesting to note that when $L = 1$ (i.e., no past observations are used) the preceding ML estimator of $\xi_k = \max(\gamma_k(m) - 1, 0)$ yields a gain function that depends only on γ_k. The resulting gain function is nearly identical to that of the power spectral subtraction method.

7.3.3.2 Decision-Directed Approach

The second method, which was called the "decision-directed" approach [6], was based on the definition of ξ_k and its relationship with the *a posteriori* SNR γ_k. We know that ξ_k is given by

$$\xi_k(m) = \frac{E\{X_k^2(m)\}}{\lambda_d(k,m)} \tag{7.52}$$

We also know that ξ_k is related to γ_k by

$$\begin{aligned}\xi_k(m) &= \frac{E\left\{Y_k^2(m) - D_k^2(m)\right\}}{\lambda_d(k,m)} \\ &= \frac{E\left\{Y_k^2(m)\right\}}{\lambda_d(k,m)} - \frac{E\left\{D_k^2(m)\right\}}{\lambda_d(k,m)} \\ &= E\{\gamma_k(m)\} - 1\end{aligned} \tag{7.53}$$

Combining the two expressions for, ξ_k, that is, Equations 7.52 and 7.53, we get

$$\xi_k(m) = E\left\{\frac{1}{2}\frac{X_k^2(m)}{\lambda_d(k,m)} + \frac{1}{2}[\gamma_k(m) - 1]\right\} \tag{7.54}$$

The final estimator for ξ_k is derived by making the preceding equation recursive:

$$\hat{\xi}_k(m) = a\frac{\hat{X}_k^2(m-1)}{\lambda_d(k,m-1)} + (1-a)\max[\gamma_k(m)-1,0] \tag{7.55}$$

where $0 < a < 1$ is the weighting factor replacing the 1/2 in Equation 7.54, and $\hat{X}_k^2(m-1)$ is the amplitude estimator obtained in the past analysis frame. The max(.) operator is used to ensure the positiveness of the estimator, as $\hat{\xi}_k(m)$ needs to be nonnegative.

This new estimator of ξ_k is a weighted average of the past *a priori* SNR (given by the first term) and the present *a priori* SNR estimate (given by the second term). Note that the present *a priori* SNR estimate is also the ML estimate of the SNR (Equation 7.51). Equation 7.55 was called the decision-directed estimator because $\hat{\xi}_k(m)$ is updated using information from the previous amplitude estimate. The decision-directed approach for estimating the *a priori* SNR was found not only important for MMSE-type algorithms but also in other algorithms [16].

Equation 7.55 needs initial conditions for the first frame, that is, for $m = 0$. The following initial conditions were recommended [6] for $\hat{\xi}_k(n)$:

$$\hat{\xi}_k(0) = a + (1-a)\max[\gamma_k(0)-1,0] \tag{7.56}$$

Good results were obtained with $a = 0.98$.

7.4 IMPROVEMENTS TO THE DECISION-DIRECTED APPROACH

Following Ephraim and Malah's work, several improvements were made to the decision-directed approach [10,13–15,17–22]. The first improvement suggested [17] was to limit the smallest allowable value for $\hat{\xi}_k(m)$ in Equation 7.55. This can be easily done as follows:

$$\hat{\xi}_k(m) = \max\left[a\frac{\hat{X}_k^2(m-1)}{\lambda_d(k,m-1)} + (1-a)\max[\gamma_k(m)-1,0], \xi_{\min}\right] \tag{7.57}$$

where $\xi_{\min}$ is the minimum value allowed for ξ_k. As indicated in [17], the flooring of $\hat{\xi}_k(m)$ to a small value is important for reducing low-level musical noise. A value of $\xi_{\min} = -15\,\text{dB}$ was suggested in [17].

Other improvements to the decision-directed approach focused on reducing the bias and improving the speed of adaptation, which is controlled by the smoothing constant in Equation 7.55.

7.4.1 Reducing the Bias

Suppose that the value $a = 1$ is used in the decision-directed approach (Equation 7.55) for estimating $\hat{\xi}_k(m)$. For this value of a, the estimate of $\xi_k(m)$ is determined primarily by $\hat{\xi}_k(m) = \hat{X}_k^2(m-1)/\lambda_d(k,m-1)$ (for values of $a \approx 1$, we have

$\hat{\xi}_k(m) \approx \hat{X}_k^2(m-1)/\lambda_d(k,m-1))$. The fact that the square of the estimator of the amplitude is used (i.e., $(E[X_k])^2 = \hat{X}_k^2(m)$) rather than the estimator of the square (i.e., $E[X_k^2]$) causes a bias in the estimate of *a priori* SNR, particularly for small values of $\xi_k(\xi_k \ll 1)$. To see that, consider the square of the MMSE amplitude $\hat{X}_k$ (Equation 7.37) computed using the estimated *a priori* SNR $\hat{\xi}_k$, that is,

$$\hat{X}_k^2 = \frac{\pi}{4\gamma_k} \frac{\hat{\xi}_k}{1+\hat{\xi}_k} \{\Phi(-0.5, 1; -\hat{v}_k)\}^2 Y_k^2 \tag{7.58}$$

When the *a priori* SNR is small (i.e., $\xi_k \ll 1$), $\Phi(-0.5, 1; -\hat{v}_k) \approx 1$ and the preceding equation simplifies to

$$\begin{aligned} \hat{X}_k^2 &= \frac{\pi}{4\gamma_k} \hat{\xi}_k Y_k^2 \\ &= \frac{\pi}{4} \hat{\xi}_k \lambda_D(k) \end{aligned} \tag{7.59}$$

Assuming that we know ξ_k exactly, we have

$$\begin{aligned} \hat{X}_k^2 &= \frac{\pi}{4} \frac{\lambda_x(k)}{\lambda_D(k)} \lambda_D(k) \\ &= \frac{\pi}{4} \lambda_x(k) \end{aligned} \tag{7.60}$$

Hence, from the preceding equation we see that $\hat{X}_k^2$ is a biased estimator of $\lambda_X(k)$ because of the factor $\pi/4$ (note that the true value of $\lambda_x(k)$ is given by $\lambda_x(k) \triangleq E[X_k^2]$, which is not equivalent to $(E[X_k])^2$). As a result, at low SNRs, the decision-directed approach (Equation 7.55) will underestimate the true value of the *a priori* SNR and cause too much suppression.

To correct for this bias, Erkelens et al. [19] suggested inserting the factor $4/\pi$ in the first term of Equation 7.55. Furthermore, following [18], they let the max operator, which was used originally in the second term of Equation 7.55, to work on both terms together. The modified decision-directed approach had the following form [19]:

$$\hat{\xi}_k(m) = \max\left[a \frac{4}{\pi} \frac{\hat{X}_k^2(m-1)}{\lambda_d(k,m-1)} + (1-a)[\gamma_k(m)-1], \xi_{\min}\right] \tag{7.61}$$

where $\xi_{\min}$ is the minimum value allowed for ξ_k (set to $\xi_{\min} = -15\,\text{dB}$ in [19]). As indicated in [19], the correction factor $4/\pi$ introduces a bias at high SNRs; however, the influence of overestimating the value of ξ_k is smaller than the influence of underestimating it [6].

As pointed out in [18], the clipping of the second term in Equation 7.55 to zero (via the max operator) can cause a bias in the estimation of the *a priori* SNR, and for that reason the following modification to the decision-directed approach was recommended [18]:

$$\hat{\xi}_k(m) = \max\left[a\frac{\hat{X}_k^2(m-1)}{\lambda_d(k,m-1)} + (1-a)[\gamma_k(m)-1], \xi_{\min}\right] \tag{7.62}$$

where $\xi_{\min}$ is the minimum value allowed for ξ_k.

7.4.2 Improving the Adaptation Speed

The value of the smoothing a constant in Equation 7.55 controls the trade-off between the degree of smoothing of ξ_k during speech-absent segments and the level of transient distortion incurred during signal onsets. As indicated in [17], small values of a can produce significant amounts of musical noise. For that reason, the value of a needs to be close to one to counter the musical noise effect (more on this in Section 7.6). When a is close to 1, however, and a signal onset occurs, it takes a longer time for $\hat{\xi}_k(n)$ to reach its final value. This results in undesirable attenuation of weak signal components in the first frames following the transient. Therefore, the smoothing constant controls the adaptation speed of the decision-directed approach with regard to responding to signal onsets.

Ideally, the smoothing constant a should be small during the transient parts of speech so that it can respond faster to sudden changes in the signal and should be large during the steady-state segments of speech. This suggests, then, that a should not be constant but, rather, adaptive. An adaptive scheme for updating the value of a was proposed in [14] based on the assumption that the additive noise did not change significantly from frame to frame. The value of a was adapted from frame to frame based on the difference in signal energy between consecutive frames. Hasan et al. [13] proposed the following modification to the decision-directed approach:

$$\hat{\xi}_k(m) = a_k(m)\bar{\xi}_k(m-1) + (1-a_k(m))\max[\gamma_k(m)-1, 0] \tag{7.63}$$

where $\bar{\xi}_k(m-1) \triangleq \hat{X}_k^2(m-1)/\lambda_d(k,m-1)$, and the smoothing constant, $a_k(m)$, is now both *time* and *frequency dependent*. The smoothing constants $a_k(m)$ were determined in the MMSE sense by minimizing the following error:

$$J = E\left\{\left(\hat{\xi}_k(m) - \xi_k(m)\right)^2 \mid \bar{\xi}_k(m-1)\right\} \tag{7.64}$$

That is, $a_k(m)$ was obtained by minimizing the squared error between the estimated and true *a priori* SNR ($\xi_k(m)$) conditioned on $\bar{\xi}_k(m-1)$, that is, the estimate obtained in the previous frame. Substituting Equation 7.63 into Equation 7.64, we get the following expression for J:

$$J = a_k^2(m)(\overline{\xi_k}(m-1) - \xi_k(m))^2 + \left(1 - a_k^2(m)\right)^2 (\xi_k(m)+1)^2 \tag{7.65}$$

After differentiating J with respect to $a_k(m)$, we get the following expression for the optimum value of $a_k(m)$:

$$a_k(m) = \frac{1}{1 + \left(\dfrac{\xi_k(m) - \bar{\xi}_k(m-1)}{\xi_k(m)+1}\right)^2} \tag{7.66}$$

Unfortunately, $\xi_k(m)$ is unknown and, therefore, Equation 7.66 cannot be used directly. We can, however, obtain an estimate of $a_k(m)$ by substituting $\max(\gamma_k(m) - 1, 0)$ for $\xi_k(m)$ in Equation 7.66. Defining $\overline{\gamma}_k(m) \triangleq \max(\gamma_k(m) - 1, 0)$, we obtain the following estimate of the optimum smoothing constant $a_k(m)$:

$$\hat{a}_k(m) = \frac{1}{1 + \left(\dfrac{\overline{\gamma}_k(m) - \bar{\xi}_k(m-1)}{\overline{\gamma}_k(m)+1}\right)^2} \tag{7.67}$$

Experiments in [13] indicated that the objective performance of the preceding smoothing constant, when incorporated in Equation 7.63, was found to be better than the performance of the energy-based smoothing constant derived in [14].

A different method was proposed in [10,15] for deriving the *a priori* SNR. This method was based on deriving an expression of the *conditional* variance of the signal (given past noisy measurements) and dividing that by the noise variance. The resulting estimator of the *a priori* SNR was called the *conditional* SNR estimator as it was conditioned on past measurements.

Suppose we have an estimate of the signal variance based on past information up to frame $m - 1$. We refer to this variance as the conditional signal variance and denote it by $\hat{\lambda}_x(m \mid m-1)$. When a new noisy spectral measurement $Y^{(m)}(\omega_k)$ arrives at frame m, we can update the estimate of the signal variance at frame m, $\hat{\lambda}_x(m)$, by computing the conditional variance of $X^{(m)}(\omega_k)$ given $Y^{(m)}(\omega_k)$ and $\hat{\lambda}_x(m \mid m-1)$, that is,

$$\hat{\lambda}_x(m) = E\left\{X_k^2(m) \mid \hat{\lambda}_x(m \mid m-1), Y^{(m)}(\omega_k)\right\} \tag{7.68}$$

The preceding signal variance was derived in [23] (see also derivation in Section 7.8) and expressed in terms of the *a priori* and posterior SNR values. After substituting the derived equation from [23] in Equation 7.68, we obtain the following expression for $\hat{\lambda}_x(m)$:

$$\hat{\lambda}_x(m) = \frac{\hat{\xi}_k(m \mid m-1)}{1+\hat{\xi}_k(m \mid m-1)}\left(\frac{1}{\gamma_k(m)} + \frac{\hat{\xi}_k(m \mid m-1)}{1+\hat{\xi}_k(m \mid m-1)}\right)Y_k^2(m) \tag{7.69}$$

where $\hat{\xi}_k(m \mid m-1)$ denotes the estimate of the conditional *a priori* SNR at frame m given the noisy spectral observations up to frame $m-1$. Dividing both sides of Equation 7.69 by the noise variance, $\lambda_d(m)$, and after using Equation 7.35, we get the following equation for the *a priori* SNR:

$$\hat{\xi}_k(m) = \frac{\hat{\xi}_k(m \mid m-1)}{1+\hat{\xi}_k(m \mid m-1)}\left(1+\frac{\hat{\xi}_k(m \mid m-1)}{1+\hat{\xi}_k(m \mid m-1)}\gamma_k(m)\right) \tag{7.70}$$

The preceding equation requires an estimate of $\hat{\xi}_k(m \mid m-1)$, which can be obtained using a recursive equation similar to the decision-directed approach:

$$\hat{\xi}_k(m \mid m-1) = \max\left\{(1-\alpha)\hat{\xi}_k(m-1 \mid m-1)+\alpha\frac{X_k^2(m-1)}{\lambda_d(m-1)}, \xi_{\min}\right\} \tag{7.71}$$

where $\hat{\xi}_k(m-1 \mid m-1)$ denotes the conditional *a priori* SNR obtained in the previous frame (for bin k), $\alpha = 0.9$, and $\xi_{\min}$ is a lower bound on the *a priori* SNR (set to $\xi_{\min} = -25$ dB in [10]).

To summarize, the algorithm proposed in [10] for estimating the *a priori* SNR requires two steps.

Step 1 ("propagation"):

$$\hat{\xi}_k(m \mid m-1) = \max\left\{(1-\alpha)\hat{\xi}_k(m-1 \mid m-1)+\alpha\frac{X_k^2(m-1)}{\lambda_d(m-1)}, \xi_{\min}\right\} \tag{7.72}$$

Step 2 ("update"):

$$\hat{\xi}_k(m) = \frac{\hat{\xi}_k(m \mid m-1)}{1+\hat{\xi}_k(m \mid m-1)}\left(1+\frac{\hat{\xi}_k(m \mid m-1)}{1+\hat{\xi}_k(m \mid m-1)}\gamma_k(m)\right)$$

and is initialized at frame $m = -1$ with $X_k(-1) = 0$ and $\hat{\xi}_k(-1 \mid -1) = \xi_{\min}$. The preceding algorithm uses two steps, a "propagation" step and an "update" step, as in Kalman filtering, to recursively predict and update the estimate of the *a priori* SNR.

It is interesting to note that Equation 7.70, that is, the "update" step of the algorithm, can be written in the following form [10]:

$$\hat{\xi}_k(m) = \bar{\alpha}_k(m)\hat{\xi}_k(m \mid m-1) + (1-\bar{\alpha}_k(m))(\gamma_k(m)-1) \tag{7.73}$$

where $\bar{\alpha}_k(m)$ is defined by

$$\bar{\alpha}_k(m) = 1 - \frac{\hat{\xi}_k^2(m \mid m-1)}{\left(1+\hat{\xi}_k(m \mid m-1)\right)^2} \tag{7.74}$$

Equation 7.73 resembles the *a priori* SNR estimator given in Equation 7.63 that uses a time- and frequency-dependent smoothing factor.

The preceding *a priori* SNR estimator is causal as it was derived using only present and past spectral measurements. A noncausal *a priori* SNR estimator was also derived in [10] based on a Gaussian speech model (this estimator was extended in [20] for gamma and Laplacian speech models). The derived SNR estimator made use of future noisy measurements up to frame $m + L$, where L denotes the number of future frames and was based on computing the following conditional signal variance:

$$\bar{\lambda}_x(m \mid m+L) = E\left\{X_k^2(m) \mid \hat{\lambda}_x(m \mid m+L), Y^{(m)}(\omega_k)\right\} \tag{7.75}$$

where $Y^{(m)}(\omega_k)$ denotes the complex noisy speech spectrum at frame m, and $\hat{\lambda}_x(m \mid m + L)$ denotes the conditional spectral variance of $X^{(m)}(\omega_k)$ given the noisy observations $Y^{(0)}(\omega_k),\ldots, Y^{(m+L)}(\omega_k)$ excluding the measurement at frame m. The derived *a priori* SNR estimator was similar to that given in Equation 7.72, but required three steps and computation of the *a priori* and *a posteriori* SNRs of future frames, $m + 1, \ldots, m + L$. Experimental results in [10] indicated that the noncausal *a priori* SNR estimator yielded significantly better performance than the causal estimator and the decision-directed estimator (Equation 7.55) for all tested noise conditions. Listening tests revealed that the benefit of using the noncausal estimator was particularly more evident during onsets of speech. Good results were reported with a three-frame (i.e., $L = 3$) delay. Comparisons between the causal estimator and the decision-directed estimator revealed that the two estimators performed equally well in terms of objective measures. Experiments, however, showed that the causal estimator responded to onsets of speech faster than the decision-directed estimator. The latter estimator lags typically by one frame when responding to sudden onsets of speech.

7.5 IMPLEMENTATION AND EVALUATION OF THE MMSE ESTIMATOR

We now turn our attention to the implementation and evaluation of the MMSE estimator. The MMSE algorithm can be implemented using the following four steps. For each windowed speech frame, do as follows:

Step 1: Compute the DFT of the noisy speech signal: $Y(\omega_k) = Y_k \exp(j\theta_y(k))$.

Step 2: Estimate the *a posteriori* SNR γ_k as $\gamma_k = Y_k^2/\lambda_d(k)$, where $\lambda_d(k)$ is the power spectrum of the noise signal computed during nonspeech activity (e.g., during initial silence periods* or during speech pauses). Then, estimate ξ_k using either Equation 7.51 or Equation 7.55. Alternatively, any of the equations derived in the previous section (e.g., Equation 7.57, Equation 7.72) can be used to estimate $\hat{\xi}_k$.

Step 3: Estimate the enhanced signal magnitude $\hat{X}_k$ using Equation 7.39.

* In [6], $\lambda_d(k)$ was computed only once from an initial noise segment having a duration of 320 ms. Estimating $\lambda_d(k)$ once was sufficient as stationary white noise was used.

Step 4: Construct the enhanced signal spectrum as $\hat{X}(\omega_k) = \hat{X}_k \exp(j\theta_y(k))$, and compute the inverse DFT of $\hat{X}(\omega_k)$ to get the enhanced time-domain signal $\hat{x}(n)$ corresponding to a given input speech frame.

In [6], the speech signal was Hamming-windowed prior to the DFT analysis. Each analysis frame consisted of 32 ms of noisy speech with 75% overlap between frames. The enhanced signal $\hat{x}(n)$ in each frame was synthesized using the overlap-and-add method.

The performance of the MMSE algorithm was evaluated in [6] and compared against the performance of the Wiener, spectral subtraction, and ML algorithms [2]. Speech was degraded by stationary white noise at −5 to +5 dB S/N, processed, and then presented to six listeners, who evaluated the quality of the various algorithms in terms of the amount of noise reduction, nature of the residual noise (e.g., musical type or uniform), and distortion in the speech signal.

Results indicated that when the *a priori* SNR was estimated using the decision-directed approach (Equation 7.55) with $\alpha = 0.98$, the enhanced speech had colorless residual noise; that is, the residual noise was not "musical," as that produced by the spectral subtraction or Wiener algorithms. In contrast, when the *a priori* SNR was estimated using the ML approach (Equation 7.51), the enhanced speech had "musical noise." Also, the Wiener estimator and the MMSE estimator with the *a priori* SNR estimated using the ML approach ($\alpha = 0.725$ and $\alpha = 2$ in $\beta = 2$ Equation 7.50) yielded similar speech quality. Implementing the Wiener algorithm using the "decision-directed" *a priori* SNR estimator with $\alpha = 0.98$ resulted in a more distorted speech than that obtained with the MMSE algorithm. Lowering the value of α reduced the distortion but increased the level of the residual noise. The parameter α was found to control the trade-off between speech distortion and residual noise. Comparison of the MMSE and the ML [2] algorithms showed that the main difference between the two enhanced speech signals was in the nature of the residual noise. Unlike the MMSE algorithm, the ML algorithm suffered from musical noise. Subjective comparison of the MMSE algorithm with other enhancement algorithms was reported in [24] and will be discussed in detail in Chapter 12.

7.6 ELIMINATION OF MUSICAL NOISE

Ephraim and Malah [6] noted that when the *a priori* SNR was estimated using the decision-directed approach (Equation 7.51), the enhanced speech had no "musical noise." But when the ML approach was used to estimate the *a priori* SNR, the enhanced signal had musical noise. Yet, in both cases the same suppression rule was used. No explanation was given in [6] as to why that was the case. Cappe [17], 10 years later, provided a detailed explanation of the mechanisms that countered the musical noise phenomenon.

Cappe [17] noted that the effectiveness of the *a priori* SNR estimator is closely coupled to the suppression rule (Equation 7.39). The suppression rule in Equation 7.39 is greatly affected by both *a priori* (ξ_k) and *a posteriori* parameters (γ_k). The influence of these two parameters on suppression is illustrated in Figures 7.3 and 7.4. Of the two parameters, the *a priori* SNR ξ_k is the dominant one in that it exerts the most influence on suppression. Strong attenuations are obtained only if ξ_k is low. Note from Figure 7.4 that the attenuation remains relatively flat for $\xi_k \geq -5\,\text{dB}$. Changes in the *a posteriori* SNR values γ_k produce only small changes in attenuation, at least for values of $\xi_k \geq -5\,\text{dB}$. For instance, when $(\gamma_k - 1)$ changes from ± 20 to $-20\,\text{dB}$ at $\xi_k = -5\,\text{dB}$, the resulting change in attenuation is less than 10 dB (see Figure 7.3). The suppression is therefore influenced primarily by the ξ_k parameter. But what then is the role of the *a posteriori* SNR estimate γ_k?

The *a posteriori* parameter γ_k acts as a correction parameter that influences attenuation only when ξ_k is low. The correction, however, is done in an intuitively opposite direction. As shown in Figure 7.4, strong attenuation is applied when γ_k is large, and not when γ_k is small as we would expect. This counterintuitive behavior is not an artifact of the algorithm, but it is actually useful when dealing with low-energy speech segments. This is illustrated in Figure 7.5, which shows estimates of γ_k and the ξ_k obtained using the decision-directed approach. In segments containing background noise, the γ_k values are in some frames unrealistically high, and those frames are assigned increased attenuation. This overattenuation is done because the suppression rule puts more "faith" in the ξ_k values, which are low in those frames compared to the γ_k values. This behavior of the MMSE suppression rule is particularly useful in dealing with nonstationary noise, where the noise level may exceed its average level from time to time.

Understanding the dominant behavior of ξ_k on suppression is critical in understanding the mechanism responsible for eliminating musical noise. The underlying mechanism

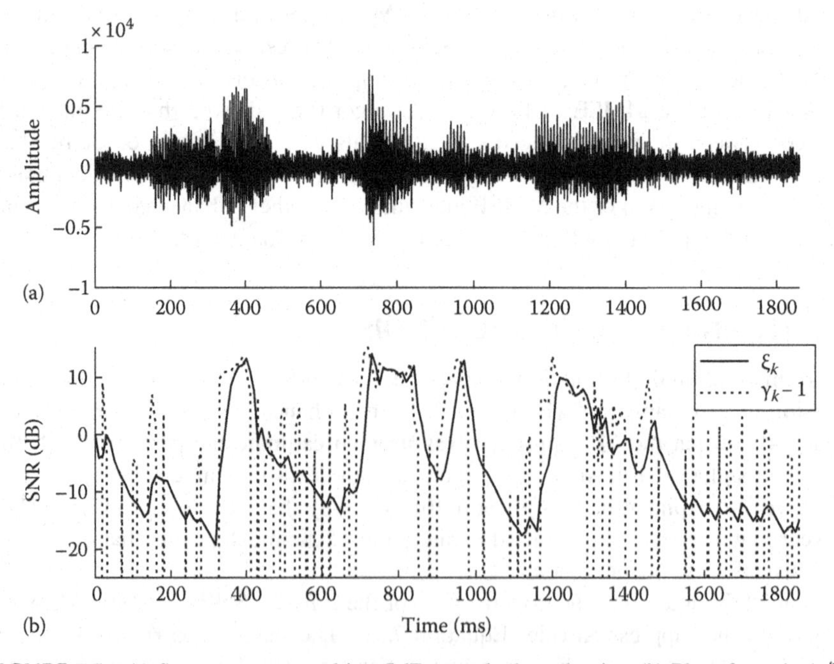

FIGURE 7.5 (a) Sentence corrupted in +5 dB speech-shaped noise. (b) Plot of *a priori*, ξ_k, and *a posteriori* SNR, γ_k. The former SNR estimate ξ_k was obtained using the decision-directed approach.

for eliminating the musical noise lies in the recursive calculation of the *a priori* SNR (Equation 7.55). The decision-directed estimator of ξ_k exhibits two different types of behaviors, depending on the value of γ_k. When γ_k stays below or is close to 0 dB, the ξ_k estimate corresponds to a smoothed version of γ_k. This is shown in Figure 7.5 in the low-energy and speech-absent segments of the signal. It is clear that the variance of the ξ_k estimate is considerably smaller than that of γ_k. When γ_k is considerably larger than 0 dB, the ξ_k estimates follow the γ_k estimates (see Figure 7.5) very closely. In fact, when γ_k is large, ξ_k can be approximated as $\hat{\xi}_k(m) \approx (1-\alpha)\gamma_k(m-1)$ [17]—that is, ξ_k follows γ_k but with a delay of one frame. Increasing the value of α increases the time delay, and that might have an adverse effect when encountering short transient segments of speech [17].

The two different aforementioned behaviors of ξ_k are shown in Figure 7.5. Note that in both cases, the decision-directed estimator of ξ_k produces smoothed estimates of the true *a priori* SNR. As the attenuation in the MMSE algorithm is primarily influenced by the smoothed value of the *a priori* SNR, the attenuation itself will not change radically from frame to frame. Consequently, the musical noise will be reduced or eliminated altogether. In contrast, the spectral subtraction algorithm depends on the estimation of the *a posteriori* SNR, which can change radically from frame to frame. As a result, musical noise is produced. In summary, it is the smoothing behavior of the decision-directed approach in conjunction with the suppression rule that is responsible for reducing the musical noise effect in the MMSE algorithm.

7.7 LOG-MMSE ESTIMATOR

In the previous section, we derived the optimal MMSE spectral amplitude estimator, which minimized the error of the spectral magnitude spectra. Although a metric based on the squared error of the magnitude spectra is mathematically tractable, it may not be subjectively meaningful. It has been suggested that a metric based on the squared error of the log-magnitude spectra may be more suitable for speech processing [24–26]. Next, we derive an estimator that minimizes the mean-square error of the log-magnitude spectra [27]:

$$E\{(\log X_k - \log \hat{X}_k)^2\} \tag{7.76}$$

The optimal log-MMSE estimator can be obtained by evaluating the conditional mean of the $\log X_k$, that is,

$$\log \hat{X}_k = E\{\log X_k \mid Y(\omega_k)\} \tag{7.77}$$

from which we can solve for $\hat{X}_k$:

$$\hat{X}_k = \exp(E\{\log X_k \mid Y(\omega_k)\}) \tag{7.78}$$

The evaluation of $E\{\log X_k \mid Y(\omega_k)\}$ is not straightforward but can be simplified if we use the moment-generating function of X_k conditioned on $Y(\omega_k)$.

Let $Z_k = \log X_k$, then the moment-generating function of Z_k conditioned on $Y(\omega_k)$ is given by

$$\begin{aligned}\Phi_{Z_k|Y(\omega_k)}(\mu) &= E\{\exp[\mu Z_k]\,|\,Y(\omega_k)\}\\ &= E\left\{X_k^{\mu}\,|\,Y(\omega_k)\right\}\end{aligned} \tag{7.79}$$

The conditional mean of $\log X_k$ can then be obtained from the moment-generating function by evaluating the derivative of $\Phi_{Z_k|Y(\omega_k)}(\mu)$ at $\mu = 0$, that is,

$$E\{\log X_k\,|\,Y(\omega_k)\} = \frac{d}{d\mu}\Phi_{Z_k|Y(\omega_k)}(\mu)\Big|_{\mu=0} \tag{7.80}$$

We are then left with the task of evaluating the moment-generating function $\Phi_{Z_k|Y(\omega_k)}(\mu)$. From Equation 7.79, we see that we need to evaluate the term $E\{X_k^{\mu}\,|\,Y(\omega_k)\}$ which is very similar (except for the power μ) to Equation 7.26, that is,

$$\begin{aligned}\Phi_{Z_k|Y(\omega_k)}(\mu) &= E\left\{X_k^{\mu}\,|\,Y(\omega_k)\right\}\\ &= \frac{\int_0^{\infty}\int_0^{2\pi} x_k^{\mu}\, p(Y(\omega_k)\,|\,x_k,\theta_x)p(x_k,\theta_x)d\theta_x dx_k}{\int_0^{\infty}\int_0^{2\pi} p(Y(\omega_k)\,|\,x_k,\theta_x)p(x_k,\theta_x)d\theta_x dx_k}\end{aligned} \tag{7.81}$$

Using the same statistical model as in derivation of the MMSE estimator, and after substituting Equations 7.30 and 7.31 into Equation 7.81, we get

$$\Phi_{Z_k|Y(\omega_k)}(\mu) = \lambda_k^{\mu/2}\Gamma\left(\frac{\mu}{2}+1\right)\Phi\left(-\frac{\mu}{2},1;-v_k\right) \tag{7.82}$$

where

- $\Gamma(\cdot)$ is the gamma function
- $\Phi(a, b; x)$ is the confluent hypergeometric function (Appendix A)
- v_k is defined in Equation 7.34
- λ_k is defined in Equation 7.33

After taking the derivative of $\Phi_{Z_k|Y(\omega_k)}(\mu)$ with respect to μ and evaluating it at $\mu = 0$, we get the conditional mean of the $\log X_k$:

$$E\{\log X_k\,|\,Y(\omega_k)\} = \frac{1}{2}\log\lambda_k + \frac{1}{2}\log v_k + \frac{1}{2}\int_{v_k}^{\infty}\frac{e^{-t}}{t}dt \tag{7.83}$$

Finally, substituting the preceding equation into Equation 7.78, we get the optimal log-MMSE estimator:

$$\hat{X}_k = \frac{\xi_k}{\xi_k + 1} \exp\left\{\frac{1}{2}\int_{v_k}^{\infty} \frac{e^{-t}}{t} dt\right\} Y_k$$

$$\triangleq G_{LSA}(\xi_k, v_k)\, Y_k \tag{7.84}$$

where

ξ_k is the *a priori* SNR
$G_{LSA}(\xi_k, v_k)$ is the gain function of the log-MMSE estimator

The integral in the preceding equation is known as the exponential integral and can be evaluated numerically. The exponential integral, $Ei(x)$, can be approximated as follows [28, Equation 8.215]:

$$Ei(x) = \int_{x}^{\infty} \frac{e^{-x}}{x} dx \approx \frac{e^{x}}{x} \sum_{k} \frac{k!}{x^{k}} \tag{7.85}$$

Other approximations to the preceding integral can be found in [29]. Figure 7.6 plots the gain function $G_{LSA}(\xi_k, v_k)$ of the log-MMSE estimator as a function of the *a posteriori* SNR and for fixed values of the *a priori* SNR. For comparative purposes, we also plot the gain function of the linear-MMSE estimator. Overall, the shape of the gain function of the log-MMSE estimator is similar to that of the gain function of the linear-MMSE estimator. The gain function of the log-MMSE estimator is shifted down for the most part by 3 dB relative to the gain function of the linear-MMSE estimator.

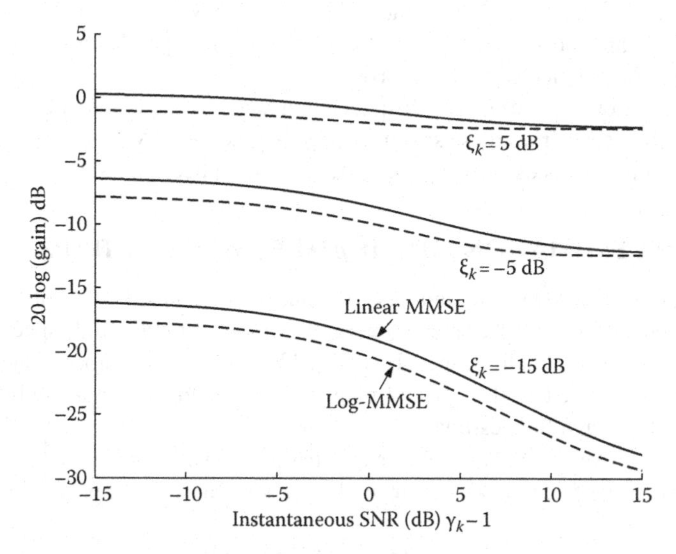

FIGURE 7.6 Attenuation curves of the log-MMSE estimator as a function of $\gamma_k - 1$.

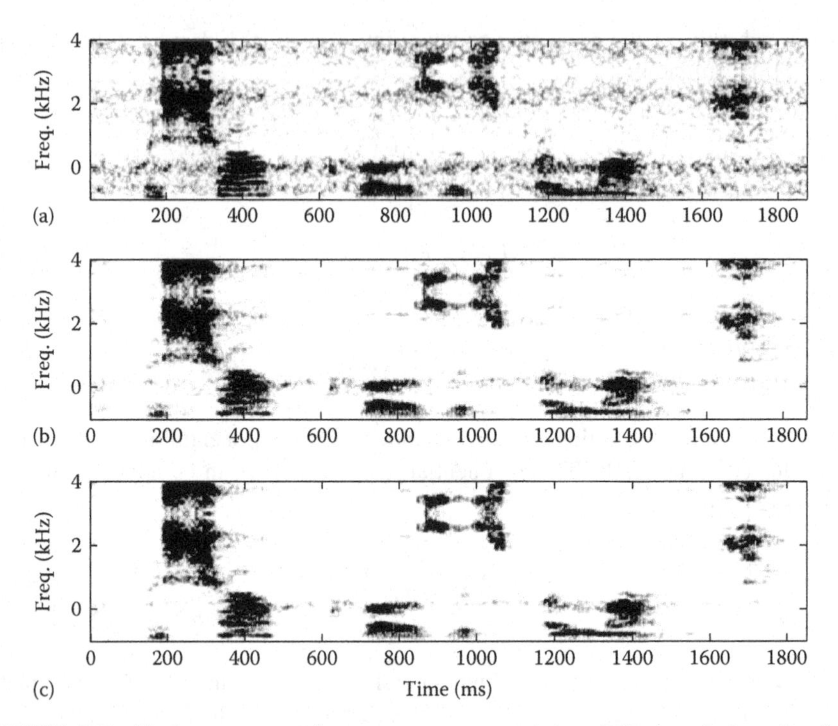

FIGURE 7.7 (a) Spectrogram of a sentence corrupted in +5 dB speech-shaped noise. (b) Enhanced speech obtained using the MMSE estimator. (c) Enhanced speech obtained using the log-MMSE estimator.

This suggests that the log-MMSE estimator provides more attenuation than the linear-MMSE estimator for the same values of the *a posteriori* and *a priori* SNRs. This was also confirmed with listening experiments [27]. The log-MMSE estimator reduces the residual noise, and most importantly, without affecting the speech signal itself, that is, without introducing much speech distortion.

Figure 7.7 shows spectrograms of speech enhanced by the log- and linear-MMSE estimators. It is clear from these spectrograms that the log-MMSE estimator reduces the residual noise considerably without affecting the speech signal.

7.8 MMSE ESTIMATION OF THE *p*TH-POWER SPECTRUM

One can extend the MMSE estimators to include optimal estimators of the magnitude-squared spectrum [30] or more general the *p*th-power magnitude spectrum [31]. In some applications such as speech coding [32], where the autocorrelation coefficients might be needed, the optimal magnitude-squared estimator might be more useful than the magnitude estimator.

First, we derive the MMSE power spectrum estimator, that is, $E\left[X_k^2 \mid Y(\omega_k)\right]$. Making use of the fact that the variance of a random variable $\mathbf{x}$ can be computed as

$$\sigma^2 = \text{var}[\mathbf{x}] = E[\mathbf{x}^2] - \{E[\mathbf{x}]\}^2 \quad (7.86)$$

we can write $E[X_k^2 \mid Y(\omega_k)]$ as

$$E\left[X_k^2 \mid Y(\omega_k)\right] = \text{var}[X(\omega_k) \mid Y(\omega_k)] + (E[X(\omega_k) \mid Y(\omega_k)])^2 \tag{7.87}$$

Note that $E[X(\omega_k)|Y(\omega_k)]$ is the Wiener estimator (assuming the Gaussian statistical model for the speech and noise Fourier transform coefficients) and is therefore equal to

$$E[X(\omega_k) \mid Y(\omega_k)] = \frac{\lambda_x(k)}{\lambda_x(k) + \lambda_d(k)} Y(\omega_k) = \frac{\xi_k}{1+\xi_k} Y(\omega_k) \tag{7.88}$$

To compute the conditional variance of $X(\omega_k)$, we need to estimate the conditional pdf of $X(\omega_k)$, that is, $p(X(\omega_k)|Y(\omega_k))$. From Bayes' rule, we know that

$$p(X(\omega_k) \mid Y(\omega_k)) \propto p(Y(\omega_k) \mid X(\omega_k)) p(X(\omega_k)) \tag{7.89}$$

and from Equation 7.30, we know that

$$p(Y(\omega_k) \mid X(\omega_k)) = \frac{1}{\pi \lambda_d(k)} \exp\left[-\frac{|Y(\omega_k) - X(\omega_k)|^2}{\lambda_d(k)} \right] \tag{7.90}$$

Assuming a Gaussian distribution for $X(\omega_k)$, that is,

$$p(X(\omega_k)) = \frac{1}{\pi \lambda_x(k)} \exp\left[-\frac{X_k^2}{\lambda_x(k)} \right] \tag{7.91}$$

and substituting Equations 7.90 and 7.91 into Equation 7.89, we get

$$p(X(\omega_k) \mid Y(\omega_k)) = \frac{1}{\pi \lambda_k} \exp\left[-\frac{|X(\omega_k) - a_k Y(\omega_k)|^2}{\lambda_k} \right] \tag{7.92}$$

where $a_k = \lambda_x(k)/(\lambda_x(k) + \lambda_d(k))$, and λ_k was defined in Equation 7.33. From the preceding equation, we can see that $p(X(\omega_k) \mid Y(\omega_k))$ is complex Gaussian with mean $a_k Y(\omega_k)$ and variance λ_k. Therefore, according to Equations 7.87 and 7.88, $E[X_k^2 \mid Y(\omega_k)]$ reduces to

$$\begin{aligned} E[X_k^2 \mid Y(\omega_k)] &= \lambda_k + \left(\frac{\xi_k}{\xi_k + 1} Y_k \right)^2 \\ &= \frac{\xi_k}{\xi_k + 1} \lambda_d(k) + \left(\frac{\xi_k}{\xi_k + 1} Y_k \right)^2 \end{aligned} \tag{7.93}$$

Substituting $\lambda_d(k) = Y_k^2/\gamma_k$ from Equation 7.35, we can further simplify the preceding equation to [30]

$$E\left[X_k^2 \mid Y(\omega_k)\right] = \frac{\xi_k}{\xi_k + 1}\left(\frac{1 + v_k}{\gamma_k}\right)Y_k^2 \tag{7.94}$$

where v_k is given by Equation 7.34. The preceding equation gives the MMSE power spectrum estimator $\hat{X}_k^2$.

More generally, one can derive the pth-power magnitude spectrum estimator that minimizes the following distance measure:

$$J = E\left[\left(X_k^p - \hat{X}_k^p\right)^2\right] \tag{7.95}$$

The MMSE estimator of the magnitude spectrum can be obtained by taking the pth root of $E[X_k^p \mid Y(\omega_k)]$, that is,

$$\hat{X}_k = \left(E\left[X_k^p \mid Y(\omega_k)\right]\right)^{1/p} \tag{7.96}$$

As shown in Equation 7.81, $E[X_k^p \mid Y(\omega_k)]$ is given by

$$E\left[X_k^p \mid Y(\omega_k)\right] = \frac{\int_0^\infty \int_0^{2\pi} x_k^p \, p(Y(\omega_k) \mid x_k, \theta_x) p(x_k, \theta_x) d\theta_x dx_k}{\int_0^\infty \int_0^{2\pi} p(Y(\omega_k) \mid x_k, \theta_x) p(x_k, \theta_x) d\theta_x dx_k} \tag{7.97}$$

Using the Gaussian statistical model (Equations 7.30 and 7.31), we have (see derivation in Appendix B for $p = 1$)

$$E\left[X_k^p \mid Y(\omega_k)\right] = \frac{\int_0^\infty x_k^{p+1} \exp(-x_k^2/\lambda_k) I_0(2x_k\sqrt{v_k/\lambda_k}) dx_k}{\int_0^\infty x_k \exp(-x_k^2/\lambda_k) I_0(2x_k\sqrt{v_k/\lambda_k}) dx_k} \tag{7.98}$$

where v_k and λ_k are given by Equations 7.34 and 7.33, respectively. Following the derivation in Appendix B (for $p = 1$), it is easy to show that

$$\hat{X}_k^p = E\left[X_k^p \mid Y(\omega_k)\right] = \lambda_k^{p/2} \Gamma\left(\frac{p}{2} + 1\right) \Phi\left(-\frac{p}{2}, 1; -v_k\right) \tag{7.99}$$

where $\Phi(\cdot)$ denotes the confluent hypergeometric function (Appendix A). Finally, the spectral magnitude can be obtained as

$$\begin{aligned}\hat{X}_k &= (E[X_k^p \mid Y(\omega_k)])^{1/p} \\ &= \sqrt{\lambda_k}\left[\Gamma\left(\frac{p}{2}+1\right)\Phi\left(-\frac{p}{2},1;-v_k\right)\right]^{1/p} \\ &= \frac{\sqrt{v_k}}{\gamma_k}\left[\Gamma\left(\frac{p}{2}+1\right)\Phi\left(-\frac{p}{2},1;-v_k\right)\right]^{1/p} Y_k \\ &= G_p(\xi_k,\gamma_k)\,Y_k \end{aligned} \tag{7.100}$$

where $G_p(\xi_k, \gamma_k)$ denotes the gain function. Note that for $p = 1$, we get the MMSE estimator of the magnitude spectrum; that is, we get Equation 7.32.

Figure 7.8 plots the gain function $G_p(\xi_k, \gamma_k)$ as a function of the instantaneous SNR ($\gamma_k - 1$) and several values of the power exponent p. As can be seen, the preceding suppression rule provides more attenuation than the linear-MMSE magnitude estimator for values of $p < 1$, and less attenuation for values of $p > 1$. When p is extremely small (i.e., $p \approx 0.01$), the resulting gain curve matches closely the gain function of the log-MMSE estimator. It is noteworthy that the difference in attenuation between the linear-MMSE magnitude estimator ($p = 1$) and the power spectrum MMSE estimator ($p = 2$) is small (≈1 dB). This suggests that Equation 7.94 can be used as a computationally simpler alternative to the MMSE estimator [6].

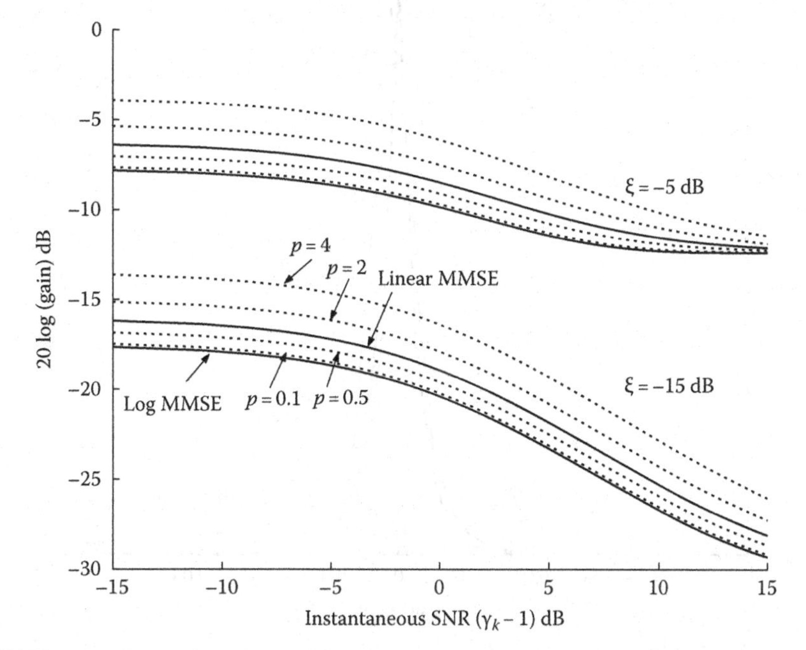

FIGURE 7.8 Attenuation curves of the pth power spectrum MMSE estimator as a function of the instantaneous SNR ($\gamma_k - 1$) and for several values of the power exponent.

It is clear from Figure 7.8 that the power exponent p influences the amount of attenuation. If p is large, then small attenuation is obtained, resulting in substantial residual noise. If p is too small, on the other hand, then heavy attenuation is obtained, possibly introducing speech distortion. Hence, it is reasonable to want to adapt p depending on the speech segment, rather than using a fixed value for p. A method for adapting p based on the segmental SNR was proposed in [31].

7.9 MMSE ESTIMATORS BASED ON NON-GAUSSIAN DISTRIBUTIONS

A key assumption made in the aforementioned MMSE algorithms is that the real and imaginary parts of the clean DFT coefficients can be modeled by a Gaussian distribution. This Gaussian assumption, however, holds asymptotically for long-duration analysis frames, in which the span of the correlation of the signal is much shorter than the DFT size. Although this assumption might hold for the noise DFT coefficients, it does not hold for the speech DFT coefficients, which are typically estimated using relatively short (20–30 ms) duration windows. For that reason, several researchers [3–5,33,34] have proposed the use of non-Gaussian distributions for modeling the real and imaginary parts of the speech DFT coefficients.

In particular, the gamma and Laplacian probability distributions can be used to model the distribution of the real and imaginary parts of the DFT coefficients. Figure 7.9 shows the histogram of the real part of the DFT coefficients (normalized

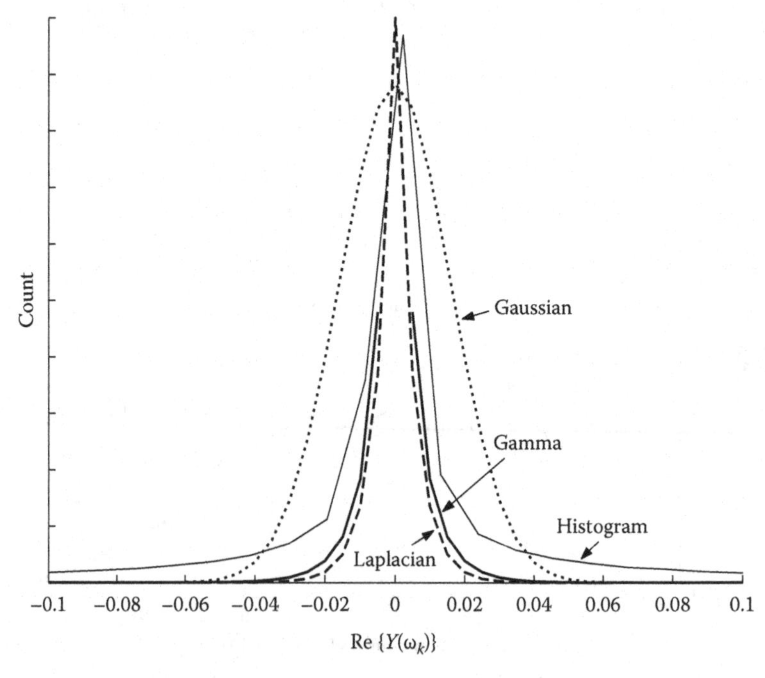

FIGURE 7.9 Histogram of the real-part of the Fourier transform coefficients obtained using 10 s of speech. The Laplacian, gamma, and Gaussian distributions are superimposed for comparison.

to have unit variance) for 10 s of speech. As can be seen, the Gaussian distribution fits the experimental data poorly. In contrast, both gamma and Laplacian distributions provide a better fit to the observed data. These two distributions provide a better fit to the experimental data than the Gaussian distribution.

It is worth mentioning here that the Gaussian and non-Gaussian models used for the distribution of the DFT coefficients might not be necessarily contradictory, as they both depend on the assumption made about the prior distribution of the variance of the DFT coefficients [29]. We can obtain, for instance, a Laplacian pdf for the DFT coefficients if we assume a conditional (on the variance) Gaussian distribution and an exponential distribution for the variance [29]. Hence, in principle, non-Gaussian models can be derived using a conditional Gaussian pdf and an appropriately chosen pdf for the variance of the DFT coefficients.

Next, we derive MMSE estimators for the real and imaginary parts of the DFT coefficients using non-Gaussian distributions for the speech DFT coefficients and a Gaussian distribution for the noise DFT coefficients. Let $Y_R(k) = \text{Re}\{Y(\omega_k)\}$ and $Y_I(k) = \text{Im}\{Y(\omega_k)\}$ denote the real and imaginary parts, respectively, of the noisy speech spectrum. For simplicity, we drop the frequency index k, and denote the complex DFT coefficients of the noisy speech signal as $Y = Y_R + jY_I$ and the complex DFT coefficients of the clean signal as $X = X_R + jX_I$.

We define the following Laplacian densities for X_R and X_I:

$$p(X_R) = \frac{1}{\sqrt{\lambda_x}} \exp\left(-\frac{2|X_R|}{\sqrt{\lambda_x}}\right), \quad p(X_I) = \frac{1}{\sqrt{\lambda_x}} \exp\left(-\frac{2|X_I|}{\sqrt{\lambda_x}}\right) \tag{7.101}$$

where $\lambda_x/2$ denotes the variance of the real and imaginary parts of the DFT coefficients of the clean signal. The gamma distributions of X_R and X_I are given by

$$p(X_R) = \frac{\sqrt[4]{1.5}}{2\sqrt{\pi}\sqrt[4]{\lambda_x}} |X_R|^{-\frac{1}{2}} \exp\left(-\frac{\sqrt{1.5}|X_R|}{\sqrt{\lambda_x}}\right)$$
$$p(X_I) = \frac{\sqrt[4]{1.5}}{2\sqrt{\pi}\sqrt[4]{\lambda_x}} |X_I|^{-\frac{1}{2}} \exp\left(-\frac{\sqrt{1.5}|X_I|}{\sqrt{\lambda_x}}\right) \tag{7.102}$$

Plots of the Laplacian and gamma distributions are given in Figure 7.10 for different values of λ_x. Assuming statistical independence between the real and imaginary parts of the DFT coefficients, we can compute the MMSE estimates of X_R and X_I separately and then combine the two to form the MMSE estimate of the complex signal spectrum $X(\omega_k)$ as follows:

$$E[X(\omega_k)\,|\,Y(\omega_k)] = E[X\,|\,Y] = E[X_R\,|\,Y_R] + j\,E[X_I\,|\,Y_I] \tag{7.103}$$

Note that if we assume that both the noise and speech DFT coefficients have a Gaussian distribution, then the preceding MMSE estimator $E[X|Y]$ becomes the

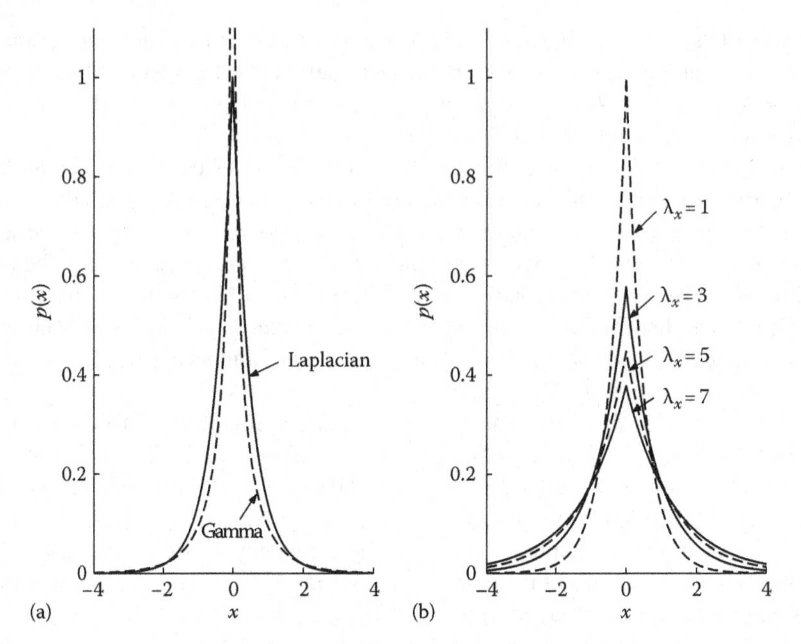

FIGURE 7.10 (a) Plots of the Laplacian and gamma distributions. (b) Plots of the Laplacian distribution for different variances (λ_x).

Wiener estimator. Next, we derive the MMSE estimate of X_R when the noise DFT coefficients are modeled by a Gaussian pdf and the speech DFT coefficients are modeled by a gamma distribution (Equation 7.102).

By definition,

$$E[X_R \mid Y_R] = \int_{-\infty}^{\infty} X_R \, p(X_R \mid Y_R) \, dX_R \tag{7.104}$$

and after using Bayes' rule we have

$$E[X_R \mid Y_R] = \frac{\int_{-\infty}^{\infty} X_R \, p(Y_R \mid X_R) \, p(X_R) \, dX_R}{p(Y_R)} \tag{7.105}$$

As the real part of the noisy speech DFT coefficients consists of the sum of the real parts of the clean and noise DFT coefficients, that is, $Y_R = X_R + D_R$, where $D_R = \text{Re}\{D(\omega_k)\}$, the conditional density $p(Y_R \mid X_R)$ is given by

$$p(Y_R \mid X_R) = p_D(Y_R - X_R) \tag{7.106}$$

where $p_D(\cdot)$ is the pdf of the noise DFT coefficients, which is assumed to be Gaussian in our case. The conditional density $p(Y_R \mid X_R)$ is therefore given by

$$p(Y_R \mid X_R) = \frac{1}{\sqrt{\pi\lambda_d}} \exp\left[-\frac{(Y_R - X_R)^2}{\lambda_d}\right] \tag{7.107}$$

The pdf of Y_R can be evaluated using

$$p(Y_R) = \int_{-\infty}^{\infty} p(Y_R \mid X_R) p(X_R)\, dX_R \tag{7.108}$$

Finally, substituting Equations 7.107 and 7.102 into Equation 7.105, we get

$$\begin{aligned}\hat{X}_R &= E\left[X_R \mid Y_R\right] \\ &= \frac{\sqrt[4]{1.5}}{2\pi\sqrt{\lambda_d\lambda_x}\; p(Y_R)} \int_{-\infty}^{\infty} X_R \mid X_R \mid^{-0.5} \exp\left[-\frac{(Y_R - X_R)^2}{\lambda_d} - \frac{\sqrt{1.5} \mid X_R \mid}{\sqrt[4]{\lambda_x}}\right] dX_R \end{aligned} \tag{7.109}$$

The preceding integral can be evaluated using the following integral relationship of the parabolic cylinder function $D_p(z)$ [28]:

$$D_p(z) = \frac{e^{-\frac{z^2}{4}}}{\Gamma(-p)} \int_0^{\infty} e^{-xz - x^2/2}\, x^{-p-1} dx \quad p < 0 \tag{7.110}$$

where $\Gamma(\cdot)$ is the gamma function. Using the preceding equation, the optimal estimator for the real part of the DFT coefficients can be shown to be equal to [4]

$$\hat{X}_R = \frac{\sqrt{\lambda_d}}{2\sqrt{2}\, Z} \left\{ \exp\left(\frac{G_2^2}{2}\right) D_{-1.5}\left(\sqrt{2}G_2\right) - \exp\left(\frac{G_1^2}{2}\right) D_{-1.5}\left(\sqrt{2}G_1\right) \right\} \tag{7.111}$$

where $D_p(z)$ denotes the parabolic cylinder function [28], G_1 and G_2 are given by

$$\begin{aligned} G_1 &= \frac{\sqrt{1.5\lambda_d}}{2\sqrt{\lambda_x}} + \frac{Y_R}{\sqrt{\lambda_d}} = \frac{\sqrt{1.5}}{2\sqrt{\xi}} + \frac{Y_R}{\sqrt{\lambda_d}} \\ G_2 &= \frac{\sqrt{1.5\lambda_d}}{2\sqrt{\lambda_x}} - \frac{Y_R}{\sqrt{\lambda_d}} = \frac{\sqrt{1.5}}{2\sqrt{\xi}} - \frac{Y_R}{\sqrt{\lambda_d}} \end{aligned} \tag{7.112}$$

and Z is given by

$$Z = \exp\left(\frac{G_2^2}{2}\right) D_{-0.5}\left(\sqrt{2}G_2\right) + \exp\left(\frac{G_1^2}{2}\right) D_{-0.5}\left(\sqrt{2}G_1\right) \tag{7.113}$$

The same estimator can be obtained for the imaginary part after substituting Y_I for Y_R in Equations 7.109 through 7.113. The final complex spectrum estimator, $E[X(\omega_k)|Y(\omega_k)]$, is obtained by substituting $\hat{X}_R$ and the corresponding $\hat{X}_I$ in Equation 7.103. Note that unlike the Wiener gain function, the resulting gain function will not be real-valued but complex. Comparisons between the Wiener estimator and the preceding estimator indicated that the two estimators behave similarly (in terms of attenuation) for high SNR values, but differ markedly for low SNRs [4].

An estimator that used a Laplacian pdf for the noise DFT coefficients and a gamma pdf for the speech DFT coefficients was also derived in [4]. The estimator that used a Laplacian pdf for the noise DFT coefficients exhibited similar behavior and performance to the estimator given in Equation 7.111. A power spectrum MMSE estimator that used a Laplacian pdf for the noise DFT coefficients and a gamma pdf for the speech DFT coefficients was also derived in [35]. The power spectrum estimator that used non-Gaussian distributions yielded a small improvement in segmental SNR when compared with the power spectrum estimator given in Equation 7.94, which used Gaussian distributions.

In summary, MMSE estimators that used non-Gaussian pdfs for the speech and noise Fourier transform coefficients yielded small improvements in performance, at least when evaluated using objective measures. Further subjective listening tests are needed to truly assess any significant benefits that could be obtained when non-Gaussian distributions are used for the Fourier transform coefficients.

7.10 MAXIMUM *A POSTERIORI* (MAP) ESTIMATORS

So far we have described speech enhancement algorithms for optimal spectral amplitude estimation based on ML and MMSE principles. Spectral magnitude estimators based on maximization of the *a posteriori* (*MAP*) pdf were also proposed [5,30]. Although the MMSE approach aims to find the average of the *a posteriori* pdf $p(X_k|Y(\omega_k))$ (i.e., $E[X_k|Y(\omega_k)]$), the MAP approach aims to find the maximum of $p(X_k|Y(\omega_k))$. Clearly, if the *a posteriori* pdf is symmetric and unimodal (e.g., Gaussian), then the MMSE and MAP estimators are identical. MAP algorithms are often used as an alternative to the MMSE algorithms in circumstances in which it is extremely difficult to derive the average *a posteriori* pdf in closed form. In some cases, it is easier to maximize the *a posteriori* pdf $p(X_k|Y(\omega_k))$ rather than to evaluate the mean of $p(X_k|Y(\omega_k))$.

In Section 7.3, we derived an MMSE estimator for the spectral magnitude and an MMSE estimator for the phase. The two estimators were derived independently, and not jointly. Using the MAP criterion, we can compute a joint maximum *a posteriori* spectral magnitude and phase estimator. More specifically, we can find the maximum of the *a posteriori* pdf $p(x_k, \theta_x|Y(\omega_k))$. The MAP estimators of the magnitude and phase can be derived as the solution to

$$(\hat{x}_k,\hat{\theta}_x) = \arg\max_{x_k,\theta_x} p(x_k,\theta_x \mid Y(\omega_k)) \tag{7.114}$$

Using Bayes' rule, we can express $p(x_k, \theta_x|Y(\omega_k))$ as

$$p(x_k,\theta_x \mid Y(\omega_k)) = \frac{p(Y(\omega_k) \mid x_k,\theta_x)p(x_k,\theta_x)}{p(Y(\omega_k))} \tag{7.115}$$

Since $p(Y(\omega_k))$ is not a function of X_k or θ_x, we can maximize $p(Y(\omega_k) \mid x_k, \theta_x)\, p(x_k, \theta_x)$. The MAP estimators of X_k and θ_x can then be obtained as the solution to

$$(\hat{X}_k,\hat{\theta}_x) = \arg\max_{x_k,\theta_x} p(Y(\omega_k) \mid x_k,\theta_x)\, p(x_k,\theta_x) \tag{7.116}$$

Assuming the Gaussian statistical model and using Equations 7.30 and 7.31, we have

$$p(Y(\omega_k) \mid x_k,\theta_x)p(x_k,\theta_x) = \frac{x_k}{\pi^2\lambda_x(k)\lambda_d(k)}\exp\left(-\frac{|Y(\omega_k)-x_k e^{j\theta_x}|^2}{\lambda_d(k)} - \frac{x_k^2}{\lambda_x(k)}\right) \tag{7.117}$$

As the log function is a monotonically increasing function, we can alternatively maximize the logarithm of the preceding equation, that is,

$$J_1 = \ln[p(Y(\omega_k) \mid x_k,\theta_x)p(x_k,\theta_x)] = -\frac{|Y(\omega_k)-x_k e^{j\theta_x}|^2}{\lambda_d(k)} - \frac{x_k^2}{\lambda_x(k)} + \ln x_k + \text{constant} \tag{7.118}$$

Differentiating J_1 with respect to the phase θ_x and setting the derivative equal to zero, we get [30]

$$\frac{\partial J_1}{\partial \theta_x} = 2j\sin(\theta_y - \theta_x) = 0 \tag{7.119}$$

and therefore

$$\hat{\theta}_x = \theta_y \tag{7.120}$$

The MAP phase estimate is therefore the noisy phase, which also happens to be the MMSE phase estimate.

Now, differentiating J_1 with respect to the magnitude X_k and setting the derivative equal to zero, we obtain the MAP magnitude estimator [30]:

$$\hat{X}_k = \frac{\xi_k + \sqrt{\xi_k^2 + 2(1+\xi_k)\xi_k/\gamma_k}}{2(1+\xi_k)} Y_k \tag{7.121}$$

Equations 7.121 and 7.120 give the MAP estimators for the magnitude and phase of $\hat{X}(\omega_k)$.

Next, we derive the MAP estimator for the magnitude X_k alone; that is, we look for the solution to

$$\hat{X}_k = \arg\max_{x_k} p(x_k \mid Y(\omega_k)) \tag{7.122}$$

Using Bayes' rule, we can express $p(x_k \mid Y(\omega_k))$ as

$$p(x_k \mid Y(\omega_k)) = \frac{p(Y(\omega_k) \mid x_k)p(x_k)}{p(Y(\omega_k))} \tag{7.123}$$

As $p(Y(\omega_k))$ is not a function of X_k, we can maximize $p(Y(\omega_k) \mid x_k)p(x_k)$, that is,

$$\hat{X}_k = \arg\max_{x_k} p(Y(\omega_k) \mid x_k)p(x_k) \tag{7.124}$$

We can use Equations 7.27 and 7.7 to evaluate $p(Y(\omega_k) \mid x_k)p(x_k)$:

$$p(Y(\omega_k) \mid x_k)p(x_k) = \frac{x_k}{\sigma_k^2}\exp\left(-\frac{x_k^2 + s_k^2}{2\sigma_k^2}\right)I_0\left(\frac{x_k s_k}{\sigma_k^2}\right) \tag{7.125}$$

where

$$\sigma_k^2 \triangleq \frac{\lambda_k}{2}, \quad s_k^2 \triangleq \lambda_k v_k \tag{7.126}$$

and v_k and λ_k were defined in Equations 7.34 and 7.33, respectively. Note that the preceding equation has the form of the Rician pdf. Substituting in Equation 7.125 the Bessel function approximation

$$I_0(|x|) \approx \frac{1}{\sqrt{2\pi |x|}}\exp(|x|) \tag{7.127}$$

we get

$$p(Y(\omega_k) \mid x_k)p(x_k) \approx \frac{1}{\sqrt{2\pi\sigma_k^2}}\sqrt{\frac{x_k}{s_k}}\exp\left(-\frac{1}{2}\left[\frac{x_k - s_k}{\sigma_k}\right]^2\right) \tag{7.128}$$

Differentiating the log of $p(Y(\omega_k) \mid x_k)p(x_k)$ with respect to x_k and setting the derivative to zero, we get the optimal MAP magnitude estimator:

$$\hat{X}_k = \frac{\xi_k + \sqrt{\xi_k^2 + (1+\xi_k)\xi_k/\gamma_k}}{2(1+\xi_k)} Y_k \tag{7.129}$$

which is different from the previously derived joint MAP estimator (Equation 7.121), by only a factor of 2 inside the square root.

The MAP estimators given in Equations 7.121 and 7.129 were compared [31] with the linear-MMSE estimator (Equation 7.39) in terms of difference in the amount of suppression applied at various SNRs. The comparisons indicated that for high ξ_k and γ_k values, the MAP and MMSE estimators were nearly the same. The difference between the two estimators was largest when both ξ_k and γ_k were very small. For very small ξ_k and γ_k, the maximum gain difference between the joint MAP estimator and the linear-MMSE estimator was 5 dB, and the maximum gain difference between the MAP estimator and the linear-MMSE estimator was roughly 2 dB.

7.11 GENERAL BAYESIAN ESTIMATORS

So far we have described two Bayesian methods for estimating the clean signal spectral magnitude: one method based on MMSE principles and another based on MAP principles. These methods are considered to be Bayesian, as they rely on Bayes' rule. More general Bayesian estimators can be derived using the concept of Bayesian risk functions. Minimization of these risk functions results in a variety of estimators, including the MMSE and MAP estimators. More importantly, the risk functions provide a mechanism by which we can incorporate some type of perceptual "weighting" in the estimator. The risk functions allow us, for instance, to incorporate psychoacoustic models in spectral magnitude estimation [36,37], something which we could not do previously.

Let $\varepsilon = X_k - \hat{X}_k$ denote the error incurred by the magnitude estimator, and let $d(X_k, \hat{X}_k)$ denote the cost function, also known as loss function. The cost function is a nonnegative function of ε and is specified by the user. Examples of $d(X_k, \hat{X}_k)$ include the squared error and the absolute value of the error. The average cost, that is, $E[d(X_k, \hat{X}_k)]$, [the expectation is with respect to the joint pdf $p(X_k, Y(\omega_k))$], is also known as the *Bayes risk* $\mathfrak{R}$, and is given by

$$\begin{aligned}\mathfrak{R} = E[d(X_k, \hat{X}_k)] &= \iint d(X_k, \hat{X}_k)\, p(X_k, Y(\omega_k)) dX_k dY(\omega_k) \\ &= \int \left[\int d(X_k, \hat{X}_k)\, p(X_k \mid Y(\omega_k))\, dX_k \right] p(Y(\omega_k))\, dY(\omega_k)\end{aligned} \tag{7.130}$$

Minimization of the Bayes risk $\mathfrak{R}$ with respect to $\hat{X}_k$ for a given cost function results in a variety of estimators. If we use the quadratic cost function $d(X_k, \hat{X}_k) = (X_k - \hat{X}_k)^2$

in Equation 7.130, and we minimize the inner integral with respect to $\hat{X}_k$ while holding $Y(\omega_k)$ fixed, we get the MMSE estimator $E[X_k|Y(\omega_k)]$ [1]. To prove that, let $\hat{\Re}$ be the inner integral in Equation 7.130, that is,

$$\hat{\Re} = \int_0^{\infty} (X_k - \hat{X}_k)^2 p(X_k \,|\, Y(\omega_k))\, dX_k \tag{7.131}$$

then

$$\begin{aligned}\frac{\partial \hat{\Re}}{\partial \hat{X}_k} &= \int_0^{\infty} \frac{\partial}{\partial \hat{X}_k}(X_k - \hat{X}_k)^2 p(X_k \,|\, Y(\omega_k)) dX_k \\ &= \int_0^{\infty} -2(X_k - \hat{X}_k) p(X_k \,|\, Y(\omega_k))\, dX_k = 0\end{aligned} \tag{7.132}$$

Solving for $\hat{X}_k$, we get

$$\hat{X}_k = \int_0^{\infty} X_k p(X_k \,|\, Y(\omega_k)) dX_k \tag{7.133}$$

which is the MMSE estimator, that is, $E[X_k|Y(\omega_k)]$. If we use the following cost function

$$d_{\log}(X_k, \hat{X}_k) = (\log X_k - \log \hat{X}_k)^2 \tag{7.134}$$

and we minimize the Bayes risk function with respect to $\hat{X}_k$, then we get the log-MMSE estimator.

Other possible cost functions can be used, leading to different estimators. The cost function $d(X_k, \hat{X}_k) = |X_k - \hat{X}_k|$ penalizes the errors proportionally, and the resulting estimator that minimizes the risk function $\Re$ gives the median of the *a posteriori* $p(X_k \mid Y(\omega_k))$. The cost function

$$d(X_k, \hat{X}_k) = \begin{cases} 0 & |X_k - \hat{X}_k| < \delta \\ 1 & |X_k - \hat{X}_k| > \delta \end{cases} \tag{7.135}$$

assigns no cost for small errors (smaller than a prescribed threshold δ) and assigns a cost of 1 for all errors larger than a threshold. The resulting estimator that minimizes this cost function (for $\delta \to 0$) gives the maximum of the *a posteriori* $p(X_k \mid Y(\omega_k))$; that is, it is the MAP estimator [1].

The quadratic cost function penalizes large errors more heavily than small ones, and makes the implicit assumption that positive errors (i.e., $\hat{X}_k < X_k$) are just as bad as negative ones (i.e., $\hat{X}_k > X_k$). But, perceptually the two errors might carry different weights. In speech enhancement, a negative error (i.e., $\hat{X}_k > X_k$) might be perceived as noise, whereas a positive error (i.e., $\hat{X}_k < X_k$) might be perceived as signal attenuation. Furthermore, a positive error might be acceptable in some cases if $\hat{X}_k$ falls below the masking threshold. Clearly, the two types of errors need to be treated differently, perhaps by taking into account a perceptual model. Next, we present a series of Bayesian estimators that make use of perceptually motivated cost functions.

7.12 PERCEPTUALLY MOTIVATED BAYESIAN ESTIMATORS

A number of Bayesian estimators of the speech magnitude spectrum have been proposed, some of which were derived in closed form [37–39] and others using numerical integration techniques [36].

7.12.1 Psychoacoustically Motivated Distortion Measure

A quadratic cost function that incorporated masking thresholds was suggested in [36]:

$$d(X_k, \hat{X}_k) = \begin{cases} \left(\hat{X}_k - X_k - \dfrac{T_k}{2}\right)^2 - \left(\dfrac{T_k}{2}\right)^2 & \text{if } \left|\hat{X}_k - X_k - \dfrac{T_k}{2}\right| > \dfrac{T_k}{2} \\ 0 & \text{otherwise} \end{cases} \tag{7.136}$$

where T_k denotes the masking threshold at frequency bin k. A nonzero cost is assigned only when the estimation error is above the masking threshold, and a cost of zero is assigned if the estimation error is below the masking threshold. The analytical minimization of the average cost given in Equation 7.136 turned out to be intractable and yielded no closed-form solution [36]. Numerical optimization techniques had to be used to minimize $E[d(X_k, \hat{X}_k)]$. Other cost functions were proposed in [37], in which the estimated masked thresholds were used to control the amount of attenuation relative to standard suppression rules.

7.12.2 Weighted Euclidean Distortion Measure

The distortion measure proposed in [38] was motivated by the perceptual weighting technique used in low-rate analysis-by-synthesis speech coders [39]. In most low-rate speech coders (e.g., CELP), the excitation used for LPC synthesis is selected in a closed-loop fashion using a perceptually weighted error criterion [40,41]. This error criterion exploits the masking properties of the auditory system. More specifically, it is based on the fact that the auditory system has a limited ability to detect quantization noise near the high-energy regions of the spectrum (e.g., near the formant peaks). Quantization noise near the formant peaks is masked by the formant peaks, and is therefore not audible. Auditory masking can be exploited by shaping the frequency spectrum of the error (estimation error in our case) so that less emphasis is placed near the formant peaks and more emphasis on the spectral valleys, where any amount of noise present will be audible.

The perceptually weighted error criterion is implemented by weighting the error spectrum with a filter that has the shape of the inverse spectrum of the original signal; that way, spectral peaks are not emphasized as much as spectral valleys. As a crude approximation of this perceptual weighting filter, one can consider weighting the estimation error by $1/X_k$. More specifically, the following cost function can be used:

$$d(X_k, \hat{X}_k) = \frac{(X_k - \hat{X}_k)^2}{X_k} \tag{7.137}$$

It is clear that the preceding distortion measure penalizes the estimation error more heavily when X_k is small (spectral valley) than when X_k is large (spectral peak). To derive a Bayesian estimator of X_k based on the preceding distortion measure, we can minimize the following Bayesian risk (corresponding to the inner integral in Equation 7.130, and denoted henceforth as $\Re$):

$$\Re = \int_0^\infty \left[\frac{(X_k - \hat{X}_k)^2}{X_k} \right] p(X_k \mid Y(\omega_k)) dX_k \tag{7.138}$$

Taking the derivative of $\Re$ with respect to $\hat{X}_k$ and setting it equal to zero, we get

$$\frac{\partial \Re}{\partial \hat{X}_k} = \int_0^\infty -2 \frac{X_k - \hat{X}_k}{X_k} p(X_k \mid Y(\omega_k)) dX_k = 0 \tag{7.139}$$

Solving for $\hat{X}_k$ we get

$$\hat{X}_k = \frac{1}{\int_0^\infty \frac{1}{X_k} p(X_k \mid Y(\omega_k)) dX_k} \tag{7.140}$$

Using the Gaussian statistical model, it can be shown [38, App. A] that $\hat{X}_k$ evaluates to

$$\hat{X}_k = \frac{\sqrt{\lambda_k}}{\Gamma(1/2)} \frac{1}{\Phi\left(1/2, 1; -v_k\right)} \tag{7.141}$$

where $\Phi(a, b; x)$ denotes the confluent hypergeometric function [28, Equation 9.210.1], $\Gamma(\cdot)$ denotes the gamma function, and $1/\lambda_k = 1/\lambda_d(k) + 1/\lambda_x(k)$. It is easy to show that λ_k can also be written as

$$\lambda_k = \frac{\sqrt{v_k}}{\gamma_k} Y_k \tag{7.142}$$

where $v_k = \xi_k\gamma_k/(1 + \xi_k)$, $\gamma_k = Y_k^2 / \lambda_d(k)$, $\xi_k = \lambda_x(k)/\lambda_d(k)$, $\lambda_x(k) \triangleq E[X_k^2]$, and $\lambda_d(k) \triangleq E[D_k^2]$. Using Equation 7.142, we can also express Equation 7.141 as

$$\hat{X}_k = \frac{\sqrt{v_k}}{\Gamma(1/2)\gamma_k} \frac{1}{\Phi\left(\frac{1}{2}, 1; -v_k\right)} Y_k \tag{7.143}$$

where $\Gamma(1/2) = \sqrt{\pi}$. The preceding confluent hypergeometric function can also be written in terms of a Bessel function [42, Equation A1.31b], and simplify the preceding estimator to

$$\hat{X}_k = \frac{\sqrt{v_k}}{\sqrt{\pi}\gamma_k} \frac{\exp(v_k/2)}{I_0(v_k/2)} Y_k \tag{7.144}$$

where $I_0(\cdot)$ denotes the modified Bessel function of order zero. It is worth noting that the preceding estimator becomes the Wiener estimator when $v_k \gg 1$. To prove that, after substituting in Equation 7.144 the approximation of the Bessel function, $I_0(v_k/2) \approx \frac{1}{\sqrt{\pi v_k}} \exp(v_k/2)$ (for $v_k \gg 1$), we get

$$\hat{X}_k \approx \frac{\sqrt{v_k}}{\gamma_k} \sqrt{v_k}\, Y_k = \frac{\xi_k}{\xi_k + 1} Y_k \quad v_k \gg 1 \tag{7.145}$$

which is the Wiener estimator.

The cost function given in Equation 7.137 can be generalized to consider weighting the estimation error by X_k raised to the power p, that is, X_k^p:

$$d_{WE}(X_k, \hat{X}_k) = X_k^p (X_k - \hat{X}_k)^2 \tag{7.146}$$

Note that the preceding distortion measure emphasizes spectral peaks when $p > 0$, but emphasizes spectral valleys when $p < 0$. For $p = -2$, this distortion measure is similar to the model distortion measure proposed by Itakura [43] for comparing two autoregressive speech models. The cost function used in Equation 7.137 is a special case of Equation 7.146 obtained by setting $p = -1$. The preceding distortion measure was called the weighted Euclidean distortion measure in [38], as it can be written as $d_{WE}(X, \hat{X}) = (X - \hat{X})^T W (X - \hat{X})$, where W is a diagonal matrix, having as the kth diagonal element, $[W]_{kk} = X_k^p$. Using Equation 7.146, we can minimize the following risk:

$$\Re = \int_0^\infty X_k^p (X_k - \hat{X}_k)^2 p(X_k \mid Y(\omega_k)) dX_k \tag{7.147}$$

Taking the derivative of $\Re$ with respect to $\hat{X}_k$ and setting it equal to zero, we get

$$\frac{\partial \Re}{\partial \hat{X}_k} = \int_0^\infty -2X_k^p (X_k - \hat{X}_k) p(X_k \mid Y(\omega_k)) dX_k = 0 \tag{7.148}$$

Solving for $\hat{X}_k$ we get

$$\hat{X}_k = \frac{\int_0^\infty X_k^{p+1} p(X_k \mid Y(\omega_k))\, dX_k}{\int_0^\infty X_k^p p(X_k \mid Y(\omega_k))\, dX_k} \tag{7.149}$$

Note that the preceding Bayesian estimator is the ratio of the $(p + 1)$ moment of the posterior pdf $p(X_k \mid Y(\omega_k))$ and the pth moment of $p(X_k \mid Y(\omega_k))$, that is, it can be written as $\hat{X}_k = E[X_k^{p+1} \mid Y(\omega_k)] / E[X_k^p \mid Y(\omega_k)]$. In our case, p is not restricted to be an integer, however. Note also that when $p = 0$, we get the traditional MMSE estimator derived in [6].

Using the Gaussian statistical model [6], it can be shown [38, App. A] that $\hat{X}_k$ evaluates to

$$\hat{X}_k = \frac{\sqrt{v_k}}{\gamma_k} \frac{\Gamma\left(\frac{p+1}{2}+1\right)}{\Gamma\left(\frac{p}{2}+1\right)} \frac{\Phi\left(-\frac{p+1}{2}, 1; -v_k\right)}{\Phi\left(-\frac{p}{2}, 1; -v_k\right)} Y_k, \quad p > -2 \tag{7.150}$$

The preceding equation allows us to express $\hat{X}_k$ in terms of a nonlinear gain function $G_p(\xi_k, \gamma_k) = \hat{X}_k / Y_k$, which is a function of both the *a priori* SNR ξ_k and *a posteriori* SNR γ_k, much like the gain function of the MMSE estimator [6]. Figure 7.11 plots the gain function $G_p(\xi_k, \gamma_k)$ as a function of the instantaneous SNR $(\gamma_k - 1)$ for a fixed value of ξ_k ($\xi_k = -5$ dB in Figure 7.11a and $\xi_k = 5$ dB in Figure 7.11b) for several values of the power exponent p. For comparative purposes, the gain functions of the MMSE [6] and log-MMSE [27] estimators are superimposed. As can be seen, the shape of the gain function $G_p(\xi_k, \gamma_k)$ is similar to that of the MMSE and log-MMSE gain functions. The amount of attenuation seems to be dependent on the value of the power exponent p. Large and positive values of p provide small attenuation, whereas large and negative values of p provide heavier attenuation.

Note that for large values of γ_k the gain function $G_p(\xi_k, \gamma_k)$ converges to the MMSE gain function. In fact, $G_p(\xi_k, \gamma_k)$ converges to the Wiener gain function for $\xi_k \gg 1$ and consequently for $v_k \gg 1$. This can be proved by substituting in Equation 7.150 the following asymptotic approximation of the confluent hypergeometric function [42, eq. A1.16b]:

$$\Phi(\alpha, \beta; -v_k) \approx \frac{\Gamma(\beta)}{\Gamma(\beta - \alpha)} (v_k)^{-\alpha} \quad v_k \gg 1 \tag{7.151}$$

In doing so, we get

$$\hat{X}_k \approx \frac{\sqrt{v_k}}{\gamma_k} \frac{(v_k)^{p+1/2}}{(v_k)^{p/2}} Y_k = \frac{\xi_k}{\xi_k + 1} Y_k \quad v_k \gg 1 \tag{7.152}$$

which is the Wiener estimator.

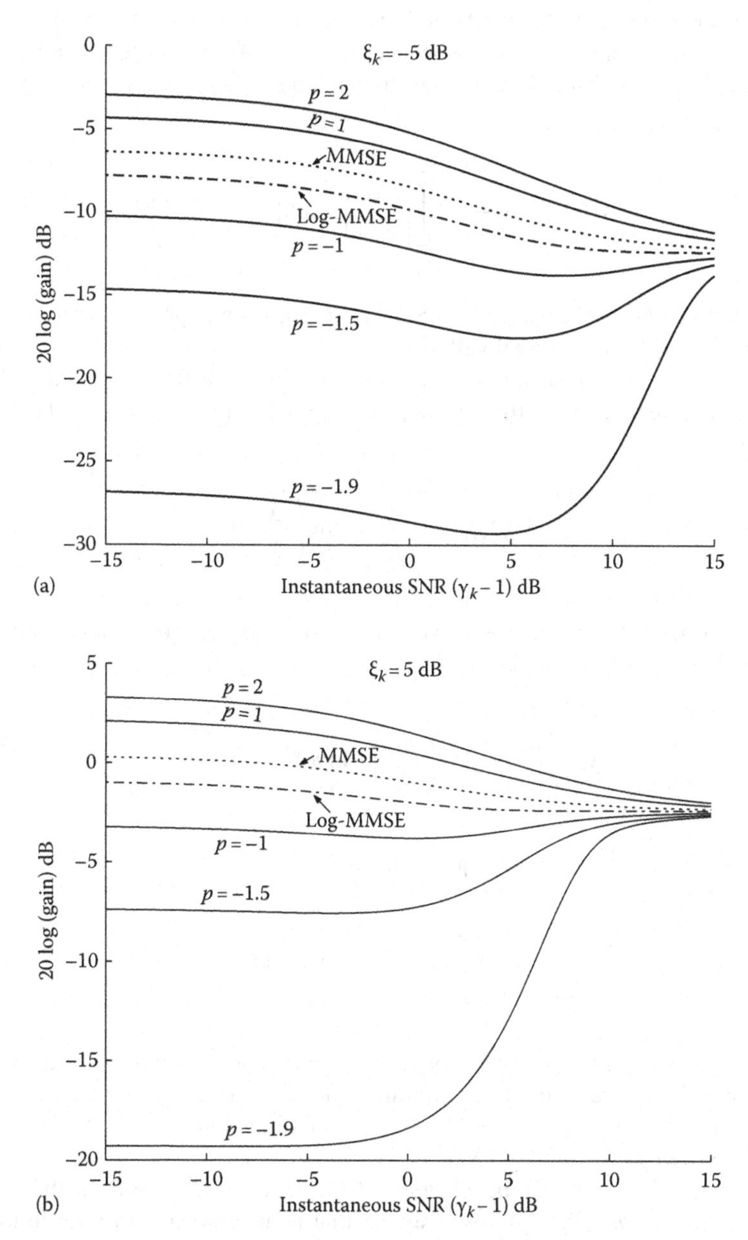

FIGURE 7.11 Gain function of the weighted-Euclidean distance estimator (Equation 7.150) as a function of the instantaneous SNR ($\gamma_k - 1$) and for several values of the power exponent p. (a) The gain function for $\xi_k = -5$ dB and (b) for $\xi_k = 5$ dB. The gain functions of the MMSE and log-MMSE estimators are also plotted for comparison.

7.12.3 Itakura–Saito Measure

A Bayesian estimator based on the Itakura–Saito (IS) measure was also proposed in [38]. The IS measure [44] has been used successfully in speech recognition for comparing a reference power spectrum $S(w)$ against a test spectrum $X(w)$ according to

$$d_{IS}(X(\omega), S(\omega)) = \frac{1}{2\pi}\int_{-\pi}^{\pi}\left[\frac{S(\omega)}{X(\omega)} - \log\left(\frac{S(\omega)}{X(\omega)}\right) - 1\right]d\omega \tag{7.153}$$

Owing to its asymmetric nature, the IS measure is known to provide more emphasis on spectral peaks than spectral valleys.

The IS distortion measure considered in [38] between the estimated and true short-time power spectra at the kth frequency bin (rather than over the whole spectrum) is given by

$$d_{IS}\left(X_k^2, \hat{X}_k^2\right) = \frac{X_k^2}{\hat{X}_k^2} - \log\left(\frac{X_k^2}{\hat{X}_k^2}\right) - 1 \tag{7.154}$$

Note that $d_{IS}(X_k^2, \hat{X}_k^2) \geq 0$, as $x - \log(x) - 1 \geq 0$. It is easy to show that minimization of the following Bayesian risk

$$\Re = \int_0^{\infty}\left[\frac{X_k^2}{\hat{X}_k^2} - \log\left(\frac{X_k^2}{\hat{X}_k^2}\right) - 1\right]p(X_k \mid Y(\omega_k))dX_k \tag{7.155}$$

yields the following magnitude-squared estimator:

$$\hat{X}_k^2 = \int_0^{\infty} X_k^2 \, p(X_k \mid Y(\omega_k))\, dX_k \tag{7.156}$$

which is also the MMSE estimator of the short-time power spectrum. So, the Bayesian estimator resulting from minimization of the IS distortion measure is the same as the MMSE estimator resulting from minimization of the following distortion measure $d(X_k, \hat{X}_k) = (X_k^2 - \hat{X}_k^2)^2$.

It is worth noting that minimization of the IS measure based on the magnitude spectra (i.e., $d_{IS}(X_k, \hat{X}_k)$) of the signal, that is, minimization of the following Bayesian risk

$$\Re = \int_0^{\infty}\left[\frac{X_k}{\hat{X}_k} - \log\left(\frac{X_k}{\hat{X}_k}\right) - 1\right]p(X_k \mid Y(\omega_k))dX_k \tag{7.157}$$

results in the MMSE estimator $\hat{X}_k = E[X_k \mid Y(\omega_k)]$. To verify this, after taking the derivative of $\Re$ given in Equation 7.157 with respect to $\hat{X}_k$, and setting it equal to zero, we get

$$\frac{\partial \Re}{\partial \hat{X}_k} = \int_0^\infty \left[-\frac{X_k}{\hat{X}_k^2} + \frac{1}{\hat{X}_k} \right] p(X_k \mid Y(\omega_k)) dX_k = 0 \tag{7.158}$$

After solving for $\hat{X}_k$, we get $\hat{X}_k = E[X_k|Y(\omega_k)]$, which is the MMSE estimator of X_k.

7.12.4 Cosh Measure

As mentioned earlier, the IS measure is asymmetric as $d_{IS}(X_k, \hat{X}_k) \neq d_{IS}(\hat{X}_k, X_k)$. A symmetric distortion measure was derived in [45] by combining the two forms of the IS measure to get a new distortion measure, which was called the cosh measure. The cosh measure considered in [38] is given by

$$d_{\cosh}(X_k, \hat{X}_k) = \cosh\left(\log \frac{X_k}{\hat{X}_k} \right) - 1 = \frac{1}{2}\left[\frac{X_k}{\hat{X}_k} + \frac{\hat{X}_k}{X_k} \right] - 1 \tag{7.159}$$

The cosh measure was shown in [45] to be nearly identical to the log-spectral distortion (Equation 7.134) for small estimation errors but to differ markedly for large errors. We can therefore infer that the cosh measure penalizes large estimation errors more heavily than the log-spectral difference measure (Equation 7.134), but penalizes small estimation errors equally.

After minimizing the cosh risk

$$\Re = \int_0^\infty \frac{1}{2}\left[\frac{X_k}{\hat{X}_k} + \frac{\hat{X}_k}{X_k} - 1 \right] p(X_k \mid Y(\omega_k)) dX_k \tag{7.160}$$

with respect to $\hat{X}_k$, we get the following magnitude-squared estimator:

$$\hat{X}_k^2 = \frac{\int_0^\infty X_k p(X_k \mid Y(\omega_k)) dX_k}{\int_0^\infty \frac{1}{X_k} p(X_k \mid Y(\omega_k)) dX_k} \tag{7.161}$$

Note that the numerator is the traditional MMSE estimator [6], and the denominator is the reciprocal of the estimator derived in Equation 7.140. Substituting Equation 7.141 for the denominator and the MMSE estimator in [6] for the numerator, we get

$$\hat{X}_k = \frac{1}{\gamma_k} \sqrt{\frac{v_k}{2} \frac{\Phi(-0.5,1;-v_k)}{\Phi(0.5,1;-v_k)}}\, Y_k \tag{7.162}$$

The preceding estimator can also be expressed in terms of Bessel functions using [42, eq. A1.31a, eq. A1.31c] as

$$\hat{X}_k = \frac{1}{\gamma_k}\sqrt{\frac{v_k + v_k^2}{2} + \frac{v_k^2}{2}\frac{I_1(v_k/2)}{I_0(v_k/2)}}\, Y_k \tag{7.163}$$

where $I_v(\cdot)$ denotes the modified Bessel function of order v.

Wanting to exploit auditory masking effects, as done with the weighted Euclidean distortion measure, we can also consider the following weighted cosh distortion measure [38]:

$$d_{W\cosh}(X_k, \hat{X}_k) = \frac{1}{2}\left[\frac{X_k}{\hat{X}_k} + \frac{\hat{X}_k}{X_k} - 1\right] X_k^p \tag{7.164}$$

Minimization of the preceding weighted-cosh-based Bayesian risk leads to the following magnitude-squared estimator:

$$\hat{X}_k^2 = \frac{\int_0^\infty x_k^{p+1} p(x_k \mid Y(\omega_k)) dx_k}{\int_0^\infty x_k^{p-1} p(x_k \mid Y(\omega_k)) dx_k} \tag{7.165}$$

It is easy to show (see derivation in [38, App. A]) that the preceding estimator evaluates to

$$\hat{X}_k = \frac{1}{\gamma_k}\sqrt{\frac{v_k\, \Gamma\left(\frac{p+3}{2}\right)\Phi\left(-\frac{p+1}{2}, 1; -v_k\right)}{\Gamma\left(\frac{p+1}{2}\right)\Phi\left(-\frac{p-1}{2}, 1; -v_k\right)}}\, Y_k, \quad p > -1 \tag{7.166}$$

Figure 7.12 plots the gain function $G_{W\cosh}(\xi_k, \gamma_k) = \hat{X}_k/Y_k$ as a function of $(\gamma_k - 1)$ for several values of p and for $\xi_k = -5$ dB. The gain function of the log-MMSE estimator is superimposed for comparative purposes. The power exponent clearly influences attenuation, with negative values providing more attenuation than positive ones. When $p = 0$, we get the "unweighted" cosh estimator given in Equation 7.162. Note that the cosh estimator given in Equation 7.162 provides slightly more attenuation than the log-MMSE estimator. Only the parametric gain curves for $\xi_k = -5$ dB were plotted in Figure 7.12. The shape of the gain functions obtained for other values of ξ_k is similar.

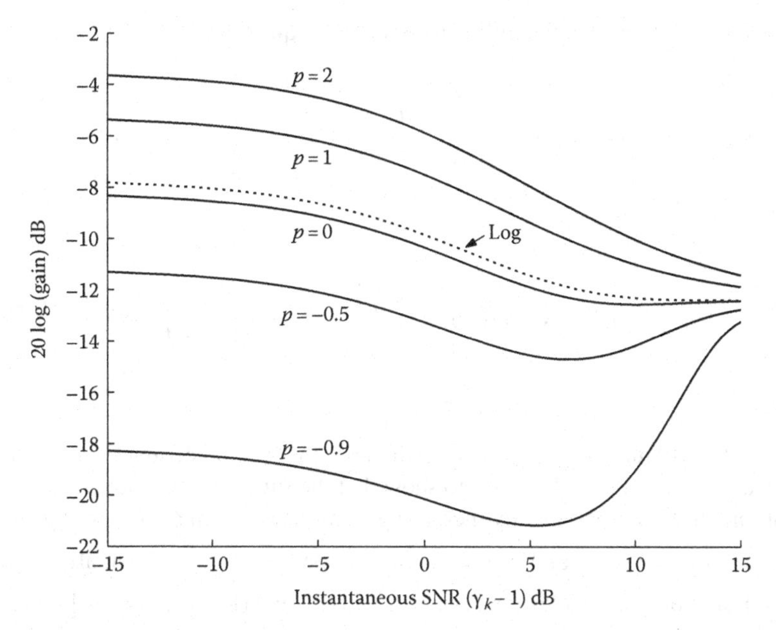

FIGURE 7.12 The gain function of the weighted-cosh estimator (Equation 7.166) as a function of the instantaneous SNR ($\gamma_k - 1$) and for several values of the power exponent p. The *a priori* SNR is fixed at $\xi_k = -5$ dB. The gain function of the log-MMSE estimator is also plotted for comparison.

7.12.5 Weighted Likelihood Ratio

As mentioned earlier, the IS measure weights spectral peaks more than spectral valleys. A different measure that places even more emphasis on spectral peaks was proposed by Shikano and Sugiyama [46]. This measure, called the weighted likelihood ratio (WLR) distortion measure, has the following form:

$$d_{WLR}(X_k, \hat{X}_k) = (\log X_k - \log \hat{X}_k)(X_k - \hat{X}_k) \tag{7.167}$$

The WLR measure can be considered to be a variant of the log-spectral difference measure given in Equation 7.134. The weighting function used in $d_{WLR}(X_k, \hat{X}_k)$ is the linear spectral difference $(X_k - \hat{X}_k)$, which weights log-spectral peaks more than spectral valleys. In contrast, the $d_{\log}(X_k, \hat{X}_k)$ measure uses implicitly the log-spectral difference, $(\log X_k - \log \hat{X}_k)$, as the weighting function, thereby weighting spectral peaks and valleys equally.

After differentiating the Bayesian risk

$$\Re = \int_0^\infty d_{WLR}(X_k, \hat{X}_k) p(X_k \mid Y(\omega_k)) dX_k \tag{7.168}$$

with respect to $\hat{X}_k$, we get the following nonlinear equation in $\hat{X}_k$:

$$\log \hat{X}_k + a_k - \frac{b_k}{\hat{X}_k} = 0 \tag{7.169}$$

where

$$a_k = 1 - E[\log X_k \mid Y(\omega_k)] = 1 - \frac{1}{2}\left[\log \lambda_k + \log v_k + \int_{v_k}^{\infty} \frac{e^{-t}}{t} dt\right] \tag{7.170}$$

and $b_k = E[X_k \mid Y(\omega_k)]$ are the MMSE estimators [6]. The preceding $E[\log X_k \mid Y(\omega_k)]$ term was derived in [27]. It is easy to show that the function $g(x) = \log x + a - b/x$ in Equation 7.169 is monotonically increasing in $(0, \infty)$ with $\lim_{x \to 0+} g(x) = -\infty$ (given that $b \geq 0$) and $\lim_{x \to \infty} g(x) = \infty$, and therefore has a single zero; that is, the nonlinear equation in Equation 7.169 yields a unique estimator. Numerical techniques [47] can be used to find the single zero of $g(x)$.

7.12.6 Modified IS Distortion Measure

With the exception of the asymmetric IS measure, the other distortion measures discussed so far were symmetric. The symmetry property is certainly desirable in pattern recognition applications, where we would like the distortion measure to yield the same value regardless of whether we compare the reference spectrum (or parametric model) against the test spectrum or the test spectrum against the reference spectrum. In speech enhancement applications, however, the distortion measure need not be symmetric, as we may want to penalize positive errors more than negative errors or vice versa. A positive estimation error ($X_k - \hat{X}_k > 0$) would suggest that the estimated spectral amplitude is attenuated as $\hat{X}_k < X_k$, whereas a negative error ($X_k - \hat{X}_k < 0$) would suggest that the estimated amplitude is amplified, as $\hat{X}_k > X_k$. The perceptual effects of these two types of errors, however, are not equivalent and therefore the positive and negative errors need not be weighted equally. Wanting to prevent attenuation of the weak speech segments (e.g., stops, fricatives), one may consider a distortion measure that penalizes the positive errors more heavily than the negative errors.

The following distortion measure can be considered [38]:

$$d_{MIS}(X_k, \hat{X}_k) = \exp(X_k - \hat{X}_k) - (X_k - \hat{X}_k) - 1 \tag{7.171}$$

which is referred to as the modified IS (MIS) measure. Note that the original IS measure had the form $d_{IS}(x, \hat{x}) = \exp(V) - V - 1$ where $V = \log x - \log \hat{x}$, whereas V is given by $V = x - \hat{x}$ in Equation 7.171. Figure 7.13 plots the preceding measure as a function of $V_k = X_k - \hat{X}_k$. As can be seen, this distortion measure is indeed

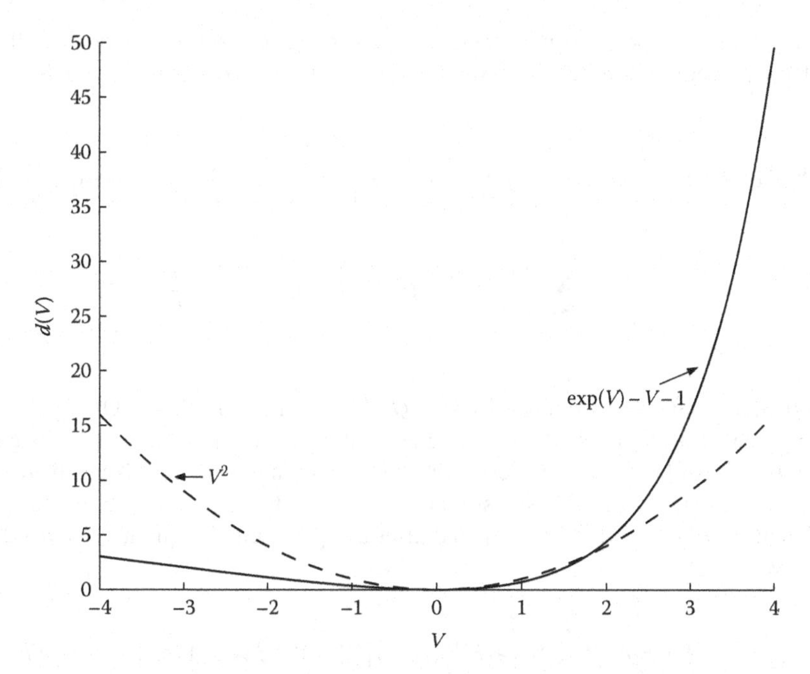

FIGURE 7.13 Plot of the modified Itakura–Saito distortion measure $d_{MIS}(V) = \exp(V) - V - 1$, where $V = X_k - \hat{X}_k$. The squared error measure (V^2) used in the MMSE estimator is also plotted (dashed line) for comparison.

nonsymmetric in that it penalizes the positive errors ($V_k > 0$ or equivalently, $\hat{X}_k < X_k$) more heavily than the negative ones. After minimizing the Bayesian risk

$$\Re = \int_0^\infty [e^{X_k - \hat{X}_k} - X_k + \hat{X}_k - 1]\, p(X_k \mid Y(\omega_k))dX_k \tag{7.172}$$

with respect to $\hat{X}_k$, we get the following estimator:

$$\hat{X}_k = \log\left[\int_0^\infty e^{X_k}\, p(X_k \mid Y(\omega_k))\, dX_k\right] \tag{7.173}$$

The integral in the preceding equation evaluates to (see derivation in [38, App. B])

$$\int_0^\infty e^{x_k} p(x_k \mid Y(\omega_k))dx_k = \exp(-v_k)\sum_{m=0}^\infty \frac{1}{m!}(v_k)^m F\left(-m, -m, \frac{1}{2}; \frac{Y_k^2}{4\gamma_k^2}\right) + \exp(-v_k)\frac{\sqrt{v_k}}{\gamma_k}Y_k$$
$$\times \sum_{m=0}^\infty \frac{\Gamma(m+1.5)}{m!\Gamma(m+1)}(v_k)^m F\left(-m, -m, \frac{3}{2}; \frac{Y_k^2}{4\gamma_k^2}\right) \tag{7.174}$$

where $F(a, b, c; x)$ denotes the Gaussian hypergeometric function [28, eq. 9.100]. In [38], the preceding infinite series was truncated to the first Q terms as follows:

$$\int_0^{\infty} e^{x_k} p(x_k \mid Y(\omega_k))dx_k \approx \exp(-v_k)\sum_{m=0}^{Q-1} \frac{1}{m!}(v_k)^m F\left(-m,-m,\frac{1}{2};\frac{Y_k^2}{4\gamma_k^2}\right) + \exp(-v_k)\frac{\sqrt{v_k}}{\gamma_k} Y_k$$

$$\times \sum_{m=0}^{Q-1} \frac{\Gamma(m+1.5)}{m!\Gamma(m+1)}(v_k)^m F\left(-m,-m,\frac{3}{2};\frac{Y_k^2}{4\gamma_k^2}\right) \tag{7.175}$$

Good performance was obtained using Q in the range of 30–40. Owing to the highly nonlinear nature of the resulting estimator, it is not possible to plot its gain function. It can be proved, however, that the preceding estimator always provides less attenuation than the MMSE estimator. Acknowledging the fact that the integral in Equation 7.173 is $E[e^{X_k} \mid Y(\omega_k)]$, and after using Jensen's inequality [48, p. 428], we have

$$\log E[e^{X_k} \mid Y(\omega_k)] \geq E[\log(e^{X_k}) \mid Y(\omega_k)] = E[X_k \mid Y(\omega_k)] \tag{7.176}$$

The proposed estimators were evaluated [38] using both objective measures and subjective listening tests, and compared against the performance of the MMSE and log-MMSE estimators. Bayesian estimators, which overemphasize spectral peak information, performed the worst. These include the traditional MMSE estimator [6], the WLR estimator (Equation 7.169), and the estimators given in Equations 7.150 and 7.166 with $p > 0$. The enhanced speech signal produced by these estimators (including the traditional MMSE estimator) had a significant amount of residual noise, which was audible. This was confirmed by listening tests. Bayesian estimators that emphasize spectral valleys more than the spectral peaks performed the best in terms of having less residual noise and better speech quality. These include the estimator given in Equation 7.150 with $p = -1$ and the estimator given in Equation 7.166 with $p = -0.5$. Listening tests confirmed that the weighted-Euclidean estimator ($p = -1$) performed significantly better than the MMSE estimator. The weighted-cosh estimator ($p = -0.5$) performed comparably with the log-MMSE estimator, but with substantially reduced residual noise. The Bayesian estimator based on the asymmetric MIS measure seemed to perform well in preserving weak speech segments (e.g., fricatives) but not in enhancing voiced segments.

7.13 INCORPORATING SPEECH ABSENCE PROBABILITY IN SPEECH ENHANCEMENT

In the preceding methods, it was implicitly assumed that speech was present at all times. However, in reality speech contains a great deal of pauses, even during speech activity. The stop closures, for example, which are brief silent periods occurring before the burst of stop consonants, often appear in the middle of a sentence (see Chapter 3). Also, speech may not be present at a particular frequency even during voiced speech segments. This was something that was exploited in multiband speech coders [49], in which the spectrum was divided into bands, and each band was declared as being voiced or unvoiced (random-like). The voiced bands were assumed to be generated by a periodic excitation, whereas the unvoiced bands were assumed to be generated by random noise. Such a mixed-source excitation model was shown to produce better speech quality than the traditional voiced/unvoiced models [50]. It follows then that a better noise suppression rule may be produced if we assume a two-state model for speech events; that is, that either speech is present (at a particular frequency bin) or it is not. Next, we present methods that incorporate the fact that speech might not be present at all frequencies and at all times. Intuitively, this amounts to multiplying the noise suppression rule (e.g., Equation 7.37) by a term that provides an estimate of the probability that speech is present at a particular frequency bin.

7.13.1 Incorporating Speech-Presence Uncertainty in Maximum-Likelihood Estimators

The two-state model for speech events can be expressed mathematically using a binary hypothesis model [2]:

$$\begin{aligned} H_0^k &: \text{ Speech absent: } \; |Y(\omega_k)| = |D(\omega_k)| \\ H_1^k &: \text{ Speech present: } \; |Y(\omega_k)| = |X(\omega_k) + D(\omega_k)| \\ &\qquad\qquad\qquad\qquad\quad = |X_k e^{j\theta_x} + D(\omega_k)| \end{aligned} \tag{7.177}$$

where

H_0^k denotes the null hypothesis that speech is absent in frequency bin k
H_1^k denotes the hypothesis that speech is present

To incorporate the preceding binary model into, say, a Bayesian estimator, we can use a weighted average of two estimators: one that is weighted by the probability that speech is present, and another that is weighted by the probability that speech is absent. So, if the original MMSE estimator of the magnitude X_k had the form $\hat{X}_k = E(X_k \mid Y_k)$, then the new estimator has the form

$$\hat{X}_k = E(X_k \mid Y_k, H_1^k)P(H_1^k \mid Y_k) + E(X_k \mid Y_k, H_0^k)P(H_0^k \mid Y_k) \tag{7.178}$$

where $P(H_1^k \mid Y_k)$ denotes the conditional probability that speech is present in frequency bin k given the noisy speech magnitude Y_k. Similarly, $P(H_0^k \mid Y_k)$ denotes the probability that speech is absent given the noisy speech magnitude. The term $E(X_k \mid Y_k, H_0^k)$ in the preceding equation is zero as it represents the average value of X_k given the noisy magnitude Y_k and the fact that speech is absent. Therefore, the MMSE estimator in Equation 7.178 reduces to

$$\hat{X}_k = E(X_k \mid Y_k, H_1^k) P(H_1^k \mid Y_k) \tag{7.179}$$

So, the MMSE estimator of the spectral component at frequency bin k is weighted by the probability that speech is present at that frequency.

The estimator in the preceding example denotes the MMSE estimate X_k and not the ML estimate of X_k. Using the fact that the ML estimator is asymptotically efficient for high SNR (i.e., it asymptotically attains the Cramer–Rao bound [1, p. 167]), we can approximate $E(X_k \mid Y_k, H_1^k)$ by the derived ML estimator given in Equation 7.10. Hence, Equation 7.179 becomes

$$\hat{X}_k \approx \frac{1}{2}\left[Y_k + \sqrt{Y_k^2 - D_k^2}\right] P(H_1^k \mid Y_k) \tag{7.180}$$

To compute $P(H_1^k \mid Y_k)$, we use Bayes' rule:

$$\begin{aligned} P(H_1^k \mid Y_k) &= \frac{p(Y_k \mid H_1^k)P(H_1)}{p(Y_k)} \\ &= \frac{p(Y_k \mid H_1^k)P(H_1)}{p(Y_k \mid H_1^k)P(H_1) + p(Y_k \mid H_0^k)P(H_0)} \end{aligned} \tag{7.181}$$

Under hypothesis H_0, $Y_k = |D(\omega_k)| = D_k$, and since the noise is complex Gaussian with zero mean and variance $\lambda_d(k)$, it follows that $p(Y_k \mid H_0^k)$ will have a Rayleigh probability distribution, that is,

$$p(Y_k \mid H_0^k) = \frac{2Y_k}{\lambda_d(k)} \exp\left(-\frac{Y_k^2}{\lambda_d(k)}\right) \tag{7.182}$$

Under hypothesis H_0, $Y_k = |X(\omega_k) + D(\omega_k)|$, and $p(Y_k \mid H_1^k)$ has a Rician pdf:

$$p(Y_k \mid H_1^k) = \frac{2Y_k}{\lambda_d(k)} \exp\left(-\frac{Y_k^2 + X_k^2}{\lambda_d(k)}\right) I_0\left(\frac{2X_kY_k}{\lambda_d(k)}\right) \tag{7.183}$$

where $I_0(\cdot)$ is the modified Bessel function of the first kind. Substituting Equations 7.182 and 7.183 into Equation 7.181 and assuming that the speech and noise states are equally likely to occur (the worst-case scenario), that is,

$$P(H_1) = P(H_0) = \frac{1}{2} \tag{7.184}$$

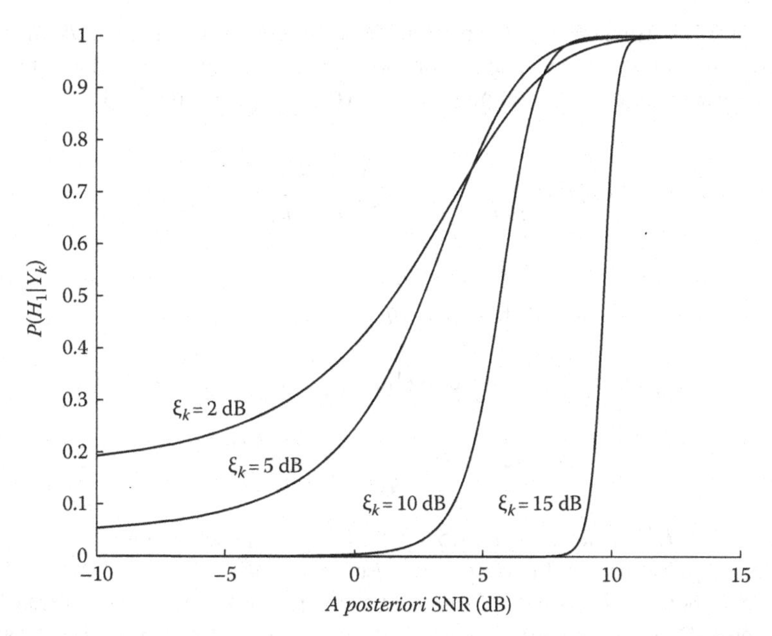

FIGURE 7.14 Plot of the *a posteriori* probability of speech presence, $p(H_1^k \mid Y_k)$, as a function of the *a posteriori* SNR γ_k.

we get

$$P\left(H_1^k \mid Y_k\right) = \frac{\exp(-\xi_k) I_0\left(2\sqrt{\xi_k \gamma_k}\right)}{1 + \exp(-\xi_k) I_0\left(2\sqrt{\xi_k \gamma_k}\right)} \tag{7.185}$$

where ξ_k is defined here as $\xi_k = X_k^2 / \lambda_d(k)$ (as opposed to $\xi_k = E[X_k^2]/\lambda_d(k)$ in Equation 7.36) and $\gamma_k = Y_k^2 / \lambda_d(k)$. This equation gives the *a posteriori* probability of speech presence at frequency ω_k, and is plotted in Figure 7.14 as a function of the *a posteriori* SNR γ_k. As shown, when the *a posteriori* SNR is large, $P(H_1^k \mid Y_k)$ is equal to one, suggesting that speech is most likely present. When the *a posteriori* SNR is small, the value of $P(H_1^k \mid Y_k)$ depends on the value of the *a priori* SNR ξ_k. If ξ_k is large but the *a posteriori* SNR is small, then $P(H_1^k \mid Y_k)$ is close to zero.

In the preceding derivation of $P(H_1^k \mid Y_k)$, the term $E(X_k \mid Y_k, H_0)$ in Equation 7.178 was assumed to be zero. Alternatively we can assume that this term is not zero, but very small. Such an approach was proposed in [51] for ML estimators and will be discussed in more detail in Section 7.13.3.

7.13.2 Incorporating Speech-Presence Uncertainty in MMSE Estimators

The linear-MMSE estimator that takes into account the uncertainty of signal presence can be derived in a similar way. The new estimator is given by

$$\hat{X}_k = E\left(X_k \mid Y(\omega_k), H_1^k\right) P\left(H_1^k \mid Y(\omega_k)\right) \tag{7.186}$$

Note that this estimator is different from the estimator in Equation 7.179 in that it is conditioned on the noisy speech (complex) spectrum $Y(\omega_k)$, rather than the noisy magnitude spectrum Y_k. To compute $P(H_1^k \mid Y(\omega_k))$, we use Bayes' rule:

$$P\left(H_1^k \mid Y(\omega_k)\right) = \frac{p\left(Y(\omega_k) \mid H_1^k\right)P(H_1)}{p\left(Y(\omega_k) \mid H_1^k\right)P(H_1) + p\left(Y(\omega_k) \mid H_0^k\right)P(H_0)}$$

$$= \frac{\Lambda(Y(\omega_k), q_k)}{1 + \Lambda(Y(\omega_k), q_k)} \tag{7.187}$$

where $\Lambda(Y(\omega_k), q_k)$ is the generalized likelihood ratio defined by

$$\Lambda(Y(\omega_k), q_k) = \frac{1-q_k}{q_k} \frac{p(Y(\omega_k) \mid H_1)}{p(Y(\omega_k) \mid H_0)} \tag{7.188}$$

where $q_k \triangleq P(H_0^k)$ denotes the *a priori* probability of speech absence for frequency bin k. The *a priori* probability of speech presence, that is, $P(H_1^k)$, is given by $(1 - q_k)$.

Under hypothesis H_0, $Y(\omega_k) = D(\omega_k)$, and as the pdf of the noise Fourier transform coefficients, $D(\omega_k)$, is complex Gaussian with zero mean and variance $\lambda_d(k)$, it follows that $p(Y(\omega_k) \mid H_0^k)$ will also have a Gaussian distribution with the same variance, that is,

$$p(Y(\omega_k) \mid H_0^k) = \frac{1}{\pi \lambda_d(k)} \exp\left(-\frac{Y_k^2}{\lambda_d(k)}\right) \tag{7.189}$$

Under hypothesis H_1, $Y(\omega_k) = X(\omega_k) + D(\omega_k)$, and because the pdfs of $D(\omega_k)$ and $X(\omega_k)$ are complex Gaussian with zero mean and variances $\lambda_d(k)$ and $\lambda_x(k)$, respectively, it follows that $Y(\omega_k)$ will also have a Gaussian distribution with variance $\lambda_d(k) + \lambda_x(k)$ (since $D(\omega_k)$ and $X(\omega_k)$ are uncorrelated):

$$p\left(Y(\omega_k) \mid H_1^k\right) = \frac{1}{\pi\left[\lambda_d(k) + \lambda_x(k)\right]} \exp\left(-\frac{Y_k^2}{\lambda_d(k) + \lambda_x(k)}\right) \tag{7.190}$$

Substituting Equations 7.189 and 7.190 into Equation 7.188, we get an expression for the likelihood ratio:

$$\Lambda(Y(\omega_k), q_k, \xi_k') = \frac{1-q_k}{q_k} \frac{\exp\left[(\xi_k'/1+\xi_k')\gamma_k\right]}{1+\xi_k'} \tag{7.191}$$

where ξ_k' indicates the conditional *a priori* SNR:

$$\xi_k' \triangleq \frac{E\left[X_k^2 \mid H_1^k\right]}{\lambda_d(k)} \tag{7.192}$$

Note that the original definition of ξ_k was unconditional, in that it gave the *a priori* SNR of the kth spectral component regardless of whether speech was present or absent at that frequency. In contrast, ξ'_k provides the conditional SNR of the kth spectral component, assuming that speech is present at that frequency. The conditional SNR is not easy to estimate, but can be expressed in terms of the unconditional SNR ξ_k as follows:

$$\begin{aligned} \xi_k &= \frac{E\left[X_k^2\right]}{\lambda_d(k)} \\ &= P\left(H_1^k\right)\frac{E\left[X_k^2 \mid H_1^k\right]}{\lambda_d(k)} \\ &= (1-q_k)\xi'_k \end{aligned} \tag{7.193}$$

Therefore, the conditional SNR ξ'_k is related to the unconditional SNR ξ_k by

$$\xi'_k = \frac{\xi_k}{1-q_k} \tag{7.194}$$

Substituting Equation 7.191 in Equation 7.187 and after some algebraic manipulations, we express the *a posteriori* probability of speech presence as

$$P\left(H_1^k \mid Y(\omega_k)\right) = \frac{1-q_k}{1-q_k+q_k(1+\xi'_k)\exp(-v'_k)} \tag{7.195}$$

where

$$v'_k = \frac{\xi'_k}{\xi'_k+1}\gamma_k \tag{7.196}$$

It is interesting to note that when ξ'_k is large, suggesting that speech is surely present, $P(H_1^k \mid Y(\omega_k)) \approx 1$, as expected. On the other hand, when ξ'_k is extremely small, $P(H_1^k \mid Y(\omega_k)) \approx 1-q_k$, that is, it is equal to the *a priori* probability of speech presence, $P(H_1^k)$.

Figure 7.15a plots $P(H_1^k \mid Y(\omega_k))$ as a function of the *a posteriori* SNR γ_k for different values of ξ'_k and for $q_k = 0.5$. The probability curves (Figure 7.14) derived for the MMSE and ML estimators are similar, except for large values of ξ'_k (it should be noted that Figure 7.14 is plotted as a function of ξ_k whereas Figure 7.15 is plotted as a function of ξ'_k). Figure 7.15b shows the influence of the value of q_k on $P(H_1^k \mid Y(\omega_k))$ for a fixed value of the conditional *a priori* SNR, $\xi'_k = 5$ dB. As q_k gets smaller, suggesting that the speech state is more likely to occur, $P(H_1^k \mid Y(\omega_k))$ gets larger and approaches one, independent of the value of the *a posteriori* SNR.

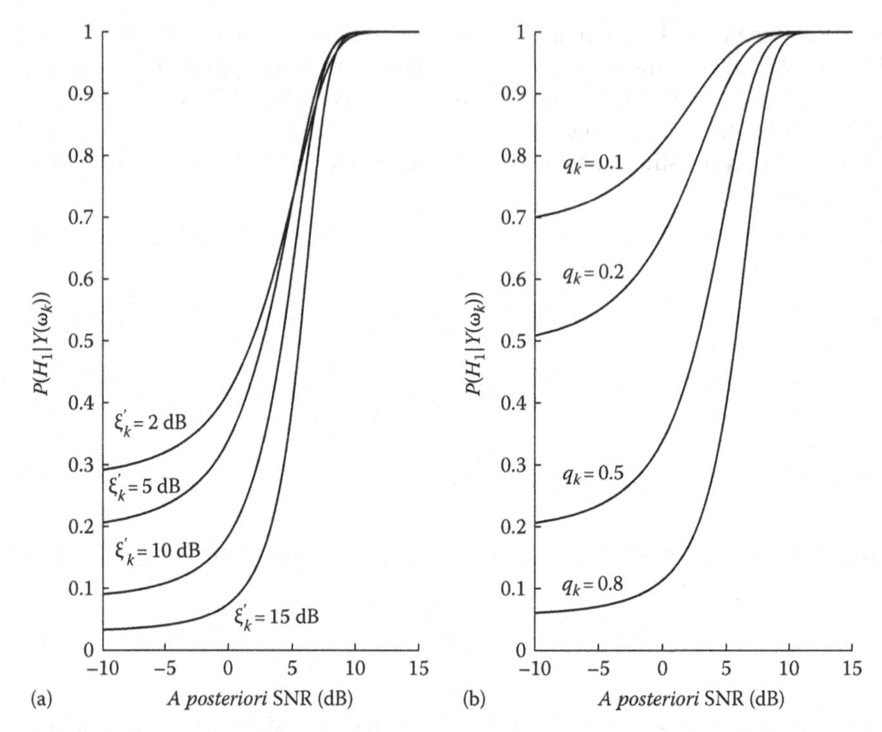

FIGURE 7.15 (a) Plot of the *a posteriori* probability of speech presence, $p(H_1^k\,|\,Y(\omega_k))$, as a function of the *a posteriori* SNR γ_k. (b) Plot of $p(H_1^k\,|\,Y(\omega_k))$ for different values of q_k.

Figure 7.16 plots the estimated $P(H_1^k\,|\,Y(\omega_k))$ for a sentence corrupted by ±5dB speech-shaped noise. The *a priori* SNR, which was estimated using the decision-directed approach, is also plotted for comparison. It is evident that $P(H_1^k\,|\,Y(\omega_k))$ follows for the most part the *a priori* SNR estimate. When ξ'_k is large, $P(H_1^k\,|\,Y(\omega_k))$ is close to 1, and when ξ'_k is small $P(H_1^k\,|\,Y(\omega_k))$ is close to $1-q_k$, which in this example is 0.5.

The final linear-MMSE estimator that incorporates signal presence uncertainty has the form

$$\hat{X}_k = P\left(H_1^k\,|\,Y(\omega_k))G(\xi_k,\gamma_k)\right|_{\xi_k=\xi'_k} Y_k$$

$$= \frac{1-q_k}{1-q_k+q_k(1+\xi'_k)\exp(-v'_k)} G(\xi'_k,\gamma_k)\, Y_k \tag{7.197}$$

where $G(\xi'_k,\gamma_k)$ is the gain function defined in Equation 7.40 but with ξ_k replaced with ξ'_k (Equation 7.194). Note that if $q_k = 0$ (i.e., speech is present all the time), then $P(H_1^k\,|\,Y(\omega_k)) = 1$ and the preceding estimator reduces to the original linear-MMSE estimator.

This linear-MMSE estimator was evaluated in [6] and compared to the ML estimator proposed in [2]. The *a priori* probability of speech absence, q_k, was fixed to $q_k = 0.2$. Subjective listening tests showed that the main difference between the quality of

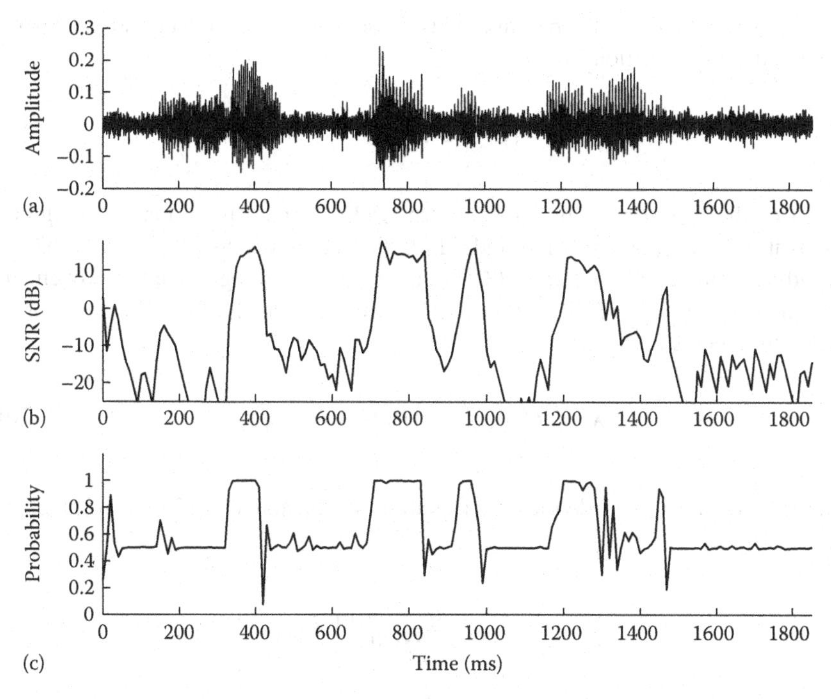

FIGURE 7.16 (a) Sentence corrupted in +5 dB speech-shaped noise. (b) *A priori* SNR estimate obtained using the decision-directed approach. (c) Plot of $p(H_1^k \mid Y(\omega_k))$ obtained using Equation 7.195.

speech produced by the two estimators was the nature of the residual noise. When the linear-MMSE estimator was used, the residual noise was colorless, but when the ML estimator was used the residual noise was "musical." A comparison between the MMSE estimator that incorporated signal-presence uncertainty (Equation 7.197) with the original MMSE estimator indicated that the former estimator resulted in better speech quality and lower residual noise.

7.13.3 Incorporating Speech-Presence Uncertainty in Log-MMSE Estimators

Using a similar procedure, we can derive the log-MMSE estimator that takes into account signal-presence uncertainty. Following Equation 7.186, we have

$$\log \hat{X}_k = E\left[\log X_k \mid Y(\omega_k), H_1^k\right] P\left(H_1^k \mid Y(\omega_k)\right) \tag{7.198}$$

and after solving for $\hat{X}_k$, we obtain

$$\begin{aligned}\hat{X}_k &= e^{E[\log X_k \mid Y(\omega_k), H_1^k] P(H_1^k \mid Y(\omega_k))} \\ &= \left(e^{E[\log X_k \mid Y(\omega_k), H_1^k]}\right)^{P(H_1^k \mid Y(\omega_k))}\end{aligned} \tag{7.199}$$

The exponential term in the parenthesis is the log-MMSE estimator and can also be expressed using Equation 7.84 as

$$\hat{X}_k = \left[G_{LSA}(\xi_k, v_k)Y_k\right]^{P(H_1^k|Y(\omega_k))} \tag{7.200}$$

Note that the *a posteriori* probability term $P(H_1^k \mid Y(\omega_k))$ is no longer multiplicative as it was in Equations 7.197 and 7.180. Simulation results [27] showed that the preceding estimator (Equation 7.200) did not result in any significant improvements over the original log-MMSE estimator. For this reason, the following multiplicatively modified estimator was suggested [52]:

$$\hat{X}_k = \left[G_{LSA}(\xi'_k, v'_k)\right] P\left(H_1^k \mid Y(\omega_k)\right) Y_k \tag{7.201}$$

where $P(H_1^k \mid Y(\omega_k))$ is defined in Equation 7.195, and $G_{LSA}(\xi'_k, v'_k)$ is given by Equation 7.84:

$$G_{LSA}(\xi'_k, v'_k) = \frac{\xi'_k}{\xi'_k + 1} \exp\left\{\frac{1}{2}\int_{v'_k}^{\infty} \frac{e^{-t}}{t} dt\right\} \tag{7.202}$$

and ξ'_k, v'_k are given by Equations 7.194 and 7.196, respectively.

The foregoing approach was suboptimal because the probability term $P(H_1^k \mid Y(\omega_k))$ was forced to be multiplicative. An optimally modified estimator was proposed in [53,54]. Starting from the original binary speech model given in Equation 7.178, we have

$$\begin{aligned}\log \hat{X}_k = {} & E\left[\log X_k \mid Y(\omega_k), H_1^k\right] P\left(H_1^k \mid Y(\omega_k)\right) \\ & + E\left[\log X_k \mid Y(\omega_k), H_0^k\right] P\left(H_0^k \mid Y(\omega_k)\right)\end{aligned} \tag{7.203}$$

where $P(H_0^k \mid Y(\omega_k)) = 1 - P(H_1^k \mid Y(\omega_k))$ denotes the *a posteriori* probability of speech absence. The second term $(E[\log X_k \mid Y(\omega_k), H_0^k])$ was previously assumed to be zero under hypothesis H_0^k. If we now assume that this term is not zero but very small [51,53], then we get

$$\begin{aligned}\hat{X}_k &= e^{E[\log X_k|Y(\omega_k),H_1^k]P(H_1^k|Y(\omega_k))} e^{E[\log X_k|Y(\omega_k),H_0^k]P(H_0^k|Y(\omega_k))} \\ &= \left(e^{E[\log X_k|Y(\omega_k),H_1^k]}\right)^{P(H_1^k|Y(\omega_k))} \left(e^{E[\log X_k|Y(\omega_k),H_0^k]}\right)^{P(H_0^k|Y(\omega_k))}\end{aligned} \tag{7.204}$$

The first exponential in parenthesis is the original log-MMSE estimator and can be expressed as $G_{LSA}(\xi_k, v_k)Y_k$ (see Equation 7.84), and the second exponential in parenthesis is assumed to be small and is set to $G_{\min} Y_k$, where $G_{\min}$ is a small value. The preceding estimator then becomes

$$\begin{aligned}
\hat{X}_k &= \left[G_{LSA}(\xi_k, v_k)Y_k\right]^{P(H_1^k|Y(\omega_k))}\left[G_{\min}Y_k\right]^{P(H_0^k|Y(\omega_k))} \\
&= \left[G_{LSA}(\xi_k, v_k)^{P(H_1^k|Y(\omega_k))} G_{\min}^{1-P(H_1^k|Y(\omega_k))}\right] Y_k^{P(H_1^k|Y(\omega_k))}\, Y_k^{1-P(H_1^k|Y(\omega_k))} \\
&= \left[G_{LSA}(\xi_k, v_k)^{P(H_1^k|Y(\omega_k))} G_{\min}^{1-P(H_1^k|Y(\omega_k))}\right] Y_k \\
&\triangleq G_{OLSA}(\xi_k, v_k)\, Y_k
\end{aligned} \tag{7.205}$$

Note that the new gain function, denoted by $G_{OLSA}(\xi_k, v_k)$, is now multiplicative. Comparisons between the preceding optimally modified log-spectrum amplitude (OLSA) estimator and the multiplicatively modified LSA estimator proposed in [52] showed that the OLSA estimator yielded better performance in terms of objective segmental SNR measures [53,54]. The advantage was more significant at low SNR levels.

7.13.4 Implementation Issues regarding *A Priori* SNR Estimation

In Section 7.3.3.2, we presented the decision-directed approach for estimating the *a priori* SNR $\xi_k(m)$ (Equation 7.55). Under speech-presence uncertainty, we showed (see Equation 7.194) that the estimated ξ_k needs to be divided by $(1 - q_k)$. Several studies [53,55] have noted, however, that this division might degrade the performance. In [53], it was shown that it is always preferable to use $\hat{\xi}_k(m)$ rather than $\hat{\xi}_k(m)/(1 - q_k)$. For that reason, the original estimate $\hat{\xi}_k(m)$ (Equation 7.55) is often used in both the gain function (e.g., $G_{LSA}(\xi_k, \gamma_k)$) and the probability term $p(H_1^k \mid Y(\omega_k))$ (Equation 7.195).

Alternatively, a different approach can be used to estimate ξ_k and γ_k under speech-presence uncertainty [56]. The *a priori* SNR estimate $\hat{\xi}_k(m)$ is first obtained using the decision-directed approach and then weighted by $p(H_1^k \mid Y(\omega_k))$ as follows:

$$\tilde{\xi}_k(m) = p\left(H_1^k \mid Y(\omega_k)\right)\hat{\xi}_k(m) \tag{7.206}$$

Similarly, the *a posteriori* SNR estimate $\gamma_k(m)$ at frame m is weighted by $p(H_1^k \mid Y(\omega_k))$:

$$\tilde{\gamma}_k(m) = p\left(H_1^k \mid Y(\omega_k)\right)\gamma_k(m) \tag{7.207}$$

The new estimates $\tilde{\xi}_k(m)$ and $\tilde{\gamma}_k(m)$ are then used to evaluate the gain function (e.g., $G(\tilde{\xi}_k, \tilde{\gamma}_k)$). Note that the probability term $p(H_1^k \mid Y(\omega_k))$ is still based on $\hat{\xi}_k(m)$, that is, the *a priori* SNR estimate obtained using the decision-directed approach.

7.14 METHODS FOR ESTIMATING THE *A PRIORI* PROBABILITY OF SPEECH ABSENCE

In the preceding methods, the *a priori* probability of speech absence, that is, $q_k = P(H_0^k)$, was assumed to be fixed, and in most cases it was determined empirically. In [2], q was set to 0.5 to address the worst-case scenario in which speech and noise are equally likely to occur. In [6], q was empirically set to 0.2 based on listening tests. In running speech, however, we would expect q to vary with time and frequency, depending on the words spoken. Improvements are therefore expected if we could somehow estimate q from the noisy speech signal. Several algorithms have been proposed for estimating and updating q, the *a priori* probability of speech absence [52,54,55].

Two methods for estimating q were proposed in [55]. The first method was based on comparing the conditional probabilities of the noisy speech magnitude, assuming that speech is absent or present. Using the conditional probabilities $P(Y_k \mid H_1^k)$ and $P(Y_k \mid H_0^k)$ from Equations 7.182 through 7.183, respectively, a binary decision b_k was made for frequency bin k according to

$$\begin{aligned}
&\text{if } P\left(Y_k \mid H_1^k\right) > P\left(Y_k \mid H_0^k\right) \text{ then} \\
&\quad b_k = 0 \quad \text{(speech present)} \\
&\text{else} \\
&\quad b_k = 1 \quad \text{(speech absent)} \\
&\text{end}
\end{aligned} \tag{7.208}$$

After making the approximation $\xi_k \approx X_k^2/\lambda_d(k)$ in Equation 7.183, the preceding condition can be simplified and expressed in terms of ξ_k and γ_k alone. More precisely, Equation 7.208 becomes

$$\begin{aligned}
&\text{if } \exp(-\xi_k) I_0\left(2\sqrt{\gamma_k \xi_k}\right) > 1 \text{ then} \\
&\quad b_k = 0 \quad \text{(speech present)} \\
&\text{else} \\
&\quad b_k = 1 \quad \text{(speech absent)} \\
&\text{end}
\end{aligned} \tag{7.209}$$

The *a priori* probability of speech absence for frame m, denoted as $q_k(m)$, can then be obtained by smoothing the values of b_k over past frames:

$$q_k(m) = cb_k + (1-c)q_k(m-1) \tag{7.210}$$

where c is a smoothing constant which was set to 0.1 in [55]. This method for determining the probability of speech absence can be considered as a hard-decision approach, in that the condition in Equation 7.209 yields a binary value—speech is either present or absent. Figure 7.17 shows as an example the estimated values of q_k for a sentence corrupted in ±5 dB speech-shaped noise. The estimated probability values of $P(H_1^k \mid Y_k)$ are also plotted for reference. As can be seen, the estimated q_k values are small in speech-present segments and are comparatively larger in speech-absent segments. Figure 7.18 shows another example of speech enhanced by the MMSE and log-MMSE estimators, with the latter estimator incorporating speech-presence uncertainty with: (a) q_k fixed to $q_k = 0.5$ and (b) q_k estimated using the preceding hard-decision approach (Equation 7.210). As shown, the residual

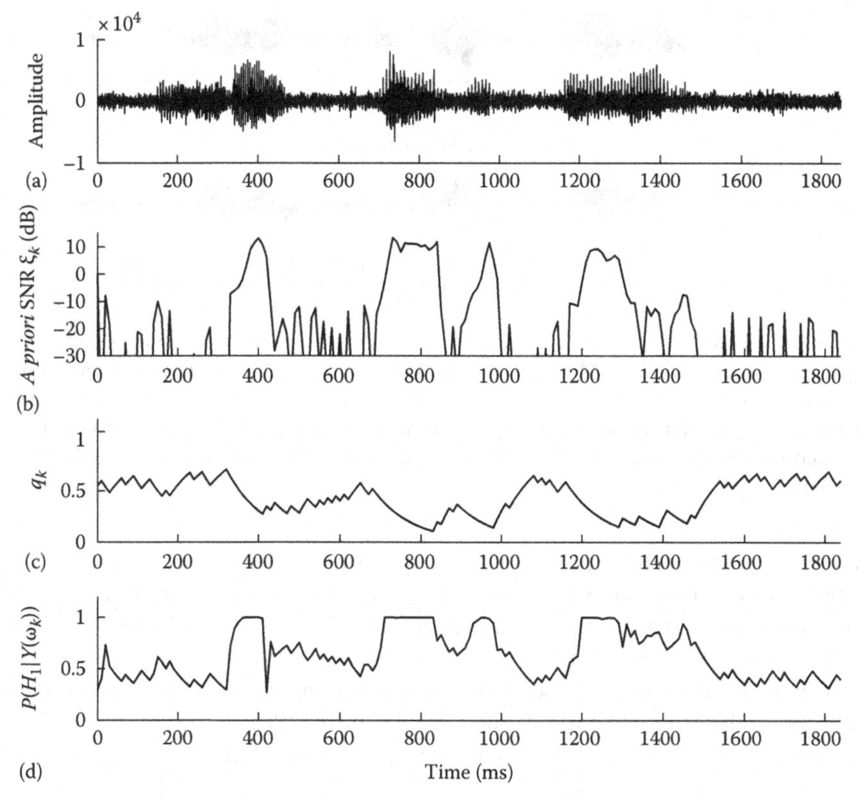

FIGURE 7.17 (a) Sentence corrupted in +5 dB speech-shaped noise. (b) *A priori* SNR estimate obtained using the decision-directed approach. (c) Estimate of q_k obtained using the hard-decision approach according to Equation 7.210. (d) Plot of $p(H_1^k \mid Y(\omega_k))$ obtained using Equation 7.195.

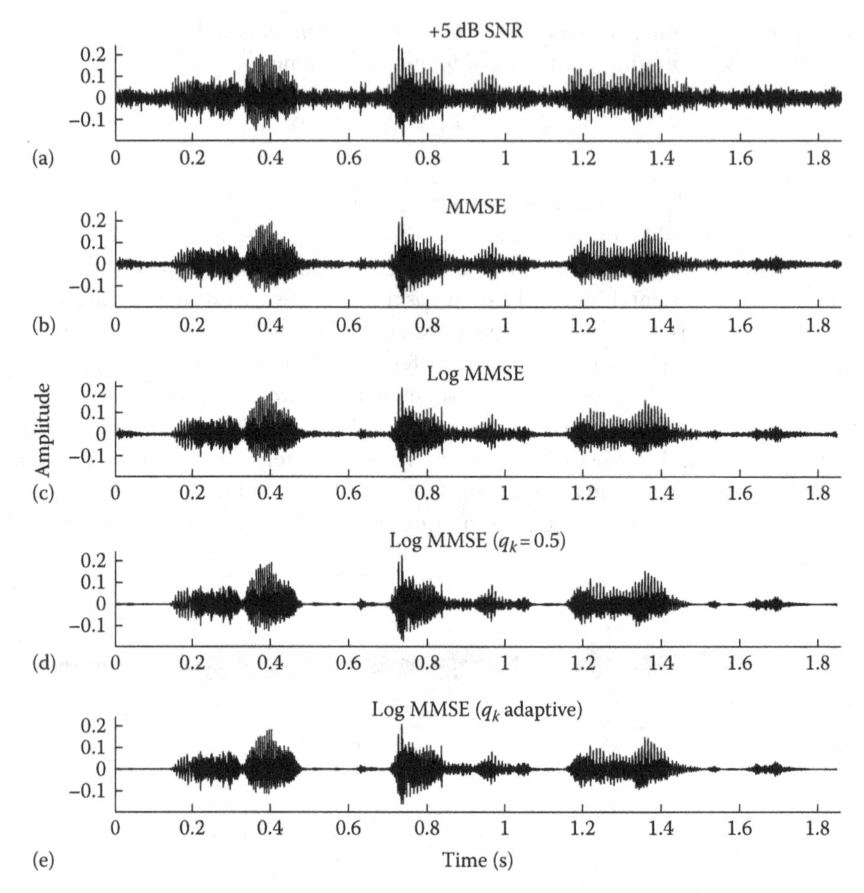

FIGURE 7.18 (a) Waveform of a sentence corrupted in +5 dB speech-shaped noise. (b and c) Speech enhanced by the MMSE and the log-MMSE estimators. (d) The enhanced waveform produced by a log-MMSE estimator that incorporated speech-presence uncertainty using $q_k = 0.5$. (e) The enhanced waveform produced by a log-MMSE estimator that incorporated speech-presence uncertainty with q_k estimated using the hard-decision approach (Equation 7.210).

noise is reduced substantially after incorporating speech-presence uncertainty. This, however, may come at a price: speech distortion. The study in either [24] indicated that incorporating speech-presence uncertainty in log-MMSE estimators may introduce speech distortion.

The second method proposed in [55] for determining q_k was based on a soft-decision approach. After using Bayes' theorem to estimate $P(H_0^k \mid Y_k)$ and after making the assumption that $P(H_0^k) = P(H_1^k)$, we can approximate $P(H_0^k \mid Y_k)$ as follows:

$$P\left(H_0^k \mid Y_k\right) \approx \frac{P\left(H_0^k \mid Y_k\right)}{P\left(H_0^k \mid Y_k\right) + P\left(H_1^k \mid Y_k\right)} \tag{7.211}$$

Substituting Equations 7.182 and 7.183 in the preceding equation, we obtain the following approximation to $P(H_0^k \mid Y_k)$:

$$\hat{P}(H_0^k \mid Y_k) \approx \frac{1}{1+\exp(-\xi_k)I_0\left(2\sqrt{\xi_k \gamma_k}\right)} \tag{7.212}$$

The *a priori* probability of speech absence for frame m is then obtained by smoothing the values of $\hat{P}(H_0^k \mid Y_k)$ over past frames:

$$q_k(m) = c\,\hat{P}(H_0^k \mid Y_k) + (1-c)q_k(m-1) \tag{7.213}$$

where c is a smoothing constant that was set to 0.1 in [55]. Note that the preceding method implicitly assumes that the *a posteriori* probability of speech absence (i.e., $P(H_0^k \mid Y_k)$ is equal (or close) to the *a priori* probability of speech absence, that is, $p(H_0^k)$).

The preceding two methods for estimating q_k were incorporated into an MMSE estimator and compared against the MMSE estimator that used a fixed $q_k = 0.2$ [55]. Results obtained, in terms of segmental SNR, indicated that both methods (hard- and soft-decision based) yielded about 2–3 dB SNR improvement over the estimator that used a fixed $q_k = 0.2$. The hard- and soft-decision methods yielded comparable improvement in terms of segmental SNR [55].

A different, and simpler, method for obtaining q_k was proposed in [52] based on the *a posteriori* SNR values γ_k. The decision on speech absence was based on a comparison of the estimated *a posteriori* SNR γ_k against a threshold:

$$\begin{aligned}
&\text{if } \gamma_k > \gamma_{th} \text{ then} \\
&\qquad I_k = 0 \quad \text{(speech present)} \\
&\text{else} \\
&\qquad I_k = 1 \quad \text{(speech absent)} \\
&\text{end}
\end{aligned} \tag{7.214}$$

where the threshold value γ_{th} was set to 0.8 to satisfy a desired significance level. The *a priori* probability of speech absence for frame m was obtained by smoothing the values of I_k over past frames:

$$q_k(m) = c\,q_k(m-1) + (1-c)I_k \tag{7.215}$$

where c is a smoothing constant that was set to 0.98 in [53]. The smoothing was performed only for frames containing speech based on a decision made by a voice activity detection (VAD) algorithm. A simple VAD detector was adopted in [53], based on the method proposed in [51]. A given frame was declared to contain speech when the average γ_k (averaged over all frequency bins in that frame) was larger than a threshold. Good threshold values were suggested to be in the range between 1.3 and 2.

A different method for estimating the probability of speech absence was proposed in [53,54]. This method exploited the strong correlation of speech presence in neighboring frequency bins of consecutive frames. The proposed estimate of speech-absence probability for frequency bin k had the following form:

$$q_k = 1 - P_{LOC}(k)\, P_{GLOB}(k)\, P_{FRAME} \tag{7.216}$$

where the terms $P_{LOC}(k)$ and $P_{GLOB}(k)$ represent the likelihood of speech presence within a local (small bandwidth) or global (larger bandwidth) neighborhood in the frequency domain. These terms are computed by applying local and global averaging of the *a priori* SNR values in the frequency domain. More specifically, if $\zeta_\lambda(k)$ denotes the smoothed *a priori* SNR, then $P_{LOC}(k)$ and $P_{GLOB}(k)$ are computed as follows:

$$P_\lambda(k) = \begin{cases} 0 & \text{if } \zeta_\lambda(k) \le \zeta_{\min} \\ 1 & \text{if } \zeta_\lambda(k) \ge \zeta_{\max} \\ \dfrac{\log(\zeta_\lambda(k)/\zeta_{\min})}{\log(\zeta_{\max}/\zeta_{\min})} & \text{else} \end{cases} \tag{7.217}$$

where $\zeta_{\min} = 0.1$ and $\zeta_{\max} = 0.3162$ corresponding to −10 and −5 dB, respectively. The subscript λ in $P_\lambda(k)$ designates local or global averaging of the *a priori* SNR values, yielding, respectively, $P_{LOC}(k)$ and $P_{GLOB}(k)$. Local averaging uses two adjacent frequency bins, that is, $(k-1, k, k+1)$ when smoothing the *a priori* SNR value at frequency bin k (ξ_k), whereas global averaging uses 30 adjacent frequency bins encompassing $k-15$ to $k+15$.

Note that Equation 7.217 is based on normalization of the smoothed *a priori* SNR to values between 0 and 1. The fact that we can estimate the likelihood of speech presence based on ξ_k alone is based on the observation that $P(H_1^k \mid Y(\omega_k))$ heavily depends on ξ_k and follows for the most part the *a priori* SNR (see Figure 7.14).

The third likelihood term, P_{FRAME}, is based on the average (across all frequency bins) of the smoothed *a priori* SNR values and is used for further attenuation of noise in noise-only frames. The P_{FRAME} term is also used for delaying the transition from speech-dominant frames to noise-dominant frames.

Note that according to Equation 7.216, when either of the three likelihood terms ($P_{LOC}(k)$, $P_{GLOB}(k)$, or P_{FRAME}) is small, suggesting that the previous frames or neighboring frequency bins do not contain speech, the resulting product of these terms will be small, and therefore $q_k \approx 1$. So, it only requires one of the three likelihood terms to be small for q_k to be close to one. Figure 7.19 shows, as an example, the estimated probability of speech absence, q_k, for a sentence corrupted

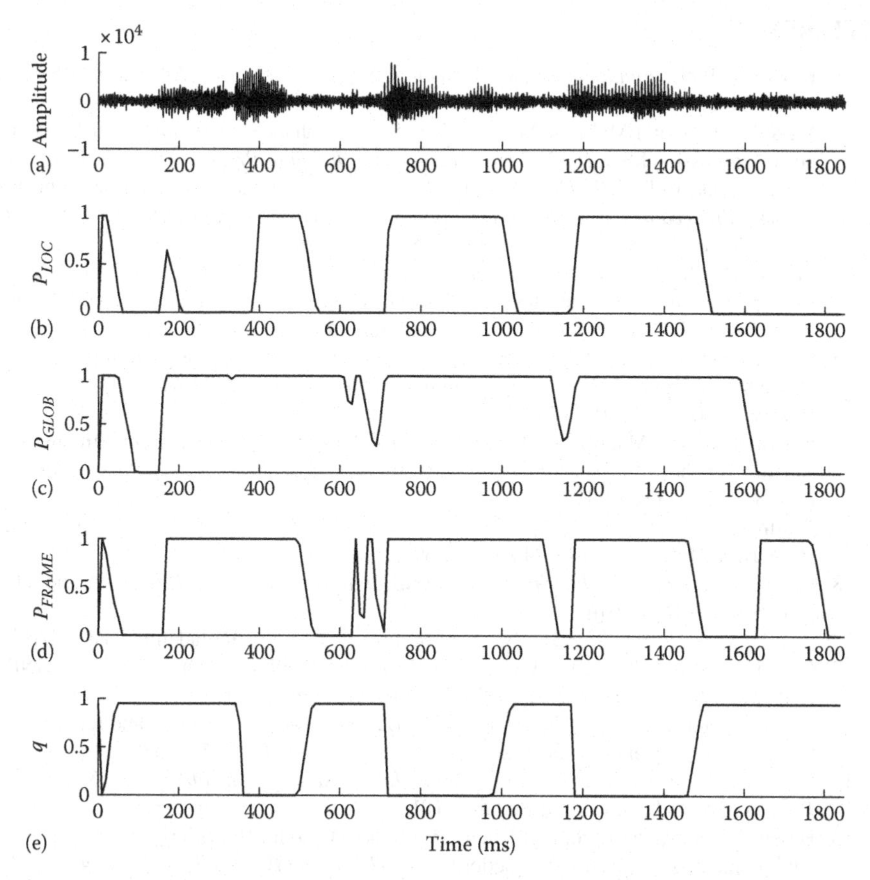

FIGURE 7.19 (a) Time-domain waveform of a sentence corrupted in +5 dB speech-shaped noise. (b–d) Estimates of the likelihood terms $P_{LOC}(k)$, $P_{GLOB}(k)$, and P_{FRAME}. (e) The estimated probability of speech absence, q_k, where k corresponds to 500 Hz.

in +5 dB speech-shaped noise. Note that the estimated q_k is for the most part equal to 0 or 1, that is, it is pseudo-binary, except in the transition regions. Estimates of the likelihood terms $P_{LOC}(k)$, $P_{GLOB}(k)$, and P_{FRAME} are also plotted in Figure 7.19 for completeness.

7.15 SUMMARY

In this chapter, we discussed several statistical-model-based methods for optimal spectral magnitude estimation. We presented an ML estimator, an MMSE magnitude estimator, and a log-MMSE estimator. Bayesian estimators of the magnitude spectrum based on perceptually motivated distortion measures were also described. MAP estimators of the magnitude and phase spectra were presented. We also discussed several methods of incorporating speech-presence uncertainty in the preceding estimators. These methods, when combined with the statistical estimators, substantially reduce the residual noise.

REFERENCES

1. Kay, S. (1993), *Fundamentals of Statistical Signal Processing: Estimation Theory,* Upper Saddle River, NJ: Prentice Hall.
2. McAulay, R. J. and Malpass, M. L. (1980), Speech enhancement using a soft-decision noise suppression filter, *IEEE Trans. Acoust. Speech Signal Process.,* 28, 137–145.
3. Porter, J. and Boll, S. F. (1984), Optimal estimators for spectral restoration of noisy speech, *Proceedings of IEEE International Conference on Acoustics, Speech, and Signal Processing,* San Diego, CA, pp. 18A.2.1–18A.2.4.
4. Martin, R. (2002), Speech enhancement using a MMSE short time spectral estimation with Gamma distributed speech priors, *IEEE International Conference on Speech, Acoustics, and Signal Processing,* Vol. I, Orlando, FL, pp. 253–256.
5. Lotter, T. and Vary, P. (2005), Speech enhancement by maximum a posteriori spectral amplitude estimation using a supergaussian speech model, *EURASIP J. Appl. Signal Process.,* 2005(7), 1110–1126.
6. Ephraim, Y. and Malah, D. (1984), Speech enhancement using a minimum mean-square error short-time spectral amplitude estimator, *IEEE Trans. Acoust. Speech Signal Process.,* 32(6), 1109–1121.
7. Pearlman, W. and Gray, R. (1978), Source coding of the discrete Fourier transform, *IEEE Trans. Inform. Theory,* 24(6), 683–692.
8. Papoulis, A. (1984), *Probability, Random Variables and Stochastic Processes,* 2nd ed., New York: McGraw-Hill.
9. Brillinger, D. (2001), *Time Series: Data Analysis and Theory,* Philadelphia, PA: SIAM.
10. Cohen, I. (2005), Relaxed statistical model for speech enhancement and a priori SNR estimation, *IEEE Trans. Speech Audio Process.,* 13(5), 870–881.
11. Wolfe, P., Godsill, S., and Ng, W.-J. (2004), Bayesian variable selection and regularisation for time-frequency surface estimation, *J. R. Stat. Soc. B,* 66, 575–589.
12. Papoulis, A. and Pillai, S. (2002), *Probability, Random Variables and Stochastic Processes,* 4th ed., New York: McGraw-Hill.
13. Hasan, M., Salahuddin, S., and Khan, M. (2004), A modified a priori SNR for speech enhancement using spectral subtraction rules, *IEEE Signal Process. Lett.,* 11(4), 450–453.
14. Soon, I. and Koh, S. (2000), Low distortion speech enhancement, *IEE Proc—Vision Image Signal Process.,* 147(3), 247–253.
15. Cohen, I. (2004), On the decision-directed estimation approach of Ephraim and Malah, *Proceedings of IEEE International Conference on Acoustics, Speech, and Signal Processing,* Vol. I, Montreal, Quebec, Canada, pp. 293–296.
16. Scalart, P. and Filho, J. (1996), Speech enhancement based on a priori signal to noise estimation, *Proceedings of IEEE International Conference on Acoustics, Speech, and Signal Processing,* Atlanta, GA, pp. 629–632.
17. Cappe, O. (1994), Elimination of the musical noise phenomenon with the Ephraim and Malah noise suppressor, *IEEE Trans. Speech Audio Process.,* 2(2), 346–349.
18. Martin, R. (2005), Statistical methods for the enhancement of noisy speech, in Benesty, J., Makino, S., and Chen, J. (Eds.), *Speech Enhancement,* Berlin, Germany: Springer, pp. 43–64.
19. Erkelens, J., Jensen, J., and Heusdens, R. (2007), A data-driven approach to optimizing spectral speech enhancement methods for various error criteria, *Speech Commun.,* 49(7–8), 530–541.
20. Cohen, I. (2005), Speech enhancement using super-Gaussian speech models and noncausal a priori SNR estimation, *Speech Commun.,* 47, 336–350.
21. Cohen, I. (2005), From volatility modeling of financial time-series to stochastic modeling and enhancement of speech signals, in Benesty, J., Makino, S., and Chen, J. (Eds.), *Speech Enhancement,* Berlin, Germany: Springer, pp. 97–113.

22. Plapous, C., Marro, C., Mauuary, L., and Scalart, P. (2004), A two-step noise reduction technique, *Proceedings of IEEE International Conference on Acoustics, Speech, and Signal Processing,* Vol. I, Montreal, Quebec, Canada, pp. 289–292.
23. Wolfe, P. and Godsill, S. (2003), Efficient alternatives to the Ephraim and Malah suppression rule for audio signal enhancement, *EURASIP J. Appl. Signal Process.,* 2003(10), 1043–1051.
24. Hu, Y. and Loizou, P. (2006), Subjective comparison of speech enhancement algorithms, *Proceedings of IEEE International Conference on Acoustics, Speech, and Signal Processing,* Vol. I, Toulouse, France, pp. 153–156.
25. Gray, R., Buzo, A., Gray, A., and Matsuyama, Y. (1980), Distortion measures for speech processing, *IEEE Trans. Acoust. Speech Signal Process.,* 28(4), 367–376.
26. Klatt, D. (1982), Prediction of perceived phonetic distance from critical band spectra, *Proceedings of IEEE International Conference on Acoustics Speech Signal Processing,* Vol. 7, Paris, France, 1278–1281.
27. Ephraim, Y. and Malah, D. (1985), Speech enhancement using a minimum mean-square error log-spectral amplitude estimator, *IEEE Trans. Acoust. Speech Signal Process.,* 23(2), 443–445.
28. Gradshteyn, I. and Ryzhik, I. (2000), *Table of Integrals, Series and Products*, 6th ed., San Diego, CA: Academic Press.
29. Ephraim, Y. and Cohen, I. (2006), Recent advancements in speech enhancement, in Dorf, R. C. (Ed.), *The Electrical Engineering Handbook,* Boca Raton, FL: CRC Press.
30. Wolfe, P. and Godsill, S. (2001), Simple alternatives to the Ephraim and Malah suppression rule for speech enhancement, *Proceedings of the 11th IEEE Workshop on Statistical Signal Processing,* Orchid Country Club, Singapore, pp. 496–499.
31. You, C., Koh, S., and Rahardja, S. (2003), Adaptive b-order MMSE estimation for speech enhancement, *Proceedings of IEEE International Conference on Acoustics, Speech, and Signal Processing,* Vol. I, Hong Kong, Hong Kong, pp. 900–903.
32. Accardi, A. and Cox, R. (1999), A modular approach to speech enhancement with an application to speech coding, *Proceedings of IEEE International Conference on Acoustics, Speech, and Signal Processing,* Phoenix, AZ, pp. 201–204.
33. Martin, R. (2005), Speech enhancement based on minimum mean-square error estimation and supergaussian priors, *IEEE Trans. Speech Audio Process.,* 13(5), 845–856.
34. Chen, B. and Loizou, P. (2007), A Laplacian-based MMSE estimator for speech enhancement, *Speech Commun.,* 49, 134–143.
35. Breithaupt, C. and Martin, R. (2003), MMSE estimation of magnitude-squared DFT coefficients with supergaussian priors, *Proceedings of IEEE International Conference on Acoustics, Speech, and Signal Processing,* Vol. I, Hong Kong, Hong Kong, pp. 896–899.
36. Wolfe, P. and Godsill, S. (2000), Towards a perceptually optimal spectral amplitude estimator for audio signal enhancement, *Proceedings of IEEE International Conference on Acoustics, Speech, and Signal Processing,* Vol. 2, Istanbul, Turkey, pp. 821–824.
37. Wolfe, P. and Godsill, S. (2003), A perceptually balanced loss function for short-time spectral amplitude estimation, *Proceedings of IEEE International Conference on Acoustics, Speech, and Signal Processing,* Vol. V, Hong Kong, Hong Kong, pp. 425–428.
38. Loizou, P. (2005), Speech enhancement based on perceptually motivated Bayesian estimators of the speech magnitude spectrum, *IEEE Trans. Speech Audio Process.,* 13(5), 857–869.
39. Kroon, P. and Atal, B. (1992), Predictive coding of speech using analysis-by-synthesis techniques, in Furui, S. and Sondhi, M. (Eds.), *Advances in Speech Signal Processing,* New York: Marcel Dekker, pp. 141–164.
40. Atal, B. and Schroeder, M. (1979), Predictive coding of speech and subjective error criteria, *IEEE Trans. Acoust. Speech Signal Process.,* 27, 247–254.

41. Schroeder, M., Atal, B., and Hall, J. (1979), Optimizing digital speech coders by exploiting masking properties of the human ear, *J. Acoust. Soc. Am.,* 66(6), 1647–1651.
42. Middleton, D. (1996), *An Introduction to Statistical Communication Theory,* New York: IEEE Press.
43. Itakura, F. (1975), Minimum prediction residual principle applied to speech recognition, *IEEE Trans. Acoust. Speech Signal Process.,* 23(1), 67–72.
44. Itakura, F. and Saito, S. (1968), An analysis-synthesis telephony based on maximum likelihood method, *Proceedings of 6th International Conference on Acoustics,* Tokyo, Japan, pp. 17–20.
45. Gray, A. and Markel, J. (1976), Distance measures for speech processing, *IEEE Trans. Acoust. Speech Signal Process.,* 24(5), 380–391.
46. Shikano, K. and Sugiyama, M. (1982), Evaluation of LPC spectral matching measures for spoken word recognition, *Trans. IECE,* 565-D(5), 535–541.
47. Brent, R. (1973), *Algorithms for Minimization without Derivatives*, Upper Saddle River, NJ: Prentice Hall.
48. Blahut, R. (1990), *Principles and Practice of Information Theory*, Reading, MA: Addison-Wesley Publishing Company.
49. Griffin, D. and Lim, J. (1988), Multiband excitation vocoder, *IEEE Trans. Acoust. Speech Signal Process.,* 36(8), 1223–1235.
50. Makhoul, J., Viswanathan, R., Schwartz, R., and Huggins, A. (1978), A mixed-source excitation model for speech compression and synthesis, *Proceedings of IEEE International Conference on Acoustics, Speech, and Signal Processing,* Tulsa, OK, pp. 163–166.
51. Yang, J. (1993), Frequency domain noise suppression approaches in mobile telephone systems, *Proceedings of IEEE International Conference on Acoustics, Speech, and Signal Processing,* Vol. II, Minneapolis, MN, pp. 363–366.
52. Malah, D., Cox, R., and Accardi, A. (1999), Tracking speech-presence uncertainty to improve speech enhancement in non-stationary environments, *Proceedings of IEEE International Conference on Acoustics, Speech, and Signal Processing,* Phoenix, AZ, pp. 789–792.
53. Cohen, I. and Berdugo, B. (2001), Speech enhancement for non-stationary noise environments, *Signal Process.,* 81, 2403–2418.
54. Cohen, I. (2002), Optimal speech enhancement under signal presence uncertainty using log-spectra amplitude estimator, *IEEE Signal Process. Lett.,* 9(4), 113–116.
55. Soon, I., Koh, S., and Yeo, C. (1999), Improved noise suppression filter using self-adaptive estimator of probability of speech absence, *Signal Process.,* 75, 151–159.
56. Kim, N. and Chang, J. (2000), Spectral enhancement based on global soft decision, *IEEE Signal Process. Lett.,* 7(5), 108–110.

8 Subspace Algorithms

The speech enhancement algorithms described so far were based on theory from signal processing and statistical estimation. In this chapter, we present a different class of algorithms that are largely based on linear algebra theory. More specifically, these algorithms are based on the principle that the clean signal might be confined to a subspace of the noisy Euclidean space. Consequently, given a method for decomposing the vector space of the noisy signal into a subspace that is occupied primarily by the clean signal and a subspace occupied primarily by the noise signal, we could estimate the clean signal simply by nulling the component of the noisy vector residing in the "noise subspace." The decomposition of the vector space of the noisy signal into "signal" and "noise" subspaces can be done using well-known orthogonal matrix factorization techniques from linear algebra and, in particular, the singular value decomposition (SVD) or eigenvector–eigenvalue factorizations. By computing the SVD of a matrix, for instance, we can obtain orthonormal bases for four fundamental subspaces: the column space of the matrix (in the context of speech enhancement, this corresponds to the signal subspace), the left nullspace, the row space, and the nullspace. In engineering, the orthogonal matrices obtained from the SVD or eigenvalue decomposition can be viewed as signal-dependent transforms that can be applied to either a matrix containing the signal or to a speech vector. In fact, the eigenvector matrix of the signal covariance matrix is often called the Karhunen–Loève transform (KLT).

We briefly note that the subspace approach can be traced back to early work in multivariate analysis involving principal components. The ideas were brought into engineering sciences by Pisarenko [1] in the early 1970s with his work on parameter estimation of sinusoidal signals and later by Schmidt [2,3], who extended Pisarenko's work with his multiple signal characterization (MUSIC) algorithm. The subspace approach has been widely used in spectral estimation, system identification, image processing, array processing, and speech recognition applications [4–6], just to name a few. In this chapter, we focus on the various SVD- and KLT-based algorithms proposed for speech enhancement.

8.1 INTRODUCTION

As much of the theory of the subspace algorithms is heavily rooted in linear algebra concepts, we start with a review of subspaces, projections, and properties of the SVD.

8.1.1 DEFINITIONS

The $\mathbb{R}^n$ vector space includes all column vectors with n components. Within each vector space there exist subspaces. For example, the vector space $\mathbb{R}^1$ is a line, whereas $\mathbb{R}^2$ is a plane, and both are subspaces of $\mathbb{R}^3$. More generally, if a matrix **A**

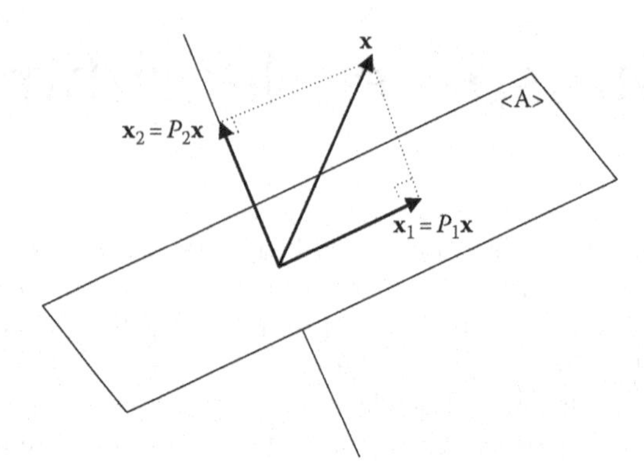

FIGURE 8.1 Decomposition of the vector **x** into its orthogonal components $\mathbf{x}_1$ and $\mathbf{x}_2$.

consists of p linearly independent column vectors of dimension N $(p < N)$, that is, $\mathbf{A} = [a_1, a_2, \ldots, a_p]$, then we say that the column vectors lie in a p-dimensional subspace spanned by the columns of A. This subspace is often called the *range* or *column space* of the matrix A, and we denote it by <A>. Subspaces satisfy the vector space properties. Specifically, the addition of two vectors in a subspace results in another vector in the same subspace, and multiplication of any vector in the subspace results in a vector in the same subspace.

We say that two subspaces <V> and <W> are orthogonal if every vector **v** in <V> is orthogonal to every vector **w** in <W>, that is, $\mathbf{v}^T\mathbf{w} = 0$ for all $\mathbf{v} \in$ <V> and $\mathbf{w} \in$ <W>. Examples of two orthogonal subspaces in $\mathbb{R}^3$ consist of a line and a plane perpendicular to the line (see Figure 8.1). Note that the sum of the dimensions of these two subspaces is equal to 3 (a line has a dimension of 1, and a plane has a dimension of 2), and we therefore say that the subspaces are *orthogonal complements* to each other.

The division of $\mathbb{R}^n$, in general, into two orthogonal subspaces is of great value to us because we can represent any vector **x** in $\mathbb{R}^n$ as a sum of two components: $\mathbf{x} = \mathbf{v} + \mathbf{w}$, where **v** lies in the <V> subspace, and **w** lies in the <W> subspace, orthogonal to <V>. The orthogonal subspace representation of vectors generally provides us with an excellent tool for decoupling a vector occupying an n-dimensional space into two components, each occupying a different subspace. In the context of speech enhancement, **x** could correspond to the noisy speech vector, **v** to the clean signal, and **w** to the noise signal. Ideally, we would like to decouple the noisy speech space into a subspace occupied primarily by the signal and a different subspace occupied primarily by the noise.

8.1.2 Projections

But, how can we decouple an arbitrary vector in $\mathbb{R}^n$ into its orthogonal components? To do that, we first note in Figure 8.1 that the line connecting the vectors $\mathbf{x}_1$ and **x** is orthogonal to the subspace <A>. The vector $\mathbf{x}_1$ is in fact the closest, in the least-squares sense, vector in <A> to **x** and can be obtained by *projecting* orthogonally the vector **x** onto the subspace <A>. The projection can be carried out by using a *projection matrix*, which can be easily derived using least-squares arguments [7, p. 156]. For a rectangular matrix A ($N \times m$), the projection matrix P has the form

$$P = A(A^T A)^{-1} A^T \tag{8.1}$$

Note that P often appears in normal equations. The preceding matrix P generally projects a vector $\mathbf{x}$ in $\mathbb{R}^n$ onto the column space of the matrix A. Note that if the matrix A has n linearly independent columns, then A^TA in Equation 8.1 will be positive definite and therefore nonsingular.

Figure 8.1 shows an example decomposition of a vector $\mathbf{x}$ into two orthogonal components, $\mathbf{x}_1$ and $\mathbf{x}_2$. The projected vector $\mathbf{x}_1$ is obtained by $\mathbf{x}_1 = P \cdot \mathbf{x}$ and lies in the column space of A, that is, <A>. In other words, $\mathbf{x}_1$ is the component of $\mathbf{x}$ in the column space of A. The other component of $\mathbf{x}$ can be obtained by using $(I - P)$ as the projection matrix, where I is the identity matrix. The matrix $(I - P)$ is also a projection matrix and projects the vector $\mathbf{x}$ onto the orthogonal subspace, the line perpendicular to <A> in this example. So, the vector $\mathbf{x}$ in Figure 8.1 can be decomposed into two orthogonal components as follows:

$$\begin{aligned}\mathbf{x} &= P\mathbf{x} + (I - P)\mathbf{x} \\ &= P_1\mathbf{x} + P_2\mathbf{x} \\ &= \mathbf{x}_1 + \mathbf{x}_2\end{aligned} \tag{8.2}$$

where the projection matrix $P_1 = P$ is given by Equation 8.1, and $P_2 \triangleq I - P$. In the example shown in Figure 8.1, the projection matrix P_2 projects the vector $\mathbf{x}$ onto a line perpendicular to <A>.

The projection matrices share two basic properties:

$$P^T = P(\text{symmetry})$$

$$P^2 = P(\text{idempotent})$$

Also, the projection matrices P_1 and P_2 in Equation 8.2 satisfy

$$P_1 + P_2 = I, \quad P_1P_2 = P_2P_1 = 0 \tag{8.3}$$

The first property in Equation 8.3 simply says that the two projection matrices decompose $\mathbb{R}^n$. The second property says that the two projection matrices are orthogonal to each other, in the sense that the rows of P_1 are orthogonal to the columns of P_2. Similarly, the rows of P_2 are orthogonal to the columns of P_1. In summary, projection matrices allow us to decompose a vector into two orthogonal components, each lying in a different subspace.

Although the equation describing the projection matrix in Equation 8.1 seems complex, it can be simplified a great deal by using the SVD decomposition of the matrix A. Let

$$A = U\Sigma V^H \tag{8.4}$$

be the SVD decomposition of the matrix A assumed to be full column rank (that is, rank(A) = m), where U ($N \times N$) and V ($m \times m$) are unitary matrices, and Σ is a diagonal matrix ($N \times m$) containing the singular values of A (which are also the square roots of the eigenvalues of A^TA and AA^T). Substituting Equation 8.4 into Equation 8.1, we get

$$P = UU^H \tag{8.5}$$

The preceding matrix P projects a vector onto the space spanned by the first r columns of U, where r = rank(A). But the span of the first r columns of the matrix U is the same as the span of A [8, eq. 2.5.5], and therefore P projects a vector onto the space spanned by the column vectors of A, that is, onto <A>.

Now, if we assume that the matrix A ($N \times m$) is not full rank, that is, rank(A) = r and $r \leq m$, then the SVD of the matrix A in Equation 8.4 simplifies to

$$A = U\Sigma V^H = [U_1 \quad U_2]\begin{bmatrix} \Sigma_1 & 0 \\ 0 & 0 \end{bmatrix}\begin{bmatrix} V_1^H \\ V_2^H \end{bmatrix} = U_1\Sigma_1 V_1^H \tag{8.6}$$

where the matrix U_1 is $N \times r$, U_2 is $N \times (N - r)$, Σ_1 is $r \times r$, and V_1^H is $r \times m$. The projection matrix in Equation 8.5 now becomes

$$P = U_1 U_1^H \tag{8.7}$$

The matrix projecting onto the complement (orthogonal) subspace is given by $I - P = I - U_1U_1^H$. As the matrix U is unitary, we have

$$UU^H = I = [U_1 \quad U_2]\begin{bmatrix} U_1^H \\ U_2^H \end{bmatrix} = U_1U_1^H + U_2U_2^H \tag{8.8}$$

and therefore the matrix projecting onto the complement subspace simplifies to

$$I - U_1U_1^H = U_2U_2^H \tag{8.9}$$

To summarize, we can use the SVD to decompose a vector y as follows:

$$\begin{aligned} \mathbf{y} &= U_1U_1^H\mathbf{y} + U_2U_2^H\mathbf{y} \\ &= \mathbf{y}_1 + \mathbf{y}_2 \end{aligned} \tag{8.10}$$

The vector $\mathbf{y}_1$ is the component of $\mathbf{y}$ that lies in the space spanned by the columns of U_1, that is, the subspace $<U_1>$. Likewise, the vector $\mathbf{y}_2$ is the component of $\mathbf{y}$ lying in the space spanned by the columns of U_2, the subspace $<U_2>$. Note that the vector $\mathbf{y}_1$ is orthogonal to $\mathbf{y}_2$, since $<U_1>$ is orthogonal to $<U_2>$. The subspace $<U_1>$ is often called the *signal* subspace, and the subspace $<U_2>$ is called the *orthogonal subspace* or *noise subspace*. The latter terminology, although in common use, is not precise as the true noise signal might (and usually does) occupy both spaces, as it spans the whole space. In the context of speech enhancement, the preceding equation tells us that if $\mathbf{y}$ represents the noisy speech vector, then we can use the projection matrices $U_1U_1^H$ and $U_2U_2^H$ to separate in some sense the speech and noise vectors.

Equation 8.10 summarizes the main principle underlying the majority of the subspace methods proposed for speech enhancement. Specifically, the idea is to project the noisy speech vector onto the "signal" subspace using $U_1U_1^H$, and retain only the projected vector, $\mathbf{y}_1$, lying in the signal subspace. We discard $\mathbf{y}_2$ as it occupies the orthogonal subspace, which we assume contains noise. In practice, however, projecting the noisy vector onto the signal subspace might not be sufficient, from the standpoint of noise reduction. For that reason, as we will see later (Section 8.6.2), the projected vector is typically modified in some way once in the signal subspace.

Example 8.1

Suppose that the signal vector $\mathbf{x}$ is corrupted by noise $\mathbf{n}$ to produce the vector $\mathbf{y} = \mathbf{x} + \mathbf{n}$, given by $\mathbf{y}^T = [1, 1, 1]$. The noisy signal occupies $\mathbb{R}^3$. Furthermore, suppose that we know that the signal vector $\mathbf{x}$ lies in the subspace spanned by the columns of the matrix X given by

$$X = \begin{bmatrix} 1 & 2 & 3 \\ 3 & 2 & 5 \\ 0 & 0 & 0 \end{bmatrix} \tag{8.11}$$

and the noise vector $\mathbf{n}$ lies in the subspace spanned by the columns of the matrix N:

$$N = \begin{bmatrix} 0 & 0 & 0 \\ 0 & 0 & 0 \\ 1 & 3 & 2 \end{bmatrix} \tag{8.12}$$

Find the orthogonal projections of the noisy vector $\mathbf{y}$ onto the signal and noise subspaces.

To find the orthogonal projections, we first compute the SVD of the matrix X:

$$X = U\Sigma V^H = \begin{bmatrix} -0.51 & -0.86 & 0 \\ -0.86 & 0.51 & 0 \\ 0 & 0 & 1 \end{bmatrix} \begin{bmatrix} 7.14 & 0 & 0 \\ 0 & 0.97 & 0 \\ 0 & 0 & 0 \end{bmatrix} \begin{bmatrix} -0.43 & 0.69 & -0.57 \\ -0.38 & -0.72 & -0.57 \\ -0.81 & -0.02 & 0.57 \end{bmatrix} \tag{8.13}$$

We note from the preceding equation, that the rank of X is 2 (as we have two nonzero singular values), and therefore we can partition the matrix U as $U=[U_1,U_2]$, where the matrix U_1 contains the first two columns of U, and U_2 contains the last column of U. Using Equation 8.7, the signal projection matrix can be constructed as

$$P_x = U_1U_1^H$$
$$= \begin{bmatrix} -0.51 & -0.86 \\ -0.86 & 0.51 \\ 0 & 0 \end{bmatrix} \begin{bmatrix} -0.51 & -0.86 & 0 \\ -0.86 & 0.51 & 0 \end{bmatrix}$$
$$= \begin{bmatrix} 1 & 0 & 0 \\ 0 & 1 & 0 \\ 0 & 0 & 0 \end{bmatrix}$$

The projection of the noisy vector y onto the signal subspace is accomplished by

$$\mathbf{x} = P_x\mathbf{y} = \begin{bmatrix} 1 \\ 1 \\ 0 \end{bmatrix} \tag{8.14}$$

Similarly, the projection of the noisy vector $\mathbf{y}$ onto the noise subspace is given by

$$\mathbf{n} = (I - P_x)\mathbf{y} = \begin{bmatrix} 0 \\ 0 \\ 1 \end{bmatrix}$$

Therefore, the noisy vector $\mathbf{y}$ can be decomposed as

$$\mathbf{y} = \mathbf{x} + \mathbf{n} = \begin{bmatrix} 1 \\ 1 \\ 0 \end{bmatrix} + \begin{bmatrix} 0 \\ 0 \\ 1 \end{bmatrix}$$

It should be clear from Equations 8.11 and 8.12 that the signal vector $\mathbf{x}$ lies in the x–y plane, whereas the noise vector lies in the subspace spanned by the z-axis. The x–y plane is perpendicular to the line (coinciding with the z-axis), and the two subspaces (x–y plane and line) are orthogonal subspace complements, as the union of the two subspaces spans $\mathbb{R}^3$. This simple example demonstrates that it is possible to estimate the signal $\mathbf{x}$ from the noisy data, $\mathbf{y}$, simply by projecting the noisy vector onto the signal subspace (Equation 8.14). We had to make one assumption, however: the signal resided in the subspace spanned by the columns of X. That assumption allowed us to construct the appropriate projection matrix.

Going back to Equation 8.10, we can view $U_1U_1^H\mathbf{y}$ as a sequence of transform operations. The matrix U_1^H first transforms the vector $\mathbf{y}$ to $\mathbf{y}_a = U_1^H\mathbf{y}$. This constitutes the "analysis" part of the operation. Then, the matrix U_1 transforms $\mathbf{y}_a$ to $\mathbf{y}_1 = U_1\mathbf{y}_a$, which constitutes the "synthesis" part. Assuming that the transforms are unitary (i.e., $U_1U_1^H = I$), we can view U_1^H as the forward transform and U_1 as the inverse transform. If, for instance, U_1^H were the (square) discrete Fourier transform (DFT) matrix, then U_1 would have been the inverse Fourier transform matrix.

In Equation 8.4, we used the SVD to decompose the matrix A. Alternatively, assuming that the matrix A is square ($N \times N$) and symmetric, we can use the following eigen-decomposition of A:

$$A = U\Lambda U^H \tag{8.15}$$

where

U is now the unitary eigenvector matrix ($N \times N$)
Λ is a diagonal matrix ($N \times N$) containing the eigenvalues of A

Assuming similar partitioning of the eigenvector matrix U as in Equation 8.8, the projection matrices will have the same form and will be $U_1U_1^H$ for the signal subspace and $U_2U_2^H$ for the orthogonal subspace. The main difference between the projection matrix constructed using the SVD decomposition (i.e., Equation 8.7) and the projection matrix constructed by Equation 8.15 is that the columns of the matrices U_1 and U_2 now contain the eigenvectors of the matrix A.

The eigenvector matrix U is also known as the Karhunen–Loève transform (KLT), which, unlike other transforms (e.g., discrete-time Fourier or cosine transforms), is signal dependent. The columns of the discrete Fourier and cosine transform matrices are fixed and are not dependent on the input signal, whereas the columns of the KLT matrix (i.e., the eigenvectors) change with the input signal. In this regard, the KLT is regarded as the optimum (signal-matched) transform. The computation of the KLT, however, is computationally intensive. For that reason, some have opted to use the discrete cosine transform (DCT) in place of the KLT [9,10]. This was motivated by the fact that the DCT provides a good approximation to the KLT, at least for autoregressive processes [9].

Figure 8.2 illustrates the preceding transform interpretation of the subspace approach. In addition to the forward and inverse transform operations, we generally consider using a gain matrix (typically diagonal) in between the two transform operations. The block

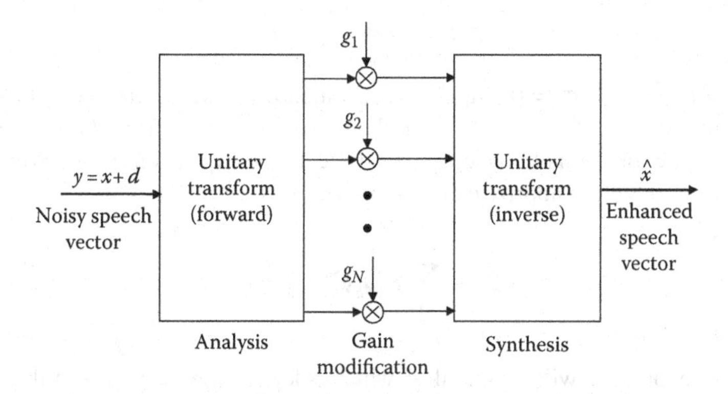

FIGURE 8.2 General structure of subspace algorithms.

diagram in Figure 8.2 describes the majority of the subspace algorithms proposed for speech enhancement and discussed in this chapter. It also describes the general family of spectral modification algorithms, for example, spectral subtraction algorithm [11]. In fact, what differentiate the various algorithms from one another are the contents of the diagonal gain matrix and the choice of the unitary transform U. Most subspace algorithms use the KLT and a Wiener-type gain matrix, whereas the spectral-subtractive type of algorithms use the DFT with a different gain matrix [11].

8.1.3 Low-Rank Modeling

In the previous section, we assumed that the signal was contained in a vector consisting of, for instance, N samples of speech (i.e., a frame of speech). In some applications, however, the input data might be arranged in a matrix. In image processing applications, for instance, the image information is represented as an $m \times n$ matrix containing the color intensities. Similarly, in speech applications we may choose to arrange the input data in a Hankel or Toeplitz matrix [12,13]. In such cases, the subspace projection approach described previously might not be appropriate, but we can consider an alternative approach that is equivalent in many respects.

Consider the SVD decomposition of a rectangular matrix A ($N \times m$), which is rank deficient, that is, rank(A) = r and $r < m$. We know that the SVD decomposition of the matrix A can also be written as

$$A = \sum_{k=1}^{r} \sigma_k u_k \mathbf{v}_k^T \tag{8.16}$$

where

r ($r \leq m$) is the rank of the matrix A
u_k is the kth column of the matrix U
$\mathbf{v}_k$ is the kth column of the matrix V

The matrix A is therefore composed of a sum of r rank-1 matrices $\left(\mathbf{u}_k \mathbf{v}_k^H\right)$ weighted by the singular values σ_k, which are arranged in descending order:

$$\sigma_1 > \sigma_2 > \sigma_3 > \cdots > \sigma_r \tag{8.17}$$

with $\sigma_{r+1} = \sigma_{r+2} = \cdots = \sigma_m = 0$. Suppose that somehow we know that the last $r - p$ singular values, that is, $\sigma_{p+1}, \sigma_{p+2}, \ldots, \sigma_r$, at the tail end of Equation 8.17 are very small. Then, we can exploit this knowledge and truncate the expansion in Equation 8.16 at $k = p$. We can therefore approximate the matrix A as

$$\hat{A}_p = \sum_{k=1}^{p} \sigma_k u_k \mathbf{v}_k^T, \quad p < r \tag{8.18}$$

The new matrix $\hat{A}_p$ will have rank p, which is lower than the rank r of the original matrix A. For this reason, we refer to $\hat{A}_p$ as the *low-rank* approximation of the matrix A.

This approximation is also the optimal (in the least-squares sense) rank p approximation of the matrix A [8, p. 73]; that is, it solves the following least-squares problem:

$$\min_{\text{rank}(\hat{A})=p} \| A-\hat{A} \|_F = \sum_i \sum_j \left(a_{ij} - \hat{a}_{ij}\right)^2 \tag{8.19}$$

where $\|\cdot\|_F$ denotes the Frobenius norm of a matrix, which is equal to the sum of squares of all elements. It is worth noting that when $p = r$, the space spanned by the columns of the low-rank matrix $\hat{A}_p$ (Equation 8.18) is identical to the signal subspace $<U_1>$ in Equation 8.10. So, the low-rank approximation of the matrix A implicitly discards the orthogonal subspace spanned by the last $N - r$ columns of U.

Similarly, using the eigen-decomposition of the matrix A, we can write A as

$$A = \sum_{k=1}^{N} \lambda_k u_k u_k^H \tag{8.20}$$

where
λ_k are the eigenvalues of A
u_k are the eigenvectors of A

The low-rank approximation of the matrix A is given by

$$\hat{A}_p = \sum_{k=1}^{p} \lambda_k u_k u_k^H, \quad p < N \tag{8.21}$$

It is easy to show that the squared error, expressed by the Frobenius norm $\|A - \hat{A}_p\|_F$, between the true-rank and low-rank ($p < N$) approximation of the matrix A is given by

$$\begin{aligned} e^2 &= \| A - \hat{A}_p \|_F \\ &= \text{tr}\left[\left(A - \hat{A}_p\right)^H \left(A - \hat{A}_p\right)\right] \\ &= \sum_{k=p+1}^{N} \lambda_k \end{aligned} \tag{8.22}$$

Hence, the smaller the tail-end eigenvalues of A are (or singular values in Equation 8.18), the smaller the error will be.

So far we focused primarily on linear algebra concepts crucial to the understanding of subspace techniques, and have not talked much about speech enhancement. Having finished presenting the general theory underlying the subspace approach, we now describe the implementation of the various subspace algorithms proposed for speech enhancement. We will start with the low-rank modeling methods, as those methods were proposed first, and continue with the subspace projection methods.

8.2 USING SVD FOR NOISE REDUCTION: THEORY

8.2.1 SVD Analysis of "Noisy" Matrices

Suppose that the matrix Y contains the noisy observations and is expressed as

$$Y = X + D \tag{8.23}$$

where

X is the matrix containing the clean (noise free) signal data
D contains the noise data

As we will see later, the input data (say a frame of speech) could be arranged in the matrix X in Toeplitz form. The objective is to recover the signal contained in X given the "noisy" matrix Y. Equivalently, we can ask the following questions: Is it possible to recover the signal subspace from Y using the SVD? Is it possible to recover the rank of the signal matrix X needed to determine the signal subspace? These questions are addressed in [14].

Suppose that the signal matrix X ($N \times m$) is rank deficient, that is, rank(X) = r ($r < m$), and has the following SVD decomposition:

$$X = U_x \Sigma_x V_x{}^H = [U_{x1} \quad U_{x2}] \begin{bmatrix} \Sigma_{x1} & 0 \\ 0 & 0 \end{bmatrix} \begin{bmatrix} V_{x1}^H \\ V_{x2}^H \end{bmatrix} \tag{8.24}$$

where

U_{x1} is $N \times r$
U_{x2} is $N \times (N - r)$
Σ_{x1} is $r \times r$
V_{x1}^H is $r \times m$
V_{x2}^H is $(N - r) \times m$

Recall that the span of U_{x1} is the column space of X and is therefore the signal subspace. The columns of V_{x1} span the row space of X while the columns of V_{x2} span the nullspace of X [7, app. A]. Using the matrices V_{x1} and V_{x2}, and the fact that $V_{x1}V_{x1}^H + V_{x2}V_{x2}^H = I$ (similar to Equation 8.8), we can write the matrix Y in Equation 8.23 as follows:

$$\begin{aligned} Y &= X + D \\ &= X + D\left(V_{x1}V_{x1}^H + V_{x2}V_{x2}^H\right) \\ &= \left(XV_{x1} + DV_{x1}\right)V_{x1}^H + \left(DV_{x2}\right)V_{x2}^H \\ &= \left(P_1 S_1 Q_1^H\right)V_{x1}^H + \left(P_2 S_2 Q_2^H\right)V_{x2}^H \\ &= \left(P_1 P_2\right)\begin{pmatrix} S_1 & 0 \\ 0 & S_2 \end{pmatrix}\begin{pmatrix} Q_1^H V_{x1}^H \\ Q_2^H V_{x2}^H \end{pmatrix} \end{aligned} \tag{8.25}$$

where $P_1S_1Q_1^H$ and $P_2S_2Q_2^H$ are the SVDs of the matrices in the parenthesis, that is, $XV_{x1} + DV_{x1} = P_1S_1Q_1^H$ and $DV_{x2} = P_2S_2Q_2^H$. The preceding equation is a valid SVD of Y provided that $P_1^HP_2 = 0$, that is, the column spaces of the matrices P_1 and P_2 are orthogonal. But, we know that the column spaces of P_1 and P_2 are identical to the column spaces of the matrices $XV_{x1} + DV_{x1}$ and DV_{x2}, respectively. Therefore, for $P_1^HP_2 = 0$, we need

$$V_{x1}^H(X^H + D^H)DV_{x2} = 0 \tag{8.26}$$

The preceding condition is a necessary condition for Equation 8.25 to be an SVD of Y. We can split this condition into two conditions:

$$X^HD = 0 \tag{8.27}$$

and

$$V_{x1}^HD^HDV_{x2} = 0 \tag{8.28}$$

Clearly, one could choose other conditions (e.g., $X = -D$) that would satisfy Equation 8.26, but the preceding two conditions are more realistic and more likely to appear in engineering applications. Equation 8.25 suggests that we can obtain from the SVD of Y the subspaces generated by V_{x1} and V_{x2} corresponding to the row space and null space of X, respectively [7, app. A], if the following conditions are satisfied:

1. The signal matrix is orthogonal to the noise matrix in the sense that $X^HD = 0$. For zero-mean random signals, this suggests that the signal is uncorrelated with the noise.
2. We know that $V_{x1}^HV_{x2} = 0$ since the row space of X is orthogonal to the null space. Hence, to satisfy the condition in Equation 8.28, we need D^HD to be a scalar multiple of the identity, that is, $D^HD = cI$. For random signals, this suggests that the noise is uncorrelated and white.
3. The smallest singular value of S_1 in Equation 8.25 needs to be larger than the largest singular value of S_2. This is necessary to be able to separate the subspace generated by V_{x1} from that generated by V_{x2}.

The last condition allows us to estimate the true rank of the matrix X. As we observe from Equation 8.25, however, we are not able to recover the signal subspace of X, since $P_1 \neq U_{x1}$. In fact, we cannot recover the signal subspace even asymptotically [14].

Assuming now that the following conditions are satisfied

$$D^HD = \sigma^2I, \quad X^HD = 0 \tag{8.29}$$

where σ^2 is the noise variance, we will next derive the SVD of Y in terms of the SVD of X. Substituting the SVD of X (Equation 8.24) in Equation 8.23, we get

$$\begin{aligned} Y &= X + D \\ &= U_{x1}\Sigma_{x1}V_{x1}^H + D\left(V_{x1}V_{x1}^H + V_{x2}V_{x2}^H\right) \\ &= \left[(U_{x1}\Sigma_{x1} + DV_{x1})\left(\Sigma_{x1}^2 + \sigma^2 I_r\right)^{-1/2} \quad DV_{x2}\sigma^{-1}\right] \\ &\times \begin{pmatrix} \sqrt{\Sigma_{x1}^2 + \sigma^2 I_r} & 0 \\ 0 & \sigma I_{m-r} \end{pmatrix} \begin{pmatrix} V_{x1}^H \\ V_{x2}^H \end{pmatrix} \\ &= (U_{y1} \quad U_{y2}) \begin{pmatrix} \Sigma_{y1} & 0 \\ 0 & \Sigma_{y2} \end{pmatrix} \begin{pmatrix} V_{y1}^H \\ V_{y2}^H \end{pmatrix} \end{aligned} \tag{8.30}$$

where I_r denotes an $r \times r$ identity matrix. We can make the following observations regarding Equation 8.30:

1. The row space of X can be recovered, since $V_{y1} = V_{x1}$.
2. The r largest left singular vectors of Y are contained in $U_{y1} = (U_{x1}\Sigma_{x1} + DV_{x1})(\Sigma_{x1}^2 + \sigma^2 I_r)^{-1/2}$. The signal subspace, that is, the column space of X, cannot be recovered consistently, since $U_{y1} \neq U_{x1}$.
3. The last $m - r$ singular values of Y are all equal, since $\Sigma_{y2} = \sigma I_{m-r}$, and can be used to estimate the "noise threshold" σ, which in turn can be used to estimate the signal-to-noise ratio (SNR). One possible definition of the SNR expressed in terms of the singular values of X is as follows:

$$\text{SNR} = \frac{\| X \|_F}{\| D \|_F} = \frac{\sigma_1^2 + \sigma_2^2 + \cdots + \sigma_r^2}{m \cdot \sigma^2}$$

where σ_i are the singular values of X and σ^2 is the noise variance.
4. The smallest singular value in Σ_{y1} is larger than the (single) singular value in Σ_{y2}. We can therefore determine the rank of the signal matrix X simply by counting the number of identical singular values in Σ_{y2}.
5. As $\Sigma_{y1} = \sqrt{\Sigma_{x1}^2 + \sigma^2 I_r}$, we can estimate the singular values of X from

$$\Sigma_{x1} = \sqrt{\Sigma_{y1}^2 - \sigma^2 I_r} \tag{8.31}$$

The preceding observations were made assuming that the conditions in Equation 8.29 are satisfied. In practice, however, these conditions are never satisfied exactly. Consequently, the singular values in Σ_{y2} will not be identical, and we cannot estimate the rank of X with absolute certainty. Practical methods for determining the effective rank of X will be presented in Section 8.3.2.

Although we cannot recover the noise-free signal subspace, it is noteworthy that we can compute the angles between the signal subspace (i.e., the column space of U_{x1}) and the noisy-data subspace (i.e., the column space of U_{y1}). The cosines of the angles between the column spaces of two orthogonal matrices, U_{x1} and U_{y1} in our case, are generally given by the singular values of their product $U_{x1}^H U_{y1}$ [8, p. 585]. After using U_{y1} from Equation 8.30, we get

$$\begin{aligned} U_{x1}^H U_{y1} &= U_{x1}^H \left(U_{x1}\Sigma_{x1} + DV_{x1}^H \right) \left(\Sigma_{x1}^2 + \sigma^2 I_r \right)^{-1/2} \\ &= \Sigma_{x1} \left(\Sigma_{x1}^2 + \sigma^2 I_r \right)^{-1/2} \\ &= \Sigma_{x1}\Sigma_{y1}^{-1} \end{aligned} \tag{8.32}$$

which itself is a diagonal matrix. So, the angles between the noise-free and noisy subspaces depend on the ratios of the clean and noisy singular values. As noted in [14], these angles are a function of the SNR. The larger the SNR, the smaller the angles. In the noise-free case, that is, when $\sigma^2 = 0$, the angles are zero.

8.2.2 Least-Squares and Minimum-Variance Estimates of the Signal Matrix

Given the noisy matrix Y, how can we estimate the signal matrix X? There are at least two methods for estimating the signal matrix X. The first method is based on the low-rank modeling approach, mentioned earlier, which is a least-squares approach. Specifically, this approach seeks the best, in the least-squares sense, rank r ($r < \text{rank}(X)$) matrix that minimizes the following squared error:

$$\min_{X} \| \hat{X} - X \|_F^2 \tag{8.33}$$

where $\|\cdot\|_F$ indicates the Frobenius norm. Note that $\| \hat{X} - X \|_F^2 = \text{tr}[(\hat{X} - X)^T (\hat{X} - X)]$. The solution to this problem is given by [8]

$$\hat{X}_{LS} = U_{y1}\Sigma_{y1}V_{y1}^H = \sum_{k=1}^{r} \sigma_k u_k \mathbf{v}_k^H \tag{8.34}$$

where

- u_k and $\mathbf{v}_k$ are the left and right singular vectors, respectively, of the noisy matrix Y
- Σ_{y1} is a diagonal matrix ($r \times r$) containing the r largest singular values of Y (i.e., $\sigma_1 > \sigma_2 > \cdots > \sigma_r$)

We are assuming for now that the effective rank r of the matrix X is known and that $r < \text{rank}(X)$.

The second method seeks the best estimate of the signal matrix X that could be obtained by linearly combining the noisy data vectors in the matrix Y. This is a minimum-variance estimate and is formulated as follows [14,15]. Given the noisy matrix Y, find the matrix H that minimizes the following squared error:

$$\min_{H} \| YH - X \|_F^2 \tag{8.35}$$

The optimum H is given by

$$H = (Y^H Y)^{-1} Y^H X \tag{8.36}$$

and the minimum-variance estimate of X, indicated by $\hat{X}_{MV}$, is given by

$$\hat{X}_{MV} = YH = Y(Y^H Y)^{-1} Y^H X \tag{8.37}$$

We know from Equation 8.1 that $Y(Y^H Y)^{-1} Y^H$ is an orthogonal projector, and therefore the minimum-variance estimate of X is an orthogonal projection of X onto the column space of Y. Because X is unknown, we cannot obtain the preceding solution from Y alone. However, after making the assumptions in Equation 8.29 (i.e., $D^H D = \sigma^2 I$ and $X^H D = 0$) and using the fact (see Section 8.1) that

$$Y(Y^H Y)^{-1} Y^H = U_y U_y^H = [U_{y1} \quad U_{y2}] \begin{bmatrix} U_{y1}^H \\ U_{y2}^H \end{bmatrix} \tag{8.38}$$

we can simplify Equation 8.37 to [14]

$$\begin{aligned} \hat{X}_{MV} &= HY \\ &= U_{y1} U_{y1}^T Y \\ &= U_{y1} U_{y1}^T \left(U_{y1} \Sigma_{y1} V_{y1}^H \right) \\ &= [U_{y1}] \Sigma_{x1}^2 \left(\Sigma_{x1}^2 + \sigma^2 I_r \right)^{-1/2} \left[V_{y1}^H \right] \end{aligned} \tag{8.39}$$

where

Σ_{x1} is an $r \times r$ diagonal matrix containing the singular values of X
σ^2 is the noise variance

The $\hat{X}_{MV}$ estimate is a function of the singular values of X, which are not available. We can use, however, the relationship in Equation 8.31 and express $\hat{X}_{MV}$ in terms of the singular values of Y:

$$\begin{aligned} \hat{X}_{MV} &= [U_{y1}] \left(\Sigma_{y1}^2 - \sigma^2 I_r \right) \Sigma_{y1}^{-1} \left[V_{y1}^H \right] \\ &= U_{y1} \Sigma_{MV} V_{y1}^H \end{aligned} \tag{8.40}$$

where $\Sigma_{MV} \triangleq \left(\Sigma_{y1}^2 - \sigma^2 I_r\right)\Sigma_{y1}^{-1}$ is a diagonal matrix. Comparing Equation 8.40 with Equation 8.34, we observe that the least-squares and minimum-variance estimates of X have the same singular vectors, but different singular values.

To summarize, the least-squares estimate of the signal matrix X can be computed from the noisy matrix Y according to

$$\hat{X}_{LS} = U_{y1}\Sigma_{y1}V_{y1}^H = \sum_{k=1}^{r} \sigma_k u_k \mathbf{v}_k^H \tag{8.41}$$

where σ_k are the singular values (in descending order) of Y. The minimum-variance estimate of the signal matrix X can be computed according to

$$\begin{aligned}\hat{X}_{MV} &= U_{y1}\Sigma_{MV}V_{y1}^H \\ &= \sum_{k=1}^{r} \frac{\sigma_k^2 - \sigma^2}{\sigma_k} u_k \mathbf{v}_k^H\end{aligned} \tag{8.42}$$

where

σ_k are the singular values of Y
σ^2 is the noise variance

Next, we present the SVD-based methods proposed for speech enhancement for white and colored noise. Note that when the additive noise is not white, we violate the assumption that $D^H D = \sigma^2 I$ (Equation 8.29). Consequently, we will treat the colored noise scenario differently.

8.3 SVD-BASED ALGORITHMS: WHITE NOISE

Dendrinos et al. [12] were among the first to apply the SVD approach to speech enhancement using a low-rank approximation of the noisy speech matrix (Equation 8.18). The basic idea of their proposed approach is that the singular vectors corresponding to the largest singular values contain speech information, whereas the remaining singular vectors contain noise information. Noise reduction is therefore accomplished by discarding the singular vectors corresponding to the smallest singular values.

8.3.1 SVD Synthesis of Speech

Assume that the noise-free signal $x(n)$, $0 \le n \le N-1$ is arranged in the matrix X in the following way:

$$X = \begin{bmatrix} x(L-1) & x(L-2) & \cdots & x(0) \\ x(L) & x(L-1) & \cdots & x(1) \\ \vdots & \vdots & \vdots & \vdots \\ x(N-1) & x(N-2) & \cdots & x(N-L) \end{bmatrix} \tag{8.43}$$

where $L < N$. The elements across all diagonal are all the same; that is, the matrix X is Toeplitz. Note, however, that X is not symmetric. This particular arrangement of the data in the matrix X was chosen because it has been used to express linear prediction equations [16], with L being the prediction order. Experimental results in [12] showed that a good choice for L is $L = N/3$, where N is the number of samples in a frame.

Alternatively, the signal $x(n)$can be arranged in a Hankel-structured matrix X, in which all the elements in the antidiagonals are identical:

$$X_h = \begin{bmatrix} x(0) & x(1) & \cdots & x(L-1) \\ x(1) & x(2) & \cdots & x(L) \\ \vdots & \vdots & \vdots & \vdots \\ x(N-L) & x(N-L+1) & \cdots & x(N-1) \end{bmatrix} \tag{8.44}$$

The Hankel arrangement of the signal matrix was used in [13]. Hankel matrices are closely related to the Toeplitz matrices in that JX_h or X_hJ are Toeplitz matrices, where J is the reflection matrix that has ones along the main antidiagonal [17]. The Hankel matrix X_h in Equation 8.44 is unitarily equivalent to the Toeplitz matrix X in Equation 8.43, in that they are related by $X = LX_hR$ for some unitary matrices L and R. In our case, $L = I_{N-L+1}$ is the $(N - L + 1) \times (N - L + 1)$ identity matrix, and $R = J_L$ is the $L \times L$ reflection matrix. Consequently, the left and right singular vectors of X_h will be unitarily invariant [18], and the two matrices (X and X_h) will have identical singular values [19, p. 193]. Hence, in regard to the SVD decomposition, it makes no difference whether we use the Toeplitz matrix arrangement (Equation 8.43) or the Hankel matrix arrangement (Equation 8.44).

Consider now a low-rank approximation of the matrix X as described in Section 8.1.3:

$$\hat{X}_p = \sum_{k=1}^{p} \sigma_k u_k \mathbf{v}_k^T, \quad p < L \tag{8.45}$$

where σ_k are the singular values, with u_k and $\mathbf{v}_k$ being the left and right singular vectors, respectively, of X obtained from SVD. Of great interest is the answer to the question: How many singular vectors are sufficient to represent speech or, equivalently, what should be the value of p? To answer this question, we can easily vary the value of p and observe the synthetic signal obtained from the corresponding low-rank approximation of X. It should be noted that the resulting low-rank matrix $\hat{X}_p$ in Equation 8.45 will not be Toeplitz. A simple technique for transforming $\hat{X}_p$ into a Toeplitz matrix is to arithmetically average the elements in all the diagonals of $\hat{X}_p$ [16,20]. Putting each average in the corresponding diagonal, we form a new matrix of the following form:

$$\hat{X}_p = \begin{bmatrix} x_p(L-1) & x_p(L-2) & \cdots & x_p(0) \\ x_p(L) & x_p(L-1) & \cdots & x_p(1) \\ \vdots & \vdots & \vdots & \vdots \\ x_p(N-1) & x_p(N-2) & \cdots & x_p(N-L) \end{bmatrix} \tag{8.46}$$

From the first row and the first column, we can obtain the synthesized signal based on a p-order rank approximation, that is, $x_p(n)$, for $n = 0, 1, 2,\ldots, N-1$. Interestingly enough, the averaging operation is equivalent [21] to finding the least-squares estimate of a Toeplitz structured matrix.

Similarly, if we arrange the data in a Hankel matrix X as in Equation 8.44, the resulting low-rank matrix $\hat{X}_p$ in Equation 8.45 will not be Hankel. But we can easily transform $\hat{X}_p$ into a Hankel matrix by arithmetically averaging the elements in all the antidiagonals of $\hat{X}_p$. This averaging operation was shown in [22] to be equivalent to subtracting zero-phase filtered versions of the original signal from itself.

In the following, we give a numerical example illustrating the Toeplitz and Hankel arrangements and averaging operations given in Equations 8.43 and 8.46.

Example 8.2

Consider the following time-domain signal $x(n) = \{1,3,2,-1,5,2\}$. Assuming that $L = 3$, we can arrange this signal in a Toeplitz matrix as per Equation 8.43:

$$X = \begin{bmatrix} 2 & 3 & 1 \\ -1 & 2 & 3 \\ 5 & -1 & 2 \\ 2 & 5 & -1 \end{bmatrix}$$

The rank of X is 3, and we can consider approximating X by a lower rank matrix, say a rank-2 matrix. After computing the SVD of X and using Equation 8.45 with $p = 2$, we get

$$\hat{X}_2 = \sum_{k=1}^{2} \sigma_k u_k \mathbf{v}_k^T$$

$$= \begin{bmatrix} 2.13 & 2.98 & 0.61 \\ 0.06 & 1.87 & -0.06 \\ 5.07 & -1.01 & 1.80 \\ 1.54 & 5.05 & 0.32 \end{bmatrix}$$

where $\sigma_k = \{6.8,5.3,3.5\}$ are the singular values of X. The matrix $\hat{X}_2$ is a low-rank approximation to the matrix X and was obtained by discarding the singular vectors corresponding to the smallest singular value (i.e., $\sigma_3 = 3.5$). Note that $\hat{X}_2$ is not Toeplitz, but we can make it Toeplitz by averaging the elements across each diagonal to obtain

$$X_{2t} = \begin{bmatrix} 1.93 & 1.46 & 0.61 \\ -0.21 & 1.93 & 1.46 \\ 5.06 & -0.21 & 1.93 \\ 1.54 & 5.06 & -0.21 \end{bmatrix}$$

The $X_{2t}(1, 2) = 1.46$ element (first row, second column), for example, was obtained by averaging 2.98 and −0.06. From the preceding matrix, we can extract the approximation to the original signal $x(n)$: $\hat{x}(n) = \{0.61, 1.46, 1.93, -0.21, 5.06, 1.54\}$.

Consider now arranging the same signal $x(n)$in a Hankel matrix:

$$X_h = \begin{bmatrix} 1 & 3 & 2 \\ 3 & 2 & -1 \\ 2 & -1 & 5 \\ -1 & 5 & 2 \end{bmatrix}$$

As mentioned earlier, Hankel matrices are unitarily equivalent to Toeplitz matrices. For this example, $X = X_h J_3$, where J_3 is a 3×3 reflection matrix that has 1's along the main antidiagonal. The left and right singular vectors of X_h are unitarily invariant [18], that is, they are related to the corresponding singular vectors of the Toeplitz matrix X by

$$u_h = \alpha u, \quad \mathbf{v}_h = \alpha J_3 \mathbf{v}$$

where $(u_h, \mathbf{v}_h)$ are the left and right singular vectors of X_h, respectively, $(u, \mathbf{v})$ are the left and right singular vectors of the Toeplitz matrix X, and α is a unit magnitude scalar. Note that the elements of the right singular vectors of X_h will be in reverse order owing to the reflection operation by J_3. The rank-2 approximation of X_h will be identical to the rank-2 approximation of the Toeplitz matrix X, and for this example is given by

$$\hat{X}_{2h} = \begin{bmatrix} 0.61 & 2.98 & 2.13 \\ -0.06 & 1.87 & 0.06 \\ 1.80 & -1.01 & 5.07 \\ 0.32 & 5.05 & 1.54 \end{bmatrix}$$

The estimated signal obtained by averaging the antidiagonals of the preceding matrix will be the same as the signal obtained earlier with the Toeplitz matrix. Therefore, from the standpoint of the low-rank approximations, it makes no difference whether we use the Toeplitz or the Hankel arrangement.

Next, we give some examples with speech signals. Consider the voiced speech segment in Figure 8.3 taken from the vowel/iy/. After arranging the signal in a Toeplitz matrix X as shown in Equation 8.43 with $N = 320$ (20 ms in duration for a 16 kHz sampling frequency) and $L = 106 (= N/3)$, we can obtain low-rank approximations to X according to Equation 8.45 for various rank orders ranging from $p = 2$ to $p = 50$. The reconstructed signals, obtained after averaging the diagonals of the low-rank matrices, are shown in Figure 8.3. Shown also are the SNRs of the reconstructed signals. Note that the SNR is used here as an objective measure assessing how closely the synthesized signal matches the original signal, with high SNR values indicating a small difference between the synthesized and original signals. As can

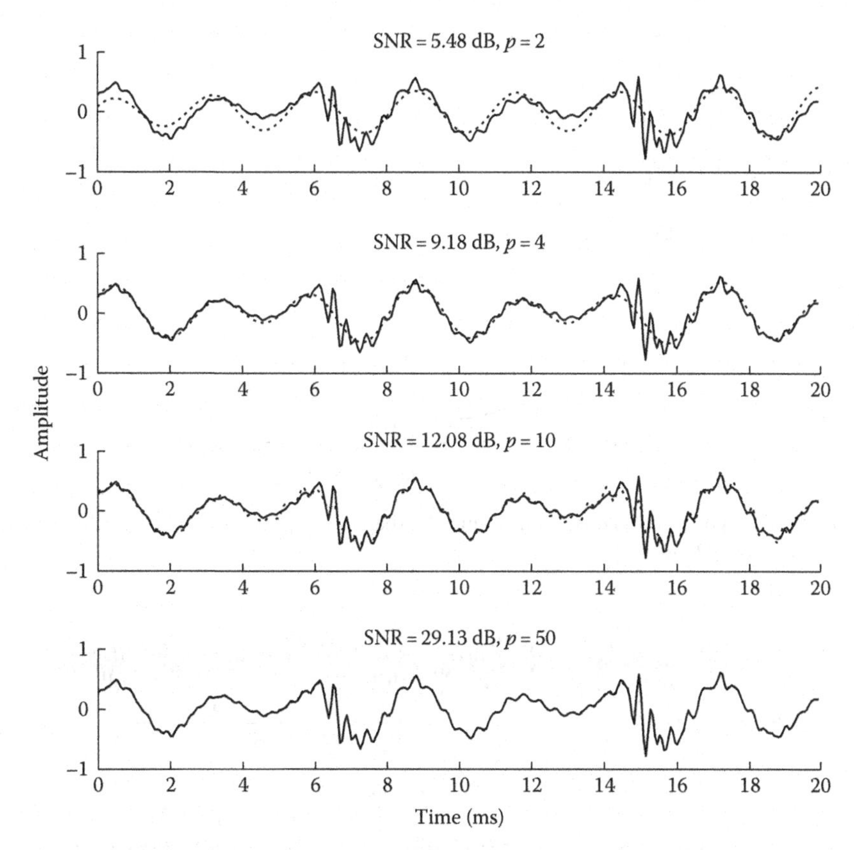

FIGURE 8.3 SVD synthesis of a voiced speech segment, taken from the vowel/iy/, as a function of the number (p) of singular vectors retained. The reconstruction SNR is indicated. The original signal is shown in thick lines and the synthesized signal in dashed lines.

be seen, retaining only 10 singular vectors corresponding to the 10 largest singular values seems to be sufficient for achieving good speech synthesis. The reason why 10 singular vectors are sufficient for this example is evident from Figure 8.4, which shows the distribution of the singular values. It is clear that the 10 largest singular values are the dominant singular values. The signal matrix X in this example had a full rank (rank(X) = 106); however, as we observe in Figure 8.4, the effective rank is approximately 50, which explains why the $p = 50$ rank approximation achieved such a high SNR (bottom panel in Figure 8.3). The synthesized signal was in fact indistinguishable from the original when $p = 50$. In [12], four to nine singular vectors were sufficient to synthesize vowels with a 15 dB SNR, consistent with the example given in Figure 8.3. In brief, good speech synthesis can be achieved even with a low-rank (p ranging from 4 to 10) approximation, at least for voiced speech segments.

For comparative purposes, Figure 8.5 shows an unvoiced segment taken from/s/ synthesized using low-rank approximations. The distribution of singular values for this segment is shown in Figure 8.6. We observe now that the singular values decay down to zero very slowly compared to the singular values obtained from a voiced

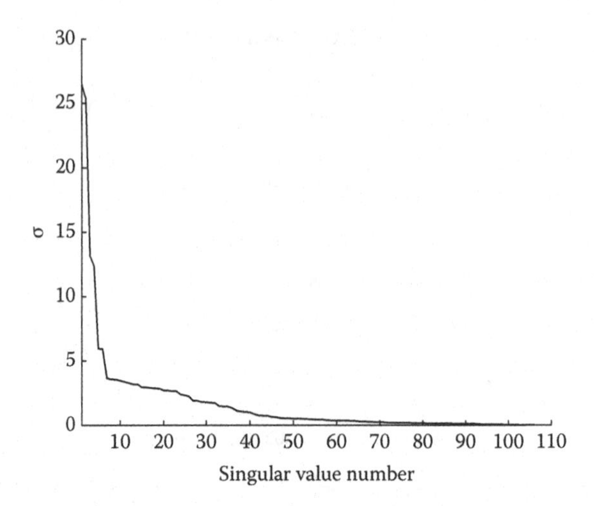

FIGURE 8.4 Distribution of singular values for the voiced speech segment (vowel/iy/) used in the example in Figure 8.3.

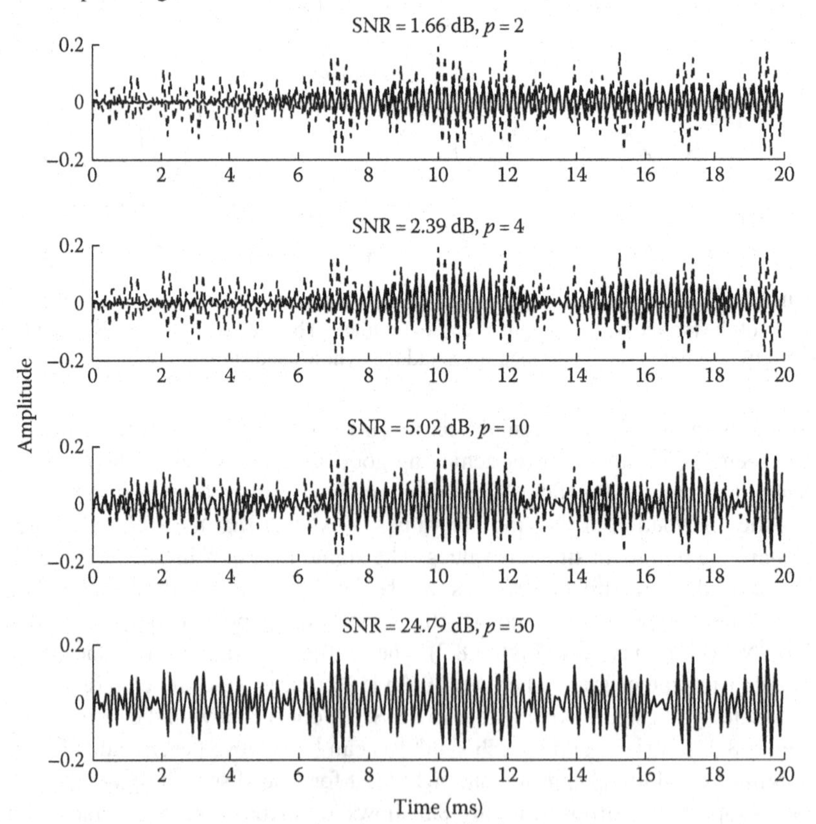

FIGURE 8.5 SVD synthesis of an unvoiced speech segment, taken from the fricative/s/, as a function of the number (p) of singular vectors retained. The reconstruction SNR is indicated. The original signal is shown in thick lines and the synthesized signal in dashed lines.

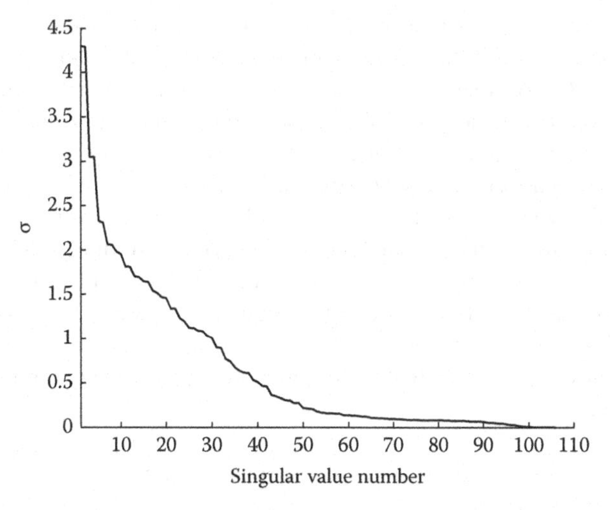

FIGURE 8.6 Distribution of singular values for the unvoiced speech segment (/s/) used in the example in Figure 8.5.

segment (see Figure 8.4). For that reason, retaining only 10 singular vectors in an unvoiced speech segment achieved only 5 dB SNR reconstruction compared to 12 dB achieved for a voiced segment (see Figure 8.3). It is clear from this example that the effective rank depends largely on the speech segment at hand, with voiced segments requiring a small number of singular vectors and unvoiced segments requiring a relatively larger number of singular vectors.

8.3.2 Determining the Effective Rank

In the preceding example we assumed that the signal matrix X contains noise-free speech samples. In noise, we have

$$Y = X + D$$

where Y, X, and D are $(N - L + 1) \times L$ data matrices containing the noisy speech, clean speech, and noise signals, respectively. The preceding matrices are arranged in a Toeplitz matrix in the same manner as in Equation 8.43. The problem of determining the effective rank of X becomes more difficult given the noisy data matrix Y. As the noise matrix D is typically full rank, the matrix Y will also be full rank, even if the signal matrix X is rank deficient, that is, rank $(X) = p < L$.

Several methods have been proposed for determining the effective rank of a matrix [8,18,23]. One method [18] chooses p as the effective rank if the following ratio of singular values is larger than a prescribed threshold δ:

$$\left(\frac{\sigma_1^2 + \sigma_2^2 + \cdots \sigma_p^2}{\sigma_1^2 + \sigma_2^2 + \cdots \sigma_L^2} \right)^{1/2} > \delta, \quad p < L \tag{8.47}$$

Note that the preceding ratio is always smaller than 1 since $p < L$. This criterion, though simple, was found to be highly dependent on the SNR, data length, and threshold value δ [24]. No unique threshold value δ was found in [24] that would lead to the correct order selection in all signal conditions. Threshold bounds based on the statistical characterization of the noise (assumed to be normally distributed with zero mean and unit variance) were proposed in [25].

An analysis-by-synthesis approach was taken in [12,24] for determining the effective rank of the matrix X. The idea was to synthesize the signal with increasingly larger number of singular vectors (Equation 8.45) and choose the value p as the effective rank when the energy of the synthesized signal (based on p singular vectors) is closest to the energy difference of the noisy speech and noise signals. This idea is based on the fact that if the signal and noise are uncorrelated and zero mean, we have

$$E[y^2(n)] = E[x^2(n)] + E[d^2(n)] \tag{8.48}$$

or equivalently

$$\sigma_y^2 = \sigma_x^2 + \sigma_d^2 \tag{8.49}$$

where
$d(n)$ denotes the noise signal
σ_d^2 the noise variance

Note that for zero-mean signals the signal variance σ_x^2 is equal to the energy of the signal. Let $x_k(n)$ denote the signal synthesized using a k-rank approximation and define the following difference in energies for the kth rank approximation:

$$E_k = E[y^2(n)] - E\left[x_k^2(n)\right] \tag{8.50}$$

If the synthesized signal $x_k(n)$ is close to the original signal $x(n)$, that is, $x_k(n) \approx x(n)$, then according to Equation 8.48 we should have $E_k \approx E[d^2(n)]$, which is the noise variance. Equivalently, the difference $(E_k - E[d^2(n)])$ should get closer to zero as $x_k(n)$ approximates more closely the signal $x(n)$. We can therefore use the difference $(E_k - E[d^2(n)])$ as the criterion for determining the effective rank of the matrix X.

By substituting Equation 8.50 into Equation 8.48, we can also express this difference as

$$E_k - \sigma_d^2 = E[x^2(n)] - E\left[x_k^2(n)\right] \tag{8.51}$$

The energy of the synthesized signal increases as we include more singular vectors, that is, $E\left[x_{k+1}^2(n)\right] > E\left[x_k^2(n)\right]$, and therefore the difference $\left(E_k - \sigma_d^2\right)$ will decrease monotonically. When k crosses the true rank p, that is, $k > p$, the energy of the synthesized signal will be larger than the signal energy $\left(\text{i.e., } E\left[x_k^2(n)\right] > E\left[x^2(n)\right]\right)$ owing to the intruded portion of the noise, and therefore the difference $\left(E_k - \sigma_d^2\right)$ will be negative. This suggests that the difference $\left(E_k - \sigma_d^2\right)$ must be close to zero at $k = p$, the true rank. To summarize, we can determine the effective rank of the matrix X by observing when the difference $\left(E_k - \sigma_d^2\right)$ crosses the zero axis. Alternatively, we can define

$$\Delta(k) = |E_k - \sigma_d^2|, \quad k = 1,2,\ldots,L \tag{8.52}$$

and seek for the minimum of $\Delta(k)$. The preceding criterion for rank-order selection was proposed in [12] and termed the *parsimonious order selection* method.

Figure 8.7 shows an example of the estimation of $\Delta(k)$ for a voiced speech segment (10 ms) embedded in +10 dB white noise. The function $\Delta(k)$ achieves a minimum at $p = 11$, and therefore $p = 11$ is selected as the effective rank for this example. Figure 8.8 shows example synthesized signals for the same speech segment using $p = 3$, 11, and 40. As the figure shows, underestimating the true order produces an oversmoothed time-domain signal (second panel from top), whereas overestimating the true order produces a more noisy signal (bottom panel). The signal synthesized using the rank estimated from the minimum of $\Delta(k)$ yields the best compromise.

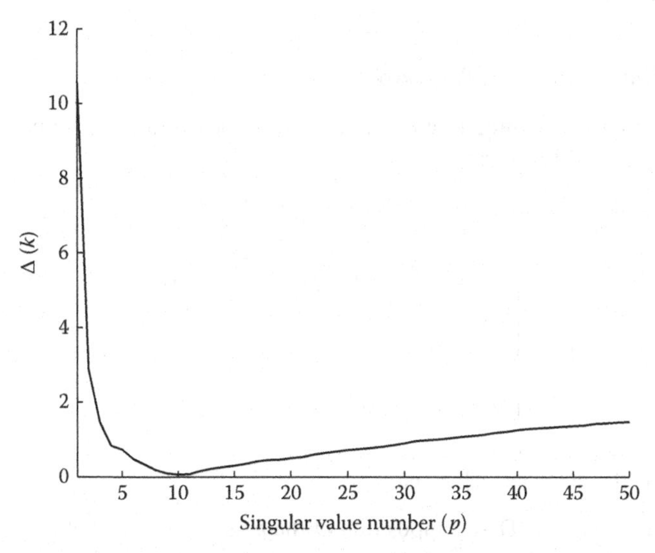

FIGURE 8.7 Plot of absolute energy difference $\Delta(k)$ (Equation 8.52) used as a criterion for rank-order selection in SVD-based methods. The rank is determined as the minimum of $\Delta(k)$, which in this example is 11. The noisy signal comprised a voiced speech segment (10 ms) embedded in +10 dB white noise.

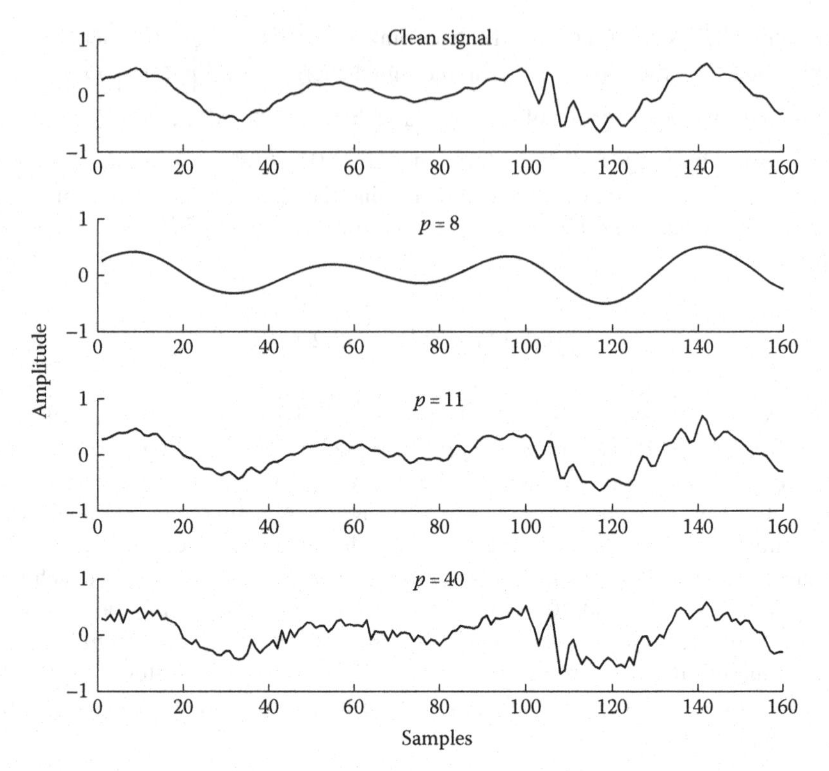

FIGURE 8.8 SVD synthesis of a noisy segment of speech as a function of the number of singular values (p) retained.

8.3.3 Noise Reduction Algorithm

We are now ready to summarize the algorithm proposed in [12]. For each frame of noisy speech, do as follows:

Step 1: Form the Toeplitz matrix Y $((N - L + 1) \times L)$:

$$Y = \begin{bmatrix} y(L-1) & y(L-2) & \cdots & y(0) \\ y(L) & y(L-1) & \cdots & y(1) \\ \vdots & \vdots & \vdots & \vdots \\ y(N-1) & y(N-2) & \cdots & y(N-L) \end{bmatrix} \tag{8.53}$$

where $y(n)$ is the noisy speech signal.

Step 2: Compute the SVD decomposition of the noisy matrix Y, that is, $Y = U\Sigma V^H$.

Step 3: Compute $\Delta(k)$ using Equations 8.52 and 8.50, for $k = 1, 2, \ldots, L$. Estimate the effective rank as: $p = \arg\min_{1 \le k \le L} \Delta(k)$.

Step 4: Compute the p-rank approximation of Y as

$$\hat{X}_p = \sum_{k=1}^{p} \sigma_k u_k \mathbf{v}_k^T$$

where u_k and $\mathbf{v}_k$ are the left and right singular vectors of Y, respectively.

Step 5: Average the diagonal elements of $\hat{X}_p$, and extract the enhanced signal $\hat{x}(n)$.

Good performance was obtained in [12] with the preceding algorithm for input SNR ≥ 10 dB. However, the enhanced signal had musical noise at lower SNR values.

8.4 SVD-BASED ALGORITHMS: COLORED NOISE

If the noise is not white, then $D^T D \neq \sigma^2 I$ and the assumption stated in Equation 8.29 is violated. We can, however, consider postmultiplying the noise matrix by some matrix W so that $(DW)^T DW$ is a scaled identity matrix. The matrix W is often referred to as the *whitening* matrix, as it whitens the transformed signal, that is, it produces a signal with a diagonal autocorrelation matrix (i.e., $E[(DW)^T DW] = I$). Next we show how to obtain the whitening matrix W.

Assuming that we estimate the noise matrix D during speech-absent segments of speech, we can factor the matrix D ($m \times n$) as

$$D = QR \tag{8.54}$$

where
- Q is a matrix ($m \times n$) with n orthonormal columns (i.e., $Q^T Q = I_n$)
- R is an upper triangular matrix ($n \times n$)

The preceding decomposition is called the "skinny" QR factorization of the matrix D [8, th. 5.2.2]. The R matrix is also the Cholesky factor of the matrix product $D^T D$, that is, $D^T D = R^T R$ [8, th. 5.2.2]. We can use the matrix R^{-1} as the whitening matrix, that is, set $W = R^{-1}$. To verify this, after postmultiplying the noise matrix by R^{-1}, we get $(DR^{-1})^T(DR^{-1}) = Q^T Q = I_n$. Therefore, the newly transformed noise matrix $\bar{D} = DR^{-1}$ satisfies the assumption in Equation 8.29.

Similarly, the noisy speech matrix Y and signal matrix X can be transformed to $\bar{Y}$ and $\bar{X}$, respectively, as follows:

$$\begin{aligned} \bar{Y} &= \bar{X} + \bar{D} \\ YR^{-1} &= XR^{-1} + DR^{-1} \end{aligned} \tag{8.55}$$

The SVD decomposition can now be done on the transformed noisy speech matrix $\bar{Y}$ given earlier. Note that if $X^H D = 0$, then

$$\bar{X}^T \bar{D} = R^{-T} X^T D R^{-1} = 0 \tag{8.56}$$

and therefore the whitening matrix preserves the orthogonality assumption between the signal and noise matrices. It can be shown [14] that the SVD of the transformed matrix $\bar{Y}$ can recover the same subspaces mentioned in Section 8.2.1.

To summarize, if the additive noise is colored we can apply the algorithm described in the previous section, but use the transformed matrix $\bar{Y} = YR^{-1}$ in place of Y. Additionally, following Step 4, we will need to "dewhiten" the low-rank matrix $\hat{X}_p$ as follows:

$$Z_p = \hat{X}_p R \tag{8.57}$$

We can obtain the enhanced signal $\hat{x}(n)$ by averaging the diagonal elements of Z_p.

The preceding implementation requires that R^{-1} be updated whenever speech is absent. The explicit computation of R^{-1}, however, followed by the computation of the matrix product $\bar{Y} = YR^{-1}$ can potentially create numerical accuracy issues. Fortunately, we can avoid these numerical accuracy issues by computing the generalized SVD (GSVD) of the matrices Y and D. The generalized SVD (also called the quotient SVD) simultaneously diagonalizes the matrices Y and D ($m \times n$) according to [8, th. 8.7.4]

$$\begin{aligned} Y &= U \Delta \Theta^{-1} \\ D &= V M \Theta^{-1} \end{aligned} \tag{8.58}$$

where

U and V are rectangular matrices ($m \times n$) with orthonormal columns
Δ and M are diagonal matrices ($n \times n$)
Θ is a nonsingular square matrix ($n \times n$)

If the matrix Y is rank deficient (i.e., $\text{rank}(Y) = r < n$), and after defining $\Phi^T = \Theta^{-1}$, we can partition the GSVD of (Y,D) as follows:

$$\begin{aligned} Y &= \begin{bmatrix} U_1 & U_2 \end{bmatrix} \begin{bmatrix} \Delta_1 & 0 \\ 0 & 0 \end{bmatrix} \begin{bmatrix} \Phi_1^T \\ \Phi_2^T \end{bmatrix} \\ D &= \begin{bmatrix} V_1 & V_2 \end{bmatrix} \begin{bmatrix} M_1 & 0 \\ 0 & 0 \end{bmatrix} \begin{bmatrix} \Phi_1^T \\ \Phi_2^T \end{bmatrix} \end{aligned} \tag{8.59}$$

where

Δ_1 is a $r \times r$ diagonal matrix
Φ_1 is an $n \times r$ matrix
U_1, V_1 are $m \times r$ matrices

Using the GSVD of Y and D, along with Equation 8.54, we can express the transformed matrix $\bar{Y}$ as follows:

$$\begin{aligned}\bar{Y} &= YR^{-1} \\ &= U\Delta\Theta^{-1}\left(Q^T D\right)^{-1} \\ &= U\Delta\Theta^{-1}\left(Q^T VM\Theta^{-1}\right)^{-1} \\ &= U\Delta M^{-1}\left(Q^T V\right)^T \\ &= U\tilde{\Sigma}\tilde{V}^T \end{aligned} \tag{8.60}$$

where
$\tilde{\Sigma} = \Delta M^{-1}$ is a diagonal matrix
$\tilde{V}$ is an orthogonal matrix

Therefore, working with the GSVD of Y and D is mathematically equivalent to working with the SVD of $\bar{Y}$. In other words, the whitening operation is implicitly embedded in the GSVD of Y and D. Hence, the GSVD reduces the two steps (computation of R^{-1} followed by the matrix product YR^{-1}) required to compute the SVD of the transformed matrix $\bar{Y}$ to a single step.

The GSVD-based algorithm for colored noise can be summarized in the following steps. For each frame of noisy speech, do as follows:

Step 1: Form the Toeplitz matrix Y (($N - L + 1) \times L$) as in Equation 8.53.

Step 2: Compute the GSVD of Y and D:

$$\begin{aligned} Y &= U\Delta\Theta^{-1} \\ D &= VM\Theta^{-1} \end{aligned} \tag{8.61}$$

Step 3: Determine the effective rank of Y either by using the analysis-by-synthesis approach described in the previous section or by choosing a fixed value for r ($r < L$).

Step 4: Form the matrix $\hat{X}_r$ as follows:

$$\hat{X}_r = U\begin{bmatrix} \Delta_1 & 0 \\ 0 & 0 \end{bmatrix}\Theta^{-1} \tag{8.62}$$

where Δ_1 is a diagonal submatrix ($r \times r$) of Δ in Equation 8.61, that is, $\Delta_1 = \text{diag}(\delta_1, \delta_2, \ldots, \delta_r)$ with $\delta_1 > \delta_2 > \cdots > \delta_r$.

Step 5: Average the diagonal elements of $\hat{X}_r$, and extract the enhanced signal $\hat{x}(n)$.

The noise matrix D, needed in Equation 8.61, can be obtained (and updated) during the speech-absent segments of speech.

Note that Equation 8.62 gives the least-squares estimate of X. Alternatively, in accordance with Equation 8.40, one can obtain the minimum-variance estimate of X as follows:

$$\Delta_{MV} = \Delta_1^{-1}\left(\Delta_1^2 - \sigma^2 I_r\right)$$

$$\hat{X}_{MV} = U\begin{bmatrix} \Delta_{MV} & 0 \\ 0 & 0 \end{bmatrix}\Theta^{-1}$$

$$= [U_1 \quad U_2]\begin{bmatrix} \Delta_{MV} & 0 \\ 0 & 0 \end{bmatrix}\begin{bmatrix} \Phi_1^T \\ \Phi_2^T \end{bmatrix} \tag{8.63}$$

where Φ_1, Φ_2 are given in Equation 8.59. The preceding algorithms were implemented and evaluated in [13,26]. Comparisons were made between the least-squares (Equation 8.62) and minimum-variance estimates (Equation 8.63) of X. Results indicated that whereas the LS approach was sensitive to the proper choice of the effective rank r, the MV approach was not as sensitive provided that r was chosen large enough [13]. Good results were obtained with the MV approach using a fixed value for r ($r = 14$). Informal listening tests showed that at low SNR levels (SNR < 10 dB) the least-squares and minimum-variance methods suffered from musical noise [13,26].

We finally note that in some applications (e.g., real-time signal processing applications) it is more desirable to update the GSVD rather than recompute it at every frame. This is an important issue that will be dealt with in more detail later on in Section 8.10. We briefly mention here that some researchers proposed the use of the rank-revealing ULLV decomposition in place of the GSVD decomposition [26,27] because it is easier to update. The ULLV decomposition of the matrices Y and D is given by [28]

$$Y = \tilde{U}L_1L_2W^T$$
$$D = \tilde{V}L_2W^T \tag{8.64}$$

where

$\tilde{U}(m \times n)$, $\tilde{V}(m \times n)$, and $W(n \times n)$ are matrices with orthonormal columns
L_1, L_2 $(n \times n)$ are lower triangular matrices

The major advantage in using the ULLV decomposition in place of the GSVD decomposition is that it can be updated efficiently as new data come in. This is because it is easier to maintain the triangular structure of L_1 and L_2 than the diagonal structure of Δ and M in Equation 8.58. Detailed analysis of the ULLV decomposition and updating schemes can be found in [29].

8.5 SVD-BASED METHODS: A UNIFIED VIEW

All SVD-based methods described so far can be summarized using the following unified notation:

$$\hat{X} = W_1 G_1 Z_1^H \tag{8.65}$$

where
$\hat{X}$ is the matrix containing the enhanced signal
G_1 is a diagonal matrix containing the gains
the matrices W_1, Z_1 are computed from either the SVD of Y or the GSVD of the matrices Y and D, depending on the noise (white or colored)

Note that the matrix Z_1 is not unitary in colored noise (see Equation 8.59). Table 8.1 summarizes the estimators described so far with the various gain matrices G_1.

8.6 EVD-BASED METHODS: WHITE NOISE

We now turn our attention to subspace methods that are based on the eigenvalue decomposition (EVD) of signal covariance matrices. The EVD methods are based on second-order statistics (covariance matrices) information, whereas the SVD methods are based on time-domain amplitude information. Unlike the methods described so far, the EVD methods operate on speech vectors rather than on matrices containing the speech signal. The general structure of the EVD-based methods is similar to that shown in Equation 8.65 with the main difference that the matrices W_1 and Z_1 are the same. We start by considering first the case when the additive noise is white.

TABLE 8.1
Summary of SVD Methods That Can Be Generally Expressed as $\hat{X} = W_1 G_1 Z_1^H$

Method	Noise	Gain Matrix G_1	W_1	Z_1	Equation
Least-squares	White	Σ_{y1}	U_{y1}	V_{y1}	8.34
Minimum-variance	White	$\left(\Sigma_{y1}^2 - \sigma^2 I_r\right)\Sigma_{y1}^{-1}$	U_{y1}	V_{y1}	8.40
Least-squares	Colored	Δ_1	U_1	Φ_1	8.59
Minimum-variance	Colored	$\Delta_1^{-1}\left(\Delta_1^2 - \sigma^2 I_r\right)$	U_1	Φ_1	8.63

Note: The various methods differ in the choice of the matrices W_1, G_1, and Z_1.

8.6.1 Eigenvalue Analysis of "Noisy" Matrices

Consider the noisy speech vector $\mathbf{y} = \mathbf{x} + \mathbf{d}$ containing K samples of speech, where $\mathbf{x}$ is the clean signal vector and $\mathbf{d}$ is the noise signal vector ($K \times 1$). The covariance matrix of $\mathbf{y}$ can be computed according to

$$\begin{aligned} R_y &\triangleq E[\mathbf{y}\mathbf{y}^T] \\ &= E[\mathbf{x}\mathbf{x}^T] + E[\mathbf{d}\mathbf{d}^T] + E[\mathbf{x}\mathbf{d}^T] + E[\mathbf{d}\mathbf{x}^T] \end{aligned} \tag{8.66}$$

The covariance matrix R_y ($K \times K$) is symmetric and positive semidefinite, assuming a stationary process. After making the assumption that the signal and noise vectors are uncorrelated and zero mean, the preceding equation reduces to

$$R_y = R_x + R_d \tag{8.67}$$

where
$R_x \triangleq E[\mathbf{x}\mathbf{x}^T]$ is the signal covariance matrix
$R_d \triangleq E[\mathbf{d}\mathbf{d}^T]$ is the noise covariance matrix

If we further make the assumption that the input noise is white, then the noise covariance matrix will be diagonal and will have the form, $R_d = \sigma^2 I$ where σ^2 is the noise variance. Equation 8.67 then reduces to

$$R_y = R_x + \sigma^2 I \tag{8.68}$$

Let $R_y = U\Lambda_y U^T$ be the eigen-decomposition of the noisy covariance matrix R_y, where U is the orthogonal eigenvector matrix, and Λ_y is the diagonal matrix containing the eigenvalues. As R_d is diagonal, the eigenvectors of R_y are also the eigenvectors of R_x and R_d, and therefore Equation 8.68 can also be written as

$$U\Lambda_y U^T = U\Lambda_x U^T + U\Lambda_d U^T \tag{8.69}$$

where $\Lambda_x = \text{diag}(\lambda_x(1), \lambda_x(2), \ldots, \lambda_x(K))$ contains the eigenvalues (assumed to be sorted in descending order) of the clean signal vector $\mathbf{x}$, and $\Lambda_d = \sigma^2 I$. From Equation 8.69, it is easy to derive the following equation relating the noisy and clean eigenvalues:

$$\lambda_y(k) = \lambda_x(k) + \sigma^2 \quad k = 1, 2, \ldots, K \tag{8.70}$$

The preceding equation holds assuming that the signal covariance matrix R_x is full rank. There is strong empirical evidence, however, which suggests that the covariance matrices of most speech vectors have eigenvalues that are near zero. It is therefore safe to make the assumption that the matrix R_x is not full rank and that the rank $(R_x) = M < K$. This implies that R_x has M positive eigenvalues and $K - M$ zero eigenvalues. Equation 8.70 then reduces to

$$\lambda_y(k) = \begin{cases} \lambda_x(k) + \sigma^2 & \text{if } k = 1,2,\ldots,M \\ \sigma^2 & \text{if } k = M+1,\ldots,K \end{cases} \tag{8.71}$$

The M largest eigenvalues of $\lambda_y(k)$ are referred to as *principal eigenvalues*, and the corresponding eigenvectors, *principal eigenvectors*. From the preceding equation we observe that we can recover the eigenvalues of the clean signal (i.e., $\lambda_x(k)$) from the noisy eigenvalues, provided we know the noise variance σ^2. A very similar equation was derived in Equation 8.31 for estimating the singular values of the clean signal matrix.

Note that to derive Equation 8.71 we had to make two assumptions: (1) the signal and noise signals were uncorrelated and zero mean, and (2) the input noise was white. Interestingly enough, those were the very assumptions we made when analyzing the SVD of noisy matrices (see Equation 8.29), the main difference being that in Section 8.3.1 we dealt with time-domain signals arranged in a Toeplitz (or Hankel) matrix, whereas here we are dealing with the covariance matrices of these signals.

Based on Equation 8.71, we can partition the eigenvector matrix as $U = [U_1\ U_2]$, where U_1 denotes the $K \times M$ matrix of principal eigenvectors corresponding to the noise eigenvalues $\{\lambda_x(k) + \sigma^2\}$, and U_2 denotes the $K \times (K - M)$ matrix of eigenvectors corresponding to the noise eigenvalues. We can therefore say that the columns of U_1 span a signal-plus-noise subspace, whereas the columns of U_2 span the noise subspace. As the signal dominates the signal-plus-noise subspace, we simply refer to the subspace spanned by U_1 as the "signal subspace." In fact, under some assumptions about the input signal, it can be shown that the subspace spanned by U_1 is the true subspace of the clean signal. More specifically, let us assume a linear model for the input clean signal of the form

$$\mathbf{x} = \sum_{m=1}^{M} c_m \mathbf{V}_m \quad M \le K \tag{8.72}$$

where

c_m are zero-mean complex random variables
$\mathbf{V}_m$ are K-dimensional complex basis vectors assumed to be linearly independent

From Equation 8.72, we note that the signal $\mathbf{x}$ lies in the subspace spanned by the vectors $\mathbf{V}_m$. Example basis vectors include the complex sinusoids:

$$\mathbf{V}_m = [1, e^{j(\omega_m + \theta_m)}, e^{j(2\omega_m + \theta_m)}, \ldots, e^{j(\omega_m(K-1) + \theta_m)}]^T \tag{8.73}$$

where

ω_m are the frequencies

θ_m are the phases, which are assumed to be statistically independent and uniformly distributed in $(0, 2\pi)$

The autocorrelation of the signal model **x** in Equation 8.72 is given by [30, p. 57]

$$R_{xx} = \sum_{k=1}^{M} c_k^2 \mathbf{s}_k \mathbf{s}_k^H \tag{8.74}$$

where $\mathbf{s}_k = [1 \ \exp(j\omega_k) \ \exp(j2\omega_k) \ \cdots \ \exp(j\omega_k(K-1))]^T$. Now, let $R_{xx} = U\Lambda U^T$ be the eigen-decomposition of R_{xx} and partition U as $U = [U_1 U_2]$, where U_1 contains the M principal eigenvectors. One can prove [30, p. 442] that the span of the M principal eigenvectors of R_{xx}, that is, the span of U_1, is the same as the span of $V \triangleq [V_1, V_2, \ldots, V_M]$, which is the true signal subspace. Therefore, for the linear signal model given in Equation 8.72, the signal subspace is the same as the subspace spanned by the principal eigenvectors of the covariance matrix R_{xx}.

The preceding observation is extremely important for speech enhancement applications, as we can use the matrix U_1 to project the noisy speech vector to the signal subspace. We can do this by first constructing the orthogonal projector matrix $U_1 U_1^T$, and then using this matrix to project the noisy speech vector onto the signal subspace. The complementary orthogonal subspace is spanned by the columns of U_2, and therefore we can use the matrix $U_2 U_2^T$ to project the noisy speech vector onto the noise subspace. In general, the noisy speech vector **y** can be decomposed as

$$\mathbf{y} = U_1 U_1^T \mathbf{y} + U_2 U_2^T \mathbf{y} \tag{8.75}$$

where

$U_1 U_1^T \mathbf{y}$ is the projection of **y** onto the signal subspace

$U_2 U_2^T \mathbf{y}$ is the projection of **y** onto the noise subspace

Based on Equation 8.75, we can enhance the noisy signal by keeping the projection onto the signal subspace (i.e., $U_1 U_1^T \mathbf{y}$) and discarding the projection onto the noise subspace. The enhanced signal $\hat{\mathbf{x}}$ is thus obtained as

$$\hat{\mathbf{x}} = U_1 U_1^T \mathbf{y} \tag{8.76}$$

The preceding equation can also be expressed as

$$\hat{\mathbf{x}} = U_1 I_M U_1^T \mathbf{y} \tag{8.77}$$

where I_M is an $M \times M$ identity matrix. We will refer to this method as the *least-squares subspace estimator* [11] as it is the estimator resulting from minimization of the following least-squares problem:

$$\min_{\hat{\mathbf{x}} = H \cdot s} \| \mathbf{y} - \hat{\mathbf{x}} \|^2 \tag{8.78}$$

where s is unknown. The solution of the preceding problem is given by $\hat{\mathbf{x}}_{LS} = H_{opt}\mathbf{y} = U_1U_1^T\mathbf{y}$ [31, p. 365], which is identical to that given in Equation 8.76.

As we will see in the next section, most subspace methods can be expressed in the general form given in Equation 8.77. What distinguish the various methods are the contents of the diagonal matrix between U_1 and U_1^T in Equation 8.77. The diagonal matrix of the basic subspace method given in Equation 8.77 is the identity matrix.

Figure 8.9 shows an example noisy speech vector enhanced using Equation 8.77 with different values of the signal subspace dimension, M. The noisy speech vector consisted of a 6.2 ms segment of the vowel/iy/embedded in white noise at 6 dB S/N.

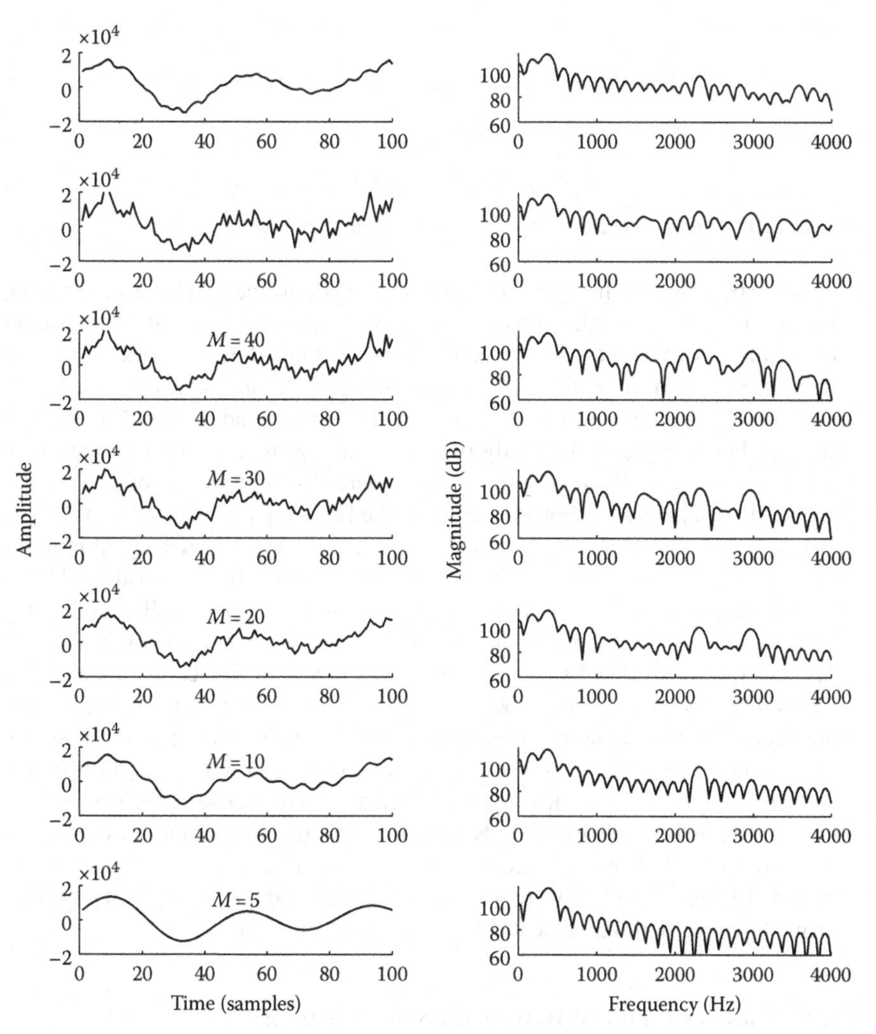

FIGURE 8.9 Synthesis of a noisy segment of speech as a function of signal subspace dimension M. Left panels show the amplitude waveforms, and right panels show the corresponding Fourier magnitude spectra. First top row shows the clean waveform and magnitude spectra, and the second top row shows the noisy waveform and magnitude spectra.

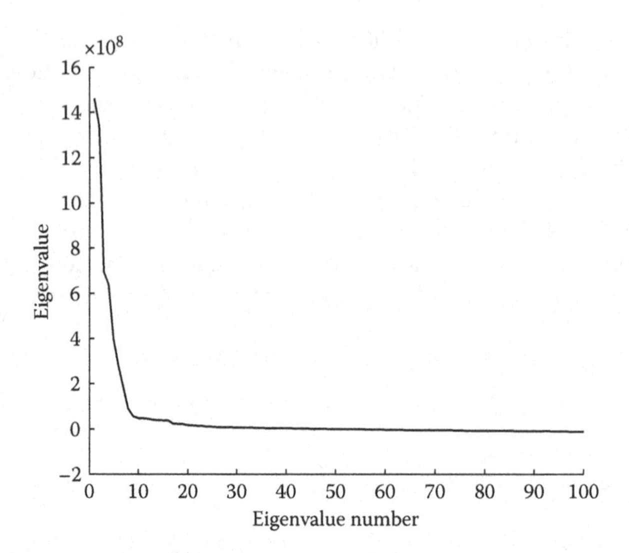

FIGURE 8.10 Eigenvalue distribution for the example shown in Figure 8.9.

To examine the effect of the signal dimension, M, on performance (in terms of reconstruction error), we show the enhanced signals synthesized using different values of M ranging from $M = 5$ to $M = 40$. Note that by varying M, we vary the dimension of the principal eigenvector matrix U_1 in Equation 8.77. For instance, if we set $M = 5$, then U_1 is a $K \times 5$ matrix, where $K = 100$ samples (corresponding to 6.2 ms for $F_s =$ 16 kHz) in this example; that is, only five principal eigenvectors are recruited with $M = 5$. It is clear from Figure 8.9 that if we underestimate the value of M, then the synthesized signal is oversmoothed (see, e.g., the bottom panel with $M = 5$). On the other hand, if we overestimate the value of M, then the synthesized signal remains noisy (see, e.g., the panel with $M = 40$). Hence, knowing the exact value of M is critically important for the subspace method given in Equation 8.77. But what is the optimal value of M for the preceding example? To answer that question, we plot in Figure 8.10 the eigenvalue distribution, from which we can deduce that the optimal M is near the value of 10. Indeed, the value of 10 gave the best results in terms of low reconstruction error and low spectral difference between the clean spectra (shown on top right panel) and synthesized spectra (shown on the right in the second from the last panel). We further quantified the reconstruction error between the synthesized and clean signals in terms of SNR. Note that a high reconstruction SNR indicates a small difference between the clean and enhanced signals. The computed SNRs for $M = 5$, 10, 20, 30, and 40 were 9.7, 12.9, 10.2, 8.2, and 7.7 dB, respectively. This confirmed that the optimal value of M was 10 in this example.

8.6.2 Subspace Methods Based on Linear Estimators

The subspace approach, as outlined earlier, is not sufficient for suppressing the additive noise, as it only projects the noisy signal onto the signal subspace without modifying it in any way. As such, as we will show shortly, it yields no signal distortion but introduces a great lot of residual noise distortion. To reduce the residual noise following projection of the noisy speech vector onto the signal subspace, the projected signal needs to be modified in some way prior to reconstruction. One method of reducing the residual noise is to derive a linear estimator that minimizes the residual error energy. As we will see next, the resulting estimator is the Wiener filter. Two alternative methods were proposed in [11] based on linear estimators that minimize the signal distortion while constraining the level of the residual noise below a preset threshold. The latter two estimators are derived using principles similar to those already presented in Chapter 6 (Section 6.9) and are presented next along with the Wiener estimator.

8.6.2.1 Linear Minimum Mean-Square Estimator (LMMSE)

Let $\hat{\mathbf{x}} = H \cdot \mathbf{y}$ be a linear estimator of the clean speech $\mathbf{x}$, where H is a $K \times K$ matrix. The residual error signal ε obtained by this estimation is given by

$$\begin{aligned} \varepsilon &= \hat{\mathbf{x}} - \mathbf{x} \\ &= H \cdot \mathbf{y} - \mathbf{x} \end{aligned} \tag{8.79}$$

After defining the energy of the residual error $\overline{\varepsilon_r^2}$ as

$$\overline{\varepsilon_r^2} = E[\varepsilon^T \varepsilon] = \mathrm{tr}(E[\varepsilon\varepsilon^T]) \tag{8.80}$$

we can obtain the optimum linear estimator by solving the following unconstrained optimization problem:

$$\min_H \overline{\varepsilon_r^2} \tag{8.81}$$

After substituting Equation 8.79 in the preceding equation, we get

$$\begin{aligned} \overline{\varepsilon_r^2} &= \mathrm{tr}\left[E\left\{ (H \cdot \mathbf{y} - \mathbf{x})(H \cdot \mathbf{y} - \mathbf{x})^T \right\} \right] \\ &= \mathrm{tr}\left[E\left\{ H \cdot \mathbf{y}\mathbf{y}^T \cdot H^T - \mathbf{x}\mathbf{y}^T H^T - H \cdot \mathbf{y}\mathbf{x}^T + \mathbf{x}\mathbf{x}^T \right\} \right] \\ &= \mathrm{tr}\left[HR_y H^T - R_{xy} H^T - HR_{yx} + R_x \right] \end{aligned} \tag{8.82}$$

where $R_{xy} \triangleq E\{\mathbf{x}\mathbf{y}^T\}$ and $R_{yx} \triangleq E\{\mathbf{y}\mathbf{x}^T\}$. Taking the derivative of $\overline{\varepsilon_r^2}$ with respect to H and setting it equal to zero, we get

$$2HR_y - 2R_{yx}^T = 0 \tag{8.83}$$

Solving for the optimal estimator, we get

$$H_{opt} = R_{xy} R_{yy}^{-1} \tag{8.84}$$

after making use of the fact that $R_{yx}^T = R_{xy}$. After substituting in the preceding equation $R_y = R_x + R_d$ (Equation 8.67) and

$$R_{xy} = E\{\mathbf{xy}^T\} = E\{\mathbf{x}(\mathbf{x}+\mathbf{d})^T\} = R_x \tag{8.85}$$

we get

$$H_{opt} = R_x(R_x + R_d)^{-1} \tag{8.86}$$

which is the Wiener matrix. For white noise, $R_d = \sigma_d^2 I$, and the preceding estimator simplifies to

$$H_{opt} = R_x\left(R_x + \sigma_d^2 I\right)^{-1} \tag{8.87}$$

This estimator can be further simplified by using the eigen-decomposition of R_x:

$$R_{\mathbf{x}} = U\Lambda_{\mathbf{x}}U^T \tag{8.88}$$

where
- U is the unitary eigenvector matrix
- $\Lambda_{\mathbf{x}}$ is the diagonal eigenvalue matrix

Substituting Equation 8.88 into Equation 8.87, we get

$$\begin{aligned}
H_W &= U\Lambda_x U^T\left(U\Lambda_x U^T + \sigma_d^2 I\right)^{-1} \\
&= U\Lambda_x U^T\left[U\left(\Lambda_x U^T + U^T\sigma_d^2 I\right)\right]^{-1} \\
&= U\Lambda_x U^T\left[\Lambda_x U^T + U^T\sigma_d^2 I\right]^{-1} U^T \\
&= U\Lambda_x U^T\left[\left(\Lambda_x + U^T\sigma_d^2 U\right)U^T\right]^{-1} U^T \\
&= U\Lambda_x U^T U\left[\Lambda_x + U^T\sigma_d^2 U\right]^{-1} U^T \\
&= U\left\{\Lambda_x\left[\Lambda_x + \sigma_d^2 I\right]^{-1}\right\}U^T \\
&= U\Lambda_W U^T
\end{aligned} \tag{8.89}$$

where Λ_W is a diagonal matrix ($K \times K$) given by

$$\Lambda_W = \Lambda_{\mathbf{x}}\left(\Lambda_{\mathbf{x}} + \sigma_{\mathbf{d}}^2 I\right)^{-1} \tag{8.90}$$

Let us now assume that the signal covariance matrix R_x has a rank M ($M < K$), so $\Lambda_\mathbf{x}$ has only M nonzeros, that is,

$$\Lambda_\mathbf{x} = \text{diag}(\lambda_x(1),\ldots,\lambda_x(M),0,\ldots,0) \tag{8.91}$$

Substituting Equation 8.91 into Equation 8.90, we can rewrite the optimal estimator as

$$H_W = U\begin{bmatrix} G_W & 0 \\ 0 & 0 \end{bmatrix}U^T \tag{8.92}$$

where G_W is a diagonal matrix ($M \times M$)

$$G_W = \Lambda_\mathbf{x}\left(\Lambda_\mathbf{x} + \sigma_\mathbf{d}^2 I_M\right)^{-1} \tag{8.93}$$

and I_M is an $M \times M$ identity matrix. Partitioning the eigenvector matrix U as $U = [U_1\ U_2]$, where U_1 denotes the $K \times M$ matrix of principal eigenvectors, we can simplify Equation 8.92 to

$$\begin{aligned} H_W &= [U_1 \quad U_2]\begin{bmatrix} G_W & 0 \\ 0 & 0 \end{bmatrix}\begin{bmatrix} U_1^T \\ U_2^T \end{bmatrix} \\ &= U_1 G_W U_1^T \end{aligned} \tag{8.94}$$

Hence, the enhanced signal $\hat{\mathbf{x}}_W = H_W\mathbf{y}$ is obtained by applying the KLT (i.e., U^T) to the noisy signal, modifying the components of $U_1^T\mathbf{y}$ by a gain function (Equation 8.93), and applying the inverse KLT (i.e., U). Figure 8.2 illustrates this process.

8.6.2.2 Time-Domain-Constrained Estimator

As in the preceding section, let $\hat{\mathbf{x}} = H \cdot \mathbf{y}$ be a linear estimator of the clean speech vector $\mathbf{x}$, where H is a $K \times K$ matrix. We can decompose the error signal ε obtained by this estimation as follows:

$$\begin{aligned} \varepsilon &= \hat{\mathbf{x}} - \mathbf{x} \\ &= (H - I)\cdot\mathbf{x} + H\cdot\mathbf{d} \\ &= \varepsilon_\mathbf{x} + \varepsilon_\mathbf{d} \end{aligned} \tag{8.95}$$

where $\varepsilon_\mathbf{x}$ represents the speech distortion, and $\varepsilon_\mathbf{d}$ represents the residual noise. After defining the energy of the signal distortion $\overline{\varepsilon_\mathbf{x}^2}$ as

$$\begin{aligned} \overline{\varepsilon_\mathbf{x}^2} &= E\left[\varepsilon_\mathbf{x}^T\varepsilon_\mathbf{x}\right] = \text{tr}\left(E\left[\varepsilon_\mathbf{x}\varepsilon_\mathbf{x}^T\right]\right) \\ &= \text{tr}[(H - I)R_x(H - I)^T] \end{aligned} \tag{8.96}$$

and the energy of the residual noise $\overline{\varepsilon_{\mathbf{d}}^2}$ as

$$\overline{\varepsilon_{\mathbf{d}}^2} = E\left[\varepsilon_{\mathbf{d}}^T \varepsilon_{\mathbf{d}}\right] = \text{tr}\left(E\left[\varepsilon_{\mathbf{d}} \varepsilon_{\mathbf{d}}^T\right]\right)$$
$$= \text{tr}(H \cdot E[\mathbf{dd}^T]H^T)$$
$$= \sigma_d^2 \,\text{tr}(HH^T) \tag{8.97}$$

we can obtain the optimum linear estimator by solving the following time-domain-constrained optimization problem:

$$\min_H \overline{\varepsilon_{\mathbf{x}}^2}$$
$$\text{subject to}: \frac{1}{K}\overline{\varepsilon_{\mathbf{d}}^2} \leq \delta \tag{8.98}$$

where δ is a positive constant. The optimal estimator in the sense of Equation 8.98 can be found using the Kuhn–Tucker necessary conditions for constrained minimization. Specifically, H is a stationary feasible point if it satisfies the gradient equation of the Lagrangian $L(H,\mu) = \overline{\varepsilon_{\mathbf{x}}^2} + \mu(\overline{\varepsilon_{\mathbf{d}}^2} - K\delta)$ and

$$\mu\left(\overline{\varepsilon_{\mathbf{d}}^2} - K\delta\right) = 0 \quad \text{for } \mu \geq 0 \tag{8.99}$$

where μ is the Lagrange multiplier. From $\nabla_H L(H, \mu) = 0$, we have $HR_{\mathbf{x}} + \mu\, HR_{\mathbf{d}} - R_{\mathbf{x}} = 0$, where $R_{\mathbf{x}}$ and $R_{\mathbf{d}}$ are the covariance matrices of the clean speech and noise, respectively. Solving for H, we get the optimal estimator:

$$H_{opt} = R_{\mathbf{x}}\left(R_{\mathbf{x}} + \mu R_{\mathbf{d}}\right)^{-1} \tag{8.100}$$

Assuming white noise, we have $R_{\mathbf{d}} = \sigma_{\mathbf{d}}^2 I$, and the optimal estimator H can be written as

$$H_{opt} = R_{\mathbf{x}}\left(R_{\mathbf{x}} + \mu\sigma_{\mathbf{d}}^2 I\right)^{-1} \tag{8.101}$$

Note that H_{opt} has the form of a parametric Wiener filter, and when $\mu = 1$, we get the Wiener estimator given in Equation 8.87. As mentioned earlier, the preceding estimator can be simplified by using the eigen-decomposition of $R_{\mathbf{x}}$ in Equation 8.88, yielding

$$H_{TDC} = U\Lambda_{TDC} U^T \tag{8.102}$$

where Λ_{TDC} is a diagonal matrix ($K \times K$) given by

$$\Lambda_{TDC} = \Lambda_{\mathbf{x}}\left(\Lambda_{\mathbf{x}} + \mu\sigma_{\mathrm{d}}^{2} I\right)^{-1} \tag{8.103}$$

Assuming that the signal covariance matrix R_x has a rank $M(M < K)$, $\Lambda_{\mathbf{x}}$ has only M nonzeros, that is,

$$\Lambda_{\mathbf{x}} = \mathrm{diag}(\lambda_x(1), \ldots, \lambda_x(M), 0, \ldots, 0) \tag{8.104}$$

and we can rewrite the optimal time-domain-constrained estimator in Equation 8.102 as

$$H_{TDC} = U \begin{bmatrix} G_{\mu} & 0 \\ 0 & 0 \end{bmatrix} U^{T} \tag{8.105}$$

where G_{μ} is a diagonal matrix ($M \times M$)

$$G_{\mu} = \Lambda_{\mathbf{x}}\left(\Lambda_{\mathbf{x}} + \mu\sigma_{\mathrm{d}}^{2} I_{M}\right)^{-1} \tag{8.106}$$

and I_M is an $M \times M$ identity matrix. Partitioning the eigenvector matrix U as $U = [U_1 \; U_2]$, where U_1 denotes the $K \times M$ matrix of principal eigenvectors, we can simplify Equation 8.105 to

$$\begin{aligned} H_{TDC} &= \begin{bmatrix} U_1 & U_2 \end{bmatrix} \begin{bmatrix} G_{\mu} & 0 \\ 0 & 0 \end{bmatrix} \begin{bmatrix} U_1^{T} \\ U_2^{T} \end{bmatrix} \\ &= U_1 G_{\mu} U_1^{T} \end{aligned} \tag{8.107}$$

Hence, the enhanced signal $\hat{\mathbf{x}}_{TDC} = H_{TDC}\mathbf{y}$ is obtained, as before, by applying the KLT to the noisy signal, modifying the components of $U^{T}\mathbf{y}$ by a new gain function (G_{μ}), and applying the inverse KLT.

As we will show shortly, the value of the Lagrange multiplier μ can influence the performance of the preceding subspace estimator. Figure 8.11 shows an example noisy speech vector enhanced using Equation 8.107 for different values of μ ranging from $\mu = 0$ to $\mu = 15$. Note that if $\mu = 0$, we get the estimator given in Equation 8.77, and if $\mu = 1$, we get the Wiener estimator given in Equation 8.94. Similar to the example given in Figure 8.9, the noisy speech vector consisted of a 6.2 ms segment of the vowel/iy/embedded in 6 dB S/N white noise (but with different realization of the noise). It is evident from this figure that we get more noise suppression as the value of μ increases. As we will show later, this is done at the expense of introducing speech distortion. The signal subspace dimension was fixed at $M = 53$ in this example for all values of μ. This value for M was computed by counting the number of positive signal eigenvalues (more on this later). We quantified the reconstruction error between the clean and enhanced signals for different values of μ. The reconstruction SNR for

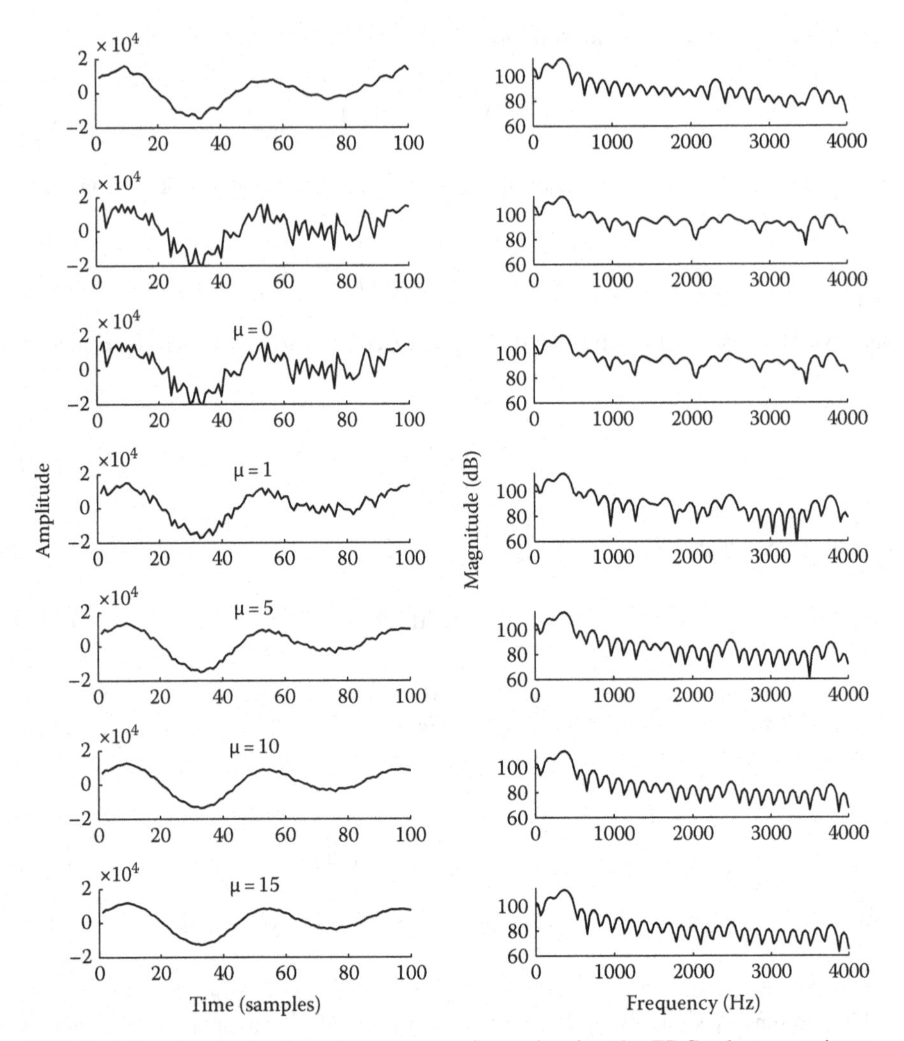

FIGURE 8.11 Synthesis of a noisy segment of speech using the TDC subspace estimator for different values of μ. Left panels show the amplitude waveforms and right panels show the corresponding Fourier magnitude spectra. First top row shows the clean waveform and magnitude spectra, and the second top row shows the noisy waveform and magnitude spectra.

$\mu = 0, 1, 5, 10$, and 15 was 5.1, 10.8, 13.9, 13.2, and 12.0 dB, respectively. The fact that the SNR does not improve monotonically with increasing values of μ suggests that there exists an optimal value of μ that yields the best compromise between speech and noise distortion (more on this in Section 8.6.3.2).

8.6.2.3 Spectral-Domain-Constrained Estimator

The basic idea of the spectral-domain-constrained estimator is to minimize the signal distortion subject to constraints on the shape of the spectrum of the residual noise. Specifically, suppose that the kth spectral component of the residual noise is given by $v_k^T \varepsilon_{\mathbf{d}}$, where v_k is the kth column vector of the eigenvector matrix of U, and ε_d is given by Equation 8.95. For $k = 1,\ldots, M$, we require the energy in $\mathbf{v}_k^T \varepsilon_{\mathbf{d}}$ to be smaller than or equal to $\alpha_k \sigma_{\mathbf{d}}^2$ ($0 < \alpha_k < 1$), whereas for $k = M + 1,\ldots, K$, we require the energy in $\mathbf{v}_k^T \varepsilon_{\mathbf{d}}$ to be zero, as the signal energy in the noise subspace is zero. Therefore, the estimator H is designed by solving the following constrained minimization problem:

$$\min_H \overline{\varepsilon_{\mathbf{x}}^2}$$

$$\text{subject to:} \begin{cases} E\{|\mathbf{v}_k^T \varepsilon_d|^2\} \leq \alpha_k \sigma_d^2 & k = 1,2,\ldots,M \\ E\{|\mathbf{v}_k^T \varepsilon_d|^2\} = 0 & k = M+1,\ldots,K \end{cases} \tag{8.108}$$

The preceding equation can be solved by following the same procedure used to derive the time-domain-constrained optimal linear estimator. The resulting gradient equation is given by

$$\begin{aligned} &J(H,\mu_1,\mu_2,\ldots,\mu_K) \\ &= \overline{\varepsilon_{\mathbf{x}}^2} + \sum_{k=1}^{K} \mu_k \left(E\{|\mathbf{v}_k^T \varepsilon_{\mathbf{d}}|^2\} - \alpha_k \sigma_{\mathbf{d}}^2 \right) = \overline{\varepsilon_{\mathbf{x}}^2} + \sum_{k=1}^{K} \mu_k \left(\mathbf{v}_k^T E\{\varepsilon_{\mathbf{d}} \varepsilon_{\mathbf{d}}^T\} \mathbf{v}_k - \alpha_k \sigma_{\mathbf{d}}^2 \right) \\ &= \text{tr}\left(HR_{\mathbf{x}}H^T - HR_{\mathbf{x}} - R_{\mathbf{x}}H^T + R_{\mathbf{x}} \right) + \sum_{k=1}^{K} \mu_k \left(\mathbf{v}_k^T H \sigma_{\mathbf{d}}^2 I H^T \mathbf{v}_k - \alpha_k \sigma_{\mathbf{d}}^2 \right) \end{aligned} \tag{8.109}$$

From $\Delta_H J(H, \mu_1,\ldots, \mu_K) = 0$, and $\nabla_H(\mathbf{v}_k^T H \sigma_{\mathbf{d}}^2 I H^T \mathbf{v}_k) = 2\sigma_{\mathbf{d}}^2 H^T \mathbf{v}_k \mathbf{v}_k^T$, we have

$$2HR_{\mathbf{x}} - 2R_{\mathbf{x}} + 2\sigma_{\mathbf{d}}^2 \left(\sum_{k=1}^{K} \mu_k \mathbf{v}_k \mathbf{v}_k^T \right) H = 0 \tag{8.110}$$

Thus, the optimal H must satisfy the following equation:

$$HR_{\mathbf{x}} + \sigma_{\mathbf{d}}^2 (U \Lambda_\mu U^T) H - R_{\mathbf{x}} = 0 \tag{8.111}$$

where $\Lambda_\mu = \text{diag}(\mu_1, \ldots, \mu_K)$ is a diagonal matrix of Lagrange multipliers. To further simplify Equation 8.111, we use the eigen-decomposition of $R_{\mathbf{x}}$:

$$HU\Lambda_{\mathbf{x}}U^T + \sigma_{\mathbf{d}}^2 (U \Lambda_\mu U^T) H - U\Lambda_{\mathbf{x}}U^T = 0 \tag{8.112}$$

After post- and premultiplying the preceding equation with U and U^T, respectively, we get

$$(I - Q)\Lambda_{\mathbf{x}} - \sigma_{\mathbf{d}}^2 \Lambda_\mu Q = 0 \tag{8.113}$$

where $Q \triangleq U^T HU$. There is no straightforward way to explicitly solve for H in Equation 8.113, but if we make the assumption that the matrix Q is diagonal, then the estimation matrix H will have the same form as the time-domain estimator (Equation 8.105), that is,

$$H = UQU^T \tag{8.114}$$

where Q is the gain matrix. Assuming that the gain matrix Q is diagonal, then from Equation 8.113 we can solve for the kth diagonal element, q_{kk}, of Q:

$$q_{kk} = \begin{cases} \dfrac{\lambda_x(k)}{\lambda_x(k) + \sigma_d^2 \mu_k} & k = 1, 2, \ldots, M \\ 0 & k = M+1, \ldots, K \end{cases} \tag{8.115}$$

Note that the preceding expression for the gains q_{kk} is similar to that used in the time-domain-constrained estimator, with the exception of the presence of the Lagrange multipliers. In Equation 8.106 one Lagrange multiplier was used for all k, whereas in Equation 8.115 a different multiplier is used for each k.

The fact that the Lagrange multipliers μ_k were frequency specific is not surprising given the spectral constraints α_k imposed in Equation 8.108. In principle, one can choose μ_k to achieve the desired spectral constraints (α_k) and shape accordingly the spectrum of the residual noise. Such an approach was proposed in [32]. A different approach was taken in [11] by finding the relationship between the gains q_{kk} and the spectral constraints α_k.

For a diagonal Q and H of the form given in Equation 8.114, we can use Equation 8.97 to compute the energy of the kth spectral component of the residual noise as

$$\begin{aligned} E\left\{| u_k^T \varepsilon_d |^2\right\} &= E\left\{| u_k^T H_{opt} u |^2\right\} \\ &= E\left\{\mathrm{tr}\left[u_k^T H_{opt} \mathbf{d} \cdot \mathbf{d}^T H_{opt}^T u_k\right]\right\} \\ &= \mathrm{tr}\left[u_k^T H_{opt} E\{\mathbf{d} \cdot \mathbf{d}^T\} H_{opt}^T u_k\right] \\ &= \mathrm{tr}\left[\sigma_d^2 u_k^T (UQU^T)(UQU^T)^T u_k\right] \\ &= \sigma_d^2 \mathbf{e}_k^T Q Q^T \mathbf{e}_k \\ &= \begin{cases} \sigma_d^2 q_{kk}^2 & k = 1, 2, \ldots, M \\ 0 & k = M+1, \ldots, K \end{cases} \end{aligned} \tag{8.116}$$

where $\mathbf{e}_k^T = [0, 0, \ldots, 1, 0, \ldots, 0]$ is the unit vector with the kth element set to one. Assuming equality in the spectral constraints in Equation 8.108, we get $\sigma_d^2 q_{kk}^2 = \alpha_k \sigma_d^2$, and therefore

$$q_{kk} = (\alpha_k)^{1/2} \quad k = 1, 2, \ldots, M \tag{8.117}$$

The preceding equation provides the relationship between the spectral constraints α_k and the gains of the estimator q_{kk}. Knowledge of α_k specifies the gains of the estimator. Two choices for α_k were suggested in [11]. The first choice for α_k was

$$\alpha_k = \left(\frac{\lambda_x(k)}{\lambda_x(k) + \sigma_d^2} \right)^{\gamma} \tag{8.118}$$

where $\gamma \geq 1$ is an experimentally determined constant that controls the suppression level of the noise, similar to the exponent in the parametric Wiener filter equation (Equation 6.51). This choice makes the spectrum of the residual noise resemble that of the clean signal and therefore could have potential masking effects. The second choice for α_k was

$$\alpha_k = \exp\left\{ -\frac{\nu \sigma_d^2}{\lambda_x(k)} \right\} \tag{8.119}$$

where $\nu \geq 1$ is an experimentally determined constant that controls the suppression level of the noise. This choice of α_k was found to provide more aggressive noise suppression than that in Equation 8.118. Large values of ν provide more suppression than small values ν. The value of $\nu = 5$ was found to work well [11]. A different method for choosing the spectral constraints based on a psychoacoustic model will be presented in Section 8.9.2.

The preceding choice of α_k (Equation 8.119) is similar to the Wiener-type function given in Equation 8.118. To see that, consider the Taylor approximation of $\exp(\sigma^2/\lambda_x(k))$ or equivalently $\exp(1/\xi_k)$, where $\xi_k \triangleq \lambda_x(k)/\sigma_d^2$. Observe that

$$\exp\left(\frac{1}{\xi_k} \right) \approx 1 + \frac{1}{\xi_k} = \frac{1 + \xi_k}{\xi_k} \quad \xi_k \gg 1 \tag{8.120}$$

and therefore the gain function in Equation 8.119 is given by

$$\exp\left(-\frac{1}{\xi_k} \right) \approx \frac{\xi_k}{1 + \xi_k} \quad \xi_k \gg 1 \tag{8.121}$$

which is the Wiener function. Figure 8.12 plots the function $\exp(-1/\xi_k)$ along with the Wiener function. As shown in Figure 8.12, the preceding approximation holds only for large values of ξ_k, particularly for $\xi_k > 10\,\text{dB}$. The shape of the function $\exp(-1/\xi_k)$ is very similar to the shape of the Wiener function, and for this reason this function was termed the *generalized Wiener* function [11]. By considering the parametric function $\exp(-\nu/\xi_k)$ we can control the steepness of the function by changing

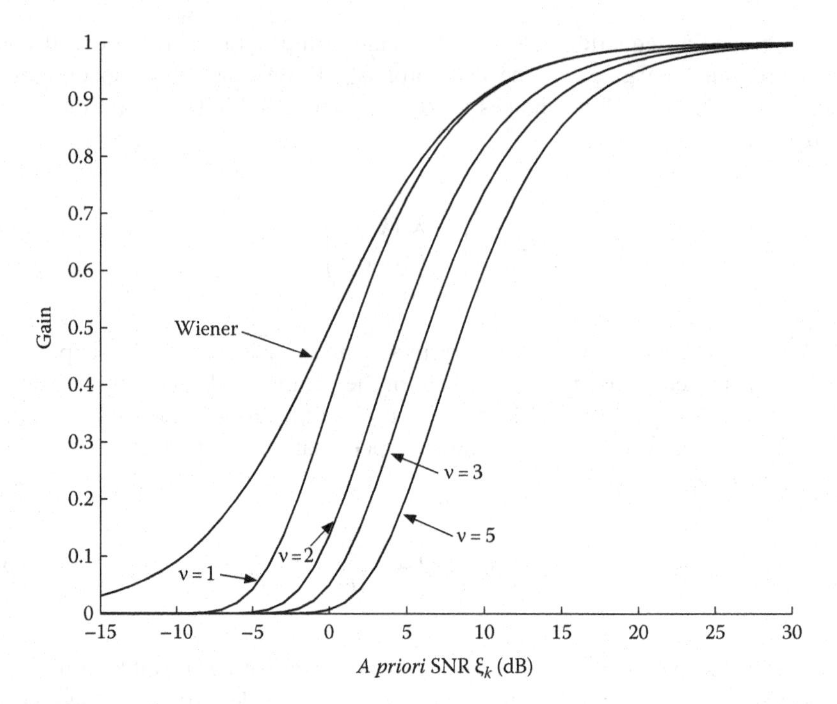

FIGURE 8.12 Generalized Wiener suppression function as a function of *a priori* SNR ξ_k and for different values of the parameter ν.

the value of ν, with large values of ν producing a steep function and small values ν producing a shallow function, similar to the Wiener function. Figure 8.12 plots the function $\exp(-\nu/\xi_k)$ for several values of ν.

To summarize, the desired estimator H that incorporates spectral constraints has the general form

$$H = UQU^T$$
$$Q = \text{diag}(q_{11}, \ldots, q_{KK}) \tag{8.122}$$
$$q_{kk} = \begin{cases} \alpha_k^{1/2}, & k = 1, \ldots, M \\ 0, & k = M+1, \ldots, K \end{cases}$$

where α_k is given by either Equation 8.118 or Equation 8.119.

Note that both time-domain- and spectral-domain-constrained estimators have the same form:

$$\begin{aligned} H &= UGU^T \\ &= U_1 G_1 U_1^T \end{aligned} \tag{8.123}$$

where

U_1 is the $K \times M$ submatrix containing the M principal eigenvectors

G_1 is an $M \times M$ diagonal matrix containing the individual gains (e.g., Equation 8.106 or Equation 8.119)

Note that the least-squares (Equation 8.77) and Wiener estimators (Equation 8.94) are special cases of the preceding estimators. The enhanced signal is obtained by

$$\hat{\mathbf{x}} = H\mathbf{y} = U_1 G_1 U_1^T \mathbf{y} \tag{8.124}$$

that is, it is obtained by first applying the KLT to the noisy speech ($U_1^T \mathbf{y}$), modifying the transformed vector by G_1, and then computing the inverse KLT $\left(U_1 \left\{G_1 U_1^T \mathbf{y}\right\}\right)$ of the transformed components.

It is interesting to note that the popular spectral subtraction approach—that half-wave rectifies the negative components—is of the form described in Equation 8.124. To see that, let F denote the $K \times K$ DFT matrix. Suppose we partition F as $F = [\underbrace{F_1}_{M} \quad \underbrace{F_2}_{K-M}]$ in a way such that the $M < K$ components of F^Hy have variance larger than the variance of the corresponding components of F^Hd; that is, the power of the M spectral components of the noisy speech is larger than the power of the corresponding noise spectral components. Then, the enhanced signal obtained by spectral subtraction is given by

$$\hat{\mathbf{x}}_{ss} = F_1 G_{ss} F_1^H \mathbf{y} \tag{8.125}$$

where G_{ss} is a diagonal ($M \times M$) matrix with the kth diagonal element given by

$$g_{ss}(k) = \frac{p_y(k) - p_d(k)}{p_y(k)} \tag{8.126}$$

where $p_y(k) \triangleq E\left\{| F^H \mathbf{y} |\right\}_k$ and $p_d(k) \triangleq E\left\{| F^H \mathbf{d} |\right\}_k$ denote the power spectral densities of the noisy speech and noise, respectively, evaluated at the kth frequency bins. So, whereas the spectral subtraction approach uses the DFT to decompose the vector space of the noisy signal, the subspace approach uses the KLT. Note that the DFT is not signal dependent and is thus computationally more efficient, whereas the KLT is signal dependent, that is, the eigenvectors (basis) need to be recomputed for each incoming frame of speech. The DFT and KLT are the same, however, when the covariance matrix is circulant [33]. Hence, asymptotically (as $K \to \infty$), the power spectral subtraction becomes optimal in the mean-square sense, and the two methods (spectral subtraction and subspace) are the same [11].

The subspace algorithms presented so far can be described by the following steps. For each frame of speech, do as follows:

Step 1: Estimate the covariance matrix R_y of the noisy speech vector **y**. Estimate the noise variance σ_d^2 using data from speech pauses or speech-absent segments of speech.

Step 2: Perform the eigen-decomposition of $R_y = U\Lambda_y U^T$, where Λ_y is the diagonal matrix $\Lambda_y = \text{diag}(\lambda_y(1), \lambda_y(1), \ldots, \lambda_y(K))$ containing the eigenvalues sorted in decreasing order.

Step 3: Estimate the dimension M of the signal subspace.

Step 4: Estimate the eigenvalues of the clean signal using

$$\lambda_{\hat{x}}(k) = \lambda_y(k) - \sigma_d^2 \quad k = 1, 2, \ldots, M$$

Step 5: Using the estimated eigenvalues $\lambda_{\hat{x}}(k)$, construct the linear estimator based on either Equation 8.107 or Equation 8.122.

Step 6: Obtain the enhanced signal vector by $\hat{\mathbf{x}} = H\mathbf{y}$.

The estimators given in [11] were evaluated and compared with the spectral subtraction approach using subjective listening tests. The estimators were applied to frames of $K = 40$ samples (sampled at 8 kHz) of speech with 50% overlap between frames. A rectangular window was used in the analysis, and a Hamming window was used in the overlap-and-add procedure. Subjective tests indicated better quality with the subspace estimators than the spectral subtraction approach, with no notable musical noise.

Note that the preceding algorithm assumes knowledge of the dimension M of the signal subspace, as well as access to the covariance matrix of the noisy speech vector. The Lagrange multiplier is assumed to be fixed but can also be estimated and updated in each frame. In the next section, we describe implementation details regarding the covariance estimation, determination of the signal subspace dimension, and computation of the Lagrange multiplier.

8.6.3 Implementation

8.6.3.1 Covariance Estimation

The subspace methods require exact knowledge of the second-order statistics (i.e., covariance) of the noisy speech and noise signals. In practice, we do not have access to this information and need to estimate the covariance matrices using finite, and limited, amounts of data. There are several methods for obtaining estimates of the covariance matrix of the speech signal. Next, we describe four of those methods reported in the literature [11,34,35].

The first method obtains an estimate of the noisy speech signal covariance matrix, denoted by $\hat{R}_y$, by computing the empirical covariance of $2L + 1$ neighboring frames of the noisy speech vector using outer products. Speech data from L past and L future frames are used in the computation. Let

$$\mathbf{y}_n = [y(n), y(n+1), \ldots, y(n+K-1)]^T \tag{8.127}$$

denote a $K \times 1$ vector of the noisy signal. Then, $\hat{R}_y$ can be obtained as follows:

$$\hat{R}_y = \frac{1}{2LK} \sum_{t=n-LK+1}^{n+LK} \mathbf{y}_t \mathbf{y}_t^T \tag{8.128}$$

Similarly, the estimate of the noise covariance matrix, $\hat{R}_d$, can be obtained using segments of the noisy signal that do not contain any speech. Assuming that the signal and noise are stationary and ergodic, it can be shown [36] that the estimated covariance matrices will asymptotically ($L \rightarrow \infty$) converge to the true covariance matrices. The covariance estimate $\hat{R}_y$ of Equation 8.128 has several important properties: (a) it is symmetric, (b) it is nonnegative definite, and (c) it has real and nonnegative eigenvalues [37, p. 396]. The matrix $\hat{R}_y$ in Equation 8.128, however, does not have a Toeplitz structure, a structure that is more suitable for speech analysis and that is easily invertible.

The second method computes an empirical Toeplitz covariance matrix $\hat{R}_y$ based on the first K biased autocorrelation estimates. The autocorrelation estimation is based on $2LK$ samples of the signal extracted from L past and L future frames. Following the estimation of K biased autocorrelations, denoted as $\{\hat{r}_y(0), \hat{r}_y(1), \ldots, \hat{r}_y(K-1)\}$, it is straightforward to construct the Toeplitz covariance matrix $\hat{R}_y$. Best results were obtained in [11] using $L = 5$ and $K = 40$ (samples) for signals sampled at 8 kHz. This is equivalent to using a total of 400 samples (50 ms) of the noisy signal to estimate the covariance matrix.

The third method [35,38] computes the covariance matrix based on a relatively larger frame length K, which is divided into smaller P-dimensional frames with 50% overlap. The frame length is chosen to be a multiple of P, yielding a total of $2K/P - 1$ vectors in one frame. The samples in the K-dimensional frame are used to construct a $P \times P$ Toeplitz covariance matrix. The noisy data in each P-dimensional subframe are enhanced using the same eigenvector matrix derived from the $P \times P$ Toeplitz covariance matrix and the same estimation matrix H. The output vectors in each subframe are windowed by a P-length Hamming window and synthesized using the overlap-and-add method. Finally, each frame is windowed by a second K-length Hamming window and the enhanced signal is reconstructed using the overlap-and-add method. The preceding covariance computation scheme yields computational savings as the EVD needs to be computed once in every frame and not for every subframe. The computational savings are proportional to K/P. In [35], $K = 256$ (32 ms) and $P = 32$ (4 ms) samples, reducing the computation of EVD by a factor of 8.

The fourth method computes the covariance matrix based on multiwindowed data [34,39]. That is, rather than using a single rectangular window to window the data in Equation 8.127, it uses multiple windows specially designed to maximize the spectral concentration in the mainlobe relative to the total energy of the window. Such windows, known as the Slepian or discrete prolate spheroidal sequences, were employed in multitaper spectral estimation [40,41]. To obtain the $K \times K$ multiwindow covariance matrix $\hat{R}_y$ from an N-dimensional ($K < N$) noisy data vector $\mathbf{y} = [y(1), y(2), \ldots, y(N)]$, we first form a $K \times (N - K + 1)$ Hankel matrix S as follows:

$$S = \begin{bmatrix} y(1) & y(2) & \cdots & y(N-K+1) \\ y(2) & y(3) & \cdots & y(N-K+2) \\ \vdots & \vdots & \ddots & \vdots \\ y(K) & y(K+1) & \cdots & y(N) \end{bmatrix} \tag{8.129}$$

Let $S = [\mathbf{s}_1, \mathbf{s}_2, \ldots, \mathbf{s}_{N-K+1}]$, where $\mathbf{s}_j$ denotes the jth column of S. Then, for each column $\mathbf{s}_j$, compute the multiwindow covariance matrix R_j as

$$R_j = \sum_{i=1}^{N_c} (E_i \cdot \mathbf{s}_j)(E_i \cdot \mathbf{s}_j)^T \quad j = 1, 2, \ldots, N-K+1 \tag{8.130}$$

where $E_i = \text{diag}(\mathbf{p}_i)$ is a diagonal matrix having in its diagonal the ith discrete prolate spheroidal sequence $\mathbf{p}_i$, and N_c is the number of prolate sequences used ($N_c = 4$ was used in [34]). The prolate sequences cannot be expressed in closed form, but are rather computed as a solution to an eigenvalue problem [41]. The final covariance estimate $\hat{R}_y$ is obtained as follows:

$$\hat{R}_y = \frac{1}{N-K+1} \sum_{j=1}^{N-K+1} R_j \tag{8.131}$$

The multiwindow estimates of the covariance matrix were shown in [39] to be superior to the conventional (single-window) covariance estimators in terms of yielding lower mean-square error.

8.6.3.2 Estimating the Lagrange Multiplier

The derived gain matrix (Equation 8.106) for the time-domain-constrained estimator was a function of the Lagrange multiplier, μ. Unfortunately, we cannot explicitly solve for μ due to the nonlinearity of the equations. Instead, we can either fix μ to a small value or find a way to adaptively estimate it in each frame. As noted in [42,43], the choice of the Lagrange multiplier, μ, can affect the quality of the enhanced speech, and in particular, it can affect the amount of noise distortion introduced. To see that, after substituting the optimal H (Equation 8.105) in Equation 8.97, we obtain the following expression for the energy of the residual noise:

$$\begin{aligned}
\overline{\varepsilon_d^2} &= \text{tr}\left(E\left[\varepsilon_d \varepsilon_d^T\right]\right) = \sigma_d^2 \,\text{tr}\{HH^T\} \\
&= \sigma_d^2 \,\text{tr}\left\{\Lambda_x^2 \left(\Lambda_x + \mu\sigma_d^2 I\right)^{-2}\right\} \\
&= \sigma_d^2 \sum_{k=1}^{K} \frac{\lambda_x^2(k)}{(\lambda_x(k) + \mu\sigma_d^2)^2}
\end{aligned} \tag{8.132}$$

Hence, the noise distortion is inversely proportional to the value of μ, with large values of μ producing smaller noise distortion (see example in Figure 8.11). Small values of μ yield distortion comparable to the noise variance (e.g., if $\mu = 0$, we get $\overline{\varepsilon_d^2} = K\sigma_d^2$). It seems then that a large value of μ would be more desirable. However, analysis of the signal distortion, similar to that done in Equation 8.132, shows that the signal distortion is directly proportional to the value of μ.

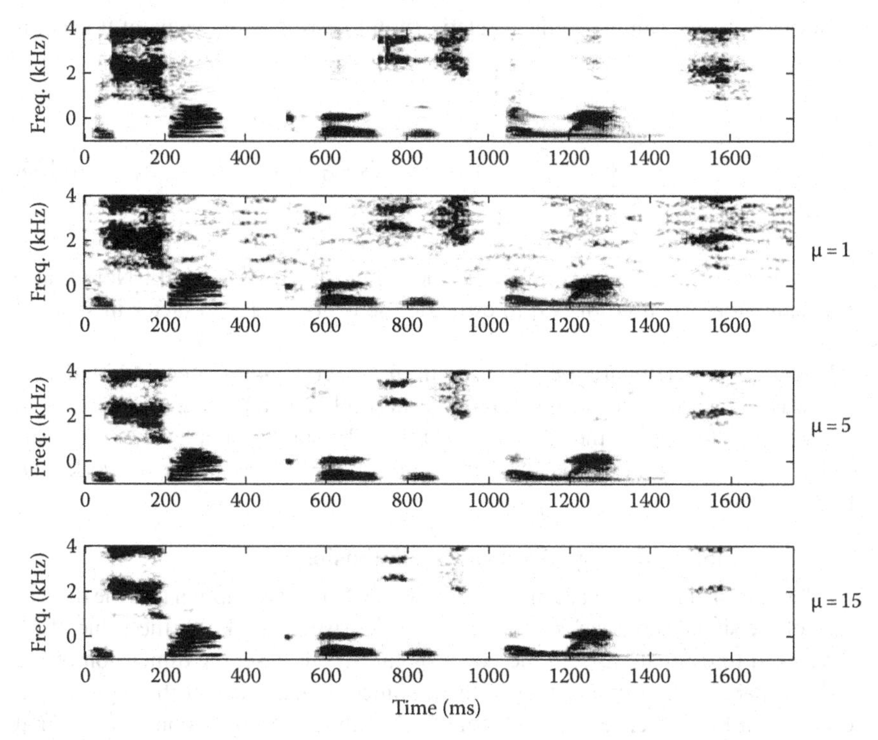

FIGURE 8.13 Spectrograms of a sentence enhanced by the TDC subspace estimator using different values of μ. Top panel shows for comparison the spectrogram of the sentence in quiet.

Therefore, the choice of μ controls the trade-off between signal and noise distortion. The value of μ needs to be chosen carefully. Figure 8.13 shows spectrograms of speech signals enhanced by the TDC estimator using $\mu = 1$, 5, and 15. The sentence was corrupted by white noise at +5 dB S/N. It is clear that the residual noise reduces significantly as the value of μ increases. However, as shown in the lower panels some portions of the spectrum are severely attenuated.

In [11], the value of μ was fixed at $\mu = 2$ and was found to work well experimentally. Methods for adjusting the value of μ were suggested in [42,44], based on the value of the *a posteriori* SNR. The proposed methods were motivated by the fact that ideally, we would like to minimize the speech distortion in speech-dominated frames as the speech signal will have a masking effect on noise. Similarly, we would like to reduce the residual noise in noise-dominated frames. To accomplish that, we can make the value of μ dependent on the short-time SNR as follows [44]:

$$\mu = 1 + \frac{1}{1 + \text{SNR}} \tag{8.133}$$

where SNR is the estimate of the *a posteriori* SNR. In Equation 8.133, μ is restricted to values in the range of $1 \le \mu \le 2$.

Alternatively, we can use a linear relationship to estimate the value of μ according to [42]:

$$\mu = \begin{cases} \mu_0 - (\text{SNR}_{dB})/s & -5 < \text{SNR}_{dB} < 20 \\ 1 & \text{SNR}_{dB} \geq 20 \\ 5 & \text{SNR}_{dB} \leq -5 \end{cases} \tag{8.134}$$

where $\mu_0 = 4.2$, $s = 6.25$, and SNR_{dB} is the *a posteriori* SNR in dB. Note that a similar equation was used in [45] to estimate the oversubtraction factor in spectral subtraction.

The gain matrix (Equation 8.119) used in the spectral-domain-constrained estimator was not dependent on the Lagrange multiplier μ but on the parameter ν. Similar to the effect of μ, the value of ν controls the suppression level of the noise and the resulting signal distortion. The value of $\nu = 5$ was found to work well in [11].

8.6.3.3 Estimating the Signal Subspace Dimension

In the derivation of the subspace algorithms, we made the assumption that the dimension M of the signal subspace is known. In practice, we do not know the value of M, and we need to estimate it from the noisy signal. In our case, the dimension of the signal subspace is the same as that of the assumed model order of the input signal (see Equation 8.72). Hence, the problem of estimating the dimension of the signal subspace is equivalent to estimating the order of the linear model in Equation 8.72. Fortunately, there is a vast literature on model order selection rules that we can use, as this is a problem frequently encountered in most parametric-based signal estimation techniques [46–50]. Order selection rules, for instance, based on maximum-likelihood principles have been found to work well, particularly in situations where we need to detect the number of sinusoidal components in a sinusoids-plus-noise signal [50].

Two different estimators of the signal subspace dimension have been investigated for subspace algorithms in speech enhancement. The first was based on the approach proposed by Merhav [49] and adapted for subspace algorithms in [11]. The second was based on minimum description length (MDL) concepts and was adapted for subspace algorithms in [10,51].

The approach by Merhav [49] was found to be particularly attractive as it guarantees minimization of the probability of underestimating the true order while maintaining an exponentially decaying probability of overestimation of the true order. For the derivation of the optimal order-selection rule, it is necessary to make the assumption that the additive noise is zero mean, Gaussian, and with unknown variance σ_d^2. The dimension of the signal subspace is selected according to [11]

$$M^* = \arg\min_{1 \leq m \leq M_u} \left\{ \frac{1}{2} \log \bar{\sigma}(m) - \frac{1}{2} \log \bar{\sigma}(M_u) < \delta \right\} - 1 \tag{8.135}$$

where the threshold δ controls the exponential rate of decay of the probability of overestimation of the true order, M_u denotes the maximum possible dimension of the signal subspace, and $\bar{\sigma}(m)$ is given by

$$\bar{\sigma}(m) = \frac{1}{K}\left\| U_m U_m^T \mathbf{y} \right\|^2 \tag{8.136}$$

where $U_m \triangleq [u_{m+1}, u_{m+2}, \ldots, u_K]$ is the $K \times (K - m)$ matrix of the eigenvectors of R_y. Note that $\bar{\sigma}(m)$ in the preceding equation computes the energy of the projected noisy vector onto the noise subspace, and as m increases (approaching K), this energy decreases. If $m = M$ in Equation 8.136, where M is the true dimension of the signal subspace, then $\bar{\sigma}(M) = \sigma_d^2$, where σ_d^2 is the noise variance.

The value of M_u is computed, according to Equation 8.71, as the number of eigenvalues of R_y that exceed the estimated noise variance, denoted as $\hat{\sigma}_d^2$. Mathematically, M_u is computed according to

$$M_u = \arg\max_{1 \le k \le K} \{\lambda_y(k) - \hat{\sigma}_d^2 > 0\} \tag{8.137}$$

where $\lambda_y(k)$ are the eigenvalues of R_y assumed to be sorted in descending order. The preceding selection rule can be used as an alternative, and simpler, rule in place of Equation 8.135. Figure 8.14 shows as an example of the estimated signal subspace dimension using Equation 8.137 for a sentence embedded in +5 dB S/N white noise (F_s = 8 kHz). Eigenvalue decomposition was performed on 40 × 40 Toeplitz covariance matrices formed using 5 ms frames of speech vectors. The estimated subspace dimension M, according to Equation 8.137, ranged from a low of 15 to a maximum of 40 for this example.

Examining Equation 8.135, we see that the optimal M^* is chosen as the smallest value of m for which the energy of the projected noisy signal in the noise subspace is close (up to δ, which in [11] was set to $\delta = 0.0025 \log \bar{\sigma}(M_u)$) to the lowest possible energy of the noisy signal in the noise subspace, which is $\bar{\sigma}(M_u)$. The preceding selection rule is based on energy differences of synthesized (projected) signals, and in this respect it is similar to the parsimonious order selection rule (see Equation 8.52) used in the SVD approach.

The MDL-based approach [47] for selecting the model order was investigated in [10,51]. Experiments in [51] indicated that the MDL estimator produced consistently lower model-order estimates compared to the Merhav's estimates obtained using Equation 8.135. Because of the low model-order estimates, the MDL estimator tended to produce distorted speech. The quality of speech produced by the Merhav estimator (Equation 8.135) and the estimator based on counting the number of positive eigenvalues (Equation 8.137) were comparable [51].

An important question regarding the estimation of the subspace dimension M is whether performance is affected by overestimation errors or underestimation

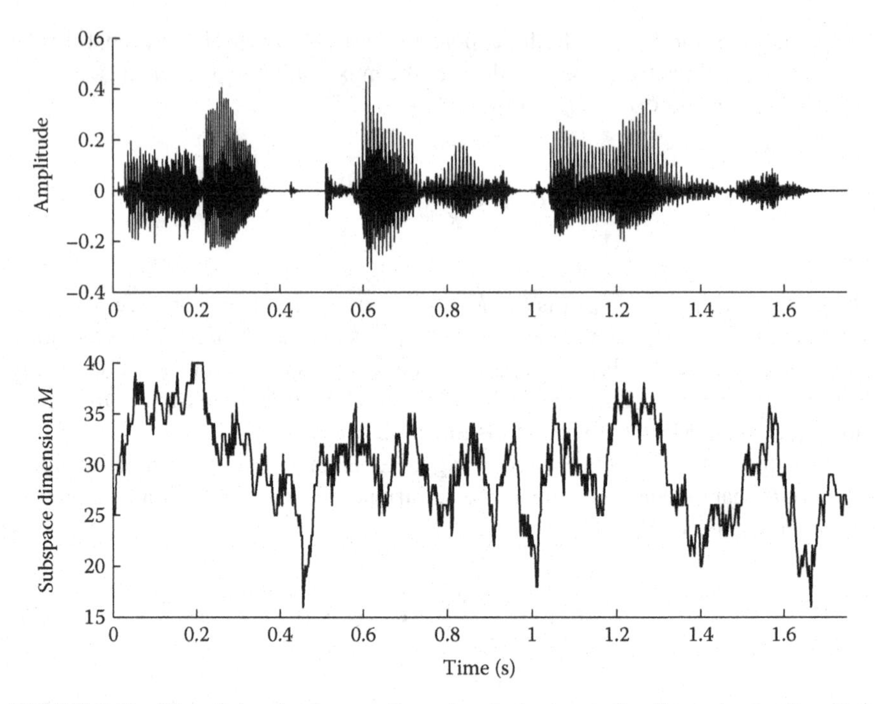

FIGURE 8.14 Plot of signal subspace dimension (bottom panel) estimated using Equation 8.137 for a sentence embedded in white noise at +5 dB S/N. The signal dimension estimation was based on the eigenvalue decomposition of a Toeplitz covariance matrix (40 × 40). The sentence in quiet is shown in the top panel.

errors and the degree at which it is affected. Figure 8.15 gives an example that demonstrates the effect of underestimating and overestimating the signal subspace dimension M. The same signal as in Figure 8.9 is used. Rather than computing the value of M using, for instance, Equation 8.137, we now fix M at a certain value varying from 5 to 40. The TDC subspace estimator given in Equation 8.106 is used with $\mu = 5$. As before, we quantify and report the reconstruction error between the clean and enhanced signals. The reconstruction SNR for M = 5, 10, 20, 30, and 40 is 11.6, 14.5, 14.1, 14.0, and 14.0 dB, respectively. The true signal dimension is roughly 10 according to Figure 8.10. Based on that, this example clearly illustrates that performance is not markedly affected when the signal dimension is overestimated (i.e., when $M > 10$) but when it is underestimated (i.e., when $M < 10$) when the TDC subspace estimator is used. This is not the case, however, when the least-squares subspace estimator is used. The example in Figure 8.9 based on the least-squares subspace estimator (Equation 8.77) demonstrated that performance degraded significantly when the signal subspace dimension was overestimated. Thus, from the examples in Figures 8.9 and 8.15 we can conclude that the TDC subspace estimator is robust to signal dimension overestimation errors, whereas the least-squares estimator is sensitive to model overestimation errors. Hence, the effect of subspace dimension overestimation or underestimation errors depends largely on the subspace estimator used.

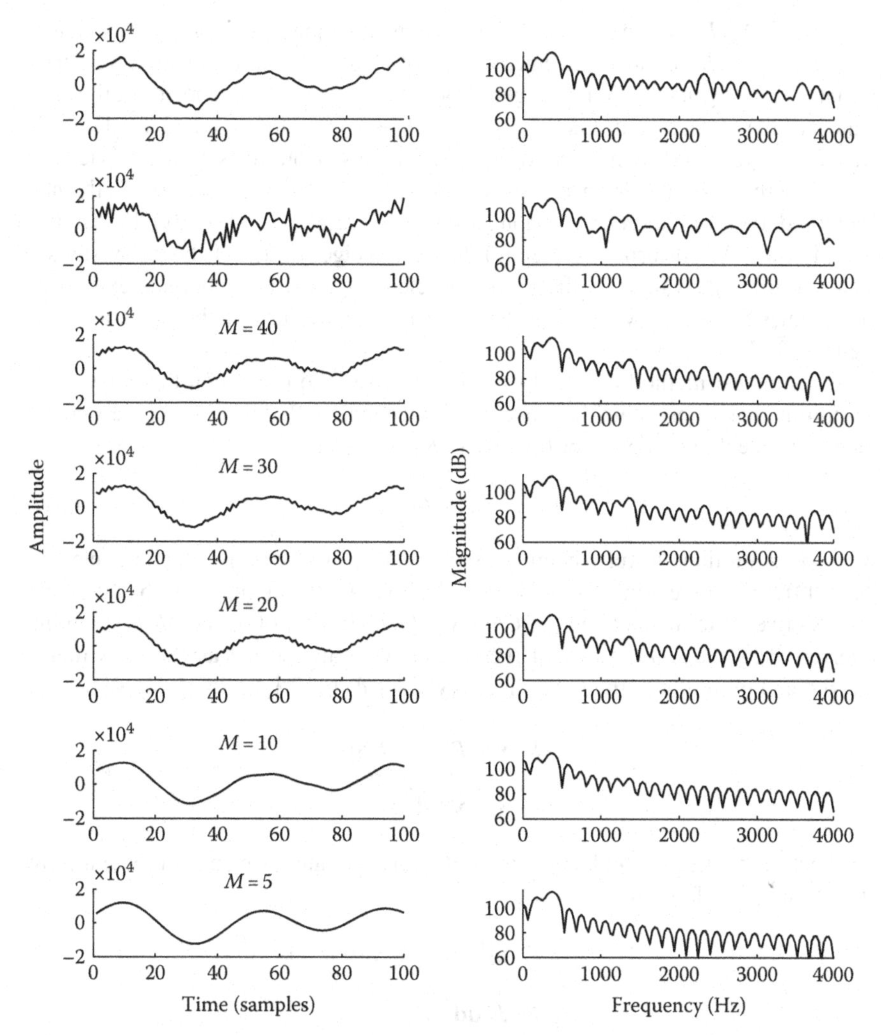

FIGURE 8.15 Synthesis of a noisy segment of speech as a function of signal subspace dimension. Left panels show the amplitude waveforms and right panels show the corresponding Fourier magnitude spectra. First top row shows the clean waveform and magnitude spectra, and the second top row shows the noisy waveform and magnitude spectra.

8.7 EVD-BASED METHODS: COLORED NOISE

Next, we turn our attention to the various subspace methods proposed for handling colored noise.

8.7.1 PREWHITENING APPROACH

One of the main assumptions made in the previous section was that the noise covariance matrix was diagonal of the form $R_d = \sigma_d^2 I$ or, equivalently, that the input noise was white. As R_d was assumed to be diagonal, we made use of the fact that the eigenvectors of R_y are also the eigenvectors of R_x and R_d. Consequently, we derived Equation 8.70, which related the eigenvalues of the noisy signal in terms of the eigenvalues of the clean signal, that is, $\lambda_y(k) = \lambda_x(k) + \lambda_d(k)$. This eigenvalue relationship was the key relationship needed to separate the noise from the signal subspaces.

If now the noise covariance matrix is not diagonal, as is the case when the noise is colored, then Equation 8.69 no longer holds and $\lambda_y(k) \neq \lambda_x(k) + \lambda_d(k)$. In fact, there is no known closed-form expression relating the eigenvalues of the noisy signal in terms of the eigenvalues of the noise and clean signals. Only bounds exist of the eigenvalues of the noisy signal in terms of the eigenvalues of the noise and clean signals [52, Equations 44.9, 48.1].

The simplest method of handling colored noise is to prewhiten the noisy signal. Assuming that we estimate the noise covariance matrix R_d during speech-absent segments of speech, we can factor the matrix R_d $(K \times K)$ as

$$R_d = R^T R \tag{8.138}$$

where R is a unique lower triangular $K \times K$ matrix with positive diagonal elements [8, p. 141]. The preceding factorization of the matrix R_d (assumed to be symmetric and positive definite) is called the *Cholesky factorization* of R_d, and R is sometimes referred to as the *square root* of the matrix. We can use R^{-1} as the prewhitening matrix, and premultiply the noisy signal ($\mathbf{y} = \mathbf{x} + \mathbf{d}$) by R^{-1}. In doing so, we get

$$\begin{aligned} R^{-1}\mathbf{y} &= R^{-1}\mathbf{x} + R^{-1}\mathbf{d} \\ \bar{\mathbf{y}} &= \bar{\mathbf{x}} + \bar{\mathbf{d}} \end{aligned} \tag{8.139}$$

To check if the transformed noise signal $\bar{\mathbf{d}}$ is uncorrelated, we can compute its covariance matrix as follows:

$$\begin{aligned} R_{\bar{d}} &= E[\bar{\mathbf{d}}\bar{\mathbf{d}}^T] = E[R^{-1}\mathbf{d}\mathbf{d}^T R^{-T}] \\ &= R^{-1}E[\mathbf{d}\mathbf{d}^T]R^{-T} \\ &= R^{-1}R_d R^{-T} \\ &= R^{-1}(RR^T)R^{-T} \\ &= I \end{aligned} \tag{8.140}$$

Hence, the transformed noise signal $\bar{\mathbf{d}}$ is indeed uncorrelated with variance $\sigma_{\bar{d}}^2 = 1$. The covariance matrix of the transformed noisy signal $\bar{\mathbf{y}}$ is given by

$$\begin{aligned} R_{\bar{y}} &= E[\bar{\mathbf{y}}\bar{\mathbf{y}}^T] \\ &= R^{-1}R_x R^{-T} + I \\ &= R_{\bar{x}} + I \end{aligned} \tag{8.141}$$

where $R_{\bar{x}} = R^{-1}R_xR^{-T}$. Therefore, the eigenvectors of $R_{\bar{y}}$ will be the same as the eigenvectors of $R_{\bar{x}}$ and I. Assuming that the rank$(R_{\bar{x}}) = M < K$, then the following eigenvalue relationship holds good:

$$\lambda_{\bar{y}}(k) = \begin{cases} \lambda_{\bar{x}}(k)+1 & k = 1,2,\ldots,M \\ 1 & k = M+1,\ldots,K \end{cases} \quad (8.142)$$

from which we can extract the principal eigenvectors of $R_{\bar{y}}$. We can then apply the subspace estimators derived in Section 8.6.2, using now the principal eigenvectors of the transformed covariance matrix $R_{\bar{y}}$.

To summarize, the prewhitening approach for handling colored noise can be implemented using the following steps:

Step 1: Based on speech-absent segments of the signal, estimate the noise covariance matrix $\hat{R}_d$, and factor it as $\hat{R}_d = RR^T$ using the Cholesky factorization.

Step 2: Apply the prewhitening matrix R^{-1} to the noisy signal to get $\bar{\mathbf{y}} = R^{-1}\mathbf{y}$.

Step 3: Compute the eigen-decomposition of the covariance matrix of $\bar{\mathbf{y}}$: $R_{\bar{y}} = U_{\bar{y}}\Lambda_{\bar{y}}U_{\bar{y}}^T$.

Step 4: Estimate the signal subspace dimension, M, using one of the methods described in Section 8.6.3.3, and construct the gain matrix $\bar{G}$ as per Equation 8.106 or Equation 8.119, using the eigenvalues $\lambda_{\bar{x}}(k)$ (Equation 8.142) and $\sigma_{\bar{d}}^2 = 1$.

Step 5: Construct the estimation matrix $\bar{H}$ using the principal eigenvectors of $R_{\bar{y}}$, that is,

$$\bar{H} = \bar{U}_1\bar{G}\bar{U}_1^T \quad (8.143)$$

where $\bar{U}_1$ contains the M principal eigenvectors of $R_{\bar{y}}$. Apply $\bar{H}$ to the transformed noisy signal: $\mathbf{x}_1 = \bar{H}\bar{\mathbf{y}}$.

Step 6: Dewhiten the signal $\mathbf{x}_1$ to get the enhanced signal vector $\hat{\mathbf{x}}$, that is, $\hat{\mathbf{x}} = R\mathbf{x}_1$.

The preceding prewhitening approach (Steps 2 through 6) can be summarized by the following equation:

$$\hat{\mathbf{x}} = R\bar{H}R^{-1}\mathbf{y} \quad (8.144)$$

where

- $\hat{\mathbf{x}}$ is the enhanced signal vector
- $\mathbf{y}$ is the noisy speech vector
- $\bar{H}$ is the estimation matrix (Step 5), which is computed using the principal eigenvectors/eigenvalues of the covariance matrix $R_{\bar{y}}$

The matrix R derived from the Cholesky factorization is not the only matrix that can whiten the noise signal. Let $R_d = U_d\Lambda_dU_d^T$ be the eigen-decomposition of the noise covariance matrix. Then, the transformation $\Lambda_{\bar{d}}^{-1/2}U_{\bar{d}}^{T}$ also whitens the noise signal, as the covariance matrix of the transformed signal $\bar{\mathbf{d}} = \Lambda_{\bar{d}}^{-1/2}U_{\bar{d}}^{T}\mathbf{d}$ is given by

$$
\begin{aligned}
R_{\bar{d}} &= E[\bar{\mathbf{d}}\bar{\mathbf{d}}^T] = E\left[\Lambda_{\bar{d}}^{-1/2}U_{\bar{d}}^{T}\mathbf{d}\mathbf{d}^T U_d \Lambda_{\bar{d}}^{-1/2}\right] \\
&= \Lambda_{\bar{d}}^{-1/2}U_{\bar{d}}^{T}E[\mathbf{d}\mathbf{d}^T]U_d\Lambda_{\bar{d}}^{-1/2} \\
&= \Lambda_{\bar{d}}^{-1/2}\left(U_{\bar{d}}^{T}R_d U_d\right)\Lambda_{\bar{d}}^{-1/2} \\
&= \Lambda_{\bar{d}}^{-1/2}\Lambda_d\Lambda_{\bar{d}}^{-1/2} \\
&= I
\end{aligned}
\tag{8.145}
$$

Hence, either $\Lambda_{\bar{d}}^{-1/2}U_{\bar{d}}^{T}$ or R^{-1} (Equation 8.138) can be used as the prewhitening matrices. Neither of the two prewhitening matrices, however, is orthogonal. Nonorthogonal transformation matrices do not preserve the Euclidean distances, that is,

$$
\|\bar{\mathbf{d}}\|^2 = \bar{\mathbf{d}}^T\bar{\mathbf{d}} = \mathbf{d}^T R^{-T}R^{-1}\mathbf{d} \neq \|\mathbf{d}\|^2 \tag{8.146}
$$

This fact has serious implications for the constrained optimization problem described in Section 8.6.2 for minimizing the signal distortion, subject to the noise distortion falling below a preset threshold. Minimizing the signal distortion of the transformed (prewhitened) signal is not equivalent to minimizing the signal distortion of the original (unmodified) signal. To see that, let

$$
\begin{aligned}
\varepsilon_x &= (H - I)\mathbf{x} \\
\varepsilon_{\bar{x}} &= (\bar{H} - I)\bar{\mathbf{x}}
\end{aligned}
\tag{8.147}
$$

denote the distortions of the original clean signal and modified signals obtained after applying the estimation matrices H and $\bar{H}$, respectively. Making use of the fact that H is related to $\bar{H}$ by $H = R\bar{H}R^{-1}$ (based on Equation 8.144), it is easy to show that the preceding two distortions are related by

$$
\varepsilon_x = R\varepsilon_{\bar{x}} \tag{8.148}
$$

We can express the energy (variance) of the signal distortion as follows:

$$
\begin{aligned}
\varepsilon_x^2 &= E\left[\varepsilon_x^T\varepsilon_x\right] \\
&= \mathrm{tr}\left(E\left[\varepsilon_x\varepsilon_x^T\right]\right) \\
&= \mathrm{tr}\left(RE\left[\varepsilon_{\bar{x}}\varepsilon_{\bar{x}}^T\right]R^T\right)
\end{aligned}
\tag{8.149}
$$

It is important to note here that had R been orthogonal, the energies of the two distortions (due to either H or $\bar{H}$) would have been equal, that is, $\varepsilon_x^2 = \varepsilon_{\bar{x}}^2$. But the prewhitening matrix R is not orthogonal.

Let $R_e R_e^T$ be the Cholesky factorization of the matrix $E\left[\varepsilon_{\bar{x}} \varepsilon_{\bar{x}}^T\right]$, that is, $E\left[\varepsilon_{\bar{x}} \varepsilon_{\bar{x}}^T\right] = R_e R_e^T$. Then, Equation 8.149 can be written as

$$\varepsilon_x^2 = \text{tr}\left(R R_e R_e^T R^T\right) = \| R R_e \|_F^2 \tag{8.150}$$

where $\| \cdot \|_F$ denotes the Frobenius norm of the matrix. Making use of the matrix-norm inequality $\| AB \|_F^2 \leq \| A \|_F^2 \| B \|_F^2$, we can obtain an upper bound on the signal distortion ε_x^2:

$$\begin{aligned} \varepsilon_x^2 &\leq \| R \|_F^2 \| R_e \|_F^2 \\ &= \text{tr}(RR^T)\,\text{tr}\left(E\left[\varepsilon_{\bar{x}} \varepsilon_{\bar{x}}^T\right]\right) \\ &= \text{tr}(R_d)\varepsilon_{\bar{x}}^2 \end{aligned} \tag{8.151}$$

Therefore, the distortion of the signal produced by the estimation matrix H (e.g., Equation 8.107) is always smaller than the distortion of the prewhitened signal produced by the estimation matrix $\bar{H}$ (obtained from the prewhitened signal). Because of this, several have proposed subspace methods for colored noise environments that avoided the use of prewhitening. These methods are described next.

8.7.2 Signal/Noise KLT-Based Method

Generally, in noise we know that the following relationship holds between the covariances of the clean and noise signals:

$$R_y = R_x + R_d \tag{8.152}$$

where the noise covariance matrix R_d is a full (not necessarily diagonal) matrix. Getting an accurate estimate of the eigenvectors of the signal covariance matrix, R_x, is extremely critical for KLT-based subspace methods. The simplest approach is to subtract the noise covariance matrix from the noisy covariance matrix, that is,

$$\hat{R}_x = R_y - \hat{R}_d \tag{8.153}$$

where $\hat{R}_d$ is the estimated noise covariance matrix, and perform the eigen-decomposition of $\hat{R}_x$. There is a problem, however, with this subtractive-based estimate of the signal covariance matrix. Owing to possible inaccuracies in estimating the noise covariance matrix (caused by say the nonstationarity of the noise), it is not guaranteed that we will get a signal covariance matrix $\hat{R}_x$ that is positive definite.

For one, the subtraction in Equation 8.153 might produce negative diagonal elements in $\hat{R}_x$ rendering the matrix nonpositive definite. This is more likely to occur in low-energy or low-SNR segments of speech. A nonpositive definite $\hat{R}_x$ might have negative eigenvalues, which will in turn affect the estimation of the signal subspace dimension, M, and consequently the estimation of the principal eigenvector matrix.

To overcome this, a selective approach was proposed in [53], in which a different eigenvector matrix was used to construct the estimation matrix H, depending on the type of frame detected, speech- or noise-dominated. If a frame was classified as a speech-dominated frame (i.e., a high-energy segment), the eigenvector matrix of the speech signal covariance matrix $\hat{R}_x$ (Equation 8.153) was used to derive the representative eigenvectors of the signal subspace. On the other hand, if a frame was classified as a noise-dominated frame, the eigenvector matrix of the noise signal covariance matrix was used to derive the representative eigenvectors for the subspace. This selective method was called the signal/noise KLT-based approach.

To account for the fact that the noise variances are no longer constant (as noise is colored) but a function of the frequency, a modification was proposed in the spectral constraints in Equation 8.108. Specifically, the following constrained minimization problem was addressed:

$$\min_{H} \overline{\varepsilon_{\mathbf{x}}^2}$$

$$\text{subject to:} \begin{cases} E\{|v_k^T \varepsilon_d|^2\} \le \alpha_k \sigma_d^2(k) & k = 1,2,\ldots,M \\ E\{|v_k^T \varepsilon_d|^2\} = 0 & k = M+1,\ldots,K \end{cases} \tag{8.154}$$

where

$\sigma_{\mathbf{d}}^2(k)$ is the kth diagonal element of $U_{\mathbf{x}}^T R_{\mathbf{d}} U_{\mathbf{x}}$

$U_{\mathbf{x}}$ is the eigenvector matrix of R_x

Note that when the noise is white, the diagonal elements of $U_{\mathbf{x}}^T R_{\mathbf{d}} U_{\mathbf{x}}$ become the eigenvalues of R_d, that is, the noise variances, σ_d^2. Restricting the estimator H to have the form

$$H = U_{\mathbf{x}} Q U_{\mathbf{x}}^T \tag{8.155}$$

where Q is a diagonal matrix with diagonal elements $q_{kk}(k = 1, \ldots, K)$, the following solution was obtained [53]:

$$q_{kk} = \min\left(1, \alpha_k^{1/2}\right) \tag{8.156}$$

which is the same solution obtained in [11]. Depending on whether the current frame was classified as speech-dominated or noise-dominated frame, different constraints (α_k) were used in Equation 8.156.

For speech-dominated frames, the following constraints were used:

$$\alpha_k = \begin{cases} \exp\left(-\dfrac{\nu\sigma_d^2(k)}{\lambda_x(k)}\right) & k = 1,2,\ldots,M \\ 0 & k = M+1,\ldots,K \end{cases} \quad (8.157)$$

where

ν is a predetermined constant

$\sigma_{\mathbf{d}}^2(k)$ is the kth diagonal element of $U_{\hat{\mathbf{x}}}^T \hat{R}_{\mathbf{d}} U_{\hat{\mathbf{x}}}$, where $U_{\hat{\mathbf{x}}}$ is the eigenvector of the estimated signal covariance matrix $\hat{R}_x$ (Equation 8.153)

Note that the preceding equation takes into account the fact that in colored noise the noise variances (i.e., $\sigma_{\mathbf{d}}^2(k)$) are no longer constant, but depend on the frequency. Equations 8.155 through 8.157 fully describe the approach taken for speech-dominated frames.

For noise-dominated frames, an assumption was made that the eigenvectors of the noise covariance matrix would provide a better approximation to the eigenvectors of $R_{\mathbf{x}}$. Therefore, the following estimation matrix H was used:

$$H = U_d Q U_d^T \quad (8.158)$$

where U_d is the eigenvector matrix of the estimated noise covariance matrix $\hat{R}_d$, that is,

$$\hat{R}_d = U_d \Lambda_d U_d^T \quad (8.159)$$

The spectral constraints were chosen according to

$$\alpha_k = \begin{cases} \exp\left(-\dfrac{2\nu\lambda_d(k)}{\lambda_{xd}(k)}\right) & k = 1,2,\ldots,M \\ 0 & k = M+1,\ldots,K \end{cases} \quad (8.160)$$

where

$\lambda_d(k)$ is the kth eigenvalue of the noise covariance matrix $\hat{R}_d$

$\lambda_{xd}(k)$ is an estimate of eigenvalue of the signal covariance matrix R_x and is obtained as the kth diagonal element of the matrix R_{xd} defined as

$$R_{xd} = \beta U_d^T R_y U_d - \Lambda_d \quad (8.161)$$

where

β is a constant

Λ_d is the diagonal eigenvalue matrix of $\hat{R}_d$ (Equation 8.159)

Note that when the noise is white (and $\beta = 1$) the covariance matrices R_x and R_d will share the same eigenvector matrix, and matrix R_{xd} in the preceding equation will be diagonal and contain the eigenvalues of $R_{\hat{x}}$. Equations 8.158 through 8.161 fully describe the approach taken for noise-dominated frames.

The speech frames were classified as speech-dominated frames if the following condition was met:

$$\text{tr}(R_y) > [\max(10^{\text{SNR}/20}, 1) + 0.3]\,\text{tr}(\hat{R}_d) \tag{8.162}$$

where SNR is the input SNR of the signal, assumed to be known *a priori*. A frame that did not meet the preceding condition was classified as a noise-dominated frame. Experiments in [53] indicated that the performance of the preceding signal/noise subspace algorithm was not sensitive to the frame classification approach described earlier as long as the estimated (or assumed) SNR value was within ±5 dB of the true SNR. Informal listening tests showed that the signal/noise subspace approach provided noise masking and exhibited better noise spectrum shaping than the subspace approach proposed in [11].

8.7.3 Adaptive KLT Approach

An adaptive KLT approach for speech enhancement was proposed in [54] to deal with nonstationary colored noise. The proposed method incorporated in the time-domain-constrained estimator (rather than the spectral-domain-constrained estimator, as done in the signal/noise KLT approach [53]) the following key observation: in colored noise environments, the noise variance is not constant but varies with frequency. Hence, they incorporated a frequency-dependent noise variance term in the time-domain-constrained estimator. No eigen-decomposition of covariance matrices was performed, but rather a projection-based subspace-tracking technique [55] was used for updating and estimating the eigenvector matrix adaptively. This technique will be described in more detail in Section 8.10.2.2.

To derive the time-domain-constrained estimator suitable for colored noise, we start from the derived optimal estimator (Equation 8.100):

$$H_{opt} = R_{\mathbf{x}}\left(R_{\mathbf{x}} + \mu R_{\mathbf{d}}\right)^{-1} \tag{8.163}$$

After substituting the eigen-decomposition of $R_{\mathbf{x}} = U_x \Lambda_{\mathbf{x}} U_x^T$ in the preceding equation, we get

$$H_{opt} = U_x \Lambda_{\mathbf{x}}\left(\Lambda_{\mathbf{x}} + \mu U_x^T R_{\mathbf{d}} U_x\right)^{-1} U_x^T \tag{8.164}$$

If we now assume that the matrix $U_x^T R_{\mathbf{d}} U_x$ is approximately diagonal containing the frequency-dependent noise variances $\sigma_d^2(k)$, that is,

$$\begin{aligned}\Lambda_{\mathbf{d}} &\triangleq \text{diag}\left(U_x^T R_d U_x\right)\\ &= \text{diag}\left(U_x^T E[\mathbf{d}\mathbf{d}^T]U_x\right)\\ &= \text{diag}\left(E\left|u_1^T\mathbf{d}\right|^2,\ E\left|u_2^T\mathbf{d}\right|^2,\ldots,E\left|u_K^T\mathbf{d}\right|^2\right)\\ &= \text{diag}\left(\sigma_d^2(1),\ldots,\sigma_d^2(K)\right)\end{aligned} \tag{8.165}$$

we can simplify the preceding estimator to

$$\begin{aligned}H_{opt} &\approx U_x\Lambda_{\mathbf{x}}\left(\Lambda_{\mathbf{x}}+\mu\Lambda_{\mathbf{d}}\right)^{-1}U_x^T\\ &= U_x G U_x^T\end{aligned} \tag{8.166}$$

where G is a diagonal matrix with the kth diagonal element given by

$$g(k)=\begin{cases}\dfrac{\lambda_x(k)}{\lambda_x(k)+\mu\sigma_d^2(k)} & k=1,2,\ldots,M\\ 0 & k=M+1,\ldots,K\end{cases} \tag{8.167}$$

Note that when the noise is white, $\sigma_d^2(k)=\sigma_d^2$ for all k and the preceding estimator reduces to that given in Equation 8.106.

An adaptive method was used in [54] to estimate $\lambda_x(k)$ and $\sigma_d^2(k)$ in Equation 8.167 that did not require the eigen-decomposition of the covariance matrices. The adaptive scheme was based on the observation that the kth diagonal element of $U_x{}^T R_{\mathrm{d}} U_x$ in Equation 8.165 can be written as

$$\sigma_d^2(k)=E\left\{\left|u_k^T\mathbf{d}\right|^2\right\} \tag{8.168}$$

where u_k is the kth eigenvector of the eigenvector matrix U_x. The expected value in the preceding equation can be approximated using the following simple recursive averaging operation:

$$\hat{\sigma}_d^{2(m)}(k)=\beta\hat{\sigma}_d^{2(m-1)}(k)+\left|u_k^T(m)\mathbf{d}(m)\right|^2 \tag{8.169}$$

where

β is a smoothing factor ($0<\beta<1$)
$\hat{\sigma}_d^{2(m)}(k)$ is the estimated noise variance at frame m
$d(m)$ is the estimated noise vector (obtained during speech-absent segments)
$u_k(m)$ is the kth eigenvector of R_y estimated at frame m

The principal eigenvectors $u_k(m)$ can generally be obtained using a subspace-tracking technique (see Section 8.10), and in [54], they used a recursive least-squares algorithm to track the principal eigenvectors $u_k(m)$ of the covariance matrix.

A similar recursive equation, as in Equation 8.169, was used to estimate the noisy signal's eigenvalues, $\lambda_y(k)$:

$$\hat{\lambda}_y^{(m)}(k) = \beta\hat{\lambda}_y^{(m-1)}(k) + \left|u_k^T(m-1)\mathbf{y}_k(m)\right|^2 \quad (8.170)$$

where

$u_k(m-1)$ are the eigenvectors estimated in the previous frame $(m-1)$

$\mathbf{y}_k(m)$ are the vectors generated by the subspace-tracking algorithm [these vectors are initialized at each frame to the noisy speech vector, that is, $\mathbf{y}_1(m) = \mathbf{y}(m)$]

Finally, after using Equations 8.169 and 8.170, we can obtain an estimate of the clean signal eigenvalues $\lambda_x(k)$ as

$$\lambda_{\hat{x}}(k) = \max\left\{\hat{\lambda}_y(k) - \hat{\sigma}_d^2(k), 0\right\} \quad (8.171)$$

To summarize, the adaptive KLT approach is implemented using the following steps. For each speech frame m, do as follows:

Step 1: Use a subspace-tracking algorithm to estimate the principal eigenvectors, $\mathbf{u}_k(m)$, of the noisy speech covariance matrix R_y.

Step 2: Estimate the clean signal eigenvalues $\lambda_x(k)$ using Equation 8.171.

Step 3: Compute the diagonal gain matrix using Equations 8.169 and 8.171.

Step 4: Construct the estimation matrix H, based on the estimated eigenvectors from Step 1 and diagonal matrix from Step 3:

$$\begin{aligned} H &= \left[u_1(m), u_2(m), \ldots, u_K(m)\right] G \left[u_1(m), u_2(m), \ldots, u_K(m)\right]^T \\ &= U_y G U_y^T \end{aligned}$$

Step 5: Apply the estimation matrix H to the noisy speech vector $\mathbf{y}(m)$ to get the enhanced signal vector at frame m: $\hat{\mathbf{x}}(m) = H \cdot \mathbf{y}(m)$.

The preceding steps were only executed if frame m was detected to contain speech, based on a voiced activity detector that utilized the maximum and minimum values of $\hat{\lambda}_y(k)$ in Equation 8.170 to make the speech/silence decision [54]. The noisy speech vector was attenuated by 30 dB if silence was detected. The noise vector $\mathbf{d}(m)$ extracted during silence segments was stored in memory and used in Equation 8.169 to estimate and update the noise variances. In the implementation of the preceding adaptive KLT method, the speech signal was processed in frames of K samples, where $K = 20$ for signals sampled at 8 kHz, and the overlap between frames was set to $(K - 1)$ samples. Listening tests in [54] showed that the majority of the listeners preferred the proposed approach over the approach in [11].

8.7.4 Subspace Approach with Embedded Prewhitening

Next, we describe other subspace methods suitable for colored noise. Unlike the previous methods described in Sections 8.7.1 through 8.7.3, these methods do not require explicit prewhitening of the covariance matrices as the prewhitening is embedded in the method.

8.7.4.1 Time-Domain-Constrained Estimator

In the previous approach, the matrix $U^T R_{\mathbf{d}} U$ was approximated by the diagonal matrix $\Lambda_{\mathbf{d}}$:

$$\Lambda_{\mathbf{d}} = \text{diag}\left(E\left(\left|u_1^T \mathbf{d}\right|^2\right), E\left(\left|u_2^T \mathbf{d}\right|^2\right), \ldots, E\left(\left|u_K^T \mathbf{d}\right|^2\right)\right) \tag{8.172}$$

where

u_k is the kth eigenvector of R_x

d is the noise vector estimated from the speech-absent segments of speech

The preceding approximation yielded the following estimator:

$$H_{opt} \approx U\Delta_{\mathbf{x}}\left(\Delta_{\mathbf{x}} + \mu\Lambda_{\mathbf{d}}\right)^{-1} U^T \tag{8.173}$$

Because of the approximation in Equation 8.165, the preceding estimator was suboptimal. Next, we present an optimal estimator suited for colored noise.

Computer simulations indicated that the matrix $U^T R_{\mathbf{d}} U$ in Equation 8.165 was not diagonal, although in some cases it was nearly diagonal. This was not surprising, as U is the eigenvector matrix of the symmetric matrix R_x and diagonalizes R_x and not R_d. Rather than approximating $U^T R_{\mathbf{d}} U$, we can look for a matrix that would simultaneously diagonalize R_x and R_d. It can be shown that such a matrix exists and can simultaneously diagonalize two matrices in the following way [7, p. 343]:

$$\begin{aligned} V^T R_{\mathbf{x}} V &= \Lambda_\Sigma \\ V^T R_{\mathbf{d}} V &= I \end{aligned} \tag{8.174}$$

where Λ_Σ and V are the eigenvalue matrix and eigenvector matrix, respectively, of $\Sigma = R_{\mathbf{d}}^{-1} R_{\mathbf{x}}$, that is,

$$\Sigma V = V\Lambda_\Sigma \tag{8.175}$$

It can be shown that Λ_Σ is a real matrix [7, p. 344], assuming that R_d is positive definite. Note that the eigenvector matrix V is not orthogonal, and that the rank of the matrix Σ is M rank $(R_x) = M$. Applying the preceding eigen-decomposition of Σ to Equation 8.163, and using Equation 8.174, we can rewrite the optimal linear estimator as [42]

$$H_{opt} = R_{\mathbf{d}} V \Lambda_\Sigma \left(\Lambda_\Sigma + \mu I\right)^{-1} V^T$$

$$= V^{-T} \Lambda_\Sigma \left(\Lambda_\Sigma + \mu I\right)^{-1} V^T \tag{8.176}$$

The enhanced $\hat{\mathbf{x}}$ signal is obtained by applying the transform V^T to the noisy signal, appropriately modifying the components of $V^T\mathbf{y}$ by a gain function, and then taking the inverse transform (V^{-T}) of the modified components. The gain matrix $G = \Lambda_\Sigma(\Lambda_\Sigma + \mu I)^{-1}$ is diagonal, and its kth diagonal element $g(k)$ can be written as

$$g(k) = \begin{cases} \dfrac{\lambda_\Sigma(k)}{\lambda_\Sigma(k) + \mu}, & k = 1, 2, \ldots, M \\ 0, & k = M+1, \ldots, K \end{cases} \tag{8.177}$$

where

$\lambda_\Sigma^{(k)}$ is the kth diagonal element of the eigenvalue matrix Λ_Σ

M is the rank of the matrix Σ and the assumed dimension of the speech signal subspace

Note that in this approach $V^T\mathbf{y}$ is not the KLT of $\mathbf{y}$. However, as we show in the following text, if the noise is white, $V^T\mathbf{y}$ becomes the KLT of $\mathbf{y}$.

Comparing the preceding estimator given in Equation 8.176 with the corresponding linear estimator obtained for white noise in [11], we can see that both estimators have the same form. In fact, the Ephraim and Van Trees' estimator [11] is a special case of the proposed estimator in Equation 8.176. When the noise is white, $R_{\mathbf{d}} = \sigma_{\mathbf{d}}^2 I$ and V becomes the unitary eigenvector matrix (U) of R_x, as $\Sigma = \frac{1}{\sigma_{\mathbf{d}}^2} R_{\mathbf{x}}$, and the diagonal matrix $\Lambda_{\mathbf{x}}$ becomes $\frac{1}{\sigma_{\mathbf{d}}^2}\Lambda_{\mathbf{x}}$, where $\Lambda_{\mathbf{x}}$ is the diagonal eigenvalue matrix of R_x. Therefore, for white noise, Equation 8.176 reduces to

$$H_{opt} = U\Delta_{\mathbf{x}}\left(\Delta_{\mathbf{x}} + \mu\sigma_{\mathbf{d}}^2 I\right)U^T \tag{8.178}$$

which is the Ephraim and Van Trees estimator [11]. The proposed approach is therefore a generalization of the subspace approach developed in [11] and can be used for both white and colored noise. In fact, the proposed approach makes no assumptions about the spectral characteristics of the noise.

For the preceding estimator, we need an estimate of the matrix Σ. Because we have no access to the covariance matrix of the clean speech signal, we can estimate

Σ from the noisy speech signal as follows. Assuming that speech is uncorrelated with noise, we have $R_{\mathbf{y}} = R_{\mathbf{x}} + R_{\mathbf{d}}$ and so

$$\Sigma = R_{\mathbf{d}}^{-1}R_{\mathbf{x}} = R_{\mathbf{d}}^{-1}(R_{\mathbf{y}} - R_{\mathbf{d}}) = R_{\mathbf{d}}^{-1}R_{\mathbf{y}} - I \tag{8.179}$$

8.7.4.2 Spectrum-Domain-Constrained Estimator

The aforementioned approach of simultaneously diagonalizing the signal and noise covariance matrices can also be extended in the spectral domain. Specifically, suppose that the kth spectral component of the residual noise is given by $\mathbf{v}_k^T\varepsilon_d$, where $\mathbf{v}_k$ is now the kth column vector of the eigenvector matrix of $\Sigma = R_{\mathbf{d}}^{-1}R_{\mathbf{x}}$. For $k = 1,\ldots,M$, we require the energy in $\mathbf{v}_k^T\varepsilon_d$ to be smaller than or equal to α_k $(0 < \alpha_k < 1)$, whereas for $k = M + 1,\ldots, K$, we require the energy in $\mathbf{v}_k^T\varepsilon_d$ to be zero, as the signal energy in the noise subspace is zero. Therefore, the estimator H is designed by solving the following constrained minimization problem:

$$\min_H \overline{\varepsilon_{\mathbf{x}}^2}$$

$$\text{subject to:} \begin{cases} E\left\{|\mathbf{v}_k^T\varepsilon_d|^2\right\} \le \alpha_k & k = 1,2,\ldots,M \\ E\left\{|\mathbf{v}_k^T\varepsilon_d|^2\right\} = 0 & k = M+1,\ldots,K \end{cases} \tag{8.180}$$

The optimal estimator can be found using the method of Lagrange multipliers as done in Section 8.6.2. The optimal H satisfies the following matrix equation:

$$HR_{\mathbf{x}} + LHR_{\mathbf{d}} - R_{\mathbf{x}} = 0 \tag{8.181}$$

where $L = \Sigma_k \mu_k \mathbf{v}_k \mathbf{v}_k^T = V\Lambda_\mu V^T$, and $\Lambda_\mu = \text{diag}(\mu_1, \ldots, \mu_K)$ is a diagonal matrix of Lagrangian multipliers. Using Equation 8.174, we can rewrite Equation 8.181 as

$$V^T HV^{-T}\Lambda_\Sigma + V^T LHV^{-T} - \Lambda_\Sigma = 0 \tag{8.182}$$

which can be further reduced to the following equation:

$$Q\Lambda_\Sigma + V^T V\Lambda_\mu Q = \Lambda_\Sigma \tag{8.183}$$

where $Q = V^T HV^{-T}$. Note that for white noise, the preceding equation reduces to the equation given in [11, p. 255], for the spectral-domain estimator. This equation is the well-known Lyapunov equation encountered frequently in control theory. The Lyapunov equation can be solved numerically using the algorithm proposed in [56]. Explicit solutions can be found in [19, p. 414] [57]. After solving for Q in Equation 8.183, we can compute the optimal H by

$$H_{opt} = V^{-T}QV^T \tag{8.184}$$

Depending on the assumptions made about the structure of the matrix Q, we can derive two different estimators [42]. In the first method, we can assume a full matrix Q having no particular structure or symmetry. In that method, we will need to solve the Lyapunov equation (Equation 8.183) for Q and from that derive the optimal estimator using Equation 8.184.

In the second method, we assume that the matrix Q is diagonal and that the matrix $V^T V$ is nearly diagonal. Making those two assumptions simplifies the solution of the Lyapunov equation in Equation 8.183 a great deal. Let $\lambda_\Sigma(k)$ be the kth diagonal element of the matrix Λ_Σ, and let q_{kk} be the kth diagonal element of Q. Then, we can simplify Equation 8.183 as

$$\left(\lambda_\Sigma(k)+\left\|\mathbf{v}_k\right\|^2\cdot\mu_k\right)\cdot q_{kk}=\lambda_\Sigma(k) \tag{8.185}$$

from which we can solve for q_{kk} as follows:

$$q_{kk}=\frac{\lambda_\Sigma(k)}{\lambda_\Sigma(k)+\left\|\mathbf{v}_k\right\|^2\cdot\mu_k}\qquad k=1,2,\ldots,K \tag{8.186}$$

Without loss of generality, we can make the norm of $\mathbf{v}_k$ equal to 1 and rewrite the preceding solution as

$$q_{kk}=\begin{cases}\dfrac{\lambda_\Sigma(k)}{\lambda_\Sigma(k)+\mu_k}, & k=1,2,\ldots,M\\ 0, & k=M+1,\ldots,K\end{cases} \tag{8.187}$$

assuming that the rank$(\Sigma)=M<K$. Comparing the preceding equation with Equation 8.177, we observe that Equation 8.187 can be interpreted as a multiband version of Equation 8.177 in that it uses a different value of μ for each spectral component. Note that Equation 8.187 is similar to the corresponding equation in [11], with the $\|\mathbf{v}_k\|^2$ term in place of the noise variance σ_w^2.

Using the preceding Q and the assumption that $V^T V$ is nearly diagonal, we have

$$E\left\{\left|\mathbf{v}_k^T\varepsilon_{\mathbf{d}}\right|^2\right\}=\begin{cases}q_{kk}^2, & k=1,\ldots,M\\ 0, & k=M+1,\ldots,K\end{cases}$$

If the nonzero constraints of Equation 8.180 are satisfied with equality, then $q_{kk}^2=\alpha_k$, suggesting that

$$q_{kk}=(\alpha_k)^{1/2},\quad k=1,\ldots,M$$

and

$$\mu_k=\begin{cases}\lambda_\Sigma(k)\left[(1/\alpha_k)^{1/2}-1\right], & k=1,\ldots,M\\ 0, & k=M+1,\ldots,K\end{cases}$$

Since $0 < \alpha_k < 1$, we have $\mu_k \geq 0$ and therefore the Kuhn–Tucker necessary conditions [58] for the constrained minimization problem are satisfied by the solution in Equation 8.187. From Equations 8.187 and 8.184, we conclude that the desired H is given by

$$q_{kk} = \begin{cases} \dfrac{\lambda_\Sigma(k)}{\lambda_\Sigma(k)+\mu_k}, & k = 1,2,\ldots,M \\ 0, & k = M+1,\ldots,K \end{cases}$$

$$Q = \mathrm{diag}\left(q_{11}, q_{22}, \ldots, q_{KK}\right) \tag{8.188}$$

$$H = V^{-T} Q V^T$$

Next, we provide the implementation details of the aforementioned two estimators based on time-domain and spectral-domain constraints.

8.7.4.3 Implementation

The aforementioned estimators (Equations 8.177 and 8.188) require knowledge of the Lagrange multipliers (μ_k). As discussed in Section 8.6.3.2, the estimation of μ_k affects the quality of speech as it controls the trade-off between residual noise and speech distortion. A large value of μ_k would eliminate much of the background noise at the expense of introducing speech distortion. Conversely, a small value of μ_k would minimize the speech distortion at the expense of introducing large residual noise. Hence, a compromise between residual noise and speech distortion needs to be made by an appropriate choice of μ_k.

As described in Section 8.6.3.2, we can make the value of μ dependent on the short-time *a posteriori* SNR:

$$\mu = \mu_0 - (\mathrm{SNR}_{dB})/s$$

where μ_0 and s are constants chosen experimentally, and $\mathrm{SNR}_{dB} = 10\log_{10}\mathrm{SNR}$. As the eigenvalues $\lambda_\Sigma(k)$ are equal to the signal energy along the corresponding eigenvector $\mathbf{v}_k$ $\left(\text{i.e., } \lambda_\Sigma(k) = E\left(|\mathbf{v}_k^T\mathbf{x}|^2\right)\right)$, we can compute the SNR value directly in the transform domain using the following equation:

$$\mathrm{SNR} = \frac{\mathrm{tr}\left(V^T R_x V\right)}{\mathrm{tr}\left(V^T R_d V\right)} = \frac{\sum_{k=1}^{M} \lambda_\Sigma(k)}{K} \tag{8.189}$$

Note that the preceding SNR definition reduces to the traditional SNR definition of SNR = $\mathrm{tr}(R_x)/\mathrm{tr}(R_d)$ for an orthonormal matrix V.

Similarly, for the spectral-domain constrained estimator (Equation 8.188), we can let μ_k vary with the estimated SNR value of each spectral component, that is,

$$\mu_k = \mu_0 - (\mathrm{SNR}_k)/s \tag{8.190}$$

where SNR_k is the SNR value of the kth spectral component. The value of SNR_k is simply $\lambda_\Sigma(k)$, since in the transform domain the noise energy along the corresponding eigenvector $\mathbf{v}_k$ is equal to one according to Equation 8.174. The μ_k values can then be computed as

$$\mu_k = \mu_0 - \lambda_\Sigma(k)/s \tag{8.191}$$

where μ_0 and s are constants chosen experimentally.

The subspace method based on time-domain constraints can be implemented using the following six steps. For each speech frame, do as follows:

Step 1: Compute the covariance matrix R_y of the noisy signal, and estimate the matrix $\Sigma = R_{\mathbf{d}}^{-1}R_{\mathbf{y}} - I$ (Equation 8.179). The noise covariance matrix R_d can be computed using noise samples collected during speech-absent frames.

Step 2: Perform the eigen-decomposition of Σ:

$$\Sigma V = V\Lambda_\Sigma$$

Step 3: Assuming that the eigenvalues of Σ are ordered as $\lambda_\Sigma(1) \geq \lambda_\Sigma(2) \geq \ldots \geq \lambda_\Sigma(K)$, estimate the dimension of the speech signal subspace as follows:

$$M = \underset{1\leq k\leq K}{\arg\max}\{\lambda_\Sigma(k) > 0\}$$

Step 4: Compute the μ value according to

$$\mu = \begin{cases} \mu_0 - (\text{SNR}_{dB})/s, & -5 < \text{SNR}_{dB} < 20 \\ 1 & \text{SNR}_{dB} \geq 20 \\ 5 & \text{SNR}_{dB} \leq -5 \end{cases}$$

where $\mu_0 = 4.2$, $s = 6.25$, $\text{SNR}_{dB} = 10\log_{10}\text{SNR}$, and SNR is computed as per Equation 8.189.

Step 5: Compute the optimal linear estimator as follows:

$$g(k) = \begin{cases} \dfrac{\lambda_\Sigma(k)}{\lambda_\Sigma(k)+\mu}, & k = 1,2,\ldots,M \\ 0, & k = M+1,\ldots,K \end{cases} \tag{8.192}$$

$$G_1 = \text{diag}\{g(1),\ldots,g(M)\}$$

$$H_{opt} = R_{\mathbf{d}}V\begin{bmatrix} G_1 & 0 \\ 0 & 0 \end{bmatrix}V^T$$

$$= V^{-T}\begin{bmatrix} G_1 & 0 \\ 0 & 0 \end{bmatrix}V^T$$

Step 6: Obtain the enhanced speech signal by: $\hat{\mathbf{x}} = H_{opt}\cdot\mathbf{y}$.

The subspace method based on spectral-domain constraints (Equation 8.188) is implemented the same way except that in Steps 4 and 5, the Lagrange multiplier μ is replaced by the individual multipliers μ_k, which are estimated as

$$\mu_k = \begin{cases} \mu_0 - \lambda'_k/s, & -5 < \lambda'_k < 20 \\ 1 & \lambda'_k \geq 20 \\ 20 & \lambda'_k \leq -5 \end{cases}$$

where

$\mu_0 = 16.2$
$s = 1.32$
$\lambda'_k = 10\log_{10}\lambda_\Sigma(k)$

The performance of the preceding estimators was evaluated in [42] using objective measures (segmental SNR and Itakura–Saito measures), and compared against the performance of the adaptive KLT method described in the previous section. Recall that the adaptive KLT approach used a suboptimal estimator as it assumed that the matrix $U_x R_d U_x^T$ was approximately diagonal. In contrast, no assumptions were made in the derivation of the preceding estimators. Results indicated large improvements in performance with these estimators compared to the estimator used in the adaptive KLT approach. The performance of the spectral-domain estimator that explicitly solved for the matrix Q in Equation 8.183 was not as good as the performance of the time-domain estimator or the spectral-domain estimator, which assumed that Q was diagonal (Equation 8.188). This finding was surprising given that no assumptions were made regarding Q, and could perhaps be attributed to the choice of μ_k values.

At first glance, the preceding estimators seemed to handle colored noise without the need for prewhitening. Closer analysis, however, revealed that these estimators have built-in prewhitening.

8.7.4.4 Relationship between Subspace Estimators and Prewhitening

The nonorthogonal matrix V used in the previous estimators was derived from simultaneous diagonalization of two symmetric matrices: the signal and noise covariance matrices. We know that joint diagonalization of two matrices involves a prewhitening step, so it is reasonable to presume that the aforementioned time-domain- and spectral-domain-constrained optimal linear estimators can be rewritten to include the prewhitening process.

We start from the optimal time domain constrained estimator given by

$$H_{TDC} = R_\mathbf{x}\left(R_\mathbf{x} + \mu R_\mathbf{d}\right)^{-1} \tag{8.193}$$

Let $R_d = RR^T$ be the Cholesky factorization of R_d (assumed to be positive definite and symmetric). Replacing R_d by its Cholesky factorization, we can rewrite the preceding equation as

$$\begin{aligned} H_{TDC} &= R_{\mathbf{x}}(R_{\mathbf{x}} + \mu R_{\mathbf{d}})^{-1} \\ &= R_{\mathbf{x}}\left(R_{\mathbf{x}} + \mu RR^T\right)^{-1} \\ &= R_{\mathbf{x}}\left(R\left(R^{-1}R_{\mathbf{x}} + \mu R^T\right)\right)^{-1} \\ &= R_x\left(R^{-1}R_{\mathbf{x}} + \mu R^T\right)^{-1}R^{-1} \\ &= R_x\left(\left(R^{-1}R_{\mathbf{x}}R^{-T} + \mu I\right)R^T\right)^{-1}R^{-1} \\ &= R \cdot R^{-1}R_{\mathbf{x}}R^{-T} \cdot \left(R^{-1}R_{\mathbf{x}}R^{-T} + \mu I\right)^{-1} \cdot R^{-1} \end{aligned} \tag{8.194}$$

Now let Ψ and Λ denote, respectively, the eigenvector and eigenvalue matrices of the symmetric matrix, $R^{-1}R_{\mathbf{x}}R^{-T}$, that is,

$$R^{-1}R_{\mathbf{x}}R^{-T} = \Psi\Lambda\Psi^T \tag{8.195}$$

After substituting this decomposition in Equation 8.194, we can rewrite H_{TDC} as

$$\begin{aligned} H_{TDC} &= R\Psi\Lambda(\Lambda + \mu I)^{-1}\Psi^T R^{-1} \\ &= \tilde{V}^{-T}\bar{G}\tilde{V}^T \end{aligned} \tag{8.196}$$

where

$$\tilde{V}^T = \Psi^T R^{-1}$$

$\bar{G}$ is diagonal, that is, $\bar{G} = \Lambda(\Lambda + \mu I)^{-1}$.

The preceding Wiener-type gain matrix $\bar{G}$ is identical to the gain matrix given in Equation 8.176 as the matrices $R^{-1}R_{\mathbf{x}}R^{-T}$ and $R_d^{-1}R_x$ are similar, and hence have the same eigenvalues—that is, Λ in Equation 8.195 is the same as Λ_Σ in Equation 8.174, and therefore $\tilde{V}^T$ in Equation 8.196 is the same as V^T in Equation 8.176. We conclude from this that the nonorthogonal matrix V^T used in the previous estimators is in effect a prewhitening transformation. The main difference between V^T and the prewhitening filter R^{-1} described in Section 8.7.1 is that V^T whitens the noise signal and decorrelates the clean signal at the same time. When H_{TDC} is applied to the noisy speech vector y, it first whitens the colored noise signal d by applying R^{-1} to d. Then the orthogonal transformation Ψ^T is applied, which diagonalizes the covariance matrix of the transformed clean signal; that is, the orthogonal transformation

Ψ^T decorrelates the clean signal vector. The transformed signal (by $\Psi^T R^{-1}$) is then modified by a diagonal Wiener-type gain matrix ($\bar{G}$), and only the components of the transformed signal that contain noise are nulled. Finally, a reverse sequence of operations is performed consisting of the inverse orthogonal transformation Ψ followed by the dewhitening operation R. The two steps (namely, the R^{-1} transformation followed by Ψ^T) can alternatively be implemented in one step by choosing V^T as the eigenvector matrix of $R_d^{-1}R_x$. Hence, the covariance matrices R_x and R_d can simultaneously be diagonalized by either using the eigenvector matrix of $R_d^{-1}R_x$ or by using the transformation $\Psi^T R^{-1}$.

Next, we give a numerical example illustrating the two steps of the whitening process.

Example 8.3

Let $\mathbf{y} = \mathbf{x} + \mathbf{d}$ denote a 3×1 noisy speech vector, and let us assume that the clean signal vector $\mathbf{x}$ and noise vector $\mathbf{d}$ have the following covariance matrices:

$$R_x = \begin{bmatrix} 4 & 1 & 2 \\ 1 & 5 & 3 \\ 2 & 3 & 6 \end{bmatrix} \quad R_d = \begin{bmatrix} 1 & 0.5 & 0.3 \\ 0.5 & 2 & 0.1 \\ 0.3 & 0.1 & 6 \end{bmatrix} \tag{8.197}$$

Note that the noise is colored as its covariance matrix is full (i.e., not diagonal). We need to find a transformation that will simultaneously diagonalize R_x and R_d. We will consider two methods to derive this transformation.

Let $R_d = RR^T$ be the Cholesky decomposition of R_d, and let us consider first the transformation R^{-1}, which for this example, evaluates to

$$R^{-1} = \begin{bmatrix} 1 & 0 & 0 \\ -0.3780 & 0.7559 & 0 \\ -0.2275 & 0.0207 & 0.7238 \end{bmatrix} \tag{8.198}$$

After applying R^{-1} to the noisy vector $\mathbf{y}$, we get

$$R^{-1}\mathbf{y} = R^{-1}\mathbf{x} + R^{-1}\mathbf{d}$$

$$\mathbf{y}_1 = \mathbf{x}_1 + \mathbf{d}_1$$

The covariance matrix of the transformed noise signal $\mathbf{d}_1$ is

$$R_{d_1} = E\left[\mathbf{d}_1\mathbf{d}_1^T\right] = E[R^{-1}\mathbf{d}\mathbf{d}^T R^{-T}] = R^{-1}R_d R^{-T} = I$$

It is easy to verify after using Equations 8.197 and 8.198 that indeed

$$R^{-1}R_d R^{-T} = \begin{bmatrix} 1 & 0 & 0 \\ 0 & 1 & 0 \\ 0 & 0 & 1 \end{bmatrix}$$

Similarly, we can compute the covariance matrix of the transformed clean signal (i.e., $\mathbf{x}_1$) as

$$R_{x_1} = E\left[\mathbf{x}_1\mathbf{x}_1^T\right] = E[R^{-1}\mathbf{x}\mathbf{x}^T R^{-T}] = R^{-1}R_x R^{-T}$$

Note that the covariance matrix R_{x_1} is not diagonal. So, although R^{-1} diagonalizes the R_{d_1} matrix, it does not diagonalize the R_{x_1} matrix.

Next, we seek for a transformation matrix that diagonalizes R_{x_1} while preserving the previous diagonalization made by R^{-1}. The simplest method of diagonalizing R_{x_1} is to use its eigenvector matrix, which will be orthogonal (because R_{x_1} is symmetric) and will preserve the previous diagonalization made by R^{-1}. Now let Ψ and Λ denote, respectively, the eigenvector and eigenvalue matrices of the symmetric matrix $R^{-1}R_{\mathbf{x}}R^{-T}$:

$$R^{-1}R_{\mathbf{x}}R^{-T} = \Psi\Lambda\Psi^T \tag{8.199}$$

The diagonal eigenvalue matrix Λ is given by Λ = diag(1.1736, 4.0646, 4.3935). The transformed signals, in the second step, will have the form

$$\Psi^T\mathbf{y}_1 = \Psi^T\mathbf{x}_1 + \Psi^T\mathbf{d}_1$$

$$\mathbf{y}_2 = \mathbf{x}_2 + \mathbf{d}_2$$

The covariance matrix of the transformed noise signal (i.e., $\mathbf{d}_2$) will be

$$R_{d_2} = E\left[\mathbf{d}_2\mathbf{d}_2^T\right] = E\left[\Psi^T\mathbf{d}_1\mathbf{d}_1^T\Psi\right] = \Psi^T R_{d_1}\Psi = \Psi^T I\Psi = I$$

because $\Psi^T\Psi = I$. Note that the previous diagonalization of the noise covariance matrix by R^{-1} is preserved because the transformation Ψ is orthonormal. Similarly, we can compute the covariance matrix of the transformed clean signal (i.e., $\mathbf{x}_2$) as

$$R_{x_2} = E\left[\mathbf{x}_2\mathbf{x}_2^T\right] = E\left[\Psi^T\mathbf{x}_2\mathbf{x}_2^T\Psi\right] = \Psi^T R_{x_2}\Psi = \Lambda$$

The overall transformation is then given by $V_1 = \Psi^T R^{-1}$, which evaluates to

$$V_1 = \Psi^T R^{-1} = \begin{bmatrix} -0.2107 & -0.4947 & 0.4855 \\ 0.1417 & 0.3854 & 0.5214 \\ 1.0631 & -0.4226 & -0.1282 \end{bmatrix} \tag{8.200}$$

It is easy to verify that

$$V_1 R_x V_1^T = (\Psi^T R^{-1})R_x(R^{-T}\Psi) = \begin{bmatrix} 1.1736 & 0 & 0 \\ 0 & 4.0646 & 0 \\ 0 & 0 & 4.3935 \end{bmatrix} = \Lambda \tag{8.201}$$

and $V_1R_dV_1^T = I$. Therefore, the transformation matrix given in Equation 8.200 simultaneously diagonalizes the matrices R_x and R_d. This diagonalization was executed in two steps. Alternatively, the transformation can be obtained in a single step.

Let $R_d^{-1}R_x = U_2\Lambda_2U_2^T$ be the eigen-decomposition of the matrix $R_d^{-1}R_x$, where U_2 is the eigenvector matrix, and Λ_2 is the eigenvalue matrix. As mentioned earlier, because the matrices $R_d^{-1}R_x$ and $R^{-1}\ R_xR^{-T}$ are similar, they have the same eigenvalues, and therefore $\Lambda_2 = \Lambda = \text{diag}(1.1736, 4.0646, 4.3935)$. The eigenvector matrix U_2 is given by

$$U_2^T = \begin{bmatrix} -0.2909 & -0.6829 & 0.6701 \\ 0.2134 & 0.5807 & 0.7856 \\ 0.9235 & -0.3671 & -0.1113 \end{bmatrix}$$

The eigenvectors of U_2 are not normalized with respect to R_d and as a result the matrix $U_2^TR_dU_2$, although diagonal, will not be equal to the identity matrix. To ensure that $U_2^TR_dU_2 = I$, we need to normalize the eigenvectors of U_2 by $\left(u_i/\sqrt{u_i^TR_du_i}\ \ i = 1, 2, 3\right)$. For this example, $\sqrt{u_i^TR_du_i} = \{1.3804, 1.5067, 0.8687\}$ for $i = 1, 2, 3$, respectively. After dividing the U_2 eigenvectors by $\sqrt{u_i^TR_du_i}$, we get a normalized eigenvector matrix, which we denote by V_2^T:

$$V_2^T = \begin{bmatrix} -0.2107 & -0.4947 & 0.4855 \\ 0.1417 & 0.3854 & 0.5214 \\ 1.0631 & -0.4226 & -0.1282 \end{bmatrix}$$

It is easy to verify that indeed $V_2^TR_dV_2 = I$ and $V_2^TR_xV_2 = \text{diag}(1.1736, 4.0646, 4.3935)$. Note that the aforementioned matrix V_2^T is the same matrix as V_1 in Equation 8.200. Therefore, we can simultaneously diagonalize two covariance matrices (R_x and R_d) either by using the eigenvector matrix of $R_d^{-1}R_x$ or by using $\Psi^T R^{-1}$.

We can derive a similar relationship to that in Equation 8.196 for the spectral-domain-constrained estimator H_{SDC}, which we know from Equation 8.182 satisfies the following equation:

$$V^THV^{-T}\Lambda_\Sigma + V^TLHV^{-T} - \Lambda_\Sigma = 0 \tag{8.202}$$

Let

$$\tilde{H} = V^THV^{-T} \quad \text{and} \quad \tilde{L} = V^TLV^{-T}$$

then Equation 8.202 can be written as

$$\tilde{L}\tilde{H} + \tilde{H}\Lambda_\Sigma = \Lambda_\Sigma \tag{8.203}$$

After solving the preceding equation for $\tilde{H}$, H_{SDC} can be obtained by

$$H_{SDC} = V^{-T}\tilde{H}V^T$$

If we choose $V^T = \Psi^T R^{-1}$, then we can find a closed-form expression for $\tilde{H}$ [57] and can express H_{SDC} as

$$\begin{aligned} H_{SDC} &= R\Psi\tilde{H}\Psi^T R^{-1} \\ &= V^{-T}\tilde{H}V^T \end{aligned} \tag{8.204}$$

which is similar in form to the time-domain-constrained estimator H_{TDC} given in Equation 8.196. The main difference between H_{TDC} and H_{SDC} is that for colored noise $\tilde{H}$ in Equation 8.204 is not diagonal, but $\bar{G}$ in Equation 8.196 is diagonal. An explicit form of $\tilde{H}$ was derived in [57], with the kth column of $\tilde{H}$ given by

$$\tilde{\mathbf{h}}_k = T\lambda_V(k)\left(L + \lambda_V(k)I\right)^{-1} T^{-1}\mathbf{e}_k \tag{8.205}$$

where $\mathbf{e}_k$ denotes the unit vector with the kth component equal to one, $L = \text{diag}(K\mu_1, K\mu_2, \ldots, K\mu_K)$, $\lambda_V(k)$ is the kth eigenvalue of V, and $T = V^T\Phi$, where Φ is the orthogonal eigenvector matrix of L. Equation 8.205 gives the unique solution to Equation 8.203 provided that $\mu_k \geq 0$ for all $k = 1,2,\ldots,K$, and R_x is positive definite [57].

8.8 EVD-BASED METHODS: A UNIFIED VIEW

All the eigen-based methods described so far can be summarized using the following unified notation:

$$\begin{aligned} \hat{\mathbf{x}} &= H\mathbf{y} \\ &= W_1^{-T} G_1 W_1^T \mathbf{y} \end{aligned} \tag{8.206}$$

where the gain matrix $G_1 = \text{diag}(g_1, g_2, \ldots, g_M)$ depends on the estimation method, and the matrix W_1 may or may not contain orthonormal columns, depending on the type of noise (white or colored). Table 8.2 tabulates the gain matrices G_1 used by the various estimators.

8.9 PERCEPTUALLY MOTIVATED SUBSPACE ALGORITHMS

To reduce the perceptual effect of the residual noise, several speech enhancement methods incorporated a human auditory model that is widely used in wideband audio coding [59,60]. This model is based on the fact that additive noise is inaudible to the human ear as long as it falls below some *masking threshold.* Methods are available to calculate the masking threshold in the frequency domain, using critical-band analysis and the excitation pattern of the basilar membrane [60]. The idea behind the perceptually based subspace methods for speech enhancement is to shape the residual noise spectrum in such a way that it falls below the masking threshold, thereby making the residual noise inaudible. To do that, however, we need to have a way of relating the Fourier transform domain to the (KLT) eigen-domain. A method for incorporating the auditory model into the subspace-based methods for speech

TABLE 8.2
List of Gain Matrices G_1 Used by the Various Subspace Estimators for White and Colored Noise

Method	Noise	Gain Matrix	W_1	Equation
Least-squares	White	I_M	U_{x1}	8.77
Linear-MMSE	White	$\Lambda_{x1}(\Lambda_{x1}+\sigma^2 I_M)^{-1}$	U_{x1}	8.93, 8.94
TDC	White	$\Lambda_{x1}(\Lambda_{x1}+\mu\sigma^2 I_M)^{-1}$	U_{x1}	8.106, 8.107
SDC	White	$\text{diag}\left(\exp\left(-\frac{\nu}{2\xi_1}\right)\ \exp\left(-\frac{\nu}{2\xi_2}\right)\ \cdots\ \exp\left(-\frac{\nu}{2\xi_M}\right)\right)$	U_{x1}	8.119, 8.122
TDC-EW	Colored	$\Lambda_{\Sigma 1}(\Lambda_{\Sigma 1}+\mu I_M)^{-1}$	V_1	8.177, 8.176
SDC-EW	Colored	$\Lambda_{\Sigma 1}(\Lambda_{\Sigma 1}+\Lambda_\mu)^{-1}$	V_1	8.187, 8.188
Spectral subtraction	Colored	$\text{diag}\left(\frac{P_y(1)-P_d(1)}{P_d(1)}\ \frac{P_y(2)-P_d(2)}{P_d(2)}\ \cdots\ \frac{P_y(M)-P_d(M)}{P_d(M)}\right)$	F_1	8.125, 8.126

enhancement was proposed in [35,61]. In this method, the eigen-decomposition of the clean signal covariance matrix (obtained by subtracting the noisy signal and noise covariance matrices) was first performed, and then the masking thresholds were estimated based on the spectrum derived from an eigen-to-frequency domain transformation. The masking thresholds were transformed back to the eigenvalue domain using a frequency-to-eigen domain transformation and then incorporated into the signal subspace approach.

8.9.1 Fourier to Eigen-Domain Relationship

In the Fourier domain, the K-dimensional vector $\mathbf{y}$ can be obtained by using the discrete inverse Fourier transform (Equation 2.51):

$$\mathbf{y} = \frac{1}{K} F^H \mathbf{c}_F$$

where F^H is the $K \times K$ unitary DFT matrix, and the $\mathbf{c}_F$ ($K \times 1$) contains the Fourier transform coefficients. In the KLT domain, the K-dimensional vector $\mathbf{y}$ can be obtained by using the inverse KLT:

$$\mathbf{y} = U\mathbf{c}_K$$

where U is the orthogonal eigenvector matrix of R_y, and $\mathbf{c}_K$ ($K \times 1$) contains the Karhunen–Loeve (KL) coefficients. Equating the previous two equations, we get an expression for the KL coefficient vector c_K in terms of both KL and Fourier transforms:

$$\mathbf{c}_K = U^T \mathbf{y} = \frac{1}{K} U^T F^H \mathbf{c}_F \tag{8.207}$$

The ith element of the KL coefficient vector $\mathbf{c}_K$, denoted as $\mathbf{c}_K(i)$, is related to the ith eigenvalue λ_i of R_y as follows:

$$\begin{aligned}
\lambda_i &= u_i^T R_y u_i \\
&= u_i^T E\left[\mathbf{y}\mathbf{y}^T\right] u_i \\
&= E\left\{\left|u_i^T \mathbf{y}\right|^2\right\} \\
&= E\left\{\left|\mathbf{c}_K(i)\right|^2\right\}
\end{aligned} \tag{8.208}$$

where u_i is the ith eigenvector of R_y. Substituting $\mathbf{c}_K(i)$ from Equation 8.207 in the preceding equation, we get

$$\begin{aligned}
\lambda_i &= E\left\{\left|u_i^T \frac{1}{K} F^H \mathbf{c}_F\right|^2\right\} \\
&= \frac{1}{K^2} E\left\{\left|\mathbf{c}_F^H F u_i\right|^2\right\} \\
&= \frac{1}{K^2} E\left|\begin{bmatrix} Y(\omega_0) & \cdots & Y(\omega_{K-1}) \end{bmatrix}^T \begin{bmatrix} V_i(\omega_0) \\ \vdots \\ V_i(\omega_{K-1}) \end{bmatrix}\right|^2 \\
&= \frac{1}{K^2} E\left\{\left|\sum_{m=0}^{K-1} Y(\omega_m) V_i(\omega_m)\right|^2\right\}
\end{aligned} \tag{8.209}$$

where $Y(\omega_m)$ is the DFT of $\mathbf{y}$, and $V_i(\omega)$ is the K-point DFT of the ith eigenvector u_i of R_y:

$$V_i(\omega_m) = \sum_{k=0}^{K-1} u_i(k) e^{-jk\omega_m} \tag{8.210}$$

and $\omega_m = 2\pi m/K$ for $m = 0,1,\ldots, K-1$ and $u_i(k)$ is the kth element of the u_i eigenvector. Assuming that the Fourier transform coefficients $Y(\omega_m)$ ($m = 0, 1,\ldots, K-1$) are zero mean and uncorrelated (see Section 7.3 for the justification), then Equation 8.209 simplifies to

$$\begin{aligned}\lambda_i &= \frac{1}{K^2}\sum_{m=0}^{K-1} E\left\{\left|Y(\omega_m)V_i(\omega_m)\right|\right\}^2 \\ &= \frac{1}{K^2}\sum_{m=0}^{K-1} E\left\{\left|Y(\omega_m)\right|^2\right\}\left|V_iY(\omega_m)\right|^2 \\ &= \frac{1}{K}\sum_{m=0}^{K-1} P_y(\omega_m)\left|V_i(\omega_m)\right|^2 \end{aligned} \tag{8.211}$$

where $P_y(\omega_m) \triangleq E\{|Y(\omega_m)|^2\}/K$ is asymptotically ($K \to \infty$) the true power spectrum of y. The preceding equation provides the discrete (in frequency) version of the Fourier to KL (eigen-domain) relationship. The continuous version of this equation is given by [37, p. 817]

$$\lambda_i = \frac{1}{2\pi}\int_{-\pi}^{\pi} P_y(\omega)\left|V_i(\omega)\right|^2 d\omega \tag{8.212}$$

Equation 8.211 or Equation 8.212 gives us the relationship between the Fourier transform domain and the KLT domain (equations that relate the KLT domain to the Fourier domain can be found in [35,61]). Given the power spectrum of the signal, we can use the preceding relationship to go to the KLT domain and compute the corresponding eigenvalues.

The preceding equation has an interesting filterbank interpretation [38,62], which is shown in Figure 8.16. In the frequency domain, the eigenvalue decomposition can be viewed as a signal-dependent filterbank design, with the number of subbands set to the number of (principal) eigenvalues. The eigenvalues are computed as the total energy of the product of each subband "filter" response with the original power spectrum; that is, the ith eigenvalue λ_i contains the energy of the output of the ith subband filter. Unlike the DFT filterbanks, which have passbands uniformly distributed over the frequency range of interest, the location of the passbands of the eigen-filters are signal dependent. Figure 8.17 shows the eigen-filters computed for a segment of the vowel/eh/embedded in +10 dB white noise. As can be seen, eigen-filters 1–4 capture the first formant of the vowel, eigen-filters 5–7 capture the second formant, and eigen-filters 9–12 capture the third formant. Eigen-filters 7–8 capture the first harmonic, and the remaining eigen-filters capture information falling between the formants.

Turning our attention to speech enhancement, if we somehow can estimate the power spectrum of the masking thresholds, we can use Equation 8.211 to convert the Fourier-based masking thresholds to eigen-based masking thresholds. Such an approach was adopted in [35,61,63] and is described next.

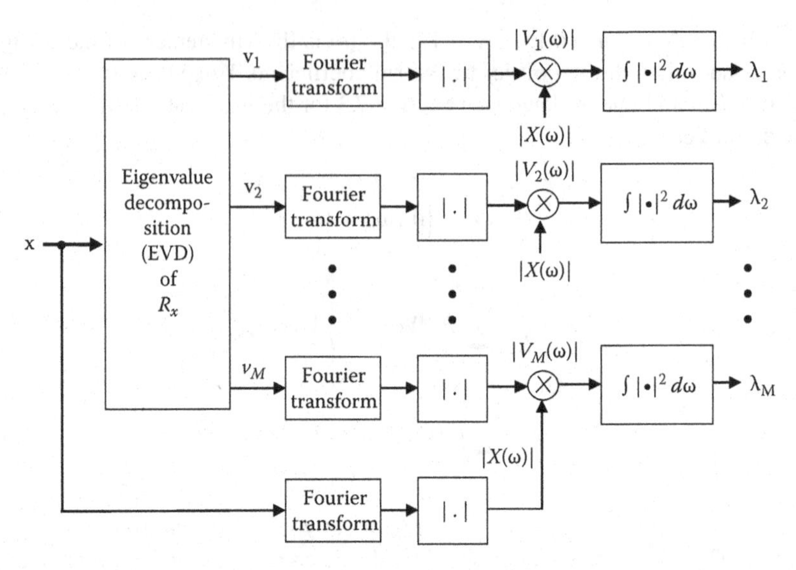

FIGURE 8.16 Schematic representation of the eigen-frequency relationship.

8.9.2 Incorporating Psychoacoustic Model Constraints

The simplest approach to incorporating psychoacoustic-based constraints is to replace the generic constraints in Equation 8.108 with the KL-based masking thresholds [63]. More specifically, we can consider solving the following constrained minimization problem:

$$\min_{H} \overline{\varepsilon_{\mathbf{x}}^2}$$

$$\text{subject to: } \begin{cases} E\left\{\left|\mathbf{v}_k^T \varepsilon_d\right|^2\right\} \leq \alpha_k T_k & k = 1,2,\ldots,M \\ E\left\{\left|\mathbf{v}_k^T \varepsilon_d\right|^2\right\} = 0 & k = M+1,\ldots,K \end{cases} \tag{8.213}$$

where $0 < \alpha_k < 1$, and T_k are the eigen-domain masking thresholds—that is, T_k can be obtained using the Fourier to eigen-domain relationship given in Equation 8.211, by substituting $P_y(\omega_m)$ with the power spectrum estimate of the masking thresholds. Similar to the derivation in Section 8.6.2, the optimal estimator H satisfies the equation

$$(I - Q)\Lambda_x - \sigma_d^2 \Lambda_\mu Q = 0 \tag{8.214}$$

where $Q \triangleq U^T H U$. If we assume a diagonal matrix $Q = \text{diag}(q_{11}, q_{22}, \ldots, q_{KK})$, then for white noise

$$E\left\{\left|\mathbf{v}_k^T \varepsilon_d\right|^2\right\} = q_{kk}^2 \sigma^2 \quad k = 1,2,\ldots,M \tag{8.215}$$

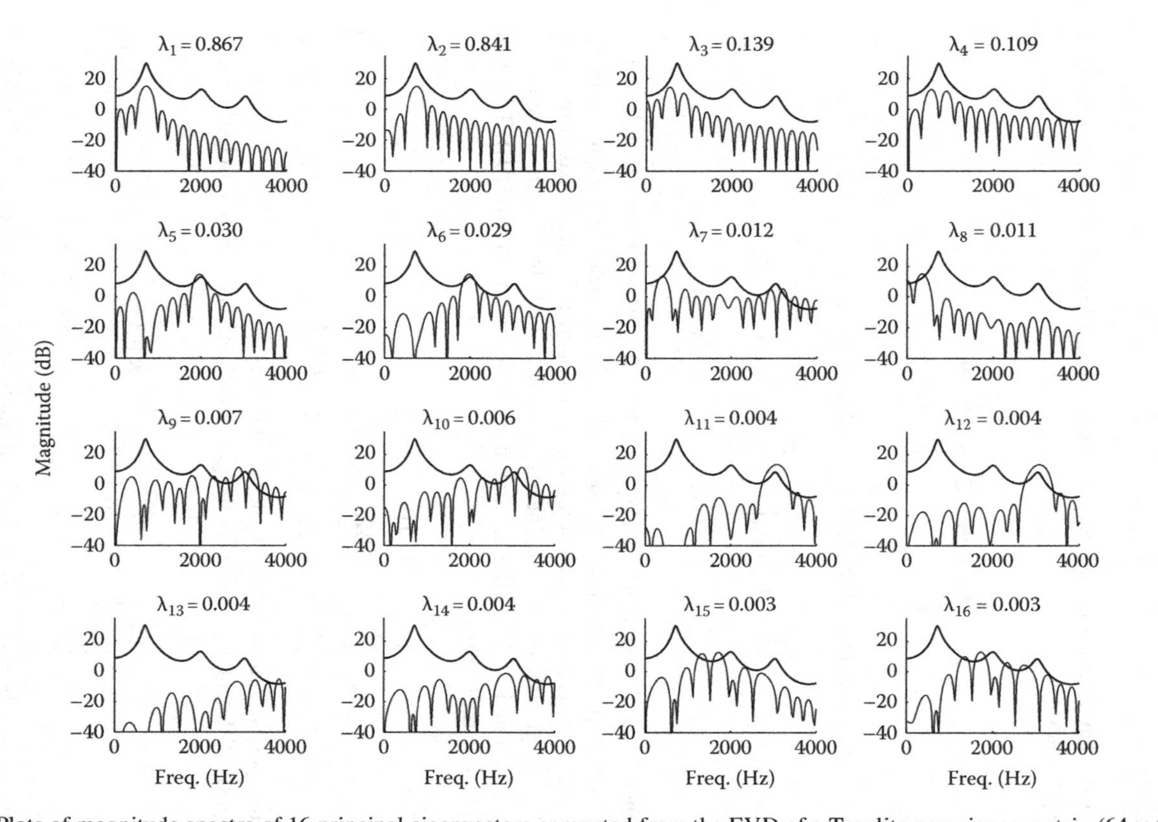

FIGURE 8.17 Plots of magnitude spectra of 16 principal eigenvectors computed from the EVD of a Toeplitz covariance matrix (64 × 64) of a short-segment (4 ms) of the vowel/eh/embedded in +10 dB white noise. The corresponding eigenvalues are indicated. Magnitude spectrum of vowel/eh/(in quiet) is superimposed (thick lines).

and after using the equality in the nonzero constraints in Equation 8.213, we get

$$q_{kk}^2 = \begin{cases} \dfrac{\alpha_k T_k}{\sigma^2} & k = 1,2,\ldots,M \\ 0 & k = M+1,\ldots,K \end{cases} \tag{8.216}$$

To ensure that α_k are smaller than one, we need q_{kk} to satisfy $0 < q_{kk} < 1$, and the preceding equation becomes

$$q_{kk}^2 = \begin{cases} \alpha_k \min\left(1, \dfrac{T_k}{\sigma^2}\right) & k = 1,2,\ldots,M \\ 0 & k = M+1,\ldots,K \end{cases} \tag{8.217}$$

The diagonal elements of the Q matrix are finally given by

$$q_{kk} = \begin{cases} (\alpha_k)^{1/2} \min\left(1, \sqrt{\dfrac{T_k}{\sigma^2}}\right) & k = 1,2,\ldots,M \\ 0 & k = M+1,\ldots,K \end{cases} \tag{8.218}$$

It is interesting to note that when $\alpha_k = 1$ (all k), the preceding equation becomes identical to the psychoacoustic filter derived in [64], except that T_k in Equation 8.218 are KL-domain-derived masking thresholds and not Fourier-based masking thresholds. In general $\alpha_k \neq 1$ and needs to be specified. In [63], they used $\alpha_k = \exp(-\nu\sigma^2/\lambda_x(k))$ and replaced the minimum operation with $\exp(-\sigma^2/\beta T_k)$. The final gain function had the form

$$q_{kk} = \begin{cases} \exp\left(-\dfrac{1}{2}\dfrac{(1+\nu)\sigma^2}{\beta T_k + \lambda_x(k)}\right) & k = 1,2,\ldots,M \\ 0 & k = M+1,\ldots,K \end{cases} \tag{8.219}$$

where the constant β took values in the range $0 \leq \beta \leq e$.

A slightly different expression for the gain function was proposed in [35]:

$$q_{kk} = \begin{cases} \exp\left[-\dfrac{\nu\sigma^2}{\min\left(\lambda_x(k), T_k\right)}\right] & k = 1,2,\ldots,M \\ 0 & k = M+1,\ldots,K \end{cases} \tag{8.220}$$

The motivation behind the use of the minimum operation in Equation 8.220 is to provide more noise suppression whenever $T_k < \lambda_x(k)$, that is, the masking threshold levels are smaller than the corresponding power spectrum amplitudes of the signal. In this way, we can achieve more noise suppression without having to increase the value of ν in Equation 8.220. The main problem with the minimum operation, however, is that during weak speech frames, the estimation of T_k might not be very accurate, and therefore not enough noise suppression will be achieved. It should be noted that Equation 8.220 was derived based on informal listening tests and not as an optimal solution to a constrained minimization problem [35].

Following estimation of the gain function, either by Equation 8.219 or Equation 8.220, we can obtain the optimal linear estimator as

$$H = U\,\mathrm{diag}\left(q_{11}, q_{22}, \ldots, q_{KK}\right) U^T \tag{8.221}$$

For the derivation of the gain functions given in Equation 8.219 or Equation 8.220, we assumed that the noise was white with variance σ^2. For colored noise, we can replace σ^2 in Equations 8.219 and 8.220 with the frequency-dependent variance $\sigma_d^2(k)$, which can be computed as described in Section 8.7.3, as the kth diagonal element of $U^T R_d U$, that is, $\sigma_d^2(k) = u_k^T R_d u_k$, where R_d is the noise covariance matrix, and u_k is the kth eigenvector of the noisy covariance matrix R_y.

For the preceding perceptually motivated subspace methods, it is necessary to estimate the masking thresholds of the speech signal from the noisy data. For more accurate estimates of the masking thresholds, the noisy speech signal is typically preprocessed by a simple, nonaggressive noise reduction algorithm (e.g., spectral subtraction algorithm) and the masking thresholds are computed using the enhanced spectra [35,65]. The estimated (Fourier-based) masking thresholds are finally converted using Equation 8.211 to the eigen-based masking thresholds, denoted as T_k in Equations 8.219 and 8.220. Hence, a preprocessing stage is almost always required with the aforementioned subspace methods to accurately estimate the masking thresholds. In low-SNR conditions, however, the estimated masking threshold levels might deviate from the true ones, leading possibly to additional residual noise caused by the inaccuracy of the estimated thresholds. Next, we present a perceptually motivated subspace method that does not rely on the accurate estimation of masking thresholds and therefore does not require preprocessing of the noisy signal.

8.9.3 Incorporating Auditory Masking Constraints

A different approach that did not rely on accurate estimation of the masking thresholds was proposed in [34]. This approach was motivated by the perceptual weighting technique used in low-rate analysis-by-synthesis speech coders [66], which takes into account the frequency-domain masking properties of the human auditory system. Analysis-by-synthesis speech coders (e.g., CELP) obtain the optimal excitation for LPC synthesis in a closed-loop manner by minimizing a perceptually weighted error criterion [67]. This criterion was motivated by frequency-masking experiments [66] that showed the auditory system has a limited ability to detect noise in frequency bands in which the speech signal has high energy, that is, near the formant peaks. Hence, to take advantage of this masking effect, we can consider distributing unevenly the quantization noise (estimation error) across the spectrum in such a way that it is masked by the speech signal. In our application, we can distribute the spectrum of the residual noise so that it gets masked by the signal spectrum. This can be done using a perceptual filter that is derived from LPC analysis of the speech signal [67,68] and has the following transfer function:

$$T(z) = \frac{A(z)}{A(z/\gamma)}$$

$$= \frac{1 - \sum_{k=1}^{p} a_k z^{-k}}{1 - \sum_{k=1}^{p} a_k \gamma^k z^{-k}} \tag{8.222}$$

where

$A(z)$ is the LPC polynomial

a_k are the short-term linear prediction coefficients

γ is a parameter ($0 \leq \gamma \leq 1$) that controls the energy of the error in the formant regions

p is the prediction order (see example in Figure 6.19)

We can use the preceding perceptual weighting filter $T(z)$ in the constrained linear estimation problem to shape the noise distortion and make it inaudible. We can do this by using a perceptually weighted error criterion in place of the squared-error criterion used in Equation 8.97. The perceptually weighted residual signal is related to the residual noise $\varepsilon_d(n)$ defined in Equation 8.95 by

$$\varepsilon_{wd}(n) = \varepsilon_d(n) * h(n)$$

$$= \sum_k h_k \varepsilon_d(n-k) \tag{8.223}$$

where h_k is the infinite-duration impulse response of $T(z)$ (Equation 8.222). In practice, a truncated impulse response is used, and the preceding equation is expressed in matrix notation as follows:

$$\varepsilon_{wd} = W \cdot \varepsilon_d \tag{8.224}$$

where W is a lower triangular matrix ($K \times K$) of the form

$$W = \begin{bmatrix} h_0 & 0 & \cdots & 0 \\ h_1 & h_0 & \cdots & 0 \\ \vdots & \vdots & \ddots & \vdots \\ h_{K-1} & h_{K-2} & \cdots & h_0 \end{bmatrix} \tag{8.225}$$

where h_k is the truncated impulse response of $T(z)$. We can now define the energy of the perceptually weighted noise distortion as

$$\varepsilon_{wd}^2 = E\left[\varepsilon_{wd}^T \varepsilon_{wd}\right] = \text{tr}\left(E\left[\varepsilon_{wd} \varepsilon_{wd}^T\right]\right)$$

$$= \text{tr}\left(W \cdot E\left[\varepsilon_d \varepsilon_d^T\right] \cdot W^T\right) \tag{8.226}$$

The new optimal linear estimator can be obtained by solving the following constrained optimization problem:

$$\min_{H} \varepsilon_{\mathbf{x}}^2$$

$$\text{subject to: } \frac{1}{K}\varepsilon_{wd}^2 \leq \delta \qquad (8.227)$$

where δ is a positive constant. The solution to the preceding problem can be found using techniques similar to those described in Section 8.6.2, and the optimal estimator H satisfies the following equation [34]:

$$\mu(W^T W)H + HR_x R_d^{-1} = R_x R_d^{-1} \qquad (8.228)$$

where μ is the Lagrange multiplier. Assuming colored noise, we can use the embedded prewhitening approach (described in Section 8.7.4) and construct a matrix V that simultaneously diagonalizes the covariance matrices R_x and R_d as per Equation 8.174. In doing so, the preceding equation becomes

$$\mu(W^T W)H + HV^{-T}\Lambda V^T = V^{-T}\Lambda V^T \qquad (8.229)$$

where Λ is the diagonal eigenvalue matrix of $R_d^{-1}R_x$. This equation has the form of the Lyapunov equation and can be solved numerically for H using the algorithm proposed in [56]. Explicit solutions can also be found in [19]. Following estimation of the estimation matrix H, the enhanced signal $\hat{\mathbf{x}}$ can be obtained as $\hat{\mathbf{x}} = H \cdot \mathbf{y}$. Simulations conducted in [34] showed that the preceding perceptually motivated approach performed better, in terms of objective measures, than the approach proposed in [42] when implemented with the same embedded prewhitening but with no perceptual filter. Informal listening tests indicated that the benefit of the perceptual weighting technique was more evident in the high-SNR than low-SNR conditions.

8.10 SUBSPACE-TRACKING ALGORITHMS

All the algorithms discussed so far in this chapter are based on the EVD of an estimated correlation matrix or the SVD of the corresponding data matrix. The explicit computation of these decompositions, however, can be prohibitively expensive for real-time processing. More precisely, direct computation of the SVD of a $K \times L$ data matrix ($K > L$) requires $O(K^2L)$ operations, and direct computation of the EVD of a square $K \times K$ correlation matrix requires $O(K^3)$ operations. This large computational load coupled with the fact that subspace algorithms do not require estimation of all eigenvectors and eigenvalues motivated researchers to develop low-cost algorithms for estimating eigenvalues and eigenvectors. Special attention has been given to algorithms that can recursively estimate and update the eigencomponents (eigenvectors and eigenvalues) as new data are received. As these algorithms attempt to continuously track the signal (or noise) subspace, they came to be known as *subspace-tracking* algorithms. In this section, we provide a brief overview of the various subspace-tracking algorithms proposed. More detailed surveys can be found in [69–71].

The subspace-tracking algorithms can be broadly classified into two categories: (a) block algorithms, which can be either iterative or direct, and (b) recursive algorithms. Block algorithms compute the EVD (or SVD) based on a block (i.e., a frame) of data, and do not utilize any previous information collected in the past. Recursive algorithms, on the other hand, update the previously computed eigen-information using newly received data. In this regard, the recursive algorithms are more suitable for real-time processing, and generally these algorithms require a significantly smaller number of computations than the block algorithms.

8.10.1 Block Algorithms

Block algorithms compute the EVD of a matrix based on a block of data and can be further subdivided into direct or iterative algorithms. The direct methods are preferred when all or the majority of the eigenvectors need to be estimated. These methods reduce the given matrix to a simpler form by applying a sequence of similarity transformations that do not alter the eigenvalues. Orthogonal transformations, such as the Givens or Householder transformations [8, p. 419], can be used for instance to reduce a symmetric matrix to a symmetric tridiagonal form and from that estimate the eigenvalues/eigenvectors efficiently.

Iterative methods are preferred when only a few eigenvectors and eigenvalues need to be estimated. The most common iterative method is the power method [8, p. 351]. Let R be a $K \times K$ symmetric covariance matrix. Then, the following iterative algorithm estimates the eigenvector corresponding to the largest eigenvalue of R:

$$
\begin{aligned}
&\text{for } k = 1, 2, \ldots \\
&\mathbf{z}^{(k)} = R \cdot u^{(k-1)} \\
&u^{(k)} = \mathbf{z}^{(k)} / \|\mathbf{z}^{(k)}\|_2 \\
&\lambda^{(k)} = [u^{(k)}]^T R \cdot u^{(k)} \\
&\text{end}
\end{aligned}
\tag{8.230}
$$

where $u^{(k)}$ and $\lambda^{(k)}$ denotes the estimate of the dominant eigenvector and eigenvalue at iteration k, respectively. The eigenvector $u^{(0)}$ can be initialized with a unit 2-norm vector. The preceding algorithm is guaranteed to converge to the principal eigenvector, provided that there is a sufficient gap between the two largest eigenvalues [8, p. 352].

The preceding power method estimates a single (i.e., the largest) eigenvalue and associated eigenvector. If we want to estimate, say, the m-dominant (principal) eigenvalues/eigenvectors, then we can either use *deflation* techniques or generalizations of the power method (see review in [72]). The deflation method replaces the given matrix by a new matrix whose largest eigenvalue becomes the second largest eigenvalue of the given matrix. The power method can then be applied to this new matrix to estimate the second largest eigenvalue/eigenvector. This procedure can be repeated m times to estimate the m principal eigenvalues/eigenvectors. One possible choice for creating the new matrix is given by

$$R' = \left(I - u_1 u_1^T\right) R \tag{8.231}$$

where u_1 is the estimated principal eigenvector. Applying the power iteration method (Equation 8.230) to the new matrix R' will yield the second largest eigenvalue and corresponding eigenvector. The deflation approach is simple; however, it introduces additional complexity. Other deflation techniques can be found in [52].

Example 8.4

Consider the following matrix R:

$$R = \begin{bmatrix} 10 & 1 & 3 \\ 1 & 5 & -1 \\ 3 & -1 & 6 \end{bmatrix}$$

Use the power method to estimate all eigenvalues and eigenvectors of R. The exact eigen-decomposition of R is given by

$$U = \begin{bmatrix} -0.3944 & 0.2459 & -0.8855 \\ 0.6277 & 0.7758 & -0.0641 \\ 0.6712 & -0.5810 & -0.4603 \end{bmatrix}, \quad \Lambda = \begin{bmatrix} 3.3023 & 0 & 0 \\ 0 & 6.0658 & 0 \\ 0 & 0 & 11.6319 \end{bmatrix} \tag{8.232}$$

where
- U is the eigenvector matrix
- Λ is the eigenvalue matrix of R

After running the power method (Equation 8.230) for 10 iterations using $\mathbf{u}_1^{(0)} = [1 \quad 0 \quad 0]^T$, we get the following eigenvalues.

Iteration k	Eigenvalue $\lambda(k)$	Error $\lVert\lambda^{(k)} - \lambda_1\rVert_2$
1	11.390909	2.409718e−001
2	11.589705	4.217630e−002
3	11.622401	9.480288e−003
4	11.629465	2.415797e−003
5	11.631237	6.438271e−004
6	11.631707	1.740241e−004
7	11.631834	4.723917e−005
8	11.631868	1.283949e−005
9	11.631877	3.491061e−006
10	11.631880	9.493273e−007

Relatively accurate estimates of the largest eigenvalue were obtained within a few iterations. The error (given in the rightmost column in the table) between the true and estimated eigenvalues is smaller than 5×10^{-3} within four iterations. The dominant eigenvector estimated in the 10th iteration is $u_1^{(10)} = [0.8856, 0.0644, 0.4600]^T$.

To compute the second largest eigenvalue, we use deflation—that is, we replace the matrix R with $(I - u_1 u_1^T)R$, and apply the power method to the new matrix $R' = (I - u_1 u_1^T)R$, where u_1 is the estimated principal eigenvector of R, which in this example corresponds to $u_1^{(10)}$. The second largest eigenvalue of R will now be the largest eigenvalue of R'. After applying the power method to R', we get the eigenvalues listed in the following table. The eigenvectors were initialized again to $u_2^{(0)} = [1 \quad 0 \quad 0]^T$.

Iteration k	Eigenvalue $\lambda^{(k)}$	Error $\|\lambda^{(k)} - \lambda_2\|_2$
1	4.866401	1.199418e+000
2	5.554045	5.117745e–001
3	5.891413	1.744066e–001
4	6.011727	5.409262e–002
5	6.049564	1.625538e–002
6	6.060982	4.837184e–003
7	6.064384	1.434762e–003
8	6.065395	4.247273e–004
9	6.065694	1.252279e–004
10	6.065783	3.644872e–005

The dominant eigenvector estimated in the 10th iteration is given by $u_2^{(10)} = [0.2470, 0.7735, -0.5837]^T$. We can use deflation one more time to estimate the third largest eigenvalue, which in this example is the minimum eigenvalue. To do that, we replace the matrix R' with the new matrix $R'' = (I - u_2 u_2^T)R'$, where u_2 is the second principal eigenvector of R, that is, it is $u_2^{(10)} = [0.2470,\ 0.7735,\ -0.5837]^T$. After applying the power method for a few iterations to R'' with $u_3^{(0)} = [1 \quad 0 \quad 0]^T$, we get the eigenvalues listed in the following table.

Iteration k	Eigenvalue $\lambda^{(k)}$	Error $\|\lambda^{(k)} - \lambda_3\|_2$
1	3.302337	3.739805e–005
2	3.302337	3.739805e–005
3	3.302337	3.739805e–005

The dominant eigenvector estimated in the third iteration is given by $u_3^{(10)} = [0.3935, -0.6305, -0.6691]^T$. Note that in the preceding example, we run the power method for a fixed number of iterations. In practice, one can use an appropriate convergence criterion to terminate the algorithm. This example illustrates that the power method is a very simple and effective method of computing the eigenvalues and eigenvectors of a matrix, and requires a significantly smaller number of operations than direct methods.

Other than the power method, there exist other iterative algorithms for computing the eigenvalues of a matrix given a block of data. Lanczos-type algorithms are recommended for symmetric matrices that are large and sparse [71,73].

For symmetric and Toeplitz matrices, different types of algorithms were proposed that exploit the Toeplitz structure [74–77]. For instance, one can make use of efficient methods to perform the matrix-vector multiplication required in the power method (Equation 8.230). By appropriately embedding a Toeplitz matrix in a circulant matrix C, we can use the FFT to efficiently perform the matrix-vector multiplication in less than $O(K^2)$ operations [78] (see Example 8.5). Let F denote the DFT matrix, and suppose that we are interested in performing $C \cdot \mathbf{x}$, where C is a circulant matrix. After making use of the fact that the DFT matrix F diagonalizes the circulant matrix C, that is, $C = F^H \Delta F$, where $\Delta = \text{diag}(F \cdot c)$ is a diagonal matrix containing the Fourier transform of the first column of C, we can express $C \cdot \mathbf{x}$ as

$$\begin{aligned} \mathbf{y} &= C \cdot \mathbf{x} \\ &= F^H \Delta F \cdot \mathbf{x} \\ &= F^H \,\text{diag}(F\mathbf{c}) F \cdot \mathbf{x} \\ &= F^H (F\mathbf{c}.{*}F\mathbf{x}) \end{aligned} \tag{8.233}$$

where

".*" denotes elementwise multiplication of two vectors

$\mathbf{c}$ is the first column of the matrix C

Thus, the Toeplitz matrix-vector multiplication $C \cdot \mathbf{x}$ mainly consists of computing the Fourier transform of three vectors of length K. This requires $O(K\log_2 K)$ operations, which is considerably smaller than $O(K^2)$ operations typically required for a matrix-vector multiplication.

Example 8.5

In this example, we illustrate how we can use the FFT to perform a Toeplitz matrix-vector multiplication. Consider the following Toeplitz matrix T:

$$T = \begin{bmatrix} 1 & 2 & 3 \\ 3 & 1 & 2 \\ 4 & 3 & 1 \\ 5 & 4 & 3 \end{bmatrix}$$

and suppose that we are interested in performing the following matrix-vector multiplication:

$$y = T \cdot \mathbf{x}$$

where $\mathbf{x}^T = [2\ 5\ 1]$. In order to make use of the relationship of the FFT to circulant matrices (i.e., Equation 8.233), we first need to embed the matrix T in a circulant matrix. To do that, we first note that the matrix T is fully described by the first column and a subset of the last column:

$$t_1 = \begin{bmatrix} 1 \\ 3 \\ 4 \\ 5 \end{bmatrix} \quad t_2 = \begin{bmatrix} 3 \\ 2 \end{bmatrix} \tag{8.234}$$

With these vectors, we can form the first column of the circulant matrix as follows:

$$\mathbf{c} = \begin{bmatrix} t_1 \\ 0 \\ t_2 \end{bmatrix} = \begin{bmatrix} 1 \\ 3 \\ 4 \\ 5 \\ 0 \\ 0 \\ 3 \\ 2 \end{bmatrix} \tag{8.235}$$

where the extra zeros were added to ensure that the dimension of $\mathbf{c}$ is power of two. The resulting circulant matrix C has the following form:

$$C = \begin{bmatrix} 1 & 2 & 3 & 0 & 0 & 5 & 4 & 3 \\ 3 & 1 & 2 & 3 & 0 & 0 & 5 & 4 \\ 4 & 3 & 1 & 2 & 3 & 0 & 0 & 5 \\ 5 & 4 & 3 & 1 & 2 & 3 & 0 & 0 \\ 0 & 5 & 4 & 3 & 1 & 2 & 3 & 0 \\ 0 & 0 & 5 & 4 & 3 & 1 & 2 & 3 \\ 3 & 0 & 0 & 5 & 4 & 3 & 1 & 2 \\ 2 & 3 & 0 & 0 & 5 & 4 & 3 & 1 \end{bmatrix} = \begin{bmatrix} T & * \\ * & * \end{bmatrix}$$

As shown earlier, the top left 4×3 corner of C contains the original matrix T. To account for the extra zeros added in Equation 8.235, we need to zero-pad the vector $\mathbf{x}$ as

$$\hat{\mathbf{x}} = \begin{bmatrix} \mathbf{x} \\ 0 \end{bmatrix}$$

We are now ready to use Equation 8.233 to perform the circulant matrix-vector multiplication $\hat{\mathbf{y}} = C \cdot \hat{\mathbf{x}}$. After computing the 8-point FFT of $\mathbf{c}$ and $\hat{\mathbf{x}}$, that is, $F \cdot \mathbf{c}$ and $F \cdot \hat{\mathbf{x}}$, we perform the inverse FFT of the elementwise product of $F \cdot \mathbf{c}$ and $F \cdot \hat{\mathbf{x}}$. The dimension of the resulting vector $\hat{\mathbf{y}}$ will be 8×1, and we obtain $\mathbf{y}$ as the top four elements of $\hat{\mathbf{y}}$, which for this example evaluates to $\mathbf{y}^T = [15\ 13\ 24\ 33]$. Hence, for this example we evaluated the Toeplitz matrix-vector multiplication of $T \cdot \mathbf{x}$ by computing the FFT of three 8×1 vectors.

Several iterative algorithms were also proposed for computing the smallest eigenvalue–eigenvector pair of symmetric Toeplitz matrices. These algorithms made use of the fact that the inverse of a symmetric Toeplitz matrix can be efficiently computed using the Levinson recursion in $O(K^2)$ operations. Algorithms based on the Levinson recursion were proposed in [75,76] for estimating the eigenvalues of Toeplitz matrices. The *Rayleigh quotient iteration* algorithm was used in [74] to compute the smallest eigenvalue–eigenvector pair of a symmetric Toeplitz matrix. This algorithm is an extension of the *inverse iteration* algorithm [8, p. 383] commonly used for computing selected eigenvector/eigenvalue pairs based on the Rayleigh quotient formula. The *Rayleigh quotient iteration* algorithm is described in the following text:

$$\begin{aligned}
&\lambda^{(0)} \quad \text{and} \quad u_0 \quad \text{given} \quad \text{and} \quad \| u_0 \| = 1 \\
&\text{for } k = 0,1,\ldots \\
&\qquad \text{Solve}\left(R - \lambda^{(k)} I\right)\mathbf{z}_k = u_k \quad \text{for } z_k \\
&\qquad u_{k+1} = \mathbf{z}_k / \| \mathbf{z}_k \|_2 \\
&\qquad \lambda^{(k+1)} = u_{k+1}^T R \cdot u_{k+1} \\
&\text{end}
\end{aligned} \tag{8.236}$$

The system of equations in the second step of the algorithm can be solved using the Levinson recursion in $O(K^2)$ operations since R is Toeplitz. Although the *Rayleigh quotient iteration* algorithm is guaranteed to converge with cubic convergence rate, it may not converge to the desired eigenvalue–eigenvector pair. In order to ensure that the preceding algorithm converges to the desired eigenvalue–eigenvector pair, it is critical that the initial eigenvector $\mathbf{u}_0$, or equivalently $\lambda^{(0)}$, be chosen properly. An efficient method for choosing $\lambda^{(0)}$ was proposed in [74] based on estimated lower and upper bounds of the desired eigenvalue. These bounds were obtained by performing the LDU factorization of the matrix $R - \lambda^{(k)} I$ at each iteration. The *Rayleigh quotient iteration* algorithm requires $O(K^2)$ operations to compute each eigenvalue–eigenvector pair.

8.10.2 Recursive Algorithms

Unlike the block algorithms, the recursive algorithms update the eigen-structure of the matrix given the current and past data received. These algorithms rely on a time-varying estimation of the correlation matrix, which involves either a moving rectangular window or an exponentially weighted window. At frame n, the estimate of the correlation matrix based on a moving rectangular window is given by

$$R(n) = R(n-1) + \frac{1}{K}(\mathbf{x}(n)\mathbf{x}^T(n) - \mathbf{x}(n-K)\mathbf{x}^T(n-K)) \tag{8.237}$$

where

$\mathbf{x}(n)$ is the current $K \times 1$ data vector
$\mathbf{x}(n-K)$ is the previous data vector
K is the length of the rectangular window

The updating of the covariance matrix $R(n)$ as shown earlier is known as the rank-2 update. The subtraction, however, of a rank-1 update (known as *downdating*) is potentially ill conditioned, and for that reason the following rank-1 update of the covariance matrix is typically used, which is based on an exponentially weighted window:

$$R(n) = \alpha R(n-1) + \mathbf{x}(n)\mathbf{x}^T(n) \tag{8.238}$$

where $0 < \alpha < 1$. Unlike the moving rectangular window that is fixed, the preceding window grows in size; however, the old data are deemphasized according to a moving decaying exponential window. The effective window size is approximately $1/(1 - \alpha)$long.

The recursive algorithms for subspace tracking make use of the previous recursive updates of the covariance matrix, and can be broadly classified as: (1) modified eigenvalue problem (MEP) algorithms and (2) adaptive algorithms. Although both types of algorithms are adaptive in that they track time-varying eigen-information as new data are received, they differ in one aspect. The MEP algorithms compute exact eigen-information at each update, whereas the adaptive algorithms, which are mostly based on gradient-descent type of algorithms, move toward the EVD at each update.

8.10.2.1 Modified Eigenvalue Problem Algorithms

The main objective in MEP algorithms is to compute the eigen-structure of $R(n)$ given the eigenstructure of $R(n - 1)$. Let the EVD of $R(n - 1)$ be

$$R(n-1) = U(n-1)\Lambda(n-1)U^T(n-1) \tag{8.239}$$

where $U(n - 1)$ and $\Lambda(n - 1)$ denote the eigenvector and eigenvalue matrices, respectively, of $R(n - 1)$. Consider now the rank-1 update of the covariance matrix:

$$R(n) = R(n-1) + \mathbf{x}(n)\mathbf{x}^T(n) \tag{8.240}$$

Combining Equations 8.239 and 8.240, we get

$$R(n) = U(n-1)\Delta(n)U^T(n-1) \tag{8.241}$$

where

$$\Delta(n) = \Lambda(n-1) + \mathbf{z}(n)\mathbf{z}^T(n) \tag{8.242}$$

and $\mathbf{z}(n) = U^T(n - 1)\mathbf{x}(n)$. Note that the matrix $\Delta(n)$ is similar to the matrix $R(n)$ since the orthogonal matrix $U(n - 1)$ is the inverse of $U^T(n - 1)$. Therefore, the matrices $\Delta(n)$ and $R(n)$ share the same eigenvalues [7, p. 304]. Rather than focusing on computing the eigen-structure of $R(n)$, we can instead focus on estimating the eigen-structure of $\Delta(n)$, which consists of the sum of a diagonal matrix ($\Lambda(n - 1)$) and a rank-1 term $\mathbf{z}(n)\mathbf{z}^T(n)$. It is thus computationally easier to work with $\Delta(n)$ than with $R(n)$. Several researchers (e.g., see [79,80]) have considered solving the preceding problem and developed algorithms with low computational complexity.

Golub [81] considered solving explicitly the eigenvalues of $\Delta(n)$. The eigenvalues of $\Delta(n)$ can be computed by solving the following characteristic equation:

$$\det[\Lambda(n-1)+\mathbf{z}(n)\mathbf{z}^T(n)-\lambda I]=0 \tag{8.243}$$

resulting in the following secular equation:

$$f(\lambda)=1+\sum_{i=1}^{K}\frac{z_i^2}{(\mu_i-\lambda)^2} \tag{8.244}$$

where

μ_i denotes the ith diagonal element of $\Lambda(n-1)$

z_i denotes the ith element of $z(n)$

The eigenvalues of $\Delta(n)$, or equivalently $R(n)$, can be computed exactly by finding the zeros of the preceding secular equation, and this can be done in $O(K)$ operations per eigenvalue. The eigenvectors can be computed using the inverse iteration algorithm [8] or, alternatively, the eigenvectors can be computed explicitly [79]. More efficient methods were proposed in [71,82] for computing the eigenvectors of $\Delta(n)$. A more thorough review of rank-1 EVD update algorithms can be found in [69,70,83].

8.10.2.2 Adaptive Algorithms

Adaptive algorithms for eigenvector estimation made use of the fact that these vectors can be obtained by minimizing a specific cost function subject to certain constraints on these vectors (e.g., orthonormality constraints). For example, it is known that the eigenvector corresponding to the minimum eigenvalue is the solution to the following constrained minimization problem [84]:

$$\begin{gathered}\min_{w}\mathbf{w}^T R\mathbf{w}\\ \text{subject to } \mathbf{w}^T\mathbf{w}=1\end{gathered} \tag{8.245}$$

More generally, the solution to the following constrained minimization problem [85]

$$\begin{gathered}\min_{W}\operatorname{tr}(W^T RW)\\ \text{subject to: } W^T W=I\end{gathered} \tag{8.246}$$

yields a matrix W ($K \times m$) containing the m eigenvectors corresponding to the m smallest eigenvalues. If we perform maximization instead of minimization in Equation 8.246, then we will get the m eigenvectors corresponding to the m largest eigenvalues. The preceding minimization problems can be solved iteratively using a constrained gradient-search type of algorithm of the form

$$W'(n) = W(n-1) - \mu\nabla(n) \tag{8.247}$$

where

μ is a small constant
n is the iteration (sample) index
$\hat{\nabla}(n)$ is an estimator of the gradient of the cost function (Equation 8.246) with respect to W

As the gradient descent algorithm does not guarantee that the columns of the matrix $W'(n)$ will be mutually orthonormal, we need to orthonormalize the columns of $W'(n)$ at the end of each iteration (update). The orthonormalization of $W'(n)$ can be done using the Gram–Schmidt procedure [7, p. 172]. Following the Gram–Schmidt procedure, the matrix $W(n)$ will contain the orthonormalized columns of $W'(n)$.

The gradient ∇ of the cost function in Equation 8.246 is given by

$$\nabla = \frac{\partial}{\partial W}\operatorname{tr}(W^T R W) = 2RW \tag{8.248}$$

Using the estimate of the covariance matrix given in Equation 8.238 and assuming that $W(n) \approx W(n-1)$, we can approximate the preceding gradient as $\hat{\nabla}(n) = 2R(n)W(n-1)$.

Alternatively, to avoid the computation involved in the update of $R(n)$ (i.e., Equation 8.238), we can use an instantaneous estimate of $R(n) = \mathbf{x}(n)\mathbf{x}^T(n)$ and get the following least mean square (LMS)-type algorithm:

$$\begin{aligned} y_i(n) &= \mathbf{x}^T(n)\mathbf{w}_i(n-1) \\ \mathbf{w}_i'(n) &= \mathbf{w}_i(n-1) - \mu\mathbf{x}(n)y_i(n), \quad i = 1,2,\ldots,m \end{aligned} \tag{8.249}$$

where $\mathbf{w}_i(n)$ indicates the ith column of the matrix W. The vectors $\mathbf{w}_i(n)$ are obtained by orthonormalizing $\mathbf{w}_i'(n)$ based on the Gram–Schmidt procedure and therefore satisfy $\mathbf{w}_j^T(n)\mathbf{w}_i(n) = 0$ for $i \neq j$ and $\mathbf{w}_j^T(n)\mathbf{w}_j(n) = 1$ for $i = j$. The preceding algorithm can be used to estimate the m eigenvectors $\mathbf{w}_i(n)$ ($i = 1,2,\ldots, m$) corresponding to the m smallest eigenvalues. To estimate the m eigenvectors $\mathbf{w}_i(n)$ ($i = 1,2,\ldots, m$) corresponding to the m largest eigenvalues, we simply make the sign in the update equation (Equation 8.249) positive. The preceding LMS-type algorithm only requires $O(Km)$ operations per cycle for the update equation and $O(Km^2)$ operations for the Gram–Schmidt orthonormalization procedure. A Gauss–Newton type recursive algorithm was proposed in [86] for computing the minimum eigenvalue–eigenvector pair without requiring the use of the Gram–Schmidt orthonormalization procedure.

The orthonormalization step, done using the Gram–Schmidt procedure, is a necessary step as it ensures that the vectors are mutually orthogonal. However, it can be costly if m, the number of principal eigenvectors, is close to K, the dimension of the data vector. We can avoid the Gram–Schmidt procedure by introducing a deflation step or, equivalently, an inflation step if we are interested in estimating the minimum eigenvectors [85]. More specifically, we can replace the data vector $\mathbf{x}(n)$ in Equation 8.249 by the vectors $\mathbf{x}_i(n)$, which are updated according to

$$\mathbf{x}_i(n) = \mathbf{x}_{i-1}(n) - \mathbf{w}_{i-1}(n) y_{i-1}(n), \quad i = 1, 2, \ldots, m \tag{8.250}$$

where $y_i(n) = \mathbf{w}_i^T(n-1)\mathbf{x}_i(n)$. To see that the preceding equation is indeed a deflation step, we first expand the $y_i(n)$ term in Equation 8.250 to get the equation:

$$\mathbf{x}_i(n) = \mathbf{x}_{i-1}(n) - \mathbf{w}_{i-1}(n)\mathbf{w}_{i-1}^T(n-1)\mathbf{x}_{i-1}(n) \tag{8.251}$$

and observe that this equation has the same form as Equation 8.231, assuming that the signal is relatively stationary and therefore $\mathbf{w}_{i-1}(n) \approx \mathbf{w}_{i-1}(n-1)$. The purpose of the deflation step is to make the ith largest eigenvalue of the original covariance matrix $R(n)$, the largest eigenvalue of the new covariance matrix $R_i(n) = E\left[\mathbf{x}_i(n)\mathbf{x}_i^T(n)\right]$. It can be shown that the vectors $\mathbf{w}_i(n)$, $i = 1, 2, \ldots, m$, converge asymptotically (assuming stationary data) to the m principal (and orthogonal) eigenvectors of $R(n)$, and therefore the explicit orthonormalization of these vectors via the Gram–Schmidt procedure is no longer required.

The modified algorithm that includes the deflation step is

$$\begin{aligned}
&\text{for } n = 1, 2, \ldots \\
&\qquad \mathbf{x}_1(n) = \mathbf{x}(n) \\
&\text{for } i = 1, 2, \ldots, m \\
&\qquad y_i(n) = \mathbf{w}_i^T(n-1)\mathbf{x}_i(n) \\
&\qquad \lambda_i(n) = \alpha\lambda_i(n-1) + |y_i(n)|^2 \\
&\qquad \hat{\mathbf{w}}_i(n) = \mathbf{w}_i(n-1) + \mu\mathbf{x}_i(n)y_i(n) \\
&\qquad \mathbf{w}_i(n) = \mathbf{w}_i(n) / \|\hat{\mathbf{w}}_i(n)\|_2 \\
&\qquad \mathbf{x}_{i+1}(n) = \mathbf{x}_i(n) - \mathbf{w}_i(n)y_i(n) \\
&\text{end}
\end{aligned} \tag{8.252}$$

where $\lambda_i(n)$ is the recursive estimate of the ith eigenvalue, assuming the covariance matrix $R(n)$ is updated according to Equation 8.238.

So far, we have considered computing adaptively the EVD by solving a constrained minimization problem. The EVD can also be computed by solving a nonconstrained minimization/maximization problem for tracking the noise/signal subspace. Nonconstrained problems are more attractive as we can use fast gradient search algorithms to solve these problems iteratively without being concerned about constraining the solution vectors to be mutually orthogonal. A nonconstrained approach was proposed in [55,86] for estimating the principal eigenvectors of the covariance matrix.

Consider the following scalar function:

$$\begin{aligned} J(W) &= E\,\|\mathbf{x} - WW^T\mathbf{x}\|^2 \\ &= \mathrm{tr}(R) - 2\,\mathrm{tr}(W^T R W) + \mathrm{tr}(W^T R W \cdot W^T W) \end{aligned} \tag{8.253}$$

where

$R \triangleq E[\mathbf{x} \cdot \mathbf{x}^T]$ is the true correlation matrix of the $K \times 1$ data vector $\mathbf{x}$

W is a $K \times m$ matrix

It can be proved that $J(W)$ has a global minimum at which the column span of W equals the signal subspace, that is, the span of the m principal eigenvectors of R [55]. It should be pointed out that the optimum W that minimizes $J(W)$ will not contain the m principal eigenvectors of R, but rather an arbitrary orthonormal basis of the signal subspace. In some applications (e.g., MUSIC algorithm), having access to an arbitrary orthonormal basis of the signal subspace is sufficient and does not require the explicit computation of eigenvectors. For our application, however, we are interested in computing explicitly the principal eigenvectors spanning the signal subspace. Such an approach was proposed by Yang in [55] based on the minimization of a modified cost function of the form

$$J'(W(n)) = \sum_{i=1}^{n} \alpha^{n-i}\,\|\mathbf{x}(i) - W(n)\mathbf{y}(i)\|^2 \tag{8.254}$$

where α is a forgetting factor

$$\mathbf{y}(i) = W^T(i-1) \cdot \mathbf{x}(i)$$

The exponentially weighted sum in the preceding equation is used to approximate the expectation in Equation 8.253. It is further assumed that the difference between $W^T(i-1) \cdot \mathbf{x}(i)$ and $W^T(n) \cdot \mathbf{x}(i)$ is very small. The main advantage in using the weighted least-squares criterion given earlier is that it is well suited for adaptive filtering applications and has been studied extensively [37, ch. 9]. The scalar function in Equation 8.254 is minimized by [37, p. 439]

$$W(n) = R_{xy}(n) R_{yy}^{-1}(n) \tag{8.255}$$

where

$$R_{xy}(n) \triangleq \sum_{i=1}^{n} \alpha^{n-i}\mathbf{x}(i)\mathbf{y}^T(i) = \alpha R_{xy}(n-1) + \mathbf{x}(n)\mathbf{y}^T(n)$$
$$R_{yy}(n) \triangleq \sum_{i=1}^{n} \alpha^{n-i}\mathbf{y}(i)\mathbf{y}^T(i) = \alpha R_{yy}(n-1) + \mathbf{y}(n)\mathbf{y}^T(n) \tag{8.256}$$

The optimum solution in Equation 8.255 requires the inversion of the matrix $R_{yy}(n)$ at each update. But since the structure of $R_{yy}(n)$ is suitable for the matrix inversion lemma [37, p. 440], we can obtain the inverse of $R_{yy}(n)$ recursively. This results in the well-known recursive least-squares (RLS) algorithm [37, ch. 9]. We can therefore use the traditional RLS algorithm to recursively update $W(n)$ in Equation 8.255, and after including a deflation step in the RLS algorithm, we get the following adaptive algorithm, called the PASTd algorithm [55], for estimating the m principal eigenvectors $\mathbf{w}_i(n)$ and corresponding eigenvalues $\lambda_i(m)$:

$$\begin{aligned}
&\text{for } n = 1, 2, \ldots \\
&\quad \mathbf{x}_1(n) = \mathbf{x}(n) \\
&\text{for } i = 1, 2, \ldots, m \\
&\quad y_i(n) = \mathbf{w}_i^T(n-1)\mathbf{x}_i(n) \\
&\quad \lambda_i(n) = \alpha\lambda_i(n-1) + |y_i(n)|^2 \\
&\quad \mathbf{e}_i(n) = \mathbf{x}_i(n) - y_i(n)\mathbf{w}_i(n-1) \\
&\quad \mathbf{w}_i(n) = \mathbf{w}_i(n-1) + \frac{y_i(n)}{\lambda_i(n)}\mathbf{e}_i(n) \\
&\quad \mathbf{x}_{i+1}(n) = \mathbf{x}_i(n) - \mathbf{w}_i(n)y_i(n) \\
&\text{end}
\end{aligned} \tag{8.257}$$

Note that aside from the deflation step, the preceding algorithm is identical to the recursive least-squares algorithm used for adaptive noise cancellation [37, p. 448] with $y_i(n)$ acting as the reference signal and $x_i(n)$ acting as the primary signal (see Figure 8.18). The vectors $\mathbf{w}_i(n)$ in Equation 8.257 will converge to the principal eigenvectors of the correlation matrix $R(n)$ (Equation 8.238), and the $\lambda_i(n)$ will converge to the corresponding principal eigenvalues. As argued in [55], the multiplication of $R_{yy}(n)$ by $R_{yy}^{-1}(n)$ in Equation 8.255 behaves like an approximate orthonormalization, and therefore the vectors $\mathbf{w}_i(n)$ do not need to be orthonormalized. The deflation step, however, introduces a slight loss of orthonormality between $\mathbf{w}_i(n)$ that depends on the SNR and the forgetting factor α. The preceding algorithm requires only 4 $Km + O(m)$ operations per update to estimate m principal eigenvectors.

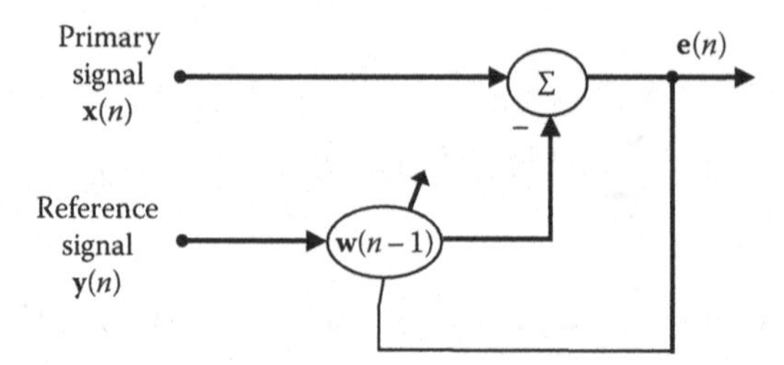

FIGURE 8.18 Schematic representation of the RLS algorithm used in the PASTd subspace-tracking algorithm.

Figure 8.19 gives an example of the estimation of the second largest eigenvalue for a short segment of speech using the PASTd algorithm (Equation 8.257). The bottom panel in Figure 8.19 shows the estimation of the second largest eigenvalue using the LMS algorithm [85] given in Equation 8.252. For comparative purposes, we superimpose the true eigenvalues of the covariance matrix $R(n)$, which are updated according to Equation 8.238. These eigenvalues are computed via an exact EVD. Both algorithms were initialized with $\lambda_i(0) = 1$ and $\mathbf{w}_i^T(0) = \mathbf{e}_i$, where $\mathbf{e}_i$ is the unit vector with one in the ith element. As can be seen in this example, the PASTd algorithm can track the second largest eigenvalues of $R(n)$ with good accuracy even when the second-order statistics of the signal change. The speech segment switched from being voiced (vowel/iy/) to being unvoiced (/s/) at about $n = 800$ samples. In contrast, the LMS algorithm failed to track accurately the eigenvalue when the speech segment switched from voiced to unvoiced. Note also that the LMS algorithm was

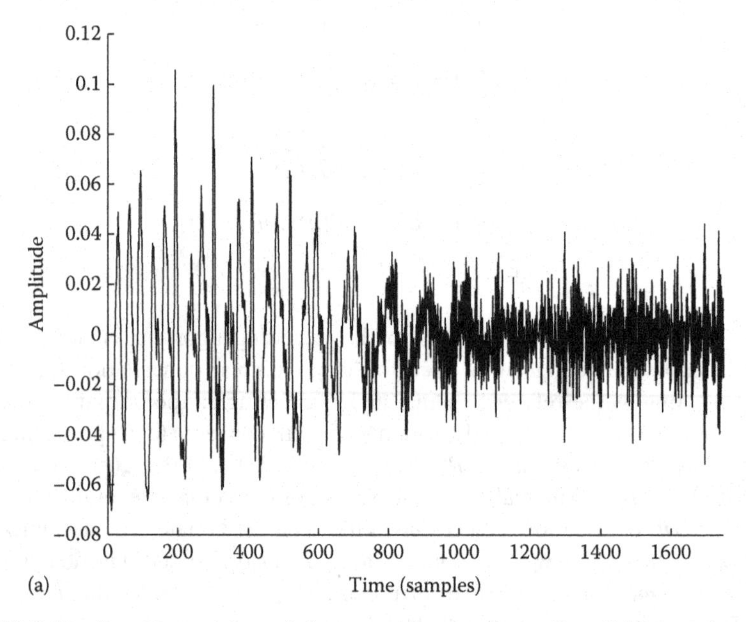

FIGURE 8.19 Running estimate of the second largest eigenvalue of the speech segment shown in panel (a) using two different subspace-tracking algorithms,

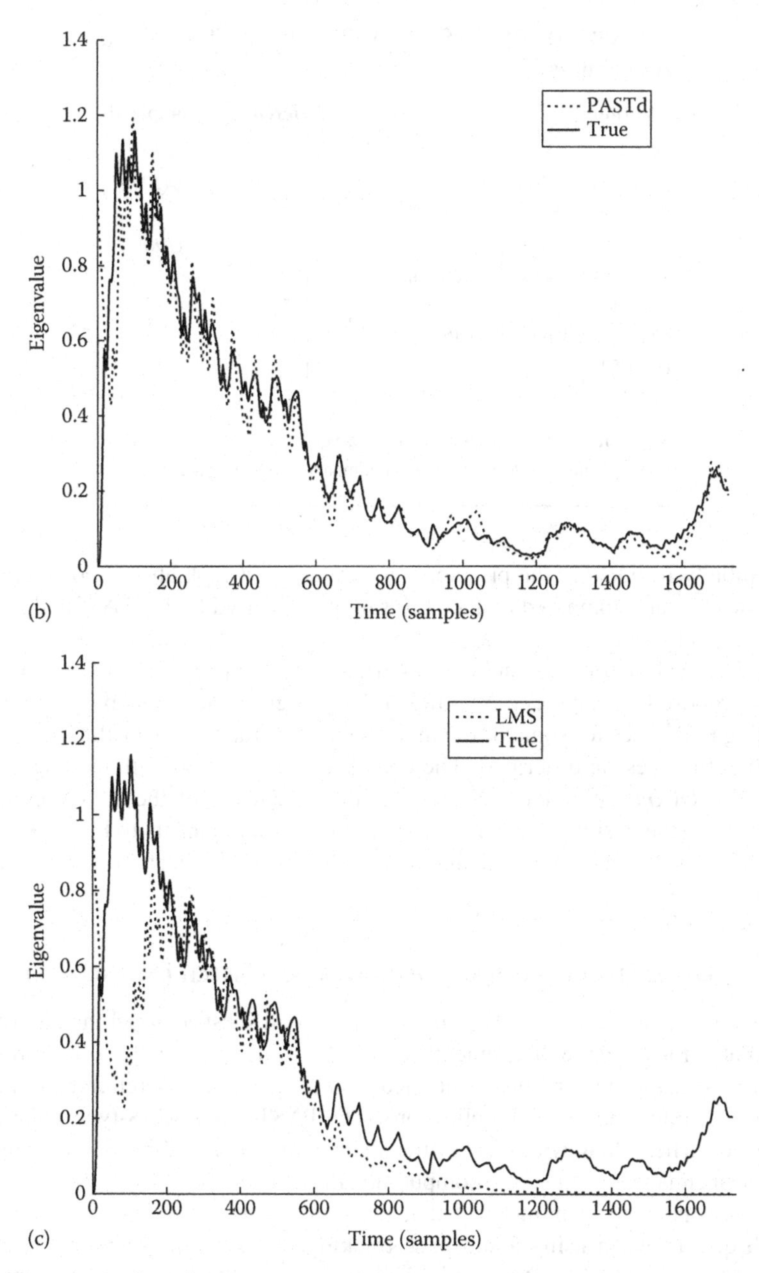

FIGURE 8.19 (continued) Running estimate of the second largest eigenvalue of the speech segment shown in panel (b) the PASTd algorithm and (c) an LMS-type algorithm. The true eigenvalues (obtained using EVD) are also shown (solid lines) for comparison.

TABLE 8.3
Complexity Involved in Various Subspace-Tracking Algorithms

Algorithm	Reference	Complexity
Direct	[8]	$O(K^3)$
Lanczos-type algorithms	[71,73]	$O(K^3m)$
Power methods	[8,72]	
FAST algorithm	[87]	$O(Km^2)$
Approximate subspace iteration	[71]	
PASTd	[55]	$O(Km)$
LMS-type adaptive algorithms	[85]	
IV-PAST	[88]	

Note: K is the dimension of the data vector, and m ($m < k$) is the number of principal eigen-components to be tracked.

slow initially in tracking the principal eigenvalue, as it took about 200 samples to reach steady state, compared to about 80 samples required for the PASTd algorithm to reach steady state.

We finally close this section by summarizing the complexity of the various algorithms proposed for subspace tracking. Table 8.3 gives the complexity and corresponding references for some of the major subspace-tracking algorithms proposed, including the ones we described. The complexity of these algorithms ranges from $O(K^2m)$ to $O(Km)$ operations, where K is the dimension of the data vector, and m ($m < K$) is the desired number of principal eigen-components to be tracked. We define one operation here to be equal to a single real multiplication or a single real addition.

8.10.3 Using Subspace-Tracking Algorithms in Speech Enhancement

As a word of caution, we need to point out that not all subspace-tracking algorithms are suitable for speech enhancement. Some algorithms (e.g., [80]) do not preserve the eigen-structure information contained in the signal, and therefore can only be used in a limited number of applications. The PASTd- and LMS-type algorithms described earlier, along with most of the algorithms listed in Table 8.3, are suitable for speech enhancement and are computationally efficient.

We also need to bear in mind that there might be a serious compromise in speech quality when using a subspace-tracking algorithm in place of the direct EVD of the covariance matrix. This is mainly due to the fact that the estimation of the covariance matrix can severely affect the quality of speech enhanced by subspace algorithms (see discussion in Section 8.6.3.1). The majority of the recursive class of subspace-tracking algorithms converge to the principal eigenvectors/eigenvalues of the matrix $R(n)$, which is updated according to Equation 8.238, that is, a covariance matrix that is based on exponentially weighted estimates of the autocorrelation. Such an estimate of the covariance matrix, however, might not be suitable for nonstationary signals such as the speech signal. The rectangular window-based estimate of the covariance matrix (see Equation 8.237) might be more appropriate for nonstationary signals. One solution to the stationarity issue, as suggested in [54], is to incorporate in the algorithm a mechanism by which the eigenvectors are only updated during speech activity. Such a mechanism would require an accurate voiced activity detector. Lastly, the rank-1 and rank-2 updates of the covariance matrix, although symmetric, do not possess a Toeplitz structure, which is more suitable for speech.

The adaptive algorithms (e.g., PASTd) proposed for subspace tracking are attractive in terms of low complexity; however, these algorithms need to be called more often compared to the direct methods for computing the EVD that are based on processing blocks of data (frames) every 5–10 ms. The update rate of adaptive algorithms needs to be on the order of a few samples rather than on the order of hundreds of samples. The requirement for a faster update rate may therefore overshadow the benefits of using an adaptive algorithm for tracking the signal subspace.

These and perhaps other issues associated with using subspace-tracking algorithms in speech enhancement have not been examined in the literature and warrant further investigation.

8.11 SUMMARY

This chapter presented subspace algorithms for speech enhancement. These algorithms were all based on the principle that the vector space of the noisy signal can be decomposed into "signal" and "noise" subspaces. The decomposition can be done using either the SVD of a Toeplitz-structured data matrix or the eigen-decomposition of a covariance matrix. Noise can be suppressed to some degree by keeping the components falling in the "signal" subspace and nulling the components falling into the "noise" subspace. Simply retaining the signal components, however, did not provide enough noise suppression, and in practice the signal components were subjected to further processing, implemented in the form of a diagonal gain matrix (see examples in Tables 8.1 and 8.2). Different methods for deriving the gain matrix were presented based on constrained or unconstrained minimization of various error criteria. Some criteria were based on the mathematically tractable square error, whereas other criteria were based on perceptually motivated measures. The majority of the subspace algorithms were originally formulated under the assumption that the additive noise is white. Extensions of the subspace algorithms to handle colored noise were also presented. The implementation of subspace algorithms requires a high computational load as an SVD or EVD needs to be performed in every frame. Subspace-tracking algorithms, which can be used to alleviate the heavy computational load, were also presented. These algorithms can recursively update and estimate the required number of eigenvectors and eigenvalues. The performance of the subspace algorithms in relation to the other speech enhancement algorithms described in the previous chapters was not presented. This performance comparison will be presented in Chapter 12.

REFERENCES

1. Pisarenko, V. (1973), The retrieval of harmonics from a covariance function, *Geophys. J. R. Astron. Soc.*, 33, 347–366.
2. Schmidt, R. (1979), Multiple emitter location and signal parameter estimation, *Proceedings of the RADC Spectrum Estimation Workshop*, Rome, NY, pp. 243–258.
3. Schmidt, R. (1981), A signal subspace approach to multiple source location and spectral estimation, PhD dissertation, Stanford University, Stanford, CA.
4. Deprettere, E. (1988), *SVD and Signal Processing: Algorithms, Applications and Architectures*, Amsterdam, the Netherlands: Elsevier Science.
5. Krim, H. and Viberg, M. (1996), Two decades of array signal processing research, *IEEE Signal Process. Mag.*, 13(4), 67–94.
6. Hermus, K., Wambacq, P., and Hamme, H. (2007), A review of signal subspace speech enhancement and its application to noise robust speech recognition, *EURASIP J. Advances Signal Process.*, Article ID 45821, 195.
7. Strang, G. (1988), *Linear Algebra and Its Applications*, 3rd ed., Orlando, FL: Harcourt.
8. Golub, G. and Van Loan, C. (1989), *Matrix Computations*, 2nd ed., Baltimore, MD: The Johns Hopkins University Press.
9. Huang, J. and Zhao, Y. (2000), A DCT-based fast signal subspace technique for robust speech recognition, *IEEE Trans. Speech Audio Process.*, 8(6), 747–751.
10. Vetter, R. (2001), Single channel speech enhancement using MDL-based subspace approach in Bark domain, *Proceedings of the IEEE International Conference on Acoustics, Speech, and Signal Processing*, Salt Lake City, UT, Vol. 1, pp. 641–644.
11. Ephraim, Y. and Van Trees, H.L. (1995), A signal subspace approach for speech enhancement, *IEEE Trans. Speech Audio Process.*, 3(4), 251–266.
12. Dendrinos, M., Bakamides, S., and Carayannis, G. (1991), Speech enhancement from noise: A regenerative approach, *Speech Commun.*, 10, 45–57.
13. Jensen, S., Hansen, P., Hansen, S., and Sorensen, J. (1995), Reduction of broadband noise in speech by truncated QSVD, *IEEE Trans. Speech Audio Process.*, 3(6), 439–448.
14. Moor, B. (1993), The singular value decomposition and long and short spaces of noisy matrices, *IEEE Trans. Signal Process.*, 41(9), 2826–2838.
15. Huffel, S. (1993), Enhanced resolution based on minimum variance estimation and exponential data modeling, *Signal Process.*, 33(3), 333–355.
16. Tufts, D. and Kumaresan, R. (1982), Estimation of frequencies of multiple sinusoids: Making linear prediction perform like maximum likelihood, *Proc. IEEE*, 70(9), 975–989.
17. Horn, R. and Johnson, C. (1985), *Matrix Analysis*, Cambridge, U.K.: Cambridge University Press.
18. Cadzow, J. (1984), SVD representation of unitarily invariant matrices, *IEEE Trans. Acoust. Speech Signal Process.*, 32(3), 512–516.
19. Lancaster, P. and Tismenetsky, M. (1985), *The Theory of Matrices*, 2nd ed., San Diego, CA: Academic Press.
20. Tufts, D., Kumaresan, R., and Kirsteins, I. (1982), Data adaptive signal estimation by singular value decomposition of a data matrix, *Proc. IEEE*, 70(6), 684–685.
21. Tufts, D. and Shah, A. (1993), Estimation of a signal waveform from noisy data using low-rank approximation to a data matrix, *IEEE Trans. Signal Process.*, 41(4), 1716–1721.
22. Dologlu, I. and Carayannis, G. (1991), Physical interpretation of signal reconstruction from reduced rank matrices, *IEEE Trans. Signal Process.*, 39(7), 1681–1682.
23. Chambers, J. (1977), *Computational Methods for Data Analysis*, New York: John Wiley & Sons.

24. Bakamides, S., Dendrinos, M., and Carayannis, G. (1991), SVD analysis by synthesis of harmonic signals, *IEEE Trans. Signal Process.*, 39(2), 472–477.
25. Konstantinides, K. and Yao, K. (1988), Statistical analysis of effective singular values in matrix rank determination, *IEEE Trans. Acoust. Speech Signal Process.*, 36(5), 757–763.
26. Hansen, P., Hansen, P., Hansen, S., and Sorensen, J. (1999), Experimental comparison of signal subspace based noise reduction methods, *Proceedings of the IEEE International Conference Acoustics, Speech, and Signal Processing*, Phoenix, AZ, Vol. I, pp. 101–104.
27. Hansen, P.S., Hansen, P.C., Hansen, S.D., and Sorensen, D. (1997), ULV-based signal subspace methods for speech enhancement, *International, Workshop on Acoustic Echo Noise Control*, London, U.K., pp. 9–12.
28. Luk, F. and Qiao, S. (1993), A new matrix decomposition for signal processing, in Moonen, M., Golub, G., and De Moor, B. (Eds.), *Linear Algebra for Large Scale and Real-Time Applications*, Amsterdam, the Netherlands: Kluwer, pp. 241–247.
29. Hansen, P. (1997), Signal subspace methods for speech enhancement, PhD thesis, Department of Mathematical Modeling, Technical University of Denmark, Kongens Lyngby, Denmark.
30. Kay, S. (1988), *Modern Spectral Estimation*, Englewood Cliffs, NJ: Prentice Hall.
31. Scharf, L. (1991), *Statistical Signal Processing*, Readings, MA: Addison-Wesley.
32. Hu, Y. and Loizou, P. (2004), Incorporating a psychoacoustical model in frequency domain speech enhancement, *IEEE Signal Process. Lett.*, 11(2), 270–273.
33. Gray, R.M. (1977), Toeplitz and circulant matrices, Technical Report 6504–1, Stanford University, Stanford, CA.
34. Hu, Y. and Loizou, P. (2003), A perceptually motivated approach for speech enhancement, *IEEE Trans. Speech Audio Process.*, 11(5), 457–465.
35. Jabloun, F. and Champagne, B. (2003), Incorporating the human hearing properties in the signal subspace approach for speech enhancement, *IEEE Trans. Speech Audio Process.*, 11(6), 700–708.
36. Marple, L. (1987), *Digital Spectral Analysis with Applications*, Englewood Cliffs, NJ: Prentice Hall.
37. Haykin, S. (2002), *Adaptive Filter Theory*, 4th ed., Englewood Cliffs, NJ: Prentice Hall.
38. Jabloun, F. and Champagne, B. (2006), Signal subspace techniques for speech enhancement, in Benesty, J., Makino, S., and Chen, J. (Eds.), *Speech Enhancement*, Berlin, Germany: Springer, pp. 135–159.
39. McWhorter, L. and Scharf, L. (1998), Multiwindow estimators of correlation, *IEEE Trans. Signal Process.*, 46(2), 440–448.
40. Thomson, D. (1982), Spectrum estimation and harmonic analysis, *Proc. IEEE*, 70(9), 1055–1096.
41. Slepian, D. (1978), Prolate spheroidal wave functions, Fourier analysis and uncertainty—V: The discrete case, *Bell Syst. Tech. J.*, 57, 1371–1430.
42. Hu, Y. and Loizou, P. (2003), A generalized subspace approach for enhancing speech corrupted by colored noise, *IEEE Trans. Speech Audio Process.*, 11, 334–341.
43. Hu, Y. (2003), Subspace and multitaper methods for speech enhancement, PhD dissertation, University of Texas-Dallas, Richardson, TX.
44. Ephraim, Y. and Van Trees, H.L. (1993), A signal subspace approach for speech enhancement, *Proceedings of the IEEE International Conference on Acoustics, Speech, and Signal Processing*, Minneapolis, MN, Vol. II, pp. 355–358.
45. Berouti, M., Schwartz, M., and Makhoul, J. (1979), Enhancement of speech corrupted by acoustic noise, *Proceedings of the IEEE International Conference on Acoustics, Speech, and Signal Processing*, Washington, DC, pp. 208–211.
46. Akaike, H. (1974), A new look at the statistical model identification, *IEEE Trans. Automat. Control*, AC-25, 996–998.

47. Rissanen, J. (1978), Modeling by shortest data description, *Automatica*, 14, 465–471.
48. Wax, M. and Kailath, T. (1985), Detection of signals by information theoretic criteria, *IEEE Trans Acoust. Speech Signal Process.*, 33, 387–392.
49. Merhav, N. (1989), The estimation of the model order in exponential families, *IEEE Trans. Inf. Theory*, 35(5), 1109–1113.
50. Stoica, P. and Selen, Y. (2004), Model-order selection, *IEEE Signal Process. Mag.*, 21(4), 36–47.
51. Klein, M. (2002), Signal subspace speech enhancement with perceptual post-filtering, MS thesis, McGill University, Montreal, Quebec, Canada.
52. Wilkinson, J.H. (1999), *The Algebraic Eigenvalue Problem*, New York: Oxford University Press.
53. Mittal, U. and Phamdo, N. (2000), Signal/noise KLT based approach for enhancing speech degraded by noise, *IEEE Trans. Speech Audio Process.*, 8(2), 159–167.
54. Rezayee, A. and Gazor, S. (2001), An adaptive KLT approach for speech enhancement, *IEEE Trans. Speech Audio Process.*, 9(2), 87–95.
55. Yang, B. (1995), Projection approximation subspace tracking, *IEEE Trans. Signal Process.*, 43(1), 95–107.
56. Bartels, R. and Stewart, G. (1972), Solution of the matrix equation AX + XB = C, *Commun. ACM*, 15(9), 820–826.
57. Lev-Ari, H. and Ephraim, Y. (2003), Extension of the signal subspace speech enhancement approach to colored noise, *IEEE Signal Process. Lett.*, 10(4), 104–106.
58. Luenberger, D. (1984), *Linear and Nonlinear Programming*, Reading, MA: Addison-Wesley.
59. Brandenburg, K. and Stoll, G. (1994), ISO-MPEG-1 audio: A generic standard for coding of high quality digital audio, *J. Audio Eng. Soc.*, 42, 780–792.
60. Johnston, J. (1988), Transform coding of audio signals using perceptual noise criteria, *IEEE J. Sel. Areas Commun.*, 6, 314–323.
61. You, C., Koh, S., and Rahardja, S. (2005), An invertible frequency eigendomain transformation for masking-based subspace speech enhancement, *IEEE Signal Process. Lett.*, 12(5), 461–464.
62. Hansen, P.C. and Jensen, S. (1998), FIR filter representations of reduced-rank noise reduction, *IEEE Trans. Signal Process.*, 46(6), 1737–1741.
63. Kim, J., Kim, S., and Yoo, C. (2003), The incorporation of masking threshold to subspace speech enhancement, *Proceedings of the IEEE International Conference on Acoustics, Speech, and Signal Processing*, Hong Kong, Vol. I, pp. 76–79.
64. Gustafsson, S., Jax, P., and Vary, P. (1998), A novel psychoacoustically motivated audio enhancement algorithm preserving background noise characteristics, *Proceedings of the IEEE International Conference on Acoustics, Speech, and Signal Processing*, Seattle, WA, pp. 397–400.
65. Klein, M. and Kabal, P. (2002), Signal subspace speech enhancement with perceptual post-filtering, *Proceedings of the IEEE International Conference on Acoustics, Speech, and Signal Processing*, Orlando, FL, Vol. I, pp. 537–540.
66. Schroeder, M., Atal, B., and Hall, J. (1979), Optimizing digital speech coders by exploiting masking properties of the human ear, *J. Acoust. Soc. Am.*, 66(6), 1647–1651.
67. Kroon, P. and Atal, B. (1992), Predictive coding of speech using analysis-by-synthesis techniques, in Furui, S. and Sondhi, M. (Eds.), *Advances in Speech Signal Processing*, New York: Marcel Dekker, pp. 141–164.
68. Atal, B. and Schroeder, M. (1979), Predictive coding of speech and subjective error criteria, *IEEE Trans. Acoust. Speech Signal Process.*, 27, 247–254.
69. Reddy, V., Mathew, G., and Paulraj, A. (1995), Some algorithms for eigensubspace estimation, *Digital Signal Process.*, 5, 97–115.

70. DeGroat, R., Dowling, E., and Linebarger, D. (1998), Subspace tracking, in Madisseti, V. and Williams, D. (Eds.), *The Digital Signal Processing Handbook*, Boca Raton, FL: CRC Press, pp. 66-1–66-15.
71. Comon, P. and Golub, G. (1990), Tracking a few extreme singular values and vectors in signal processing, *Proc. IEEE*, 78(8), 1327–1343.
72. Hua, Y. (2004), Asymptotical orthonormalization of subspace matrices without square root, *IEEE Signal Process. Mag.*, 21(4), 56–61.
73. Xu, G., Zha, M., Golub, G., and Kailath, T. (1994), Fast algorithms for updating signal subspaces, *IEEE Trans. Circuits Syst.-II*, 41(8), 537–549.
74. Hu, Y.H. and Kung, S.-Y. (1985), Toeplitz eigensystem solver, *IEEE Trans. Acoust. Speech Signal Process.*, 33(4), 1264–1271.
75. Hayes, M. and Clements, M. (1986), An efficient algorithm for computing Pisarenko's harmonic decomposition using Levinson's recursion, *IEEE Trans. Acoust. Speech Signal Process.*, 34(3), 485–491.
76. Morgera, S. and Noor, F. (1988), An eigenvalue recursion for Hermitian Toeplitz matrices, *Proc. IEEE Int. Conf. Acoust. Speech Signal Process.*, 3, 1647–1650.
77. Morgera, S. and Noor, F. (1993), Recursive and iterative algorithms for computing eigenvalues of Hermitian Toeplitz matrices, *IEEE Trans. Signal Process.*, 41(3), 1272–1280.
78. Elden, L. and Sjostrom, E. (1996), Fast computation of the principal singular vectors of Toeplitz matrices arising in exponential data modelling, *Signal Process.*, 50, 151–164.
79. Bunch, J., Nielsen, C., and Sorensen, D. (1978), Rank-one modification of the symmetric eigenvalue problem, *Numerische Mathematik*, 31, 31–48.
80. DeGroat, R. (1992), Noniterative subspace tracking, *IEEE Trans. Signal Process.*, 40(3), 571–577.
81. Golub, G. (1973), Some modified matrix eigenvalue problems, *SIAM Rev.*, 15(2), 318–334.
82. Cappe, O. (1994), Elimination of the musical noise phenomenon with the Ephraim and Malah noise suppressor, *IEEE Trans. Speech Audio Process.*, 2(2), 346–349.
83. DeGroat, R. and Roberts, R. (1988), A family of rank-one subspace updating methods, in Deprettere, E. (Ed.), *SVD and Signal Processing*, Amsterdam, the Netherlands: Elsevier Science, pp. 277–300.
84. Thompson, P. (1979), An adaptive spectral analysis technique for unbiased frequency estimation in the presence of white noise, *Proceedings of the 13th Asilomar Conference on Circuits, Systems and Computers*, Pacific Grove, CA, pp. 529–533.
85. Yang, J. and Kaveh, M. (1988), Adaptive eigensubspace algorithms for direction or frequency estimation and tracking, *IEEE Trans. Acoust. Speech Signal Process.*, 36(2), 241–251.
86. Reddy, V. and Kailath, T. (1982), Least squares type algorithm for adaptive implementation of Pisarenko's harmonic retrieval method, *IEEE Trans. Acoust. Speech Signal Process.*, 30(3), 399–405.
87. Real, E., Tufts, D., and Cooley, J. (1999), Two algorithms for fast approximate subspace tracking, *IEEE Trans. Signal Process.*, 47(7), 1936–1945.
88. Gustafsson, T. (1998), Instrumental variable subspace tracking using projection approximation, *IEEE Trans. Signal Process.*, 46(3), 669–681.

9 Noise-Estimation Algorithms

So far, we have assumed that an estimate of the noise spectrum is available. Such an estimate is critical for the performance of speech-enhancement algorithms as it is needed, for instance, to evaluate the Wiener filter in the Wiener algorithms or to estimate the *a priori* SNR in the MMSE algorithms or to estimate the noise covariance matrix in the subspace algorithms. The noise estimate can have a major impact on the quality of the enhanced signal. If the noise estimate is too low, annoying residual noise will be audible, and if the noise estimate is too high, speech will be distorted, possibly resulting in intelligibility loss. The simplest approach is to estimate and update the noise spectrum during the silent (e.g., during pauses) segments of the signal using a voice activity detection (VAD) algorithm. Although such an approach might work satisfactorily in stationary noise (e.g., white noise), it will not work well in more realistic environments (e.g., in a restaurant), wherein the spectral characteristics of the noise change constantly. This chapter focuses on a new class of algorithms that estimate the noise continuously, even during speech activity. As such, these algorithms are suitable for highly nonstationary noisy environments.

9.1 VOICE ACTIVITY DETECTION VS. NOISE ESTIMATION

The process of discriminating between voice activity (i.e., speech presence) and silence (i.e., speech absence) is called voice activity detection (VAD). VAD algorithms typically extract some type of feature (e.g., short-time energy, zero-crossings) from the input signal that is in turn compared against a threshold value, usually determined during speech-absent periods. VAD algorithms generally output a binary decision on a frame-by-frame basis, where a frame may last approximately 20–40 ms. A segment of speech is declared to contain voice activity (VAD = 1) if the measured values exceed a predefined threshold, otherwise it is declared as noise (VAD = 0).

Several VAD algorithms were proposed based on various types of features extracted from the signal [1–10]. The early VAD algorithms were based on energy levels and zero-crossings [10], cepstral features [4], the Itakura LPC spectral distance measure [9], and the periodicity measure [8]. Some of the VAD algorithms are used in several commercial applications including audioconferencing, the Pan-European digital cellular telephone (GSM) system [3], cellular networks [1], and digital cordless telephone systems [5]. VAD algorithms are particularly suited for discontinuous transmission in voice communication systems as they can be used to save the battery life of cellular phones. This is based on the fact that in a two-way telephone conversation, one party is active for only about 35% of the time [11]. A good review of VAD algorithms used in commercial voice communication standards can be found in [12, Chapter 10].

The VAD algorithms exploit the fact that there is silence not only at the beginning or end of a sentence but even in the middle of a sentence. These silent segments correspond to the closures of the stop consonants, primarily the unvoiced stop consonants, that is, /p/, /t/, /k/. Figure 9.1a shows as an example the TIMIT sentence "I'll have a scoop of that exotic, purple and turquoise sherbet" spoken by a female speaker. Note that in this sentence there are eight different individual silent segments, each of which can be used to estimate and update the noise spectrum. For this example, if we assume that the VAD algorithm correctly identifies the initial period as silence, then the next update of the noise spectrum would not occur until $t = 0.65$ s; that is, it would take 0.5 s before updating the noise spectrum. Within this 0.5 s period, however, the background noise might change. Hence, relying on the existence of a large number of stop-closures in the sentence is neither sufficient nor practical as the number of stop-closures varies depending on the sentence spoken. Different properties of the speech signal need to be exploited for better noise estimation.

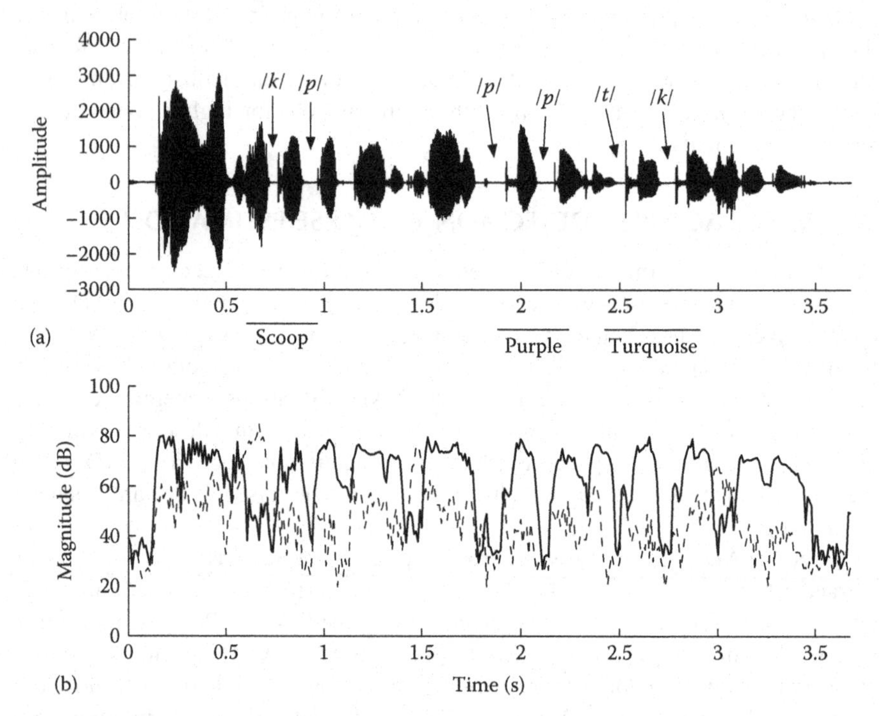

FIGURE 9.1 (a) Shows the waveform of the TIMIT sentence "I'll have a scoop of that purple and turquoise sherbet." Arrows indicate the silent intervals occurring within the sentence. These intervals correspond to the closures of the stop consonants indicated. (b) Shows a plot of the power spectral level at two frequencies, $f = 200$ Hz (solid line) and $f = 6000$ Hz (dashed line).

The majority of the VAD algorithms encounter problems in low-SNR conditions, particularly when the noise is nonstationary [1,2]. Also, some of those algorithms require tuning. Having an accurate VAD algorithm in a nonstationary environment might not be sufficient in speech-enhancement applications, as an accurate noise estimate is required at all times, even during speech activity. Noise-estimation algorithms that continuously track the noise spectrum are therefore more suited for speech-enhancement applications in nonstationary scenarios. This is a particularly challenging task, as we need to somehow estimate the noise spectrum even during speech activity. However, as we will see in this chapter, this can be accomplished by exploiting a few key properties of the speech signal.

9.2 INTRODUCTION TO NOISE-ESTIMATION ALGORITHMS

Noise-estimation algorithms are based on the following key observations:

Observation 1: The stop-closures are not the only silent segments in speech in which the spectral energy goes to zero or near the noise floor. "Silent" segments also occur during speech activity, specifically during

- Unvoiced fricatives at low frequencies, particularly below 2 kHz
- The vowels or generally during voiced sounds (semivowels, nasals), at high frequencies, above 4 kHz (see example in Figure 9.1b).

Owing to this nature of the speech signal, the noise will have a nonuniform effect on the speech spectrum. As a result, different frequency bands in the spectrum will have effectively different SNRs. If, for instance, the noise is low-pass in nature (e.g., car noise), then the high-frequency region of the spectrum will be affected the least, whereas the low-frequency region will be affected the most. Consequently, the noise spectrum can be estimated and updated more reliably based on information extracted from the high-frequency region of the noisy spectrum rather than the low-frequency region. More generally, for any type of noise we can estimate and update individual frequency bands of the noise spectrum whenever the probability of speech being absent at a particular frequency band is high or whenever the effective SNR at a particular frequency band is extremely low. These observations led to the recursive-averaging type of noise-estimation algorithms (e.g., [13–17]).

Observation 2: The power of the noisy speech signal in individual frequency bands often decays to the power level of the noise, even during speech activity. We can therefore obtain an estimate of the noise level in individual frequency bands by tracking the minimum, within a short window (0.4–1 s), of the noisy speech spectrum in each frequency band. As the minimum value is smaller than the average value, the noise estimate will always be biased toward smaller values. This observation led to the minima-tracking algorithms (e.g., [18,19]).

Observation 3: Histograms of energy values in individual frequency bands reveal that the most frequent value (i.e., the histogram maximum) corresponds to the noise level of the specified frequency band. In some cases, the histogram of spectral

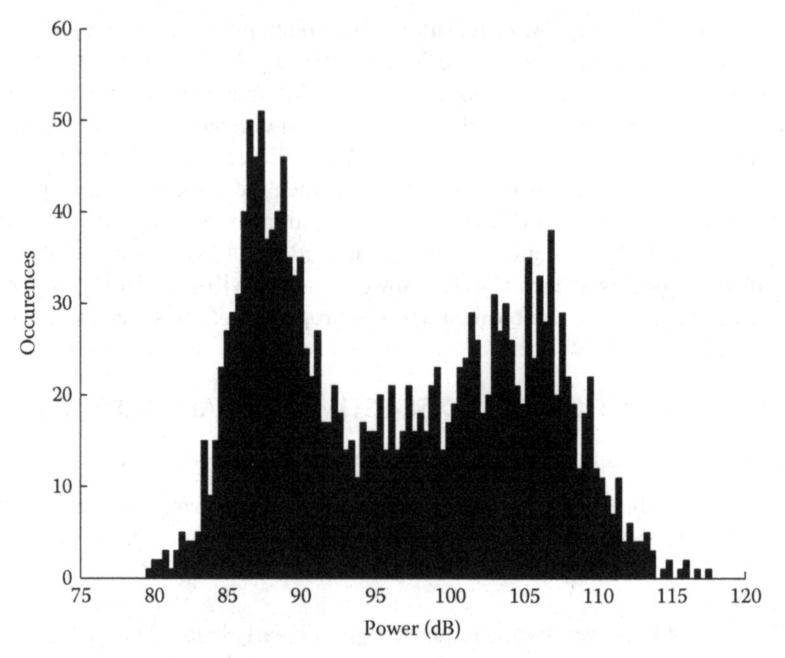

FIGURE 9.2 Histogram of power spectrum levels in the 200–400 Hz band for 18 s of speech. Power spectrum was computed using the FFT applied to 20 ms duration (nonoverlapping) frames of speech.

energy values contains two modes: (a) a low-energy mode corresponding to the silent and low-energy segments of speech, and (b) a high-energy mode corresponding to the (noisy) voiced segments of speech. The low-energy mode is larger (i.e., more frequent) than the high-energy one (see example in Figure 9.2). This pattern, however, is not consistent and depends among other things on the frequency band examined, the duration of the signal considered, and the type of noise. Our simulations indicated that the histogram is typically bimodal in the low frequencies, and monomodal in the mid to high frequencies. The observation that the maximum of the histogram of energy values of individual frequency bands is related to the noise level in the specified frequency bands led to histogram-based noise-estimation algorithms [20–22]. Algorithms based on order statistics [23] were also motivated by the preceding observations.

These three observations led to three main classes of noise-estimation algorithms:

1. Minimal-tracking algorithms
2. Time-recursive averaging algorithms
3. Histogram-based algorithms

All algorithms operate in the following fashion. First, the signal is analyzed using short-time spectra computed from short overlapping analysis frames, typically, 20–30 ms windows with 50% overlap between adjacent frames. Then, several consecutive frames, forming what we refer to as an *analysis segment*, are used in the computation of the noise spectrum. The typical time span of this segment may range from 400 ms to 1 s. The noise-estimation algorithms are based on the following assumptions:

1. The analysis segment is long enough to contain speech pauses and low-energy signal segments.
2. The noise present in the analysis segment is more stationary than speech. That is, noise changes at a relatively slower rate than speech.

The preceding assumptions impose contradictory restrictions on the duration of the analysis segment. The analysis segment has to be long enough to encompass speech pauses and low-energy segments, but it also has to be short enough to track fast changes in the noise level. As a result, the chosen duration of the analysis segment will result from a trade-off between these two restrictions.

9.3 MINIMAL-TRACKING ALGORITHMS

As mentioned earlier, the minimal-tracking algorithms are based on the assumption that the power of the noisy speech signal in individual frequency bands often decays to the power level of the noise, even during speech activity. Hence, by tracking the minimum of the noisy speech power in each frequency band, one can get a rough estimate of the noise level in that band. Two different algorithms were proposed for noise estimation. The first algorithm, called the *minimum-statistics* (MS) algorithm [18,24,25], tracks the minimum of the noisy speech power spectrum within a finite window (analysis segment), whereas the second algorithm [19] tracks the minimum continuously without requiring a window.

9.3.1 Minimum Statistics Noise Estimation

9.3.1.1 Principles

Let $y(n) = x(n) + d(n)$ denote the noisy speech signal, where $x(n)$ is the clean signal and $d(n)$ is the noise signal. We assume that $x(n)$ and $x(n)$ are statistically independent and zero mean. The noisy signal is transformed in the frequency domain by first applying a window $w(n)$ to M samples of $y(n)$ and then computing the M-point FFT of the windowed signal:

$$Y(\lambda, k) = \sum_{m=0}^{M-1} y(\lambda M + m) w(m) e^{-j2\pi mk/M} \tag{9.1}$$

where

λ indicates the frame index

k ($k = 0, 1, 2, \ldots, M-1$) indicates the frequency bin index

Note that $Y(\lambda, k)$ is the STFT of $y(n)$ (Chapter 2). Owing to the assumed independence of speech and noise, the periodogram of the noisy speech is approximately equal to the sum of the periodograms of clean speech and noise, respectively; that is,

$$|Y(\lambda,k)|^2 \approx |X(\lambda,k)|^2 + |D(\lambda,k)|^2 \tag{9.2}$$

where $|Y(\lambda, k)|^2$, $|X(\lambda, k)|^2$, and $|D(\lambda, k)|^2$ are the periodograms of noisy speech, clean speech, and noise, respectively. Because of this assumption, we can estimate the noise power spectrum by tracking the minimum of the periodogram $|Y(\lambda, k)|^2$ of the noisy speech over a fixed window length. This window length is chosen wide enough to bridge the broadest peak in the speech signal. It was found out experimentally [18,25] that window lengths (analysis segments) of approximately 0.8–1.4 s gave good results.

The periodogram $|Y(\lambda, k)|^2$ fluctuates very rapidly over time; hence, it is preferable to use a first-order recursive version of the periodogram:

$$P(\lambda,k) = \alpha P(\lambda-1,k) + (1-\alpha)|Y(\lambda,k)|^2 \tag{9.3}$$

where α is the smoothing constant. The preceding recursive equation, which can easily be recognized as an IIR low-pass filter, provides a smoothed version of the periodogram $|Y(\lambda, k)|^2$. We can obtain an estimate of the power spectrum of the noise by tracking the minimum of $P(\lambda, k)$ over a finite window. Figure 9.3 shows an example of minimal

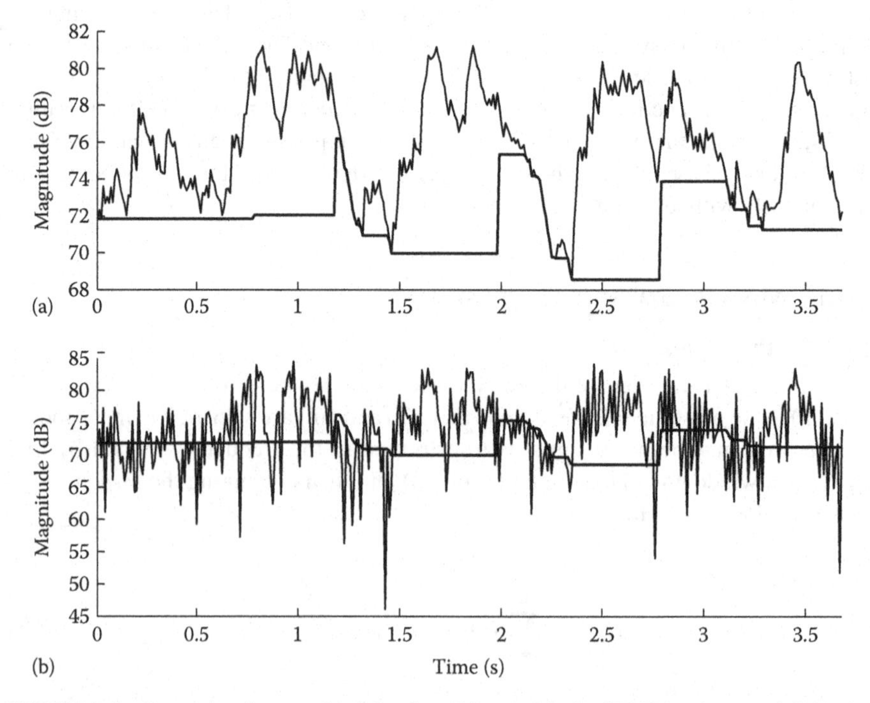

FIGURE 9.3 Example of spectral minimal tracking (at bin $f = 200$ Hz) using $\alpha = 0.8$ for the smoothing factor. (a) Shows the smoothed power spectrum of noisy speech superimposed on the spectral minima. (b) Shows the true noise power spectrum superimposed on the estimated noise power spectrum based on spectral minima tracking.

tracking using $\alpha = 0.8$ and a 400-ms window. Figure 9.3a shows $P(\lambda, k)$ along with the noise estimate (thick line) for an individual frequency bin corresponding to $f = 200$ Hz. Figure 9.3b shows the true noise spectrum at $f = 200$ Hz along with the estimated noise spectrum. It is clear from Figure 9.3b that the estimate of the noise level tends to be lower than the true noise level—see, for instance, the segment from $t = 1.5$ to 2 s or from $t = 2.4$ to 2.8 s; that is, the noise estimate tends to be biased toward lower values.

In the preceding example, we used $\alpha = 0.8$ in Equation 9.3. However, that choice is not optimal by any means. Figure 9.4 shows $P(\lambda, k)$ for three different values of the smoothing constant α. The spectrum becomes increasingly smoother as the value of the smoothing constant (α) approaches one. As a consequence, the speech peaks become broader (compare Figure 9.4a and c at $t = 0.7$–1.3 s) and the small notches in the speech spectrum are eliminated. Oversmoothing might lead to inaccurate estimates of the noise level, as the minimum might slip into the broad peak (see, for instance, the minimum estimate at $t = 1.2$ s in Figure 9.4c), thereby overestimating the true noise level. Ideally, for better noise tracking we would like α to be close to zero when speech is present. Note that when $\alpha \approx 0$, $P(\lambda, k) \approx |Y(\lambda, k)|^2$ and therefore the minimum will be extracted from the nonsmoothed periodogram.

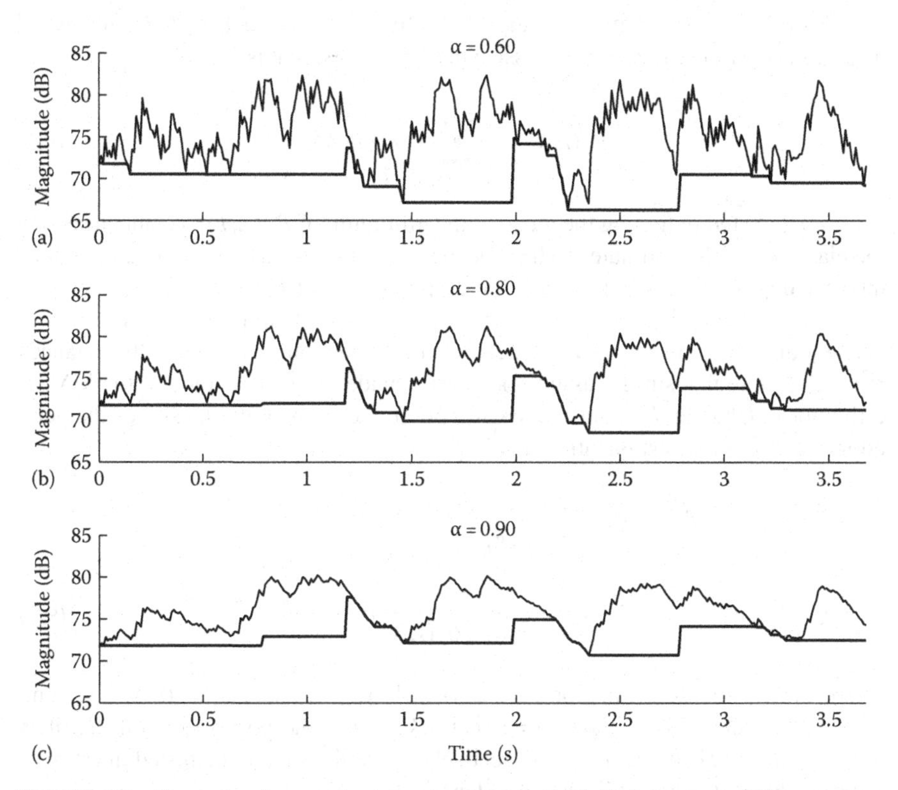

FIGURE 9.4 Example of spectral minimum tracking (thick line) for three different values of α ($f = 200$ Hz). Plot (a), (b) and (c) show the smoothed power spectrum (thin line) of noisy speech superimposed on spectral minima with different value of smoothing factor α.

The examples in Figures 9.3 and 9.4 indicate two main issues with the spectral minimal-tracking approach: the existence of a bias in the noise estimate and the possible overestimate of the noise level because of inappropriate choice of the smoothing constant. A better (more accurate) noise-estimation algorithm can be developed by (a) deriving a bias factor to compensate for the lower noise values and (b) incorporating a smoothing constant that is not fixed but varies with time and frequency.

9.3.1.2 Derivation of the Bias Factor

For nontrivial probability densities, the minimum of a set of random variables is smaller than their mean, and therefore the estimate of the noise level, based on MS, will be biased toward lower values. We can use the estimate of the mean of the minimum of a sequence of random variables to compensate for this inherent bias. More precisely, we can compensate for the bias by multiplying the noise power spectrum density (psd) estimate, computed from MS, by the reciprocal of the estimate of the mean of the minimum of sequence of random variables. In our case, the sequence of random variables corresponds to $P(\lambda, k)$ in Equation 9.3, for $\{\lambda, \lambda-1, \ldots, \lambda-D+1\}$, where D is the search window (i.e., analysis segment) given in terms of the number of past frames. To estimate the mean of the minimum of $P(\lambda, k)$ over$\{\lambda, \lambda-1, \ldots, \lambda-D+1\}$, we will first need to compute the pdf of the individual power estimate $P(\lambda, k)$.

For simplicity, let us first consider the case of computing $P(\lambda, k)$ by means of nonrecursive smoothing of L successive periodograms; that is,

$$P_{nr}(\lambda,k)=\frac{1}{L}\sum_{m=0}^{L-1}|Y(\lambda-m,k)|^2 \tag{9.4}$$

We are interested in finding the mean of the minimum of $P_{nr}(\lambda, k)$ to compensate for the bias in the noise estimate. To find the mean, we first need to determine the pdf of the periodogram $|Y(\lambda, k)|^2$ and from that derive the pdf of $P_{nr}(\lambda, k)$.

We assume that the real and imaginary parts of $Y(\lambda, k)$ in Equation 9.1 are independent and are modeled by zero-mean Gaussian random variables with variances $\sigma_y^2(\lambda,k)/2$ (note that similar assumptions were made in the derivation of the MMSE estimator in Chapter 7). Under this assumption, the probability density of the periodogram $|Y(\lambda, k)|^2$ is exponential; that is,

$$\begin{aligned} f_{|Y(\lambda,k)|^2}(x) &= \frac{u(x)}{\sigma_y^2(\lambda,k)}e^{-x/\sigma_y^2(\lambda,k)} \\ &= \frac{u(x)}{\sigma_d^2(\lambda,k)+\sigma_x^2(\lambda,k)}e^{-x/\left(\sigma_d^2(\lambda,k)+\sigma_x^2(\lambda,k)\right)} \end{aligned} \tag{9.5}$$

where $u(x)$ is the step function (i.e., $u(x) = 1$, $x \geq 1$ and $u(x) = 0$, $x < 0$), and $\sigma_x^2(\lambda,k)=E\{|X(\lambda,k)|^2\}$, $\sigma_d^2(\lambda,k)=E\{|D(\lambda,k)|^2\}$ are the power spectral densities of the clean signal and the noise, respectively. Note that we are interested in estimating $\sigma_d^2(\lambda,k)$, that is, the noise spectral density.

The pdf of $P_{nr}(\lambda, k)$ in Equation 9.4 can be derived analytically if we assume that the L successive periodogram estimates, that is, $\{|Y(\lambda,k)|^2$, $|Y(\lambda-1,k)|^2$,

$|Y(\lambda-2,k)|^2,\ldots,|Y(\lambda-L+1,k)|^2\}$, are independent and identically distributed. Under this assumption, $P_{nr}(\lambda, k)$ will have a chi-square distribution with mean $N\sigma^2(k)$:

$$f_{P_{nr}}(y)=\frac{1}{\sigma^N(k)2^{N/2}\Gamma(N/2)}y^{N/2-1}e^{-y/2\sigma^2(k)} \quad y\geq 0 \tag{9.6}$$

where $N = 2L$ is the number of degrees of freedom for all frequency bins except the DC and Nyquist frequency bins, $N = L$ otherwise, $\Gamma(\cdot)$ is the Gamma function, and $\sigma^2(k)=\sigma_y^2(k)/2=(\sigma_x^2(k)+\sigma_d^2(k))/2$ is the variance of the real and imaginary parts of $Y(\lambda,k)$. The mean of $P_{nr}(\lambda, k)$ is equal to $N\sigma^2(k)$, and the variance of $P_{nr}(\lambda, k)$ is equal to $2N\sigma^4(k)$. Note that during speech pauses, $\sigma_x^2(k)=0$ and the variance of $P_{nr}(\lambda, k)$ is equal to $N\sigma_d^4(k)/2$. The preceding chi-square distribution of $P_{nr}(\lambda, k)$ reduces to an exponential distribution when $N = 2$.

As the periodogram estimates are computed using speech segments that overlap (typically by 50%), the chi-square distribution of $P_{nr}(\lambda, k)$ will have less than N degrees of freedom. Estimates of equivalent degrees of freedom for overlapping speech segments were provided by Welch [26] for both recursive (as in Equation 9.3) and nonrecursive (as in Equation 9.4) type of smoothing. The equivalent degrees of freedom for recursive periodogram smoothing (as done in Equation 9.3) are given by the following formula [25,26]:

$$N_{rec}\approx 2\frac{1+\alpha}{(1-\alpha)f(\alpha)} \tag{9.7}$$

where
- α is the smoothing constant (Equation 9.3)
- $f(\alpha)$ are functions of L and the type of window used

So, regardless of the type of smoothing (recursive or nonrecursive) we apply to the periodograms, the resulting pdf of $P(\lambda, k)$ will be chi-square. The difference will be in the number of degrees of freedom.

We are now in a position to compute the probability density of the minimum power estimate, which we denote by $P_{\min}(\lambda, k)$, based on D independent (and identically distributed) power estimates, $P(\lambda, k)$, obtained at $\{\lambda,\lambda-1,\ldots,\lambda-D+1\}$. We define $P_{\min}(\lambda, k)$ as

$$P_{\min}(\lambda,k)=\min\{P(\lambda,k),P(\lambda-1,k),\ldots,P(\lambda-D+1,k)\} \tag{9.8}$$

Based on [27, p. 246], the pdf of $P_{\min}(\lambda, k)$ is given by

$$f_{P_{\min}}(y)=D\cdot(1-F_{P_y}(y))^{D-1}f_{P_y}(y) \tag{9.9}$$

where
- $f_{P_y}(y)$ is given by Equation 9.6
- $F_{P_y}(y)$ denotes the cumulative distribution function of the chi-square density [28, p. 42]:

$$F_{P_y}(y)=1-e^{-y/2\sigma^2(k)}\sum_{m=0}^{N/2-1}\frac{1}{m!}\left(\frac{y}{2\sigma^2(k)}\right)^m \quad y\geq 0 \tag{9.10}$$

Using Equations 9.9 and 9.10, we can evaluate the mean of the minimum power estimate $P_{min}(\lambda, k)$. Without loss of generality, we can assume that $\sigma^2(k) = 1$. We can compensate for the bias by multiplying the minimum estimate by the inverse of the mean evaluated at $\sigma^2(k) = 1$; that is, we can compute the bias of the minimum estimate as

$$B_{min} = \frac{1}{E\{P_{min}(\lambda, k)\}\,|_{\sigma^2(k)=1}} \tag{9.11}$$

Figure 9.5 shows the evaluation of $E\{P_{min}(\lambda, k)\} = 1/B_{min}$ for different values of D (i.e., the number of frames involved in the search of the minimum) and different degrees of freedom N. The mean $E\{P_{min}(\lambda, k)\}$ was evaluated numerically. As the figure shows, the bias B_{min} is influenced by both the value of D (i.e., the search window) and the degrees of freedom (i.e., the number of past periodograms used to compute the smooth power estimate $P(\lambda, k)$). For a fixed value of D ($D > 60$), the bias is inversely proportional to the degrees of freedom; that is, the larger the number of degrees of freedom, or equivalently the larger the number of past periodograms considered in the estimate of the smoothed power spectrum $P(\lambda, k)$, the smaller the bias. Speech, however, is highly nonstationary, and in practice we

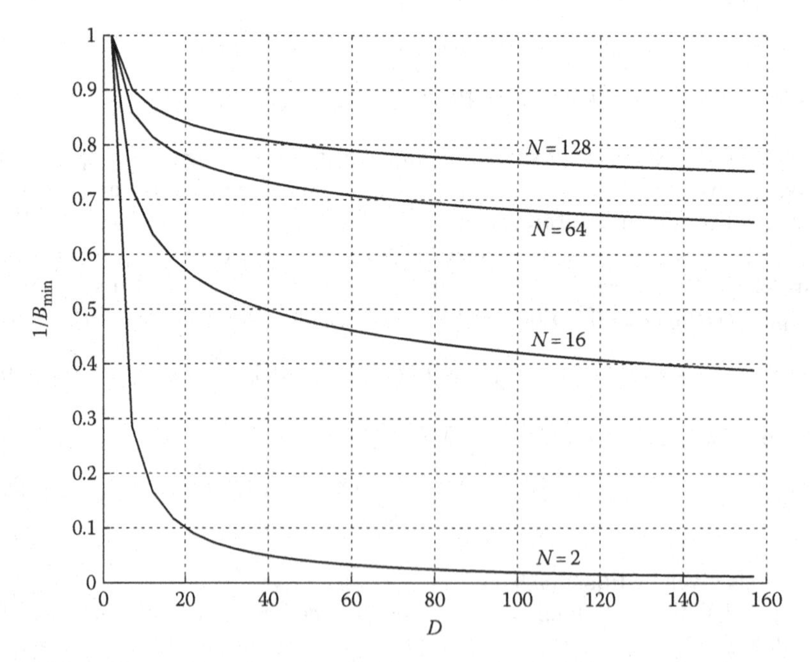

FIGURE 9.5 Plot of the reciprocal of the bias factor, that is, $1/B_{min}$, as a function of D (the number of frames involved in the search window) for different values of N, the number of past periodograms used to compute the smooth power spectrum.

cannot use an infinitely large number of past periodogram estimates to compute $P(\lambda, k)$ in Equation 9.4. In practice, exponential weighting is used in the smoothing, as in Equation 9.3, to emphasize recent power estimates and deemphasize old estimates.

The derivation of the bias in Equation 9.11 was based on the assumption that successive values of $P(\lambda, k)$ were uncorrelated. In practice, successive values of $P(\lambda, k)$ are correlated, but there is no known analytical expression for the pdf of $P_{\min}(\lambda, k)$. Consequently, we are unable to compute numerically the mean of $P_{\min}(\lambda, k)$. We can, however, use simulations to estimate the mean of the minimum of $P(\lambda, k)$ over D consecutive segments. Specifically, we can generate large amounts of exponentially distributed data with unit variance and average the minimum values for various values of D. Simulations in [18] showed that the values of the mean $E\{P_{\min}(\lambda, k)\}$ plotted as a function of D are very similar to those shown in Figure 9.5. Using an asymptotic finding in [29, Sec. 7.2], Martin [18] approximated the bias factor $B_{\min}$ using the following equation:

$$B_{\min}(\lambda,k) \approx 1 + (D-1)\frac{2}{\hat{Q}_{eq}(\lambda,k)} \tag{9.12}$$

where D is the window length (in number of frames) over which the minimum is searched, and $\hat{Q}_{eq}(\lambda, k)$ is proportional to the "equivalent degrees of freedom" and is given by

$$\hat{Q}_{eq}(\lambda,k) = \frac{Q_{eq}(\lambda,k) - M(D)}{1 - M(D)} \tag{9.13}$$

where $M(D)$ is a function of the number of frames, D, and takes values in the range of zero to one [18, p. 512]. The term $Q_{eq}(\lambda, k)$ in Equation 9.13 was defined in [18] as the normalized variance and is given by

$$Q_{eq}(\lambda,k) = 2\sigma_d^4(\lambda,k) / \mathrm{var}(P(\lambda,k)) \tag{9.14}$$

For nonrecursive smoothing of the power spectrum (i.e., according to Equation 9.4), recall that $\mathrm{var}(P(\lambda,k)) = N\sigma_d^4(\lambda,k)/2$ (during speech pauses, $\sigma_x^2(k) = 0$), and therefore $Q_{eq}(\lambda, k) = 4/N$, where N is the number of degrees of freedom.

Note that according to Equation 9.12, the bias factor is inversely proportional to the degrees of freedom, consistent with the bias found for uncorrelated data (see Figure 9.5). Because of the dependence on $Q_{eq}(\lambda, k)$, the bias factor $B_{\min}(\lambda, k)$ is no longer constant but varies across time (λ) and frequency (k). Computation of $Q_{eq}(\lambda, k)$ in Equation 9.14 requires access to the noise psd squared, that is, $\sigma_d^4(\lambda, k)$, which we do not have. In practice, we can use the noise estimate obtained in the previous frame, that is, $\hat{\sigma}_d^4(\lambda-1,k)$. Computation of $Q_{eq}(\lambda, k)$

also requires knowledge of the variance of $P(\lambda, k)$, which can be approximated according to

$$\widehat{\text{var}}\{P(\lambda,k)\} = \widehat{P^2}(\lambda,k) - \bar{P}^2(\lambda,k) \tag{9.15}$$

where

$\widehat{P^2}(\lambda,k)$ is an estimate of the second moment of $P(\lambda, k)$ (i.e., $E\{P^2(\lambda, k)\}$)
$\bar{P}^2(\lambda, k)$ is the estimate of the mean of $P(\lambda, k)$ squared (i.e., $(E\{P(\lambda, k)\})^2$), both obtained using first-order smoothing

The normalized variance $1/Q_{eq}(\lambda, k)$ in Equation 9.14 is approximated as

$$\frac{1}{Q_{eq}(\lambda,k)} \approx \frac{\widehat{\text{var}}(P(\lambda,k))}{2\hat{\sigma}_d^4(\lambda-1,k)} \tag{9.16}$$

where $\widehat{\text{var}}(P(\lambda,k))$ is given by Equation 9.15. The normalized variance $1/Q_{eq}(\lambda, k)$ was limited in [18] to a maximum of 0.5, corresponding to a minimum of $Q_{eq}(\lambda, k) = 2$. These constraints on the values of $1/Q_{eq}(\lambda, k)$ limit the range of values that the bias factor $B_{min}(\lambda, k)$ in Equation 9.12 can take to a minimum of one and a maximum of D. The bias factor $B_{min}(\lambda, k)$ attains its maximum value of D when $Q_{eq}(\lambda, k) = 2$. Figure 9.6 plots the bias factor $B_{min}(\lambda, k)$ for a single-frequency bin for a 4 s segment of speech corrupted in +5 dB noise (multitalker babble). For this example, $D = 150$ and $B_{min}(\lambda, k)$ attains sometimes the

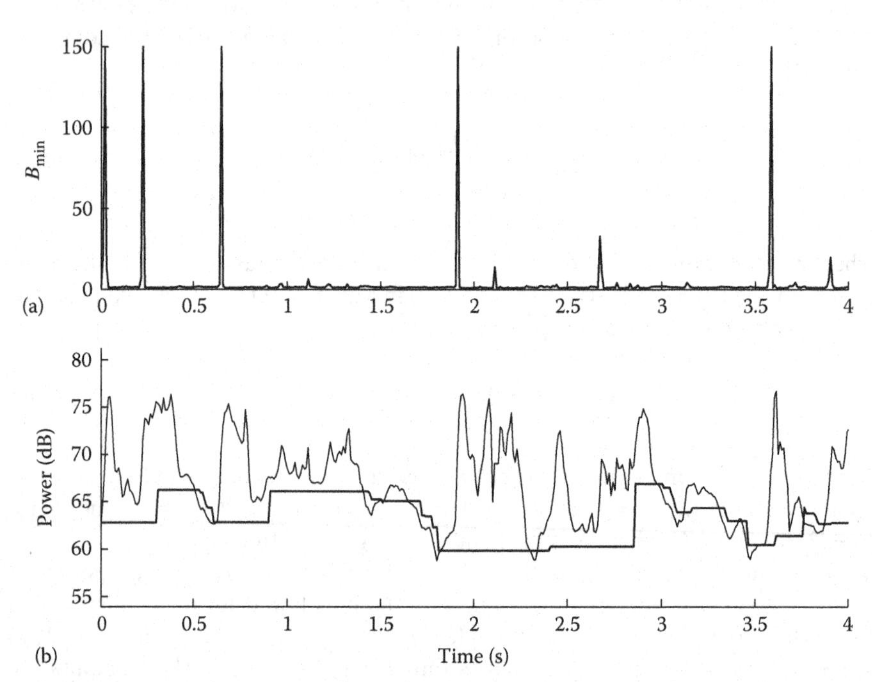

FIGURE 9.6 (a) Shows the plot of the estimated bias factor $B_{min}(\lambda, k)$, computed according to Equation 9.12 for a sentence embedded in 5-dB multitalker babble ($f = 200$ Hz). (b) Shows the smoothed power spectrum superimposed on the noise power spectrum (thick line) estimated using the MS algorithm.

maximum value of 150. Note that this situation occurs primarily when we have a sudden increase in noisy speech power $P(\lambda, k)$ (see, for instance, the segments at $t = 0.7$, 1.8, and 3.6s shown in Figure 9.6a). A sudden increase in $P(\lambda, k)$ increases the variance of $P(\lambda, k)$ in Equation 9.16, making the value of $Q_{eq}(\lambda, k)$ small (see Equation 9.14). A small value of $Q_{eq}(\lambda, k)$ in turn increases the value of $B_{\min}(\lambda, k)$ according to Equation 9.12. As a result, $B_{\min}(\lambda, k)$ attains a large value whenever $P(\lambda, k)$ increases abruptly.

Finally, following the computation of $B_{\min}(\lambda, k)$, the unbiased noise estimate at frame λ is obtained by

$$\hat{\sigma}_d^2(\lambda, k) = B_{\min}(\lambda, k) \cdot P_{\min}(\lambda, k) \tag{9.17}$$

where

$B_{\min}(\lambda, k)$ is given by Equation 9.12
$P_{\min}(\lambda, k)$ is given by Equation 9.8

9.3.1.3 Derivation of Optimal Time- and Frequency-Dependent Smoothing Factor

As discussed earlier, the smoothing parameter used in Equation 9.3 can affect the estimate of the noise level. If it is chosen too large (close to one), then the minimum might slip into a broad speech peak, resulting in overestimation of the noise level (see example in Figure 9.4). Ideally, we would like the smoothing parameter to be small only during speech activity to better track the nonstationarity of the speech signal. Hence, there is a need to make the smoothing factor time and frequency dependent, taking into account the presence or absence of speech activity.

We can derive the smoothing constant by requiring that the smoothed power spectrum $P(\lambda, k)$ be equal to the noise psd $\sigma_d^2(\lambda, k)$ during speech pauses. More specifically, we can derive an optimal smoothing parameter by minimizing the mean squared error (MSE) between $P(\lambda, k)$ and $\sigma_d^2(\lambda, k)$ as follows:

$$E\left\{\left(P(\lambda, k) - \sigma_d^2(\lambda, k)\right)^2 \mid P(\lambda - 1, k)\right\} \tag{9.18}$$

where

$$P(\lambda, k) = \alpha(\lambda, k)P(\lambda, k) + (1 - \alpha(\lambda, k))\left|Y(\lambda, k)\right|^2 \tag{9.19}$$

Note that we now use a time–frequency-dependent smoothing factor $\alpha(\lambda, k)$ in place of the fixed α in Equation 9.3. Substituting Equation 9.19 in Equation 9.18 and after taking the first derivative of the MSE with respect to $\alpha(\lambda, k)$ and setting it equal to zero, we get the optimum value for $\alpha(\lambda, k)$:

$$\begin{aligned}\alpha_{opt}(\lambda, k) &= \frac{1}{1 + \left(P(\lambda - 1, k)/\sigma_d^2(\lambda, k) - 1\right)^2} \\ &= \frac{1}{1 + (\bar{\gamma} - 1)^2}\end{aligned} \tag{9.20}$$

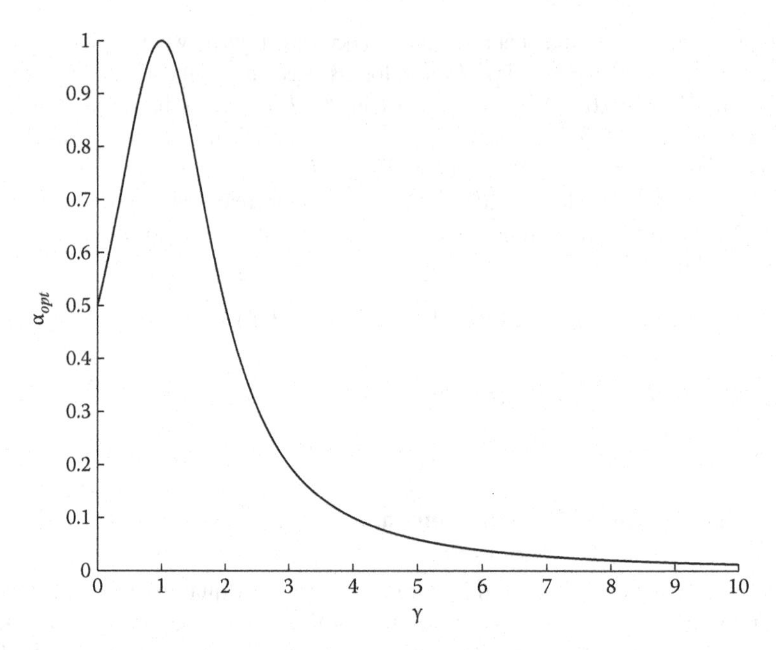

FIGURE 9.7 Plot of $\alpha_{opt}(\lambda, k)$ (Equation 9.20) as a function of the smooth *a posteriori* SNR $\bar{\gamma}$.

where $\bar{\gamma} \triangleq P(\lambda-1,k)/\sigma_d^2(\lambda,k)$ is recognized as a smoothed *a posteriori* SNR. Figure 9.7 plots $\alpha_{opt}(\lambda, k)$ as a function of the smoothed *a posteriori* SNR $\bar{\gamma}$. Note that $\alpha_{opt}(\lambda, k)$ is always positive and smaller than one, attaining a maximum at $\bar{\gamma} = 1$. The smoothing parameter $\alpha_{opt}(\lambda, k)$ gets progressively smaller for large values of $\bar{\gamma}$, which are attained typically during speech activity. Hence, the smoothing parameter $\alpha_{opt}(\lambda, k)$ possesses the desired behavior of being small when speech is present (i.e., for large $\bar{\gamma}$) for better minimum tracking. Figure 9.8 shows the smoothed power spectrum (Figure 9.8b) for a speech sentence degraded by 5 dB babble noise and the corresponding smoothing factor $\alpha_{opt}(\lambda, k)$ (Figure 9.8a). As can be seen, the smoothing constant decreases to near zero when the speech power increases, for better tracking of changes in the psd, and becomes close to one (see segments at t = 1.4–1.9 s and t = 3–3.5 s) when speech is absent, to reduce the variance of the minimum.

From Equation 9.20 we note that $\alpha_{opt}(\lambda, k)$ depends on the true noise psd $\sigma_d^2(\lambda,k)$, which we do not have. In practice, we can replace $\sigma_d^2(\lambda,k)$ with the latest estimated value $\hat{\sigma}_d^2(\lambda-1,k)$, where the $\wedge$ notation is used to indicate estimated values. The noise estimate, $\hat{\sigma}_d^2(\lambda-1,k)$, however, in general lags the true noise psd, and as a result the estimated smoothing parameter may be too small or too large. Problems may arise when $\alpha_{opt}(\lambda, k)$ is close to one because $P(\lambda, k)$ will not respond fast enough to changes of the noise. Hence, we need to somehow detect tracking errors and adjust the smoothing parameter accordingly. Tracking errors were monitored in [18] by comparing the average short-term smoothed psd estimate of the previous frame $\sum_{k=0}^{M-1} P(\lambda-1,k)$ to the average periodogram $\sum_{k=0}^{M-1} |Y(\lambda,k)|^2$. The comparison

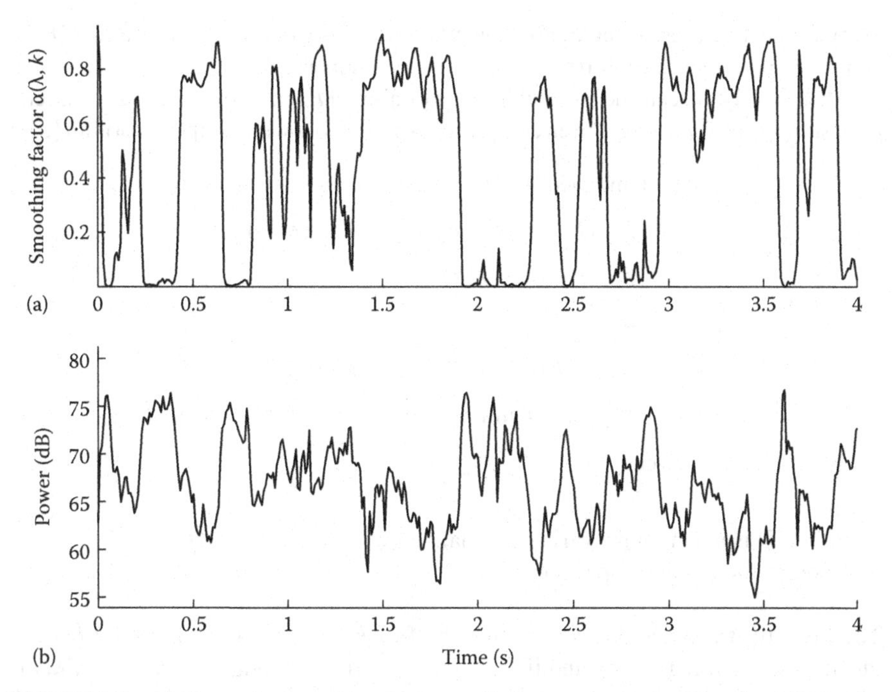

FIGURE 9.8 (a) Shows the smoothing factor $\alpha_{opt}(\lambda, k)$ computed using Equation 9.20 for the sentence given in Figure 9.6. (b) Shows the smoothed speech power spectrum.

was implemented by means of a $1/(1 + x^2)$ function, and the result of this comparison was used to modify the smoothing parameter with the following factor:

$$\alpha_c(\lambda) = \frac{1}{1+\left(\sum_{k=0}^{M-1} P(\lambda-1,k) \Big/ \sum_{k=0}^{M-1} |Y(\lambda,k)|^2 - 1\right)^2} \tag{9.21}$$

The final smoothing parameter after including the preceding correction factor $\alpha_c(\lambda)$ and after limiting the smoothing parameter to a maximum value α_{max} is as follows:

$$\alpha_{opt}(\lambda,k) = \frac{\alpha_{max} \cdot \alpha_c(\lambda)}{1+\left(P(\lambda-1,k)/\hat{\sigma}_d^2(\lambda-1,k)-1\right)^2} \tag{9.22}$$

where α_{max} was set to $\alpha_{max} = 0.96$ in [18] to avoid deadlock when $\bar{\gamma} = 1$. In [18], $\alpha_c(\lambda)$ was also smoothed over time, and the smoothing parameter was limited to a minimum value of $\alpha_{min} = 0.3$.

9.3.1.4 Searching for the Minimum

The preceding algorithm requires that we find the minimum $P_{min}(\lambda, k)$ over D consecutive smoothed psd estimates $P(\lambda, k)$. The complexity, in terms of compare operations, as well as the inherent delay associated with this algorithm depends on how often we update the minimum estimate $P_{min}(\lambda, k)$. We can update the minimum in every frame; however, the complexity would be high as we would have to make $D - 1$ compare operations at each frame and for every frequency bin.

Alternatively, we can choose to update the minimum $P_{\min}(\lambda, k)$ only after D consecutive estimates of $P(\lambda, k)$ have been computed, using the following simple algorithm [25]:

$$
\begin{aligned}
&\text{if mod}(\lambda/D) = 0\\
&\quad P_{\min}(\lambda,k) = \min\{P_{tmp}(\lambda-1,k), P(\lambda,k)\}\\
&\quad P_{tmp}(\lambda,k) = P(\lambda,k)\\
&\text{else}\\
&\quad P_{\min}(\lambda,k) = \min\{P_{\min}(\lambda-1,k), P(\lambda,k)\}\\
&\quad P_{tmp}(\lambda,k) = \min\{P_{tmp}(\lambda-1,k), P(\lambda,k)\}\\
&\text{end}
\end{aligned}
\tag{9.23}
$$

where

$P_{tmp}(\lambda, k)$ is a temporary variable initialized with $P_{tmp}(0, k) = P(0, k)$
mod(.) is the modulus operator

The first "if" statement checks whether the frame index (λ) is divisible by D (i.e., the modulus of λ/D is zero), and if it is, it updates the temporary variable $P_{tmp}(\lambda, k)$. The preceding algorithm requires only a single compare operation per frame and per frequency bin. The minimum for the noisy speech is found over D consecutive frames. In the worst-case scenario of increasing noise levels, the minimum search lags behind by $2D$ frames. This happens when the minimum, saved in the temporary variable $P_{tmp}(\lambda, k)$, occurs at the beginning of the D-frame long window. Although the preceding algorithm has low complexity, the minimum may lag by as many as $2D$ frames. This can be seen in Figure 9.3.

To reduce this lag we can divide the whole window of D frames into U subwindows of V frames each ($D = U \cdot V$) [18,25]. In this case, the maximum delay is reduced to $D + V$ frames compared to $2D$ frames in the previous algorithm (Equation 9.23). The window length D must be large enough to encompass any peak of speech activity (thereby avoiding noise overestimation) but short enough to follow nonstationary variations of the noise spectrum. Experiments have shown that window lengths of approximately 0.8–1.4 s gave good results [25]. For a sampling frequency of 8 kHz and an FFT length of 256 samples, the following values of U and V were found to work well in [18]: $U = 8$ and $V = 12$.

9.3.1.5 Minimum Statistics Algorithm

The MS algorithm was originally proposed in [25] and later refined in [18] to include a bias compensation factor and better smoothing factor. The noise-estimation algorithm [18] is summarized as follows:

Minimum-statistics algorithm:

For each frame l do

Step 1: Compute the short-term periodogram $|Y(\lambda, k)|^2$ of the noisy speech frame.

Step 2: Compute the smoothing parameter $\alpha(\lambda, k)$ using Equation 9.22.

Step 3: Compute the smoothed power spectrum $P(\lambda, k)$ using Equation 9.19.

Step 4: Compute the bias correction factor $B_{min}(\lambda, k)$ using Equations 9.12 and 9.16.

Step 5: Search for the minimum psd $P_{min}(\lambda, k)$ over a D-frame window. Update the minimum whenever V ($V < D$) frames are processed.

Step 6: Compute and update the noise psd according to Equation 9.17, that is, $\hat{\sigma}_d^2(\lambda, k) = B_{min}(\lambda, k) \cdot P_{min}(\lambda, k)$.

Implementation details, particularly pertaining to steps 4 and 5, can be found in [18, Figure 5].

Figure 9.9 shows the power spectrum (at frequency bin f = 500 Hz) of noisy speech and the estimated noise power spectrum of a 9 s speech signal (comprising 10 sentences) degraded by babble noise at 5 dB SNR. The estimated noise spectrum is compared to the true noise spectrum in the lower panel. As is evident from Figure 9.9, the MS algorithm does a good job in tracking the minimum levels of the noise psd, but for the most part it underestimates the true noise level. It also does a good job of tracking decreasing levels of noise.

The performance of the preceding noise-estimation algorithm was assessed in [18] using both objective and subjective measures. It was also assessed and compared against other noise-estimation algorithms in [30–32]. In the objective evaluation [18], the percentage relative estimation error and the error variance were calculated

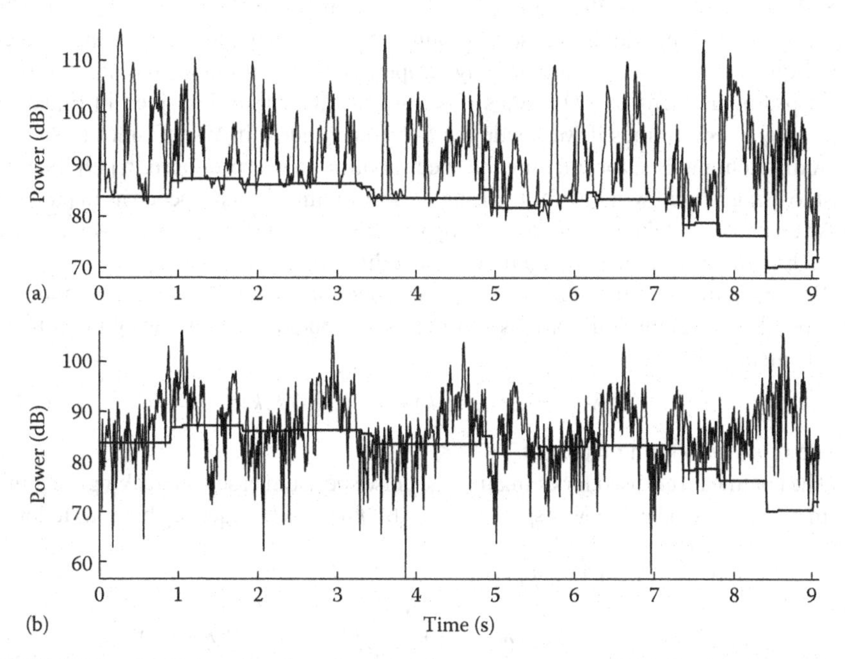

FIGURE 9.9 (a) Shows the plot of the noise power spectrum (thick line) estimated (for f = 500 Hz) using the MS algorithm for a set of sentences embedded in multitalker babble at +5 dB S/N. The smoothed power spectrum of noisy speech (thin line) is also shown for comparison. (b) Shows the true noise power spectrum (thin line) superimposed on the estimated noise psd using the MS algorithm.

between the true noise spectrum and estimated noise spectrum for white Gaussian noise, vehicular noise, and street noise, using sentences embedded in 15-dB S/N. Results indicated mean errors on the order of a few percent for the white and vehicular noises. A larger error was noted for street noise, which was attributed to the highly nonstationary nature of the noise and the inability of the algorithm to track increasing levels of noise power without a delay. In the subjective evaluation, the noise-estimation algorithm was combined with an MMSE algorithm and used as a front end to enhance the quality of the 2400 bps MELP speech coder. The performance of the MS algorithm was compared with an algorithm that estimated the noise spectrum by means of a VAD and soft-decision updating during speech activity [33]. Formal listening tests were conducted to evaluate the quality and intelligibility of the enhanced and coded speech. Compared to the algorithm that used the VAD algorithm [33], the MS approach yielded better quality (as evaluated by the DAM test) and improved speech intelligibility scores (as evaluated by the DRT test). The tracking of minimum in each frequency bin helped preserve the weak voiced consonants (e.g., /m/ and /n/), which might otherwise be classified as noise by most VAD algorithms as their energy is concentrated in a small number of frequency bins (low frequencies).

9.3.2 Continuous Spectral Minimum Tracking

As indicated earlier, one of the drawbacks of the minimal tracking employed in the MS algorithm is its inability to respond to fast changes of the noise spectrum. The tracking algorithm, which is based on samplewise comparisons of adjacent frames (see Equation 9.23) is computationally simple, but the minimum may lag the true noise psd by as many as $2D$ frames if we use the algorithm described in Equation 9.23 or by $D + V$ frames if we divide the D-frame window in V subframes [18].

A different method for tracking the spectral minima was proposed in [19]. In contrast to using a fixed window for tracking the minimum of noisy speech as in [18], the noise estimate is updated continuously by smoothing the noisy speech power spectra in each frequency bin using a nonlinear smoothing rule.

For minimum tracking of the noisy speech power spectrum, a short-time smoothed version of the periodogram of noisy speech is computed as before using the following recursion:

$$P(\lambda,k) = \alpha P(\lambda-1,k) + (1-\alpha)\,|Y(\lambda,k)|^2 \tag{9.24}$$

where α is a smoothing factor ($0.7 \le \alpha \le 0.9$).

The nonlinear rule used for estimating the noise spectrum based on tracking the minimum of the noisy speech power spectrum ($P_{min}(\lambda, k)$) in each frequency bin is as follows:

$$\begin{aligned}
&\text{if } P_{min}(\lambda-1,k) < P(\lambda,k)\\
&\quad P_{min}(\lambda,k) = \gamma P_{min}(\lambda-1,k) + \frac{1-\gamma}{1-\beta}\left(P(\lambda,k) - \beta P(\lambda-1,k)\right)\\
&\text{else}\\
&\quad P_{min}(\lambda,k) = P(\lambda,k)\\
&\text{end}
\end{aligned} \tag{9.25}$$

where $P_{min}(\lambda, k)$ is the noise estimate, and the parameter values are set to $\alpha = 0.7$, $\beta = 0.96$, and $\gamma = 0.998$. The preceding rule uses a "look-ahead" factor β in the minimum tracking, which can be adjusted if needed to vary the adaptation time of the algorithm. The typical adaptation time using the values mentioned previously is 0.2–0.4 s. Figure 9.10 shows an example of the continuous minimal tracking based on Equation 9.25. As shown, the preceding algorithm does a good job of estimating the noise spectrum (see Figure 9.10b), with a significantly low computational cost compared to the MS algorithm.

The nonlinear tracking, however, maintains continuous psd smoothing without making any distinction between speech-absent and -present segments. Hence, the noise estimate increases whenever the noisy speech power spectrum increases, irrespective of the changes in the noise power level. This is largely due to the second term in Equation 9.25, which implements a first-order differencing operation, that is, a discrete approximation of the derivative. When the noisy speech power level $P(\lambda, k)$ increases, so will the derivative, as the difference $(P(\lambda, k) - P(\lambda - 1, k))$ will be positive. Likewise, when the noisy speech power is decreasing, the slope (derivative) will be negative and the estimate of the noise level will decrease. Problems arise when very narrow peaks in the speech spectrum are encountered, as they produce large derivative values and consequently produce sudden, and large, increases in the noise

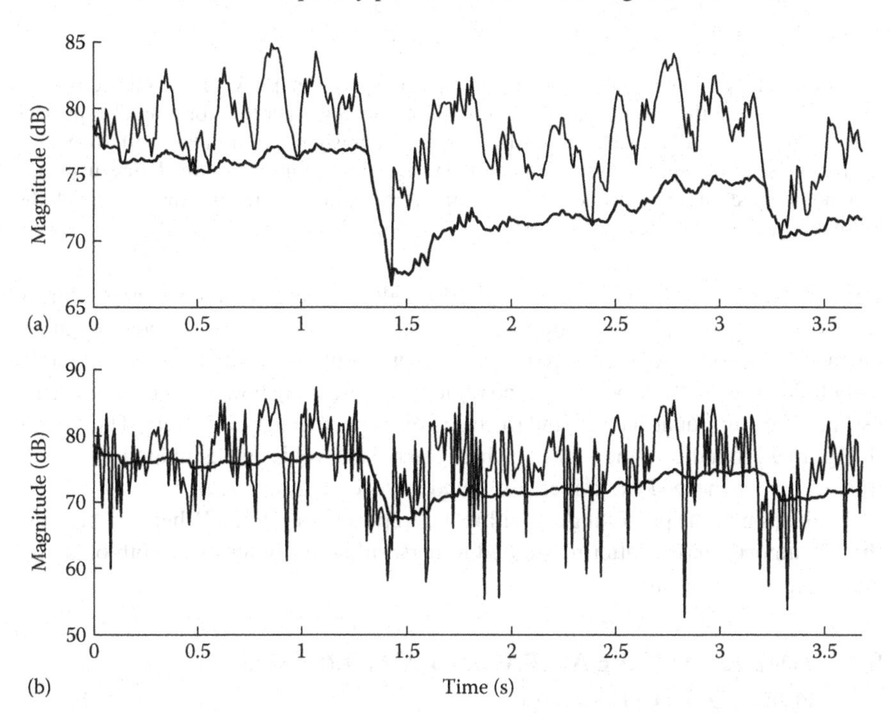

FIGURE 9.10 (a) (Thick line) shows the estimate of the noise psd at $f = 200$ Hz computed using the continuous minimal-tracking algorithm proposed in [19]. The smoothed power spectrum (with $\alpha = 0.7$) of noisy speech is superimposed (thin line). Sentence was embedded in babble at +5 dB S/N. (b) Shows the true noise power spectrum superimposed on the estimated noise psd (thick line).

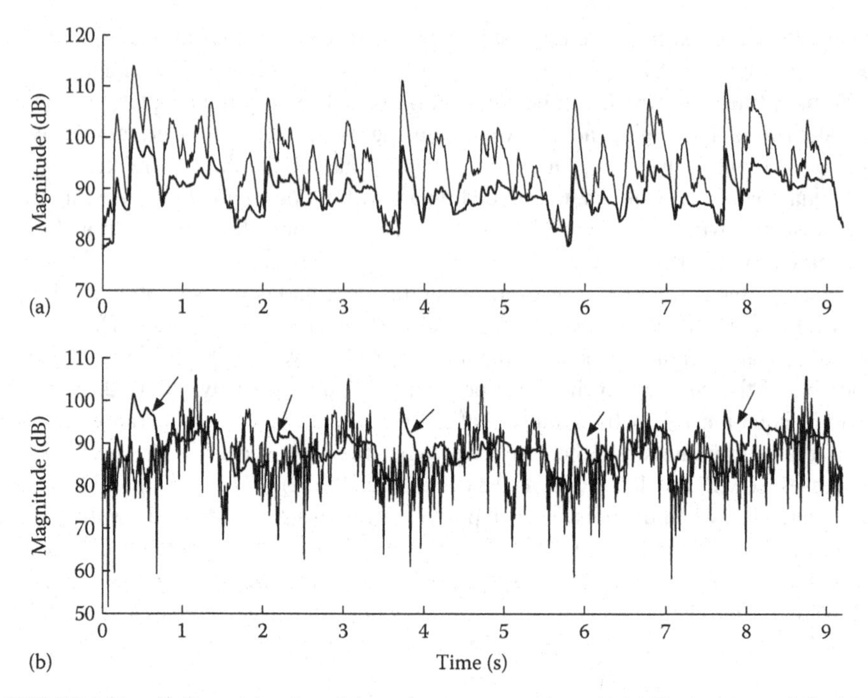

FIGURE 9.11 (a) Shows the plot of the noise power spectrum (thick line) estimated (for bin $f = 500$ Hz) using the continuous spectral minima-tracking algorithm for a set of sentences embedded in multitalker babble at +5 dB S/N (the same signal as in Figure 9.9). (b) Shows the true noise power spectrum superimposed on the estimated noise psd (thick line) using the continuous spectral minima-tracking algorithm. Arrows indicate the instances at which the noise level was overestimated.

estimate (see example in Figure 9.11). This results in overestimation of noise during speech activity and, possibly, clipping of speech. Also, the increase in noise estimate during high-energy regions may result in clipping of low-energy regions immediately following the high-power speech regions. Figure 9.11 shows the noise spectrum estimated using Equation 9.25 and the true noise spectrum at $f = 500$ Hz. The arrows in Figure 9.11b indicate the times at which the noise level is overestimated. Note that this occurs whenever $P(\lambda, k)$ increases suddenly (see Figure 9.11a).

Evaluation of the preceding algorithm was reported in [31,32]. When compared to the MS algorithm, the latter was found to perform better in terms of both objective and subjective measures.

9.4 TIME-RECURSIVE AVERAGING ALGORITHMS FOR NOISE ESTIMATION

The time-recursive averaging algorithms exploit the observation that the noise signal typically has a nonuniform effect on the spectrum of speech, in that some regions of the spectrum are affected by noise more than others. Put differently, each spectral component will typically have a different effective SNR.

Consequently, we can estimate and update individual frequency bands of the noise spectrum whenever the effective SNR at a particular frequency band is extremely low. Equivalently, we can update the individual frequency bands of the noise spectrum whenever the probability of speech being present at a particular frequency band is low. This observation led to the recursive-averaging type of algorithms in which the noise spectrum is estimated as a weighted average of the past noise estimates and the present noisy speech spectrum. The weights change adaptively depending either on the effective SNR of each frequency bin or on the speech-presence probability.

All time-recursive algorithms to be described in this section have the following general form:

$$\hat{\sigma}_d^2(\lambda,k) = \alpha(\lambda,k)\hat{\sigma}_d^2(\lambda-1,k) + (1-\alpha(\lambda,k))\,|Y(\lambda,k)|^2 \tag{9.26}$$

where

$|Y(\lambda, k)|^2$ is the noisy speech magnitude spectrum squared (periodogram)
$\hat{\sigma}_d^2(\lambda,k)$ denotes the estimate of the noise psd at frame λ and frequency k
$\alpha(\lambda, k)$ is the smoothing factor, which is time and frequency dependent

Different algorithms were developed depending on the selection of the smoothing factor $\alpha(\lambda, k)$. Some chose to compute $\alpha(\lambda, k)$ based on the estimated SNR of each frequency bin [16,34], whereas others chose to compute $\alpha(\lambda, k)$ based on the probability of speech being present/absent at frequency bin k [13,14,33,35]. These two approaches are conceptually very similar. Others chose to use a fixed value for $\alpha(\lambda, k)$, but updated $\hat{\sigma}_d^2(\lambda,k)$ only after a certain condition was met [20,30].

9.4.1 SNR-Dependent Recursive Averaging

In the recursive-averaging technique proposed in [34], the smoothing factor $\alpha(\lambda, k)$ is chosen to be a sigmoid function of the *a posteriori* SNR $\gamma_k(\lambda)$:

$$\alpha(\lambda,k) = \frac{1}{1+e^{-\beta(\gamma_k(\lambda)-1.5)}} \tag{9.27}$$

where β is a parameter with values in the range$15 \leq \beta \leq 30$, and $\gamma_k(\lambda)$ is an approximation to the *a posteriori* SNR given by

$$\gamma_k(\lambda) = \frac{|Y(\lambda,k)|^2}{\frac{1}{10}\sum_{m=1}^{10}\hat{\sigma}_d^2(\lambda-m,k)} \tag{9.28}$$

The denominator in Equation 9.28 gives the average of the estimated noise psd in the past 10 frames. Alternatively, as suggested in [34], the median rather than the average of the noise estimates of the past 5–10 frames could be used.

In [16], a different function was proposed for computing $\alpha(\lambda, k)$:

$$\alpha(\lambda,k) = 1 - \min\left\{1, \frac{1}{(\gamma_k(\lambda))^p}\right\} \tag{9.29}$$

where

p is a parameter
$\gamma_k(\lambda)$ is given by Equation 9.28

The minimum operation is used to ensure that $\alpha(\lambda, k)$ is in the range of $0 \leq \alpha(\lambda, k) \leq 1$.

Figure 9.12 shows a plot of $\alpha(\lambda, k)$ given in Equations 9.27 and 9.29 as a function of $\gamma_k(\lambda)$ and for different values of β and p. It is clear from Figure 9.12 that the shapes of the $\alpha(\lambda, k)$ functions in Equations 9.27 and 9.29 are similar, with the following common characteristics. For large values of the *a posteriori* SNR $\gamma_k(\lambda)$, $\alpha(\lambda, k) \to 1$, whereas for small values of $\gamma_k(\lambda)$, $\alpha(\lambda, k) \to 0$. The parameters β and p used in Equations 9.27 and 9.29, respectively, control the steepness of the $\alpha(\lambda, k)$ function.

The recursive algorithm given in Equation 9.26 can be explained as follows. If speech is present, the *a posteriori* estimate $\gamma_k(\lambda)$ will be large (see Figure 9.12) and therefore $\alpha(\lambda, k) \approx 1$. Consequently, because $\alpha(\lambda, k) \approx 1$, we will have

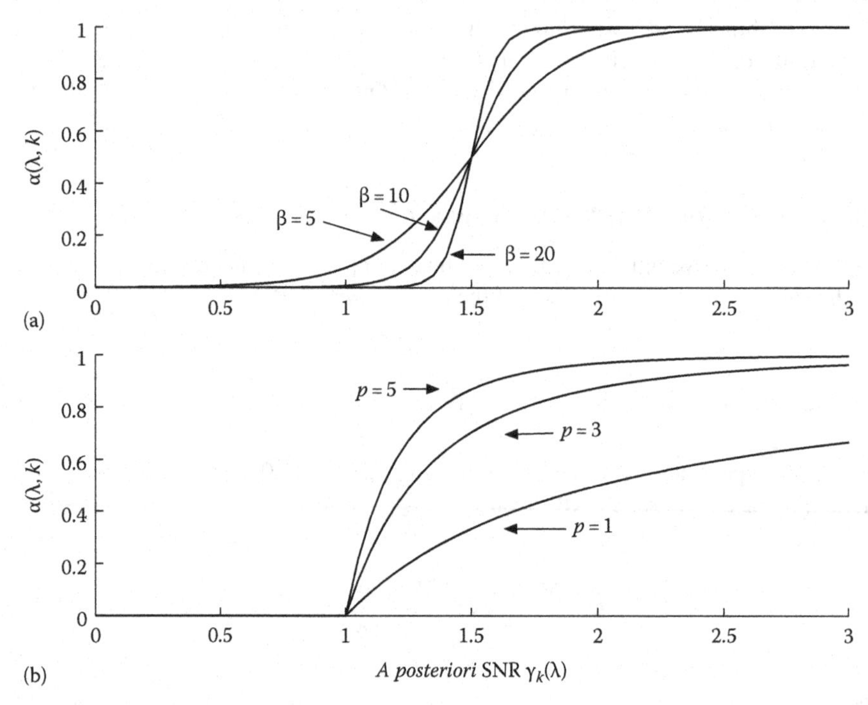

FIGURE 9.12 (a) Shows the plot of the smoothing factor $\alpha(\lambda, k)$ computed according to Equation 9.27 for different values of the parameter β. (b) Shows the smoothing factor $\alpha(\lambda, k)$ computed according to Equation 9.29 for different values of the parameter p.

$\hat{\sigma}_d^2(\lambda, k) \approx \hat{\sigma}_d^2(\lambda-1, k)$ according to Equation 9.26; that is, the noise update will cease and the noise estimate will remain the same as the previous frame's estimate. Conversely, if speech is absent, the *a posteriori* estimate $\gamma_k(\lambda)$ will be small (see Figure 9.12) and therefore $\alpha(\lambda, k) \approx 0$. As a result, $\hat{\sigma}_d^2(\lambda, k) \approx |Y(\lambda, k)|^2$; that is, the noise estimate will follow the psd of the noisy spectrum in the absence of speech. The main advantage of using the time smoothing factors given in Equation 9.27 or Equation 9.29, as opposed to using a fixed value for $\alpha(\lambda, k)$, is that these factors are time and frequency dependent. This means that the noise psd will be adapted differently and at different rates in the various frequency bins, depending on the estimate of the *a posteriori* SNR $\gamma_k(\lambda)$ in that bin. This is particularly suited in situations in which the additive noise is colored.

The parameters β and p in Equations 9.27 and 9.29 need to be chosen carefully as they can affect the estimate of the noise spectrum. This effect can best be seen in Figure 9.13, which plots the noise estimate against the true noise psd for different values of β. Note that if β is chosen too large, then the transition from $\alpha(\lambda, k) = 1$ to $\alpha(\lambda, k) = 0$ becomes very steep (see Figure 9.12), in effect making $\alpha(\lambda, k)$ a step function (i.e., $\alpha(\lambda, k)$ will assume only binary values, 0 or 1). As a result, the recursive algorithm will underestimate the true value of the noise spectrum (see Figure 9.13b). For this example, the value $\beta = 0.6$ yielded good tracking of the noise spectrum.

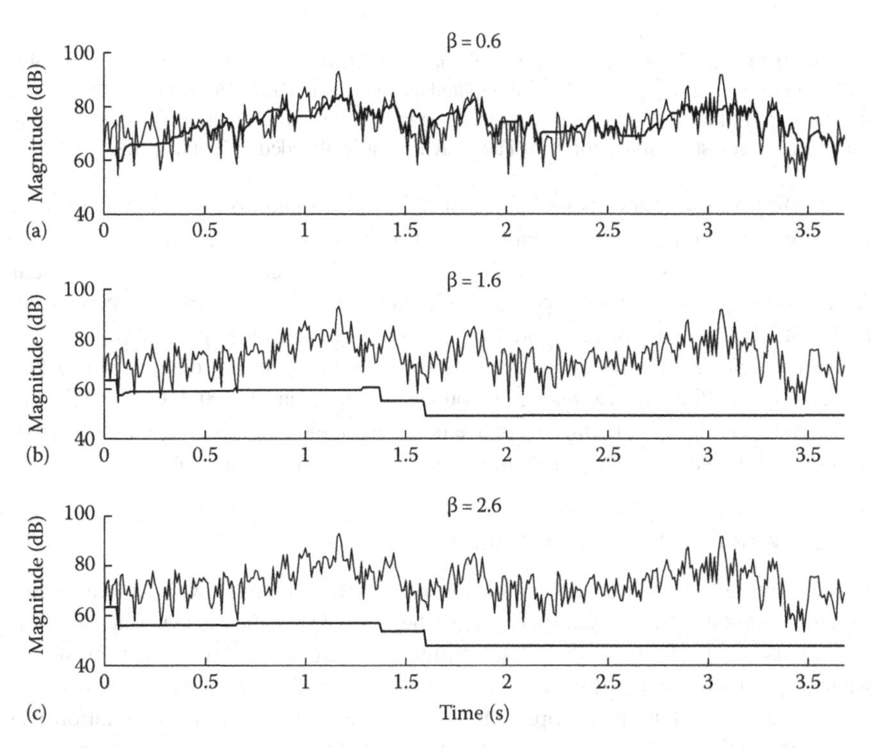

FIGURE 9.13 Plots (a), (b), and (c) show the noise psd (thick line) estimated using the recursive averaging algorithm for different values of the parameter β in Equation 9.27. The smoothed psd (thin line) of noisy speech is superimposed.

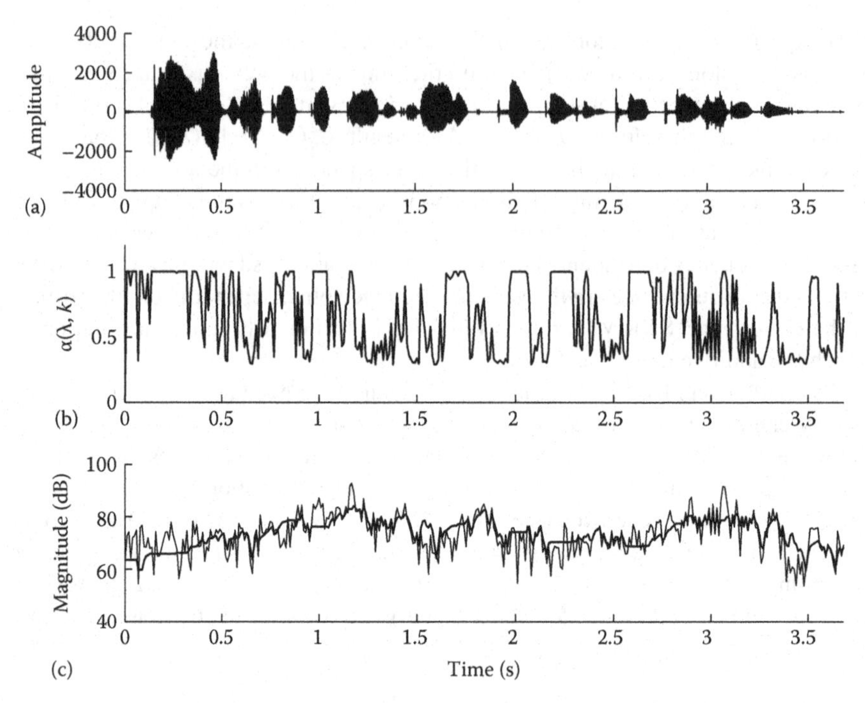

FIGURE 9.14 (a) Shows the waveform (in quiet) of a TIMIT sentence (same as in Figure 9.1). (b) Shows the smoothing factor $\alpha(\lambda, k)$ computed using Equation 9.27 with $\beta = 0.6$. (c) Shows the true noise psd (thin line) superimposed on the estimated noise psd (thick line) using the SNR-dependent noise-estimation algorithm. The sentence was embedded in babble at +5 dB S/N.

Figure 9.14 shows a plot of the values of $\alpha(\lambda, k)$ estimated over time according to Equation 9.27 with $\beta = 0.6$. As can be seen, $\alpha(\lambda, k)$ takes large values (close to or equal to one) when speech is present and takes small values when speech is absent. As a result, the noise update stops when speech is present and continues when speech is absent. This is done for each individual frequency bin in the spectrum.

Finally, Figure 9.15 shows the estimate of the noise spectrum obtained for a long speech segment (the same example as before) using Equations 9.26 and 9.27 with $\beta = 0.6$. As can be seen, this simple time-recursive noise-estimation algorithm does surprisingly well in tracking nonstationary noise (multitalker babble for this example).

9.4.2 Weighted Spectral Averaging

In the previous algorithm, the smoothing factor $\alpha(\lambda, k)$ varied with time and controlled the update of the noise spectrum. When $\alpha(\lambda, k) \approx 1$ the noise update stopped, and when $\alpha(\lambda, k) \approx 0$ the noise update continued. Therefore, knowing when to stop or when to continue updating the noise spectrum is critical for accurate noise estimation.

A different, and simpler, approach to recursive-averaging noise estimation was proposed in [20]. In their approach, called *weighted spectral averaging*, the smoothing factor is fixed but a different method is used to control the update of the noise spectrum. More specifically, the decision as to whether the noise spectrum should

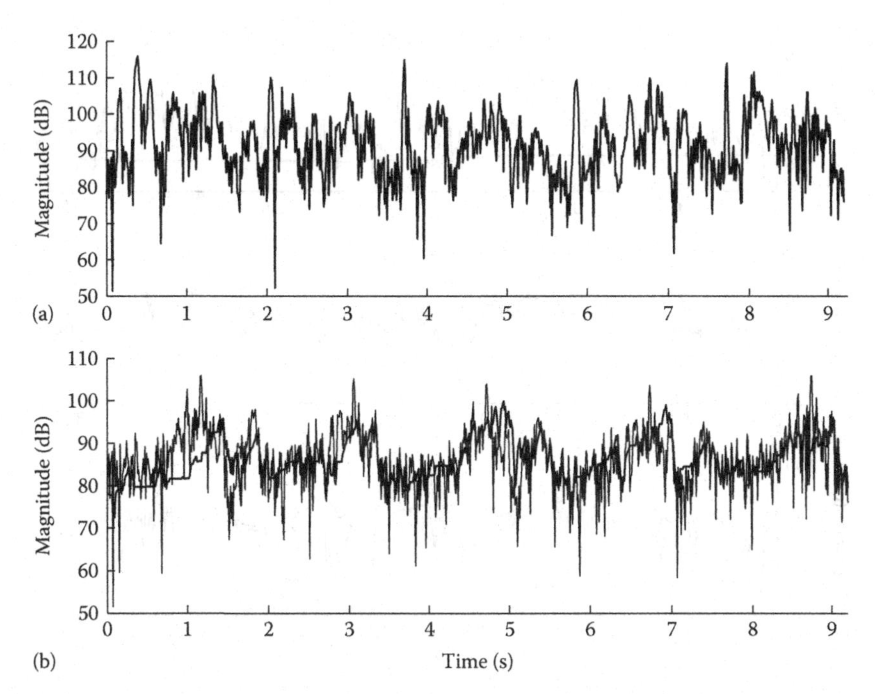

FIGURE 9.15 (a) Shows the noisy speech psd (unsmoothed) for $f = 500\,\text{Hz}$. The same set of noisy sentences was used as in Figure 9.9. (b) Shows the true noise psd (thin line) superimposed on the estimated noise psd (thick line) computed using the SNR-dependent noise-estimation algorithm. The smoothing factor $\alpha(\lambda, k)$ was computed using Equation 9.27 with $\beta = 0.6$.

be updated or not is based on the comparison of the estimated *a posteriori* SNR to a threshold. If the *a posteriori* SNR is found to be smaller than a specified threshold, suggesting speech absence, then the noise spectrum is updated. Conversely, if the *a posteriori* SNR is found to be larger than a specified threshold, suggesting speech presence, then the noise spectrum update is stopped.

The weighted-averaging technique is described as follows [20]:

$$
\begin{aligned}
&\text{if } \frac{|Y(\lambda,k)|}{\hat{\sigma}_d(\lambda-1,k)} < \beta \quad \text{then} \\
&\qquad \hat{\sigma}_d(\lambda,k) = \alpha\hat{\sigma}_d(\lambda-1,k) + (1-\alpha)\,|Y(\lambda,k)| \\
&\text{else} \\
&\qquad \hat{\sigma}_d(\lambda,k) = \hat{\sigma}_d(\lambda-1,k) \\
&\text{end}
\end{aligned}
\tag{9.30}
$$

where

$\hat{\sigma}_d(\lambda,k)$ indicates the magnitude spectrum (rather than power spectrum) of the noise
α denotes the smoothing factor (which is fixed now)
β denotes the threshold

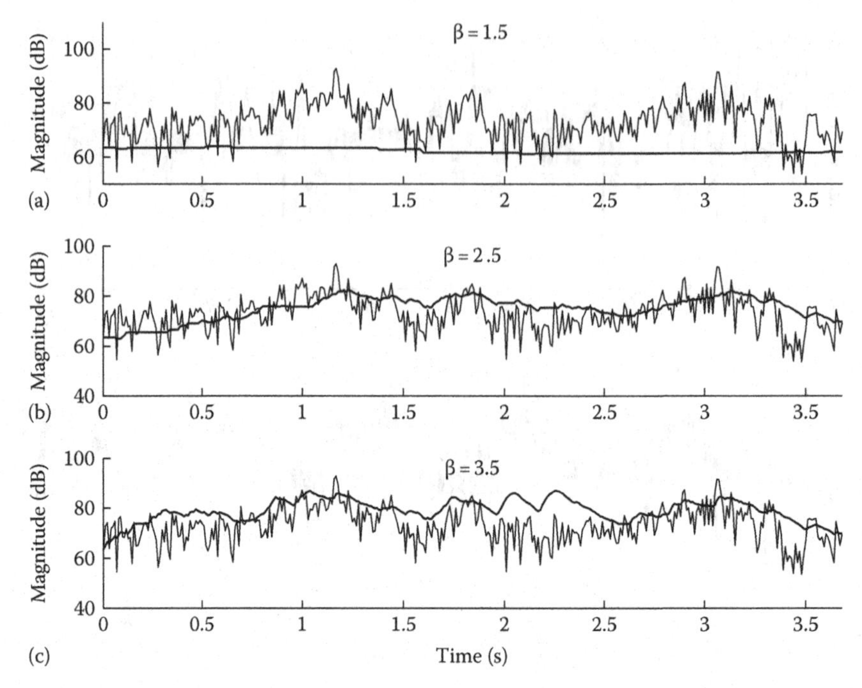

FIGURE 9.16 Plots (a), (b) and (c) show the noise psd (thick line) estimated using the weighted-averaging algorithm for different values of the threshold parameter β in Equation 9.30. The smoothed psd (thin line) of noisy speech is superimposed.

Note that the quantity $|Y(\lambda, k)|/\sigma_d(\lambda - 1, k)$ in Equation 9.30 corresponds to the square root of the *a posteriori* SNR, and it is in fact equal to $\sqrt{\gamma_k(\lambda)}$ defined in Equation 9.28, assuming that we only use the previous frame's noise estimate rather than the average of the past 10 frames. The preceding algorithm was originally defined in the magnitude-spectrum domain, but can alternatively be reformulated in the power-spectrum domain by using different threshold values.

The threshold value β in Equation 9.30 can have a significant effect on the noise spectrum estimation. Figure 9.16 shows the effect on noise estimation for three different values of β. As can be seen, if β is chosen too small, then the noise spectrum is not updated often enough and is underestimated. On the other hand, if β is chosen too large, then the noise spectrum is overestimated. For this example, the value of β = 2.5 gave a good compromise.

Figure 9.17 shows the estimate of the noise spectrum using the preceding algorithm with β = 2.5 and α = 0.9. The algorithm does moderately well; however, it occasionally overestimates the noise level (see segments indicated by the arrows). As shown in Figure 9.17a, noise overestimation occurs in low-SNR segments (e.g., unvoiced consonants), particularly the segments preceded by high-energy segments.

To overcome the preceding noise overestimation problem, Ris and Dupont [30] modified the update decision rule in Equation 9.30. Rather than updating the noise spectrum when the *a posteriori* SNR fell below a certain threshold, they updated the noise spectrum when the noisy speech magnitude spectrum fell within a fraction of

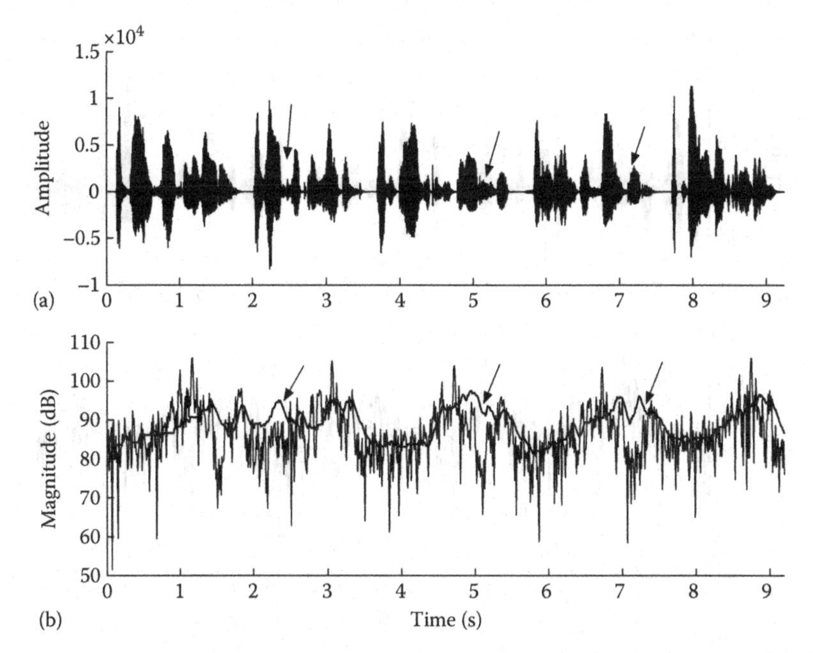

FIGURE 9.17 (a) Shows the waveform (in quiet) of a set of sentences concatenated. (b) Shows the true noise psd (thin line) superimposed on the estimated noise psd (thick line) obtained using the weighted-spectral-averaging algorithm with $\beta = 2.5$ and $\beta = 0.9$. The weighted-averaging algorithm was applied to the set of sentences shown in (a) embedded in babble at +5 dB S/N. Arrows indicate the instances at which the noise level is overestimated.

the variance of the noise estimate. More specifically, the noise spectrum was updated when the following condition was satisfied:

$$\| Y(\lambda,k) | - \hat{\sigma}_d(\lambda,k) | < \varepsilon\sqrt{\text{var}_d(\lambda,k)} \tag{9.31}$$

where $\text{var}_d(\lambda, k)$ denotes the estimate of the instantaneous variance of the noise spectrum, and ε is a tunable parameter. The variance of the noise spectrum was estimated using the following recursive equation:

$$\text{var}_d(\lambda,k) = \delta\,\text{var}_d(\lambda-1,k) + (1-\delta)\,(| Y(\lambda,k) | - \hat{\sigma}_d(\lambda,k))^2 \tag{9.32}$$

where δ is a smoothing parameter. The revised noise-estimation algorithm took the following form:

$$\begin{aligned}
&\text{if } \left| \, | Y(\lambda,k) | - \hat{\sigma}_d(\lambda-1,k) \right| < \varepsilon\sqrt{\text{var}_d(\lambda-1,k)} \\
&\qquad \hat{\sigma}_d(\lambda,k) = \alpha\hat{\sigma}_d(\lambda-1,k) + (1-\alpha)\,| Y(\lambda,k) | \\
&\qquad \text{var}_d(\lambda,k) = \delta\,\text{var}_d(\lambda-1,k) + (1-\delta)(| Y(\lambda,k) | - \hat{\sigma}_d(\lambda,k))^2 \\
&\text{else} \\
&\qquad \hat{\sigma}_d(\lambda,k) = \hat{\sigma}_d(\lambda-1,k) \\
&\text{end}
\end{aligned} \tag{9.33}$$

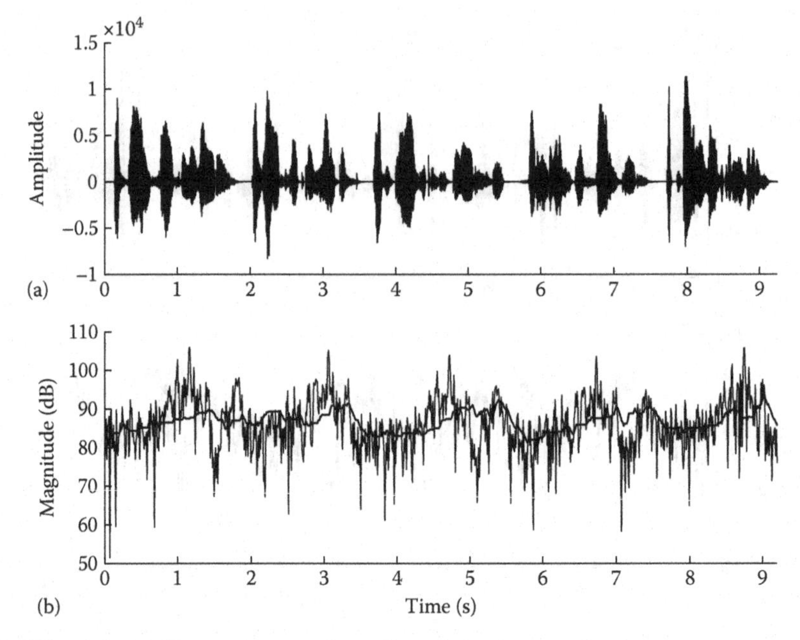

FIGURE 9.18 (a) Shows the waveform (in quiet) of a set of sentences concatenated. (b) Shows the noise psd estimate (thick line) obtained using a modified version of the weighted-averaging algorithm [30] (see Equation 9.33) for the same set of sentences as those used in Figure 9.17. The true noise psd (thin line) is superimposed.

Figure 9.18 shows the noise spectrum estimated using the preceding algorithm with $\delta = \alpha = 0.9$ and $\varepsilon = 2.5$. It is clear that the new decision rule (Equation 9.31) reduces and in most cases eliminates the overestimation error (compare Figure 9.17 with Figure 9.16).

Finally, a simple but effective algorithm similar to that described in Equation 9.30 was proposed in [36]. In the proposed algorithm, the previous noise estimate was compared with the current estimate and if it was found to lie within a specified range, the noise spectrum was updated, otherwise it was not. More specifically, the noise-estimation algorithm had the following form [36]:

$$
\begin{aligned}
&S_{tmp}(\lambda,k) = \alpha\hat{\sigma}_d(\lambda-1,k) + (1-\alpha)\,|Y(\lambda,k)| \\
&\text{if } \hat{\sigma}_d(\lambda-1,k) < \beta S_{tmp}(\lambda,k) \text{ and } \hat{\sigma}_d(\lambda-1,k) > \gamma S_{tmp}(\lambda,k) \\
&\qquad \hat{\sigma}_d(\lambda,k) = S_{tmp}(\lambda,k) \\
&\text{else} \\
&\qquad \hat{\sigma}_d(\lambda,k) = \hat{\sigma}_d(\lambda-1,k) \\
&\text{end}
\end{aligned}
\tag{9.34}
$$

where

β and γ are preset thresholds

$\hat{\sigma}_d(\lambda,k)$ is the magnitude (and not the power) of the estimated noise spectrum

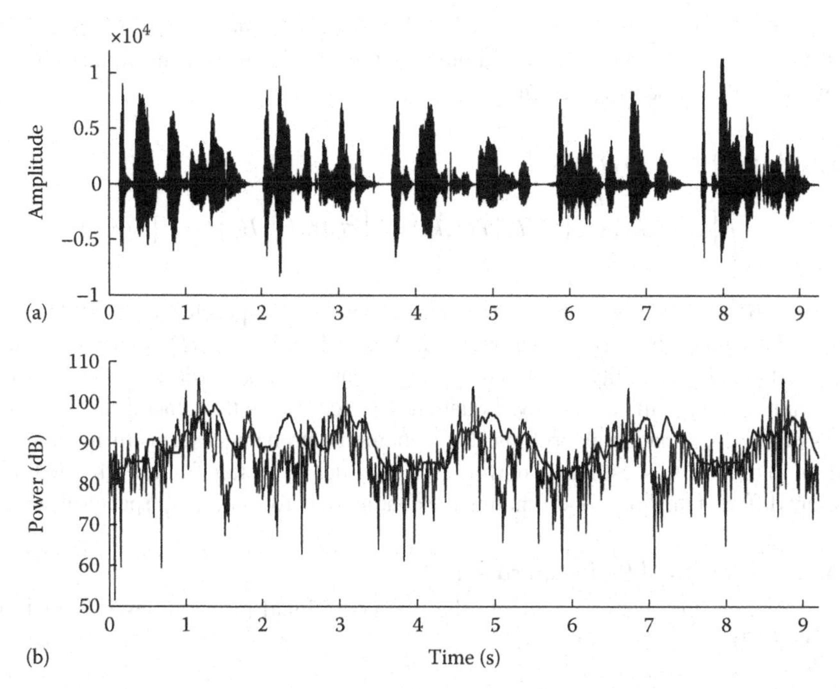

FIGURE 9.19 (a) Shows the waveform (in quiet) of a set of sentences concatenated. (b) Shows the noise psd estimate (thick line) obtained using a modified version of the weighted-averaging algorithm [36] (see Equation 9.34) for the same set of sentences as those used in Figure 9.17. The true noise psd (thin line) is superimposed.

Note that the decision rule in Equation 9.34 is similar to that of Equation 9.30 in that the noise psd is updated whenever a modified estimate of the *a posteriori* SNR falls within a specified range (i.e., $1/\beta < S_{tmp}(\lambda,k)/\hat{\sigma}_d(\lambda-1,k) < 1/\Upsilon$) rather than being smaller than a preset threshold. The thresholds β and γ can be used to control the rate of increase or decrease of the noise spectrum, and in [36] these thresholds were chosen so that the noise estimate did not increase faster than 3 dB per second or decreased faster than 12 dB per second.

Figure 9.19 shows an example of the noise psd estimation using the preceding algorithm with $\gamma = 0.85$, $\beta = 1.2$, and $\alpha = 0.9$. Aside from a few instances in which the noise was overestimated, this simple noise-estimation algorithm performed well.

9.4.3 Recursive-Averaging Algorithms Based on Signal-Presence Uncertainty

We now turn our attention to a new class of noise-estimation algorithms, which are formulated using a detection theory framework. The presence or absence of speech in frequency bin k is cast as a detection problem using the following two hypotheses:

$$\begin{aligned} &H_0^k: \text{ speech absent: } Y(\lambda,k) = D(\lambda,k) \\ &H_1^k: \text{ speech present: } Y(\lambda,k) = X(\lambda,k) + D(\lambda,k) \end{aligned} \tag{9.35}$$

where $D(\lambda, k)$ is the spectrum of the noise. The noise psd is given by $\sigma_d^2(\lambda,k) = E\{|D(\lambda,k)|^2\}$. The optimum $\sigma_d^2(\lambda,k)$, in terms of minimum MSE, estimate of the noise psd is given by

$$\begin{aligned}\hat{\sigma}_d^2(\lambda,k) &= E\left[\sigma_d^2(\lambda,k) \mid Y(\lambda,k)\right] \\ &= E\left[\sigma_d^2(\lambda,k) \mid H_0\right]P(H_0 \mid Y(\lambda,k)) + E\left[\sigma_d^2(\lambda,k) \mid H_1\right]P(H_1 \mid Y(\lambda,k)) \end{aligned} \tag{9.36}$$

where $P(H_0^k \mid Y(\lambda,k))$ denotes the conditional probability of speech being absent in frequency bin k given the noisy speech spectrum $Y(\lambda, k)$. Similarly, $P(H_1^k \mid Y(\lambda,k))$ denotes the conditional probability of speech being present in bin k, given the noisy speech spectrum. As we will see shortly, Equation 9.36 represents the general form of this class of noise-estimation algorithms. The conditional probability terms turn out to be the smoothing factors, estimated now under a statistical detection framework. Next, we present different methods for estimating the conditional probabilities of speech absence.

9.4.3.1 Likelihood Ratio Approach

As in Section 7.13, we can compute the two conditional probabilities in Equation 9.36 using Bayes' rule as follows:

$$\begin{aligned}P\left(H_0^k \mid Y(\lambda,k)\right) &= \frac{P\left(Y(\lambda,k) \mid H_0^k\right)P\left(H_0^k\right)}{P\left(Y(\lambda,k) \mid H_0^k\right)P\left(H_0^k\right) + P\left(Y(\lambda,k) \mid H_1^k\right)P\left(H_1^k\right)} \\ &= \frac{1}{1 + r\Lambda(\lambda,k)}\end{aligned} \tag{9.37}$$

where $r \triangleq P(H_1^k)/P(H_0^k)$ is the ratio of *a priori* probabilities of speech presence and speech absence, and

$$\Lambda(\lambda,k) \triangleq \frac{P\left(Y(\lambda,k) \mid H_1^k\right)}{P\left(Y(\lambda,k) \mid H_0^k\right)} \tag{9.38}$$

is the likelihood ratio. Similarly, it is easy to show that

$$P\left(H_1^k \mid Y(\lambda,k)\right) = \frac{r\Lambda(\lambda,k)}{1 + r\Lambda(\lambda,k)} \tag{9.39}$$

Substituting Equations 9.37 and 9.39 into Equation 9.36, we get the following estimate of the noise psd:

$$\hat{\sigma}_d^2(\lambda,k) = \frac{1}{1 + r\Lambda(\lambda,k)}E[\sigma_d^2(\lambda,k) \mid H_0^k] + \frac{r\Lambda(\lambda,k)}{1 + r\Lambda(\lambda,k)}E[\sigma_d^2(\lambda,k) \mid H_1^k] \tag{9.40}$$

When speech is absent in bin k, we can approximate the preceding term $E[\sigma_d^2(\lambda,k)\,|\,H_0^k]$ with the short-term power spectrum $|Y(\lambda, k)|^2$. When speech is present in bin k, we can approximate $E[\sigma_d^2(\lambda,k)\,|\,H_1^k]$ by the noise estimate of the previous frame, that is, $\hat{\sigma}_d^2(\lambda-1,k)$ (a different method for estimating $E[\sigma_d^2(\lambda,k)\,|\,H_1^k]$ was proposed in [37] and will be discussed later). After making these approximations, the noise estimate in Equation 9.40 takes the form

$$\hat{\sigma}_d^2(\lambda,k) = \frac{r\Lambda(\lambda,k)}{1+r\Lambda(\lambda,k)}\hat{\sigma}_d^2(\lambda-1,k) + \frac{1}{1+r\Lambda(\lambda,k)}|Y(\lambda,k)|^2 \tag{9.41}$$

It is interesting to note that the preceding recursion has the same form as the general form of time-recursive noise-estimation algorithms (Equation 9.26) with the time smoothing factor $\alpha(\lambda,k)$ given by

$$\alpha(\lambda,k) = \frac{r\Lambda(\lambda,k)}{1+r\Lambda(\lambda,k)} \tag{9.42}$$

Note also that $1 - \alpha(\lambda, k) = 1/(1 + r\Lambda(\lambda, k))$ consistent again with Equation 9.26. From Equations 9.36 and 9.26 we infer that $\alpha(\lambda, k)$ may be viewed as the conditional probability of speech being present in bin k, that is, $P(H_1^k\,|\,Y(\lambda,k))$. Hence, when $P(H_1^k\,|\,Y(\lambda,k))$ is high, so will be $\alpha(\lambda, k)$, and the noise update will stop. Conversely, when $P(H_1^k\,|\,Y(\lambda,k))$ is low, so will be $\alpha(\lambda, k)$, and the noise spectrum will get updated.

The smoothing factor $\alpha(\lambda, k)$ is a function of the likelihood ratio $\Lambda(\lambda, k)$. If we assume a Gaussian statistical model for the DFT coefficients, as we did in Chapter 6, then we can derive an expression for $\Lambda(\lambda, k)$. Under the Gaussian assumption, $\Lambda(\lambda, k)$ is equal to (see Section 7.13)

$$\Lambda(\lambda,k) = \frac{1}{1+\xi_k(\lambda)}\exp\left[\frac{\xi_k(\lambda)}{1+\xi_k(\lambda)}\gamma_k(\lambda)\right] \tag{9.43}$$

where

$\xi_k(\lambda)$ is the *a priori* SNR
$\gamma_k(\lambda)$ is the *a posteriori* SNR at frame λ

So, given a method to estimate ξ_k (e.g., the decision-directed approach described in Chapter 7), we can substitute Equations 9.43 and 9.42 into Equation 9.41 and update the noise spectrum.

Alternatively, rather than using $\Lambda(\lambda, k)$ in Equation 9.43, which relies on estimation of the *a priori* SNR, we can use the geometric mean of the likelihood ratios of the individual frequency bins as follows [13]:

$$\begin{aligned}\log\Lambda_G(\lambda) &= \log\left(\prod_{k=0}^{L-1}\Lambda(\lambda,k)\right)^{1/L}\\ &= \frac{1}{L}\sum_{k=0}^{L-1}\log\Lambda(\lambda,k)\end{aligned} \tag{9.44}$$

where L is the number of DFT bins. Assuming that the DFT coefficients are statistically independent and after approximating ξ_k by $\hat{\xi}_k = \gamma_k - 1$, it is easy to show that Equation 9.44 evaluates to [6,13]

$$\log \Lambda_G(\lambda) = \frac{1}{L}\sum_{k=0}^{L-1}\{\gamma_k - \log(\gamma_k) - 1\} \tag{9.45}$$

Using the preceding geometric mean of the likelihood ratios, the noise-estimation algorithm now takes the following form:

$$\begin{aligned}\hat{\sigma}_d^2(\lambda,k) &= \frac{r\Lambda_G(\lambda)}{1+r\Lambda_G(\lambda)}\hat{\sigma}_d^2(\lambda-1,k) + \frac{1}{1+r\Lambda_G(\lambda)}|Y(\lambda,k)|^2 \\ &= \alpha(\lambda)\hat{\sigma}_d^2(\lambda-1,k) + (1-\alpha(\lambda))|Y(\lambda,k)|^2 \end{aligned} \tag{9.46}$$

Note that the smoothing factors $\alpha(\lambda)$ in Equation 9.46 are no longer a function of frequency in that the same smoothing factor is applied to all frequency bins. Figure 9.20 shows the noise spectrum estimated using Equation 9.46 with $r = 0.05$. The globally estimated smoothing factors $\alpha(\lambda)$ are also plotted in the Figure 9.20b. As can be seen

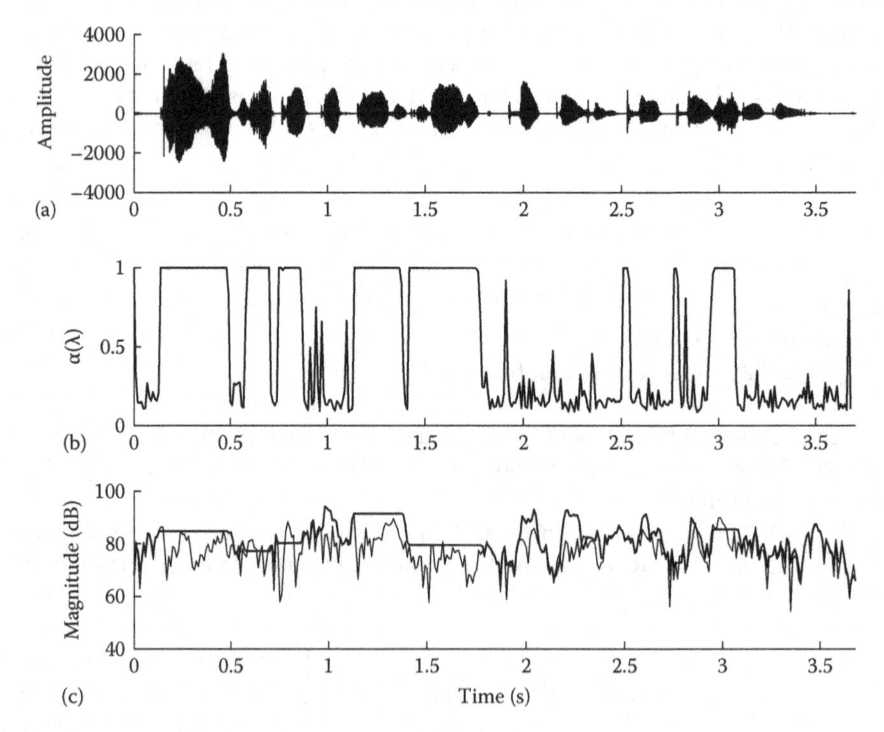

FIGURE 9.20 Noise power spectrum [(c)—thick line] estimated using the likelihood ratio approach (see Equation 9.46) with $r = 0.05$ for a sentence (Figure 9.1) embedded in babble at 5 dB S/N. The true noise spectrum is superimposed [(c)—thin line]. The estimated smoothing factors $\alpha(\lambda)$ are plotted in (b). The sentence (in quiet) is shown in (a) for reference.

from this example, the noise level is sometimes overestimated in segments where $p(H_1^k \mid Y(\lambda,k))$ (i.e., $\alpha(\lambda)$) is not very accurate (e.g., $t = 2$–2.5 s).

Note that we derived Equation 9.45 by approximating ξ_k in Equation 9.43 by $\hat{\xi}_k = \gamma_k - 1$. Alternatively, we could use the decision-directed approach [38] to estimate ξ_k. In doing so, we can derive a robust voice activity detector based on comparison of the geometric mean of the likelihood ratios (i.e., Equation 9.44) against a preset threshold [6]. The voice activity detector based on the decision-directed approach was found to perform better than the voice activity detector based on Equation 9.45 [6]. Further improvements to this voice activity detector were reported in [39,40].

In Equation 9.40, we approximated $E[\sigma_d^2(\lambda,k) \mid H_1^k]$ by the noise estimate of the previous frame, that is, by $\hat{\sigma}_d^2(\lambda-1,k)$. A different method for estimating $E[\sigma_d^2(\lambda,k) \mid H_1^k]$ was proposed in [37], based on explicit calculation of $E[\sigma_d^2(\lambda,k) \mid H_1^k]$ using the Gaussian statistical model (Chapter 7). More specifically, $E[\sigma_d^2(\lambda,k) \mid H_1^k]$ was computed according to [37] as follows:

$$E\left[\sigma_d^2(\lambda,k) \mid H_1^k\right] = \left(\frac{\xi_k}{1+\xi_k}\right)\hat{\sigma}_d^2(\lambda,k) + \left(\frac{1}{1+\xi_k}\right)^2 |Y(\lambda,k)|^2 \tag{9.47}$$

where ξ_k is the *a priori* SNR, which can be estimated using the decision-directed approach [38]. The long-term smoothed psd of the noise signal was used to update the noise psd rather than the mean-square estimate $E[\sigma_d^2(\lambda,k) \mid Y(\lambda,k)]$ (Equation 9.36). Specifically, the noise psd at frame $(\lambda + 1)$ was obtained according to [37]

$$\hat{\sigma}_d^2(\lambda+1,k) = \eta \cdot \hat{\sigma}_d^2(\lambda,k) + (1-\eta)E[\sigma_d^2(\lambda,k) \mid Y(\lambda,k)] \tag{9.48}$$

where

η is a smoothing parameter

$E[\sigma_d^2(\lambda,k) \mid Y(\lambda,k)]$ is computed as in Equation 9.36 and with $E[\sigma_d^2(\lambda,k) \mid H_1^k]$ computed now according to Equation 9.47

Note that unlike the noise-estimation algorithm given in Equation 9.46, the preceding algorithm requires an estimate of the *a priori* SNR ξ_k.

A noise-estimation algorithm similar to that in Equation 9.46 was also proposed in [33]. The smoothing factor $\alpha(\lambda)$ in [33] was computed as follows:

$$\alpha(\lambda) = 1 - 0.2\,|\,\bar{\gamma}(\lambda-1) - 1\,| \tag{9.49}$$

where $\bar{\gamma}(\lambda)$ is the average (across all bins) of the *a posteriori* SNRs of frame λ, that is, $\bar{\gamma}(\lambda) = 1/L\sum_{k=0}^{L-1}\gamma_k(\lambda)$. The two noise-estimation algorithms ([13,33]) are similar in that both algorithms rely on the average of the *a posteriori* SNR values (see Equation 9.45). The smoothing factor $\alpha(\lambda)$ in Equation 9.49 was constrained in [33] to be larger than 0.8 and smaller than 0.98.

9.4.3.2 Minima-Controlled Recursive-Averaging (MCRA) Algorithms

We showed in the previous section that the time smoothing factor $\alpha(\lambda, k)$ used in the recursive noise estimation is dependent on the conditional speech-presence probability $P(H_1^k \mid Y(\lambda,k))$. In fact, we showed that $\alpha(\lambda,k) = P(H_1^k \mid Y(\lambda,k))$. Three different methods for computing $P(H_1^k \mid Y(\lambda,k))$ and, consequently, $\alpha(\lambda,k)$ were proposed in [14,32,35,41]. In the first method [14], the probability $P(H_1^k \mid Y(\lambda,k))$ is computed by comparing the ratio of the noisy speech power spectrum to its local minimum against a threshold value. In this method, the probability estimate $P(H_1^k \mid Y(\lambda,k))$, and consequently the time smoothing factor $\alpha(\lambda,k)$, is controlled by the estimation of the spectral minimum, and for that reason the proposed algorithm is referred to as the minima-controlled recursive-averaging (MCRA) algorithm. The second method [32] computes $P(H_1^k \mid Y(\lambda,k))$ in a similar way, except that it uses a different algorithm for tracking the minimum of the noisy psd. In the third method [35], the probability $P(H_1^k \mid Y(\lambda,k))$ is computed using Equation 9.39 and an estimated *a priori* probability of speech absence $p(H_k^0)$ (recall that $p(H_k^0)$ was fixed in Equation 9.39). An elaborate method is proposed in [35] for computing the *a priori* probability of speech absence $p(H_k^0)$ needed in Equation 9.39 to evaluate $P(H_1^k \mid Y(\lambda,k))$. Details of these three methods are given next.

9.4.3.2.1 MCRA Algorithm

Following [13], the estimation of the noise power spectrum is based on the following two modified hypotheses:

$$\begin{aligned} H_0^k &: \hat{\sigma}_D^2(\lambda,k) = \alpha\hat{\sigma}_D^2(\lambda-1,k) + (1-\alpha)\,|Y(\lambda,k)|^2 \\ H_1^k &: \hat{\sigma}_D^2(\lambda,k) = \hat{\sigma}_D^2(\lambda-1,k) \end{aligned} \tag{9.50}$$

As before, Equation 9.50 is based on the principle that the noise estimate is updated whenever speech is absent, otherwise it is kept constant. The mean-square estimate of the noise psd is given as before by

$$\begin{aligned} \hat{\sigma}_d^2(\lambda,k) &= E\left[\sigma_d^2(\lambda,k) \mid Y(\lambda,k)\right] \\ &= E\left[\sigma_d^2(\lambda,k) \mid H_0\right] p(H_0 \mid Y(\lambda,k)) + E\left[\sigma_d^2(\lambda,k) \mid H_1\right] p(H_1 \mid Y(\lambda,k)) \end{aligned} \tag{9.51}$$

Based on the two hypotheses stated in Equation 9.50, we can express $\hat{\sigma}_d^2(\lambda,k)$ as

$$\begin{aligned} \hat{\sigma}_d^2(\lambda,k) &= \left[\alpha\hat{\sigma}_d^2(\lambda-1,k) + (1-\alpha)\,|Y(\lambda,k)|^2\right] p\left(H_0^k \mid Y(\lambda,k)\right) \\ &\quad + \hat{\sigma}_d^2\left(\lambda-1,k)p(H_1^k \mid Y(\lambda,k)\right) \\ &= \left[\alpha\hat{\sigma}_d^2(\lambda-1,k) + (1-\alpha)\,|Y(\lambda,k)|^2\right](1-p(\lambda,k)) \\ &\quad + \hat{\sigma}_d^2(\lambda-1,k)p(\lambda,k) \end{aligned} \tag{9.52}$$

where $p(\lambda,k) \triangleq P(H_1^k \mid Y(\lambda,k))$ denotes the conditional probability of speech presence. After simplifying Equation 9.52, we get

$$\hat{\sigma}_d^2(\lambda,k) = \alpha_d(\lambda,k)\hat{\sigma}_d^2(\lambda-1,k) + [1-\alpha_d(\lambda,k)]\left|Y(\lambda,k)\right|^2 \tag{9.53}$$

where

$$\alpha_d(\lambda,k) \triangleq \alpha + (1-\alpha)p(\lambda,k) \tag{9.54}$$

From Equation 9.54, we infer that unlike the smoothing factors used in SNR-dependent methods (e.g., see Equation 9.27), which vary in the range of zero to one, $\alpha_d(\lambda, k)$ takes values in the range of $\alpha \leq \alpha_d(\lambda, k) \leq 1$. Next, we present three time-recursive noise-estimation algorithms [14,35], of the form given in Equation 9.53, which use different methods to compute $p(\lambda, k)$ needed in Equation 9.54 to estimate the smoothing factors $\alpha_d(\lambda, k)$.

In the algorithm proposed in [14], the speech-presence probability $p(\lambda, k)$ of each frequency bin is calculated using the ratio of the noisy speech power spectrum to its local minimum [14]. The local minimum is found using a simplified version of the MS algorithm [25] by performing pairwise comparisons of the smoothed noisy speech psd, $S(\lambda, k)$. The smoothed noisy psd $S(\lambda, k)$ is estimated as follows:

$$S(\lambda,k) = \alpha_s S(\lambda-1,k) + (1-\alpha_s)S_f(\lambda,k) \tag{9.55}$$

where
- α_s is a smoothing factor
- $S_f(\lambda, k)$ is the smoothed (over frequency) noisy speech psd

$$S_f(\lambda,k) = \sum_{i=-L_w}^{L_w} w(i) \mid Y(\lambda,k-i) \mid^2 \tag{9.56}$$

where
- $w(i)$ is a windowing function (Hamming window was used in [14]
- $2L_w + 1$ is the window length

The local minimum $S_{\min}(\lambda, k)$ is found over a fixed window length of D frames by samplewise comparison of the past values of $S(\lambda, k)$ using the algorithm described in Equation 9.23.

The ratio of the smoothed noisy speech power spectra $S(\lambda, k)$ to its local minimum $S_{\min}(\lambda, k)$ is then formed as

$$S_r(\lambda,k) = \frac{S(\lambda,k)}{S_{\min}(\lambda,k)} \tag{9.57}$$

Note that the preceding ratio is similar to the definition of the *a posteriori* SNR, except that the smoothed psd $S(\lambda, k)$ is used rather than the periodogram estimate $|Y(\lambda, k)|^2$. This ratio is compared against a threshold δ to decide speech-present regions in the spectrum as follows:

$$\begin{aligned}
&\text{if } S_r(\lambda,k) > \delta \\
&\qquad p(\lambda,k) = 1 \quad \text{speech present} \\
&\text{else} \\
&\qquad p(\lambda,k) = 0 \quad \text{speech absent} \\
&\text{end}
\end{aligned} \tag{9.58}$$

Finally, the speech-presence probability $p(\lambda, k)$ is smoothed over time using the following recursion:

$$\hat{p}(\lambda,k) = \alpha_p \hat{p}(\lambda-1,k) + (1-\alpha_p)\, p(\lambda,k) \tag{9.59}$$

where

α_p is a smoothing constant
$p(\lambda, k)$ is computed according to Equation 9.58

After calculating the smoothed speech-presence probability $\hat{p}(\lambda, k)$, we compute the time–frequency-dependent smoothing factor $a_d(\lambda, k)$ using Equation 9.54 and then update the noise psd using Equation 9.53.

The MCRA noise-estimation algorithm is summarized here [14]:
MCRA algorithm:

Step 1: Compute the smooth noisy speech psd $S(\lambda, k)$ using Equation 9.55.

Step 2: Perform minimal tracking on $S(\lambda, k)$ using (9.23) to obtain $S_{\min}(\lambda, k)$.

Step 3: Determine $p(\lambda, k)$ using Equation 9.58, and use Equation 9.59 to smooth $p(\lambda, k)$ over time.

Step 4: Compute the time–frequency-dependent smoothing factor $a_d(\lambda, k)$ in Equation 9.54 using the smoothed conditional probability $\hat{p}(\lambda, k)$ from Equation 9.59.

Step 5: Update the noise psd $\hat{\sigma}_d^2(\lambda, k)$ using Equation 9.53.

Figure 9.21 shows the estimate of the noise spectrum obtained using the preceding MCRA algorithm with $\alpha = 0.95$, $\alpha_s = 0.8$, $\delta = 5$, and $\alpha_p = 0.2$ (the same parameters as employed in [14]). Note that the parameter δ used in Equation 9.58 was not found to be sensitive to the type and intensity of the noise [14]. A Hamming window was used in Equation 9.56 with $L_w = 1$. The minimum search window D was set to 1 s. Figure 9.21b shows the estimated conditional-presence probability $\hat{p}(\lambda, k)$. Note that the values of $\hat{p}(\lambda, k)$ are for the most part binary (either 1 or 0) despite the recursion in Equation 9.59. This is because $\hat{p}(\lambda, k)$ is based on the spectral minima (obtained using the MS algorithm), which may remain constant within a window of D frames. As a result, the time smoothing factor $\alpha_d(\lambda, k)$ in Equation 9.54 may take binary values, either $\alpha_d(\lambda, k) = \alpha$ or $\alpha_d(\lambda, k) = 1$, and the estimated noise psd will follow the spectral minima, similar to the MS algorithm.

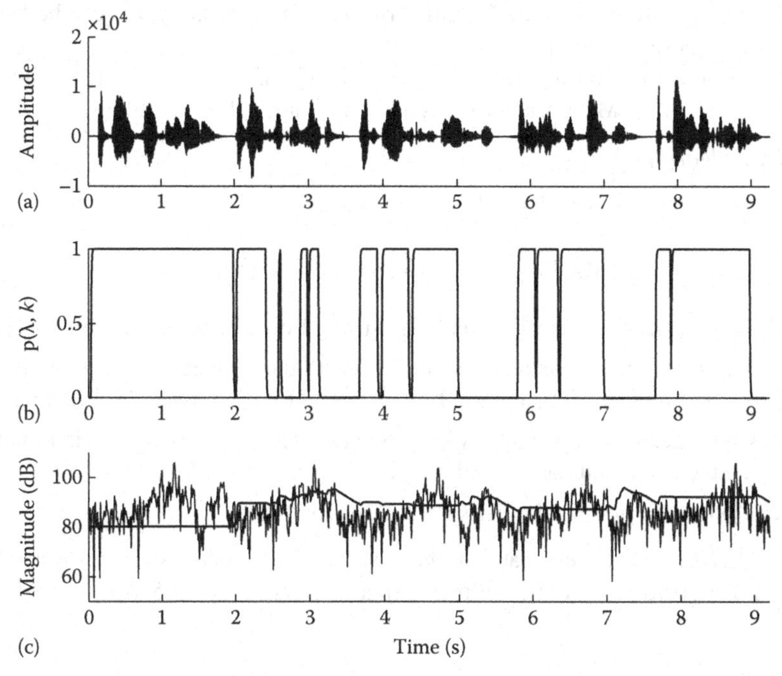

FIGURE 9.21 Noise power spectrum [(c)—thick line] estimated using the MCRA algorithm for a set of sentences embedded in babble at +5d B S/N. (b) Shows the conditional probability of speech presence computed according to Equation 9.59. The waveform (in quiet) is shown in (a) for reference.

9.4.3.2.2 MCRA-2 Algorithm

The noise psd estimate, obtained by the preceding MCRA noise-estimation algorithm, may lag, particularly when the noise power is rising, by as many as D frames from the true noise psd. To address this shortcoming, a different method was proposed in [32,42,43] for computing the ratio $S_r(\lambda, k)$ in Equation 9.57. Rather than using the MS approach for tracking the minima $S_{\min}(\lambda, k)$, the authors used the continuous spectral minima-tracking method [19] (see Section 9.3.2). Unlike the MS approach, this method tracks the minima continuously and is not constrained within a finite window.

In addition to using a different method to estimate $S_{\min}(\lambda, k)$ in Equation 9.57, a frequency-dependent threshold was used to estimate the speech-presence probability $p(\lambda, k)$ in Equation 9.58. More precisely, the fixed threshold δ in Equation 9.58 was replaced by the following frequency-dependent threshold $\delta(k)$:

$$\delta(k) = \begin{cases} 2 & 1 \leq k \leq LF \\ 2 & LF < k \leq MF \\ 5 & MF < k \leq Fs/2 \end{cases} \tag{9.60}$$

where

LF and *MF* are the bins corresponding to 1 and 3 kHz, respectively
Fs is the sampling frequency

The preceding threshold values were determined experimentally and can be potentially tuned for different types of noise [42].

The noise-estimation algorithm proposed in [32,43] is implemented using the same steps as in the MCRA algorithm and is summarized as follows:

MCRA-2 algorithm [43]:

Step 1: Smooth noisy speech psd $S(\lambda, k)$ as follows:

$$S(\lambda,k) = \alpha_s S(\lambda-1,k) + (1-\alpha_s)\,|\,Y(\lambda,k)\,|^2 \tag{9.61}$$

Step 2: Perform minimal tracking on $S(\lambda, k)$ using Equation 9.25 to obtain $S_{\min}(\lambda, k)$.

Step 3: Determine $p(\lambda, k)$ using Equation 9.58 with the frequency-dependent thresholds given by Equation 9.60, and use Equation 9.59 to smooth $p(\lambda, k)$ over time.

Step 4: Compute the time–frequency-dependent smoothing factor $a_d(\lambda, k)$ in Equation 9.54 using the smoothed conditional probability $\hat{p}(\lambda, k)$ from Equation 9.59.

Step 5: Update the noise psd $\hat{\sigma}_d^2(\lambda, k)$ using Equation 9.53.

Figure 9.22 shows the estimate of the noise psd obtained using the preceding MCRA-2 algorithm and the following parameters: α = 0.85 (Equation 9.54),

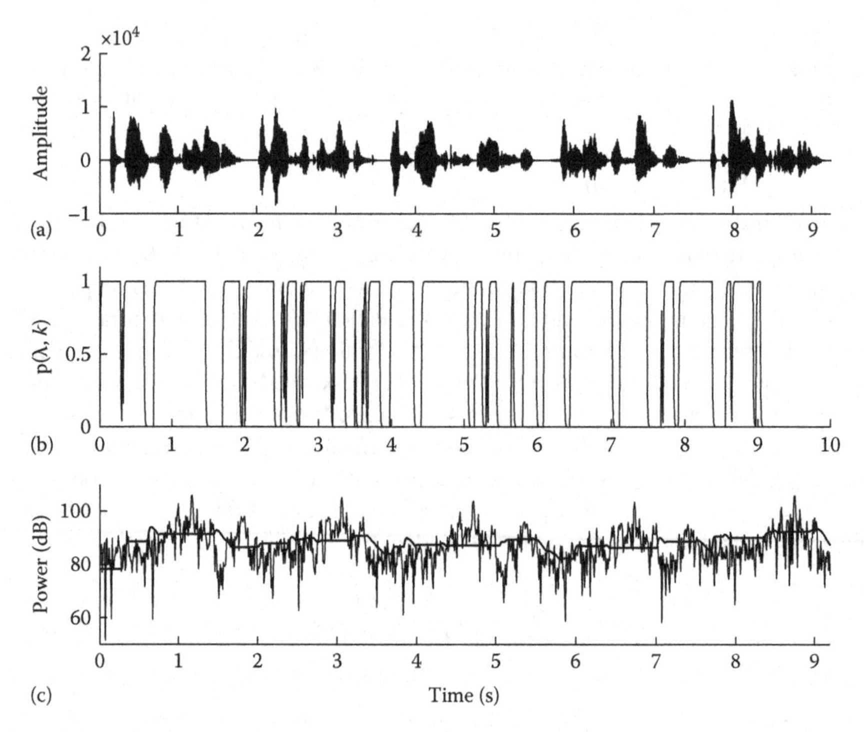

FIGURE 9.22 Noise power spectrum [(c)—thick line] estimated using the MCRA-2 algorithm [43] for a set of sentences embedded in babble at +5d B S/N. (b) Shows the conditional probability of speech presence. The waveform (in quiet) is shown in (a) for reference.

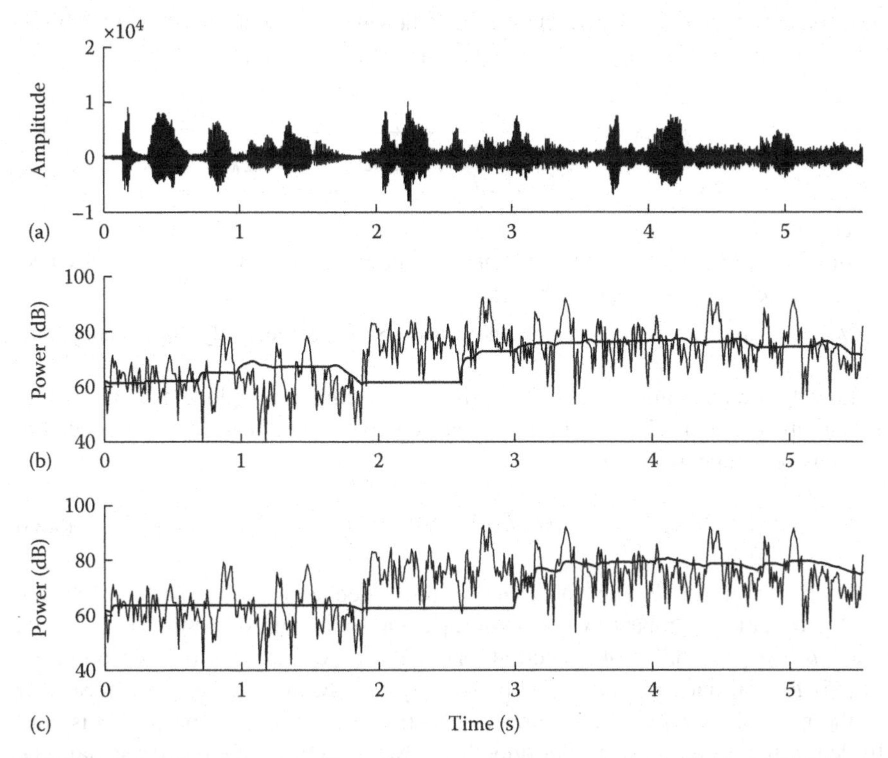

FIGURE 9.23 Comparison of noise power spectrum estimates obtained with the MCRA (c) and MCRA-2 (b) algorithms for $f = 1800$ Hz. The true noise psd (thin line) is superimposed for comparison. The noisy signal [shown in (a)] comprises three concatenated sentences, the first of which is embedded in a high S/N level (25 dB) whereas the other two are embedded in a low S/N level (5 dB).

$\alpha_s = 0.7$ (Equation 9.61), $\alpha_p = 0.2$ (Equation 9.59), $\beta = 0.9$, and $\gamma = 0.998$ (Equation 9.25). The tracking abilities of the MCRA and MCRA-2 algorithms are better compared in another example, which is shown in Figure 9.23. In this example, the signal comprises three concatenated sentences, the first of which is embedded in a high S/N level (25 dB) whereas the other two are embedded in a low S/N level (5 dB). Note that at $t = 1.8$ s, the noise power level (at $f = 1800$ Hz) increases significantly. It takes about 1 s for the MCRA algorithm (Figure 9.23c) to track the rising noise level, whereas it only requires roughly 600 ms for the MCRA-2 algorithm (Figure 9.23b) to track the noise. Objective and subjective listening evaluations of the MCRA-2 algorithm were reported in [32,42,43]. The MCRA-2 algorithm was integrated in a speech-enhancement algorithm [44] and compared using subjective preference tests against other noise-estimation algorithms including the MS and MCRA algorithms [32,42,43]. Subjective evaluations indicated that the speech quality of the MCRA-2 algorithm was better than the MCRA algorithm and comparable to that obtained with the MS algorithm.

9.4.3.2.3 Improved MCRA (IMCRA) Algorithm

Further refinements to the MCRA algorithm were reported in [35]. The conditional speech-presence probability $p(\lambda, k)$ was derived using Equation 9.39 rather than Equation 9.58.

The conditional probability $p(\lambda, k)$ takes the following form after substituting the likelihood ratio given in Equation 9.43 into Equation 9.39 (see also Section 7.13):

$$p(\lambda,k) = \frac{1}{1+\dfrac{q(\lambda,k)}{1-q(\lambda,k)}(1+\xi_k(\lambda))\exp(-v(\lambda,k))} \tag{9.62}$$

where
$q(\lambda,k) \triangleq p(H_0^k)$ is the *a priori* probability of speech absence, $v(L, k) \triangleq \gamma_k(\lambda)\xi_k(\lambda)/(1+\xi_k(\lambda))$
$\gamma_k(\lambda)$ and $\xi_k(\lambda)$ are the *a posteriori* and *a priori* SNRs, respectively, at frequency bin k

Following the computation of $p(\lambda, k)$, the noise estimation is done as before using Equations 9.53 and 9.54. In addition, a bias compensation factor β is introduced to the noise estimate as follows:

$$\tilde{\sigma}_d^2(\lambda,k) = \beta\hat{\sigma}_d^2(\lambda,k) \tag{9.63}$$

where β was set to 1.47. The bias term was introduced to minimize speech distortion.

The conditional probability $p(\lambda, k)$ in Equation 9.62 requires an estimate of $q(\lambda, k)$, the *a priori* probability of speech absence. Next, we present a method proposed in [35] for estimating the *a priori* probability of speech absence, $q(\lambda, k)$. Similar to the method described in the previous section, the estimation of $q(\lambda, k)$ is controlled by the minima values of a smoothed power spectrum of the noisy signal. The proposed method comprises two iterations of smoothing and minimum tracking. The first iteration provides rough VAD in each frequency bin. The smoothing in the second iteration excludes relatively strong speech components, thus allowing for smaller windows in minimal tracking. Recall from Section 9.2 that short windows are needed for better tracking of highly nonstationary noise.

The first iteration of smoothing is done in a similar fashion as in the previous section using Equations 9.55 and 9.56. Minimal tracking is performed over the past D frame estimates of $S(\lambda, k)$ to obtain $S_{min}(\lambda, k)$. Then, a rough speech-presence decision is made using the following rule:

$$I(\lambda,k) = \begin{cases} 1 & \text{if } \gamma_{min}(\lambda,k) < \gamma_0 \quad \text{and} \quad \zeta(\lambda,k) < \zeta_0 \text{ (speech is absent)} \\ 0 & \text{otherwise} \qquad\qquad\qquad\qquad\qquad\qquad \text{(speech is present)} \end{cases} \tag{9.64}$$

where γ_0 and ζ_0 are threshold parameters, and

$$\gamma_{min}(\lambda,k) \triangleq \frac{|Y(\lambda,k)|^2}{B_{min}S_{min}(\lambda,k)}; \quad \zeta(\lambda,k) \triangleq \frac{S(\lambda,k)}{B_{min}S_{min}(\lambda,k)} \tag{9.65}$$

and the factor B_{min} represents the bias of the minimum noise estimate. Unlike [18], a constant bias factor, B_{min} = 1.66, was used. The threshold values γ_0 and ζ_0 are chosen so that the error margin in making a wrong decision falls below a specified threshold. Equation 9.64 is based on the same principle as in Equation 9.58

except that two different ratios, $\gamma_{min}(\lambda, k)$ and $\zeta(\lambda, k)$, are used to ensure that the speech-present/-absent decisions are more reliable.

The second iteration of smoothing includes only spectral components that have been identified by Equation 9.64 to contain primarily noise. This is done using the following function, denoted $\tilde{S}_f(\lambda, k)$, which smooths (in the frequency domain) spectral components identified to contain primarily noise:

$$\tilde{S}_f(\lambda,k)=\begin{cases}\dfrac{\sum_{i=-L_w}^{L_w} w(i)I(\lambda,k-i)\,|Y(\lambda,k-i)|^2}{\sum_{i=-L_w}^{L_w} w(i)I(\lambda,k-i)}, & \text{if } \sum_{i=-L_w}^{L_w} I(\lambda,k-i)\neq 0\\ \tilde{S}(\lambda-1,k) & \text{otherwise}\end{cases} \tag{9.66}$$

where

$w(i)$ is the windowing function (applied in the frequency domain)
L_w is the length of the window (in frequency bins)
$\tilde{S}(\lambda, k)$ is defined in the following text

Following the preceding computation of $\tilde{S}_f(\lambda, k)$, the following first-order recursive averaging is performed:

$$\tilde{S}(\lambda,k)=\alpha_s\tilde{S}(\lambda-1,k)+(1-\alpha_s)\tilde{S}_f(\lambda,k) \tag{9.67}$$

Note that Equation 9.66 performs the smoothing in the frequency domain, and Equation 9.67 performs it in the time domain. Excluding strong (high-energy) speech components from the smoothing process in Equation 9.66 allows us to select larger smoothing windows (i.e., large α_s in Equation 9.67) and smaller minimum search windows (i.e., smaller D). Choosing a smaller window length D is important in minimal tracking as we can reduce the delay to responding to rising noise power. Figure 9.24 shows an example of the smoothed psd $\tilde{S}(\lambda, k)$ obtained using information from Equation 9.64. Figure 9.24a shows estimates of $S(\lambda, k)$ obtained using Equation 9.55 and Figure 9.24b shows estimates of $\tilde{S}(\lambda, k)$ obtained using Equations 9.67 and 9.66. As can be seen, the operation in Equation 9.66 indeed removes the strong speech components.

In the second iteration, minimal tracking is performed based on the values of $\tilde{S}(\lambda, k)$. Let $\tilde{S}_{min}(\lambda, k)$ be the minimum of $\tilde{S}(\lambda, k)$ in Equation 9.67 obtained over the past D frames. Then, the *a priori* speech-absence probability $q(\lambda, k)$ is computed as

$$\hat{q}(\lambda,k)=\begin{cases}1, & \text{if } \tilde{\gamma}_{min}(\lambda,k)\le 1 \text{ and } \tilde{\zeta}(\lambda,k)<\zeta_0\\ \dfrac{\gamma_1-\tilde{\gamma}_{min}(\lambda,k)}{\gamma_1-1} & \text{if } 1<\tilde{\gamma}_{min}(\lambda,k)<\gamma_1 \text{ and } \tilde{\zeta}(\lambda,k)<\zeta_0\\ 0 & \text{otherwise}\end{cases} \tag{9.68}$$

where γ_1 is a threshold parameter and

$$\tilde{\gamma}_{min}(\lambda,k)\triangleq\frac{|Y(\lambda,k)|^2}{B_{min}\tilde{S}_{min}(\lambda,k)};\quad \tilde{\zeta}(\lambda,k)\triangleq\frac{\tilde{S}(\lambda,k)}{B_{min}\tilde{S}_{min}(\lambda,k)} \tag{9.69}$$

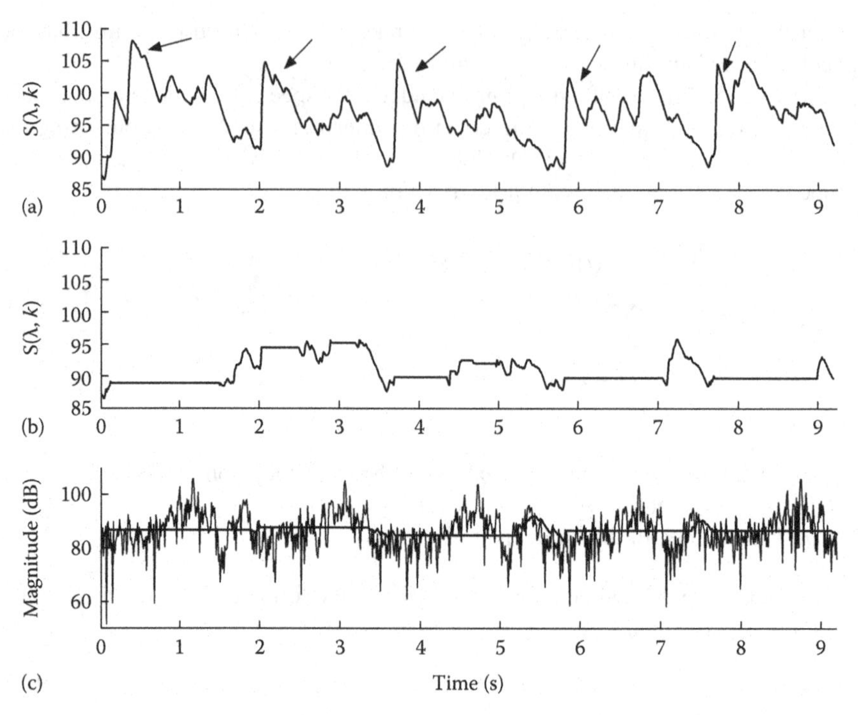

FIGURE 9.24 (a) Shows the smoothed psd obtained in the IMCRA algorithm using Equation 9.55 for a set of sentences embedded in babble at +5 dB S/N. Arrows indicate the strong speech components present. (b) Shows the smoothed psd obtained after removing the strong speech components using Equation 9.66. (c) Shows the noise psd obtained using the IMCRA algorithm. The true noise psd (thin line) is superimposed.

Note that the estimation of $q(\lambda, k)$ is similar in many respects to the estimation of $p(\lambda, k)$ in Equation 9.58. The preceding estimator assumes that speech is absent (i.e., $\hat{q}(\lambda, k) = 1$) whenever both *a posteriori* SNR measurements, based on the smoothed and instantaneous measured powers, are below a certain threshold. Similarly, speech is assumed to be present (i.e., $\hat{q}(\lambda, k) = 0$) whenever the two *a posteriori* estimators are above a certain threshold (i.e., when $\tilde{\zeta}(\lambda, k) \geq \zeta_0$ and $\tilde{\gamma}_{min}(\lambda, k) > \gamma_1$). In between, the $q(\lambda, k)$ estimator provides a soft transition between speech absence and speech presence. The use of $\zeta(\lambda, k)$ alone is not sufficient for detecting weak speech components and for that reason both $\tilde{\zeta}(\lambda, k)$ and $\tilde{\gamma}_{min}(\lambda, k)$ estimators are used. Hence, by combining conditions on both the $\tilde{\zeta}(\lambda, k)$ and $\tilde{\gamma}_{min}(\lambda, k)$ estimators, we can prevent an increase in the estimated noise level during weak speech activity, that is, during low-SNR segments.

IMCRA algorithm is summarized as follows [35, fig. 1]:

Step 1: Compute the smoothed power spectrum $S(\lambda, k)$ using Equation 9.55 and update its running minimum $S_{min}(\lambda, k)$.

Step 2: Compute the indicator function $I(\lambda, k)$ for VAT using Equation 9.64.

Step 3: Compute the smoothed psd $\tilde{S}(\lambda, k)$ using Equations 9.67 and 9.66, and update its running minimum $\tilde{S}_{min}(\lambda, k)$.

Step 4: Compute the *a priori* speech-absence probability $q(\lambda, k)$ using Equations 9.68 and 9.69.

Step 5: Compute the *a posteriori* and *a priori* SNRs $\gamma_k(\lambda)$ and $\xi_k(\lambda)$, respectively, and use those values to compute the speech-presence probability $p(\lambda, k)$ according to Equation 9.62.

Step 6: Compute the smoothing parameter $\alpha_d(\lambda, k)$ using Equation 9.54 and update the noise spectrum using Equations 9.53 and 9.63.

Note that step 5 requires the computation of the *a priori* SNR $\xi_k(\lambda)$, which can be obtained using the decision-directed approach [38]. The improved minimum-tracking algorithm proposed in [18] was used in steps 1 and 3. Recall from Section 9.3.1.4 that the tracking algorithm proposed in [18] divides the whole minimum search window of D frames into U subwindows of V frames each ($D = U \cdot V$). This was done to reduce the delay introduced when the noise power increases.

Figure 9.25c shows the estimate of the noise spectrum obtained using the preceding IMCRA algorithm with the following parameters: $\alpha_s = 0.9$, $\alpha = 0.85$, $B_{\min} = 1.66$, $\beta = 1.47$, $\gamma_1 = 3$, $\gamma_0 = 4.6$, and $\zeta_0 = 1.67$ (the same parameters as employed in [14],

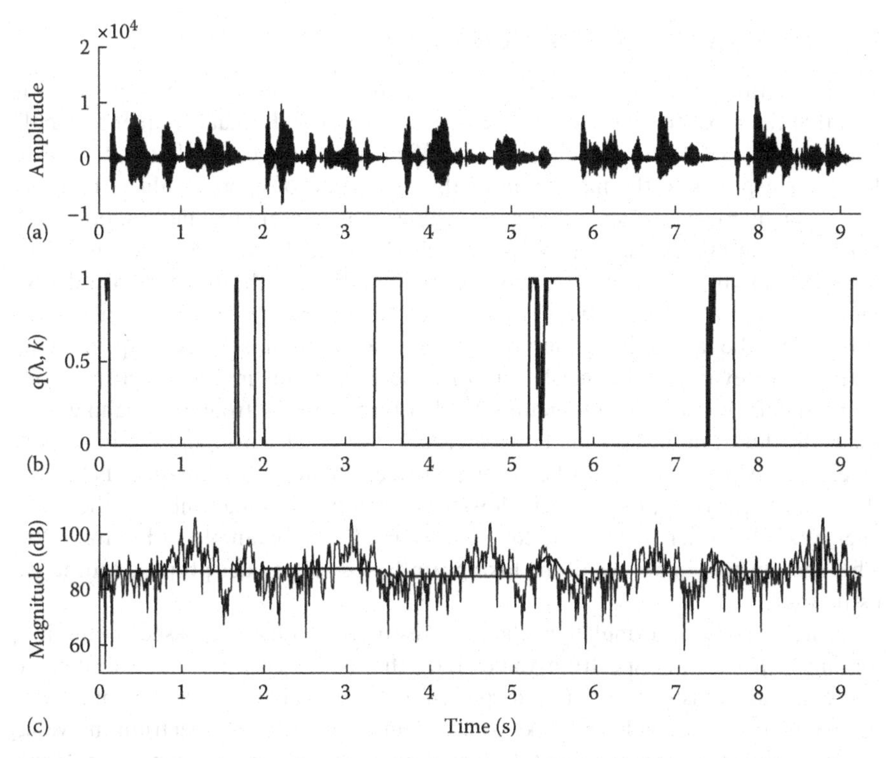

FIGURE 9.25 Plot of the estimated probability of speech absence, $q(\lambda, k)$, obtained by the IMCRA algorithm. (a) Shows the clean signal. (b) Shows the estimated speech-absence probability $q(\lambda, k)$. (c) Shows the noise psd obtained using the IMCRA algorithm. The true noise psd (thin line) is superimposed.

valid for a sampling rate of 16kHz). A Hamming window was used in Equation 9.56 with $L_w = 1$. The minimum search window D was set to 120 frames, with $V = 15$ and $U = 8$ ($D = U \cdot V$). Figure 9.25b shows the estimated speech-absence probability $q(\lambda, k)$. Note that the values of $q(\lambda, k)$ are for the most part binary (either 1 or 0). Consequently, the speech-presence probability $p(\lambda, k)$ in Equation 9.62 is also binary as the $q(\lambda, k)$ values are multiplicative to the second term in the denominator. As a result, the time smoothing factor $\alpha_d(\lambda, k)$ in Equation 9.54 will also take binary values, that is, $\alpha_d(\lambda, k) = \alpha$ or $\alpha_d(\lambda, k) = 1$, and the estimated noise psd will follow the spectral minima, similar to the MS algorithm. However, unlike the MS algorithm, which lags behind by a minimum delay of $D + V$ frames when the noise power increases, the delay of the IMCRA algorithm may be smaller because the recursive averaging (Equation 9.53) is carried out instantaneously.

The performance of this algorithm was evaluated in [35], using both subjective and objective measures. The objective evaluation involved the relative estimation error between the true and estimated noise spectra. Compared to the MS algorithm [18], the IMCRA algorithm yielded smaller estimation errors for several types of noise.

9.5 HISTOGRAM-BASED TECHNIQUES

The histogram-based noise-estimation algorithms are motivated by the observation that the most frequent value of energy values in individual frequency bands corresponds to the noise level of the specified frequency band; that is, the noise level corresponds to the maximum of the histogram of energy values. In some cases, the histogram of spectral energy values may contain two modes: (a) a low-energy mode corresponding to the speech-absent and low-energy segments of speech, and (b) a high-energy mode corresponding to the (noisy) voiced segments of speech (see example in Figure 9.2). Of the two modes, the former mode is typically the largest in the number of occurrences, that is, more frequent. This pattern, however, is not consistent in that the histograms might sometimes contain only one mode, depending among other things on the frequency band examined, the duration of the signal considered, the type of noise, and the input S/N level [30]. Also, it is not unlikely, for instance, owing to the low-pass nature of the speech spectrum, to see in the low-frequency bands a maximum in the high-energy mode rather than in the low-energy mode (see example in Figure 9.26). This section presents some of the histogram-based techniques proposed for noise estimation.

In its most basic formulation, the noise estimate is obtained based on the histogram of past power spectrum values [20]; that is, for each incoming frame, we first construct a histogram of power spectrum values spanning a window of several hundreds of milliseconds, and take as an estimate of the noise spectrum the value corresponding to the maximum of the histogram values (see example in Figure 9.26). This is done separately for each individual frequency bin. A first-order recursive smoothing may also be performed on the noise spectrum estimate to smooth out any outliers in the estimate.

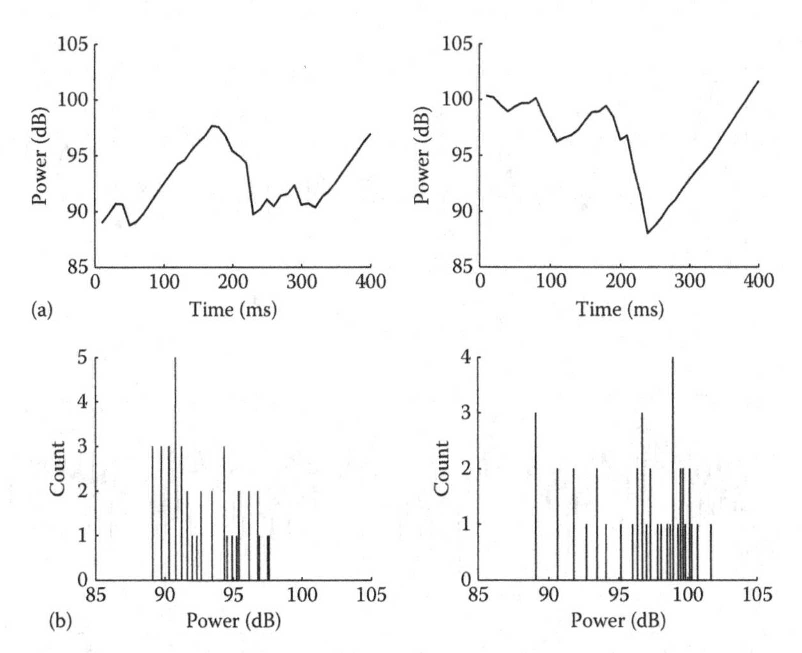

FIGURE 9.26 (a) Shows two example of the power spectrum levels (at f = 500 Hz). (b) Shows the histograms obtained from the two power spectrum forms in (a) respectively. The histograms were computed based on a 400 ms window of past spectral information.

The histogram method is summarized as follows:

For each frame λ do

Step 1: Compute the noisy speech power spectrum $|Y(\lambda, k)|^2$.

Step 2: Smooth the noisy psd using first-order recursion:

$$S(\lambda,k) = \alpha S(\lambda-1,k) + (1-\alpha)\,|\,Y(\lambda,k)\,|^2 \tag{9.70}$$

where α is a smoothing constant.

Step 3: Compute the histogram of D past psd estimates $S(\lambda, k)$ $\{S(\lambda - 1, k), S(\lambda - 2, k),\ldots, S(\lambda - D, k)\}$ using, say, 40 bins.

Step 4: Let $\mathbf{c} = [c_1, c_2, \ldots, c_{40}]$ be the counts in each of the 40 bins in the histogram and $\mathbf{s} = [s_1, s_2,\ldots, s_{40}]$ denote the corresponding centers of the histogram bins. Let $c_{\max}$ be the index of the maximum count, that is, $c_{\max} = \arg\max_{1\le i\le 40} c_i$. Then, take an estimate of the noise psd (denoted by $H_{\max}(\lambda, k)$) the value corresponding to the maximum of the histogram, that is, $H_{\max}(\lambda, k) = s(c_{\max})$.

Step 5: Smooth the noise estimate $H_{\max}(\lambda, k)$ using first-order recursion:

$$\hat{\sigma}_d^2(\lambda,k) = \alpha_m \hat{\sigma}_d^2(\lambda-1,k) + (1-\alpha_m) H_{\max}(\lambda,k)$$

where

$\hat{\sigma}_d^2(\lambda, k)$ is the smoothed estimate of the noise psd

α_m is a smoothing constant

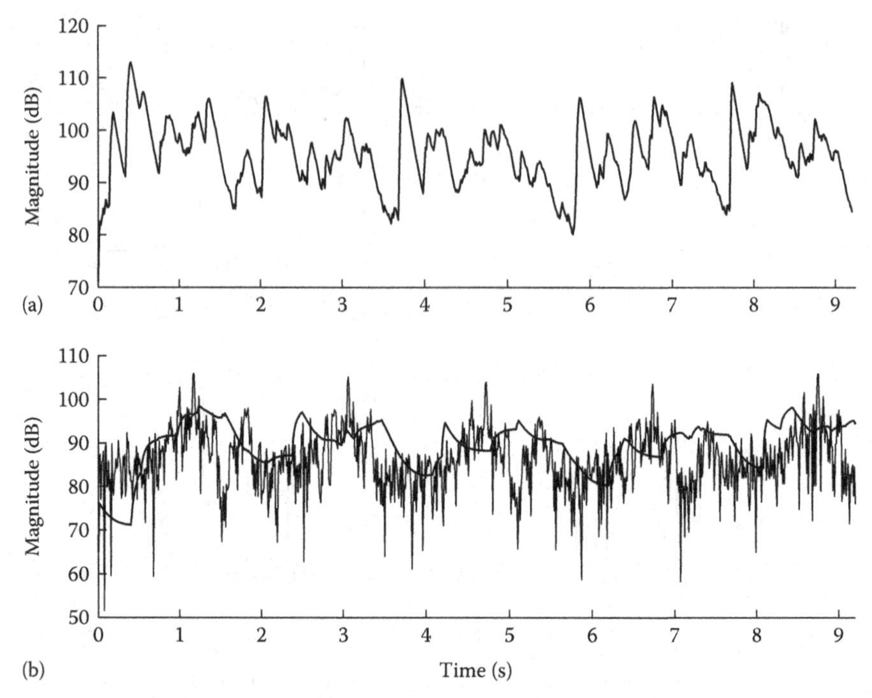

FIGURE 9.27 Noise psd [(b)—thick line] obtained (for f = 500 Hz) using the histogram method with D = 400 ms. Histogram was computed using the smoothed noisy speech psd. The true noise psd [(b)—thin line] is superimposed. (a) Shows the smoothed noisy psd.

Figure 9.27 shows an example of the noise psd estimated for a low-frequency band (f = 500 Hz) using the preceding algorithm with $\alpha = 0.8$, $\alpha_m = 0.9$, and D corresponding to 400 ms. Aside from a few instances in which the noise level is overestimated (e.g., see segments at t = 4.2 and 8.5 s), the histogram approach does a good job of tracking the noise. When compared to the weighted-averaging technique, the histogram method performed better in terms of obtaining lower relative estimation error [20].

Note that step 2 (i.e., the smoothing of the noisy speech psd) was originally omitted in [20]. Figure 9.28 shows the same example as in Figure 9.27 but without applying any smoothing on the noisy speech power spectrum, that is, using $\alpha = 0$ in Equation 9.70. As can be seen, the noise estimate is biased toward lower values and looks similar to the noise psd obtained with minimum-tracking algorithms. It is clear that the smoothing operation in step 2 influences the performance of the histogram-based noise-estimation algorithm.

The noise overestimation problem shown in Figure 9.27 is due primarily to the length of the window used for constructing the histograms. More specifically, noise overestimation occurs when the window is not long enough to encompass broad speech peaks. This can be seen in the example in Figure 9.26b, which shows the histogram of a 400 ms segment taken from broad speech activity. The maximum in the histogram is no longer at the low-energy mode but at the high-energy mode. Note that this problem is more prominent in the low-frequency bands, where the speech energy is often high. In the

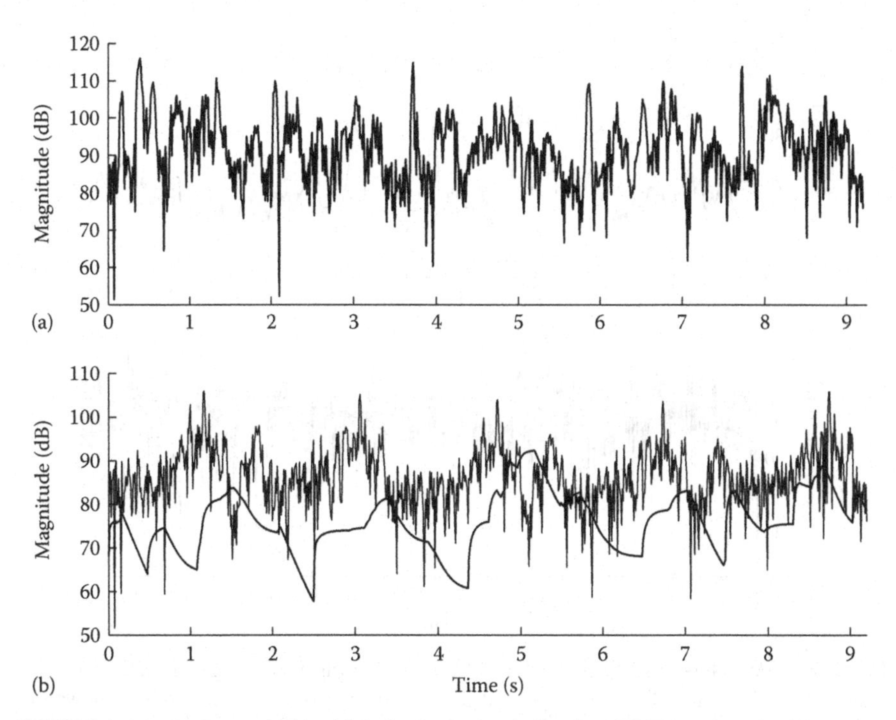

FIGURE 9.28 Noise psd [(b), thick line] obtained (for f = 500 Hz) using the histogram method (D = 400 ms) based on unsmoothed noisy speech psd [shown in (a)]. The true noise psd [(b), thin line] is superimposed.

high-frequency bands, the occurrence of strong speech peaks is not as frequent and therefore using a short window length is not an issue. This is illustrated in Figure 9.29, which shows the noise estimated for f = 4500 Hz. The noise psd is rarely overestimated.

There are at least two methods that can be used to avoid noise overestimation. The first, and easiest, approach is to simply use a longer window, that is, a larger D in Step 3 for estimating the histogram of past psd estimates. The idea is to use a window large enough to encompass broad speech activity. The effect of window length D on the estimate of the noise psd is shown in Figure 9.30. Longer windows do indeed eliminate noise overestimation, at the price, however, of diminishing the tracking ability of the estimator; that is, long windows yield noise estimators that are not capable of tracking fast changes in noise levels. This is the well-known trade-off between noise overestimation and tracking capability, not only for the histogram algorithms but also for the minimal-tracking algorithms (see Section 9.3). Note that with long windows, the pattern of noise psd estimates obtained with the histogram algorithm resembles the pattern of the minimal-tracking algorithms.

The second approach is to avoid including frames with large power values in the histogram computation; that is, to filter out the frames that most likely contain speech activity. This can be done by allowing only frames that have *a posteriori* SNR values smaller than a certain threshold, as done for instance in the weighted-averaging

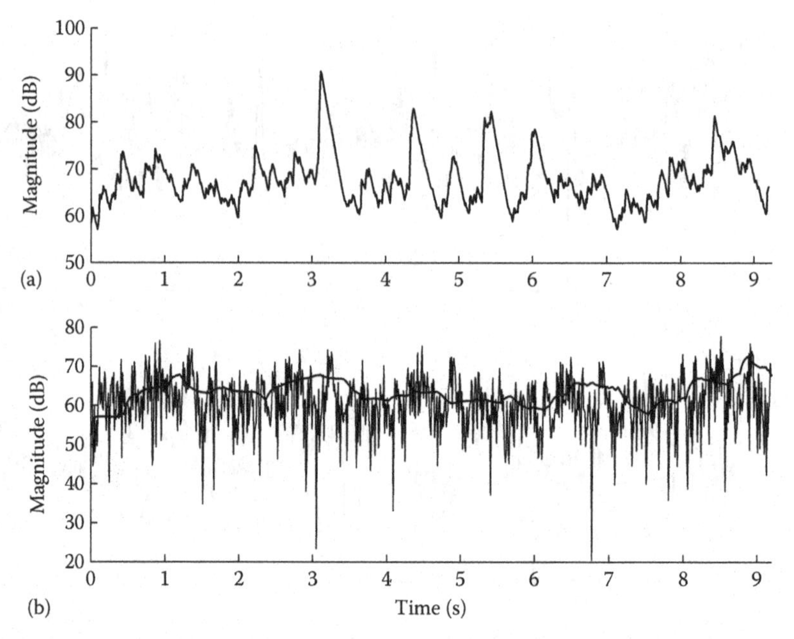

FIGURE 9.29 Noise psd [(b)—thick line] obtained using the histogram method for f = 4500 Hz (D = 400 ms). The true noise psd [(b)—thin line] is superimposed. (a) Shows the smoothed noisy speech psd.

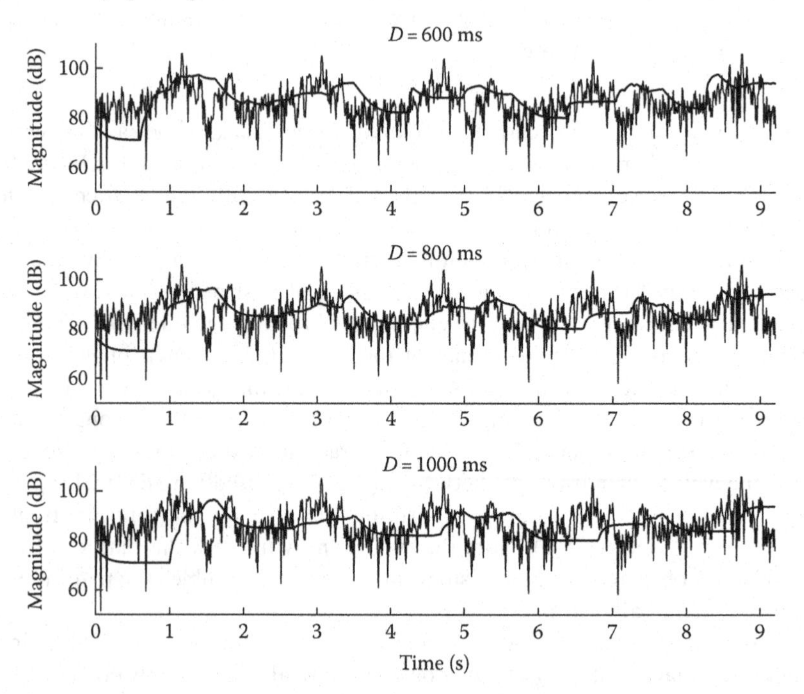

FIGURE 9.30 Effect of histogram window length (D) on the noise psd estimate (thick line). The true noise psd (thin line) is superimposed.

technique (see Equation 9.30). That is, in step 3, include in the histogram computation only past psd estimates $S(\lambda, k)$ that satisfy the following condition:

$$\frac{S(m,k)}{\sigma_d^2(\lambda-1,k)} < \delta \quad \text{for } m = \lambda-1, \lambda-2, \ldots, \lambda-D \tag{9.71}$$

where δ is a fixed threshold.

Alternatively, we can use a dynamically updated threshold and include only past psd estimates that are smaller than this threshold or smaller than the average energy of the past D frames. More specifically, in step 3, we can include in the histogram computation only past psd estimates $S(\lambda, k)$ that satisfy the following condition [30]:

$$S(m,k) < \min\{\delta(k), \bar{S}(k)\} \quad \text{for } m = \lambda-1, \lambda-2, \ldots, \lambda-D \tag{9.72}$$

where $\bar{S}(k)$ is the average energy (for frequency bin k) over the past D frames,

$$\bar{S}(k) = \frac{1}{D} \sum_{m=\lambda-1}^{\lambda-D} S(m,k) \tag{9.73}$$

and $\delta(k)$ is a dynamically updated threshold given by

$$\delta(k) = \sigma_d^2(\lambda-1,k) + r_{dB} \tag{9.74}$$

where $r_{dB} = 9$ dB. The preceding condition ensures that only frames containing noise, or low-energy speech segments, or both are included in the histogram computation.

Figure 9.31 shows the noise psd estimated using Equation 9.71 (Figure 9.31a) with $\delta = 2.5$ and Equation 9.72 (Figure 9.31b) with a value of D corresponding to 400 ms. Comparing Figure 9.31 with Figure 9.27 we see that the preceding simple modifications reduced the number of instances of noise overestimation. This was done without having to resort to larger window lengths.

Two variations to this histogram approach were proposed in [30]. The first method uses a different technique for identifying the modes in the histogram. Rather than relying on the maximum of the histogram distribution, which may lead to erroneous estimates of the noise psd, particularly in the low-frequency bands, this method uses instead a clustering algorithm to identify the two modes. More precisely, a two-centroid clustering algorithm (based on the *k-means* algorithm) is used in the first method to detect the two modes (low- and high-energy modes) of the histogram. The lower centroid value is taken to be the noise level, whereas the higher centroid value is taken to be the noisy speech level. Simulations in [30] indicated that the two-centroid clustering algorithm yielded larger noise-estimation errors than the original histogram method.

The second method [30] is based on the use of long (64 ms) analysis windows for spectral analysis. The long analysis windows yield better frequency resolution, thus allowing interharmonic components to participate in the histogram computation. Use of longer analysis windows provides a finer histogram resolution and, possibly,

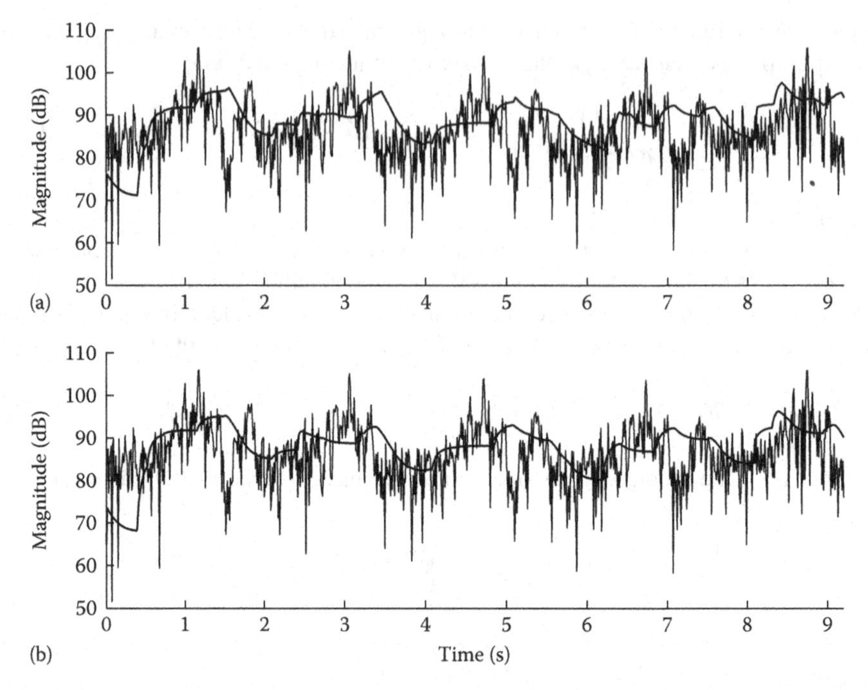

FIGURE 9.31 Noise psd estimates (f = 500 Hz) obtained using a modified histogram method that includes only past psd values satisfying certain conditions (Equations 9.71 and 9.72). (a) Shows the noise psd estimated using Equation 9.71 with $\delta = 2.5$ and (b) shows the noise psd estimated using Equation 9.72. Histogram window length was set to $D = 400$ ms.

more accurate noise psd estimates. Regions of the spectrum (200-Hz-wide frequency bands with 100-Hz overlap) are used as input to the histogram method. Simulation studies showed that the use of long analysis windows helped reduce the time segment length needed in the histogram or minimal-tracking noise-estimation algorithms and improved the noise-estimation accuracy of these algorithms.

A histogram method based on a different principle was proposed in [45]. In this method [45], the noise estimate is updated whenever a noise-only frame is detected. A chi-square test is used to detect the presence of noise-only frames. This test is based on the principle that if there is a good fit between the frequency distribution of the observed noisy speech frame and that of the estimated noise frame, the observed frame must be a noise-only frame. The noise estimate is subsequently updated whenever a noise-only frame is detected. The implementation of the chi-square noise-estimation algorithm involved the following steps [45]. The noisy speech is first band-limited to 0.2–4 kHz and then band-pass-filtered into eight subbands of equal width, using a set of IIR band-pass filters. Then, each of these subband signals is segmented into 15 ms frames. The histogram of the current frame is constructed and compared against the histogram of the previous frame using a chi-square statistic. If the value of the computed chi-square statistic is found to be smaller than a preset threshold, then the current frame is declared a noise-only frame. The noise psd estimate is finally updated using a simple first-order recursive algorithm.

9.6 OTHER NOISE-ESTIMATION ALGORITHMS

Aside from the preceding noise-estimation algorithms, several other algorithms were proposed in the literature [23,46–49] that did not quite fit in the three categories of noise-estimation algorithms described so far.

The approach proposed in [23] is motivated by the same principles as the histogram method. It is based on the observation that the low-energy spectral levels occur more frequently than the high-energy spectral levels in a given frequency band. Consider, for instance, sorting the signal energies of a specific frequency band. Figure 9.32 shows as an example the power levels (for $f = 500\,\text{Hz}$) sorted over the entire 9 s signal with the horizontal axis indicating the qth percentile, also called *quantile*. The signal energy is very low in roughly 80%–90% of the frames and is high in only 10%–20% of the frames containing high-energy (voiced segments) speech. This is also illustrated in the histogram of signal energies shown in Figure 9.32b. We can exploit this observation to estimate the noise psd from the noisy speech psd simply by taking the qth quantile in each frequency band as the noise estimate. Several values of q were investigated in [23], and the value of $q = 0.5$, that is, the median, was found to work well.

Generally, to compute the qth quantile, we first sort the noisy speech power spectrum $S_y(\lambda, k) \triangleq |Y(\lambda, k)|^2$ in each frequency bin such that

$$S_y(\lambda_0, k) \leq S(\lambda_1, k) \leq \ldots \leq S(\lambda_{D-1}, k) \quad (9.75)$$

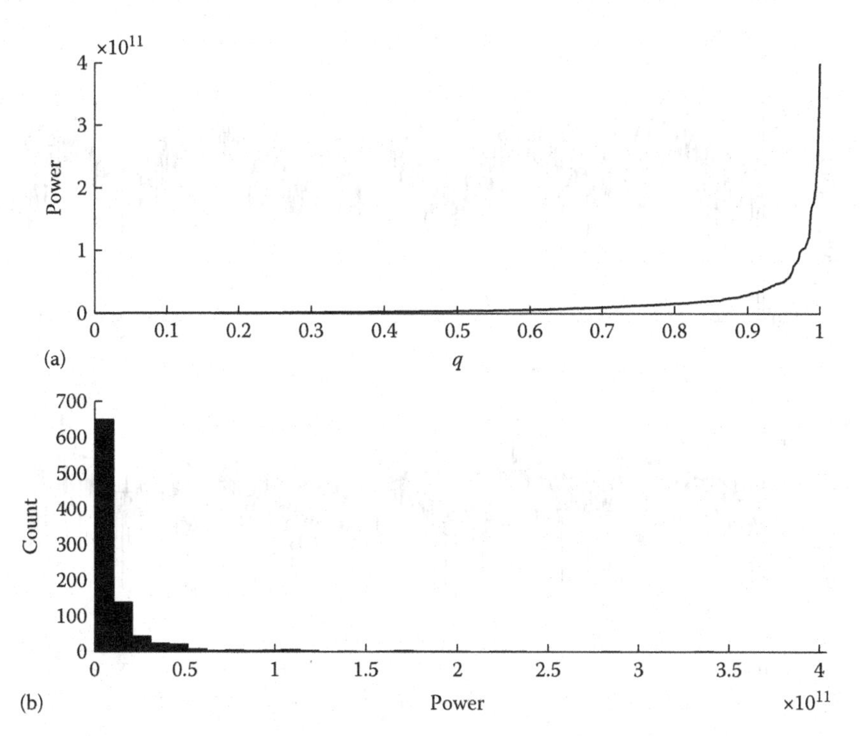

FIGURE 9.32 (a) Shows the power levels (at $f = 500\,\text{Hz}$) sorted over a 9 s duration signal with the horizontal axis indicating the qth percentile. (b) Shows the corresponding histogram of power levels.

where D is the total number of frames considered. The qth quantile noise estimate is then obtained as

$$\hat{\sigma}_d^2(\lambda, k) = S_y(\lambda_{\lfloor qD \rfloor}, k) \tag{9.76}$$

where $0 \leq q \leq 1$, $\lfloor \cdot \rfloor$ indicates the flooring operator and $S_y(\lambda, k)$ is the sorted noisy speech spectrum as per Equation 9.75. Note that $q = 0$ corresponds to the minimum of the psd estimates, $q = 1$ corresponds to the maximum and $q = 0.5$ corresponds to the median. We may consider the minimal-tracking algorithms as a special case of the preceding approach when q takes the value of $q = 0$. The minimum estimator is known to be sensitive to outliers, and it seems reasonable to consider the median estimator (i.e., $q = 0.5$), which is more robust.

The preceding quantile-based noise-estimation algorithm is summarized as follows:

Quantile-based algorithm:

For each frame λ do

Step 1: Sort the past D power spectrum estimates of the noisy speech signal, that is, $\{|Y(\lambda - 1, k)|^2, |Y(\lambda - 2, k)|^2, \ldots, |Y(\lambda - D - 1, k)|^2\}$.

Step 2: Pick the median psd estimate as the noise estimate.

Figure 9.33 shows the noise psd estimate obtained using this median-based noise-estimation algorithm, with D corresponding to 400 and 800 ms. As can

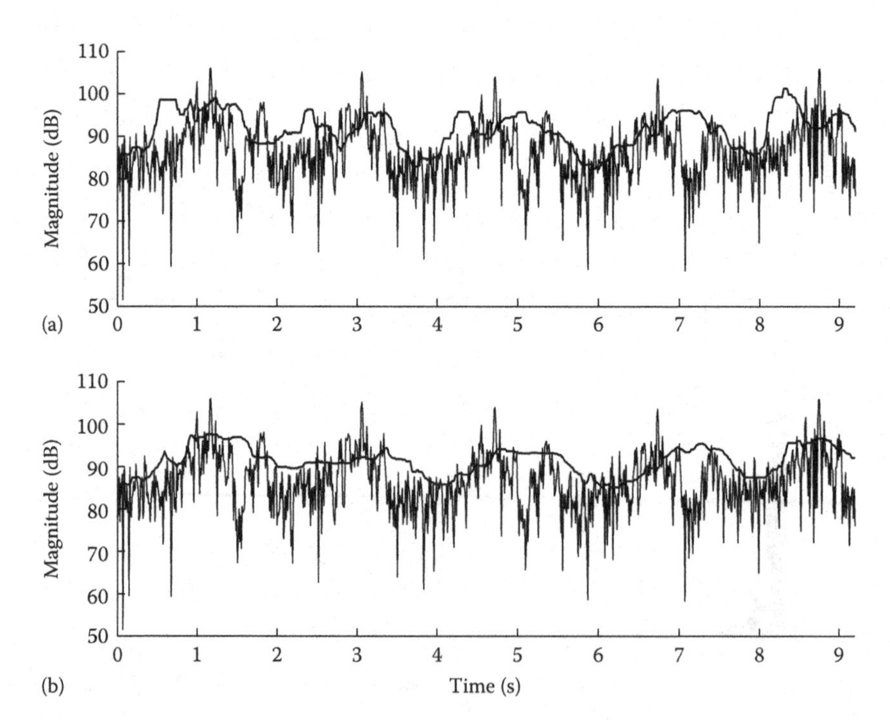

FIGURE 9.33 Noise psd estimate (thick line) obtained using the quantile-based method with $D = 400$ ms (a) and $D = 800$ ms (b). The true noise psd (thin line) is superimposed.

be seen, the window length (D) affects the accuracy of the noise estimate much like it affects the noise estimate obtained by the histogram method (see Figure 9.30). Short windows may cause noise overestimation, particularly in the low-frequency bands, where the speech peaks can be very broad. Use of longer windows, as shown in Figure 9.33, seems to reduce the number of instances of noise overestimation.

In summary, the median-based algorithm is a very simple noise-estimation algorithm. Its only drawback is that it requires sorting, which is computationally expensive.

9.7 OBJECTIVE COMPARISON OF NOISE-ESTIMATION ALGORITHMS

In this section, we compare the accuracy of the aforementioned noise-estimation algorithms using the normalized squared error between the true noise psd and the estimated noise psd. To better evaluate the ability of the noise-estimation algorithms to adapt to new types of noise, we concatenated sets of sentences, each set comprising three sentences. Each triplet set was contaminated by three different types of noise signals, one for each sentence. The three different types of noises were multitalker babble, factory noise, and white noise. Thus, a triplet test set (each of about 5 s duration) consisted of a sentence degraded by babble noise followed by a sentence degraded by factory noise and a sentence degraded by white noise without any intervening pauses (see example waveform in Figure 9.34). To better challenge the ability of the noise-estimation algorithms to track increasing noise power levels, we set the power of each of three noise signals at different levels, with the third noise signal (white noise) containing the largest power (see Figure 9.34). We used a total of 10 different triplet sets for testing. The total duration of all sentences used in the test was 50 s. The global SNR of the noisy speech (triplet set) was 5 dB; however, the individual sentence SNRs varied. On average, the first sentence of the triplet set was corrupted at about 15 dB S/N, the second at about 6 dB S/N, and the third at roughly 0 dB. The speech sentences (sampled at 20 kHz) were taken from the HINT database [50]. A 20 ms analysis rectangular window was used with 50% overlap between frames.

We used the following two objective measures for evaluating the accuracy of the noise-estimation algorithms: the mean squared error (MSE) and the median squared error (MedSE) measures. We computed the MSE as follows:

$$\text{MSE} = \frac{1}{L}\sum_{\lambda=0}^{L-1} \frac{\sum_k \left[\hat{\sigma}_d^2(\lambda,k) - \sigma_d^2(\lambda,k)\right]^2}{\sum_k \left(\sigma_d^2(\lambda,k)\right)^2} \tag{9.77}$$

where

L is the total number of frames in the signal

$\hat{\sigma}_d^2(\lambda,k)$ and $\sigma_d^2(\lambda,k)$ are the estimated and true noise power spectra, respectively

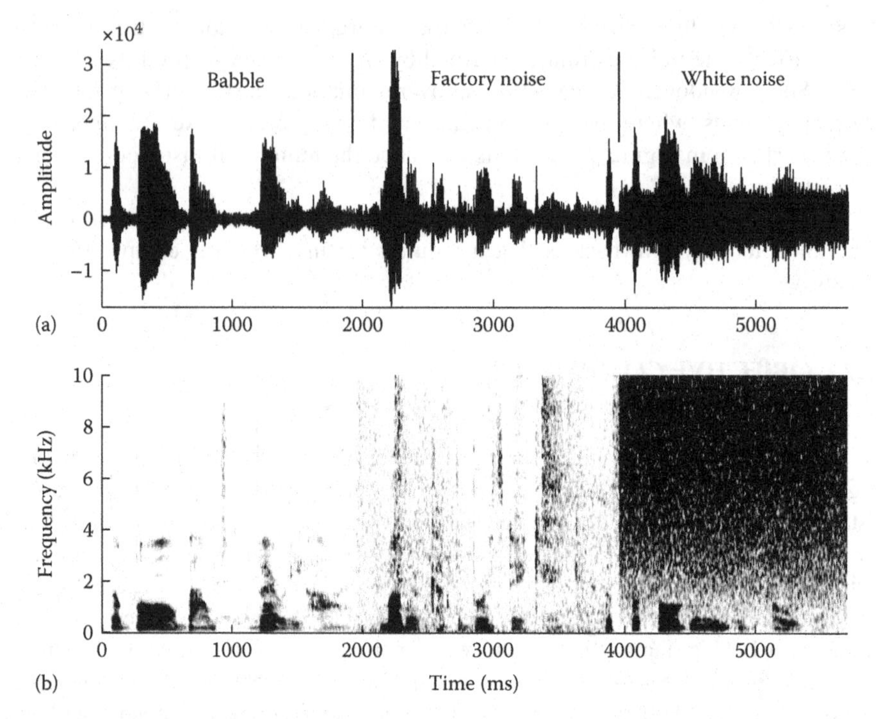

FIGURE 9.34 (a) Waveform and (b) spectrogram of a noisy signal embedded in three types of noise (babble, factory noise, and white noise). This sample signal was used in the evaluation and comparison of various noise-estimation algorithms.

The MedSE measure uses the median rather than the mean of the all normalized squared errors in the utterance. We consider using the MedSE measure since the median estimator, unlike the mean estimator, is not sensitive to outliers.

In addition to the squared error measure, we also report two measures of variability: the standard deviation (across the 10 triplet sets) of the MSE values and the average interquartile range (IQR) of the squared error values. The IQR is defined to be the difference between the upper and lower quartiles, that is, the difference between 75th percentile and 25th percentile values [51, p. 45]. IQR is often used as a measure of variability, with large values suggesting large variability and small ones suggesting low variability. The IQR of the normalized squared-error values was computed for each triplet set, and then averaged across all 10 triplets. It is adopted here as a measure of consistency within and across utterances and types of noise. A small IQR value is indicative of reliable and robust performance.

A total of 13 noise-estimation algorithms were tested. Table 9.1 gives the list of the algorithms tested along with the parameters used for each algorithm and corresponding equation. Three different weighted-average algorithms based on Equations 9.30, 9.33, and 9.34, respectively, are evaluated. Two different sets of histogram-based algorithms are tested. The first set of algorithms are based on computing histograms of unsmoothed noisy speech psd (i.e., $\alpha = 0$ in Equation 9.70) and are labeled in Table 9.1 as the HIST1 and HIST2 algorithms. The second set of algorithms are

TABLE 9.1
Objective Comparison of Representative Noise-Estimation Algorithms

Method	Parameters	Equations	MSE	MedSE	Std	IQR	Ref.
Minimum statistics	Same as in [18]		0.960	0.955	0.079	0.102	[18]
Spectral-minima	$\alpha = 0.7$, $\beta = 0.96$ $\gamma = 0.998$	(9.25)	25.640	0.966	12.463	2.735	[19]
MCRA	Same as in [14]		2.318	0.919	0.304	0.363	[14]
MCRA-2	$\delta(k) = \{1,1,5\}$	(9.60)	1.524	0.890	0.446	0.319	[32,42]
IMCRA	Same as in [35]		0.961	0.941	0.087	0.138	[35]
Weighted-average 1	$\alpha = 0.9$, $\beta = 2.5$	(9.30)	3.780	0.858	5.040	0.426	[20]
Weighted-average 2	$\boldsymbol{\varepsilon = 2.5, \alpha = \delta = 0.9}$	(9.33)	0.984	0.881	0.099	0.214	[30]
Weighted-average 3	$\boldsymbol{\alpha = 0.9, \beta = 1.2, \gamma = 0.9}$	(9.34)	0.990	0.888	0.095	0.160	[36]
SNR-dependent	$\beta = 20$	(9.26), (9.27)	0.981	0.998	0.003	0.019	[34]
SNR-dependent	$\beta = 0.6$	(9.26), (9.27)	4.906	0.856	7.186	0.342	PB
Likelihood ratio	$r = 0.5$	(9.46), (9.45)	685.247	0.965	1075.478	2.093	[13]
Histogram-1 (HIST1)	$\boldsymbol{\alpha = 0, D = 800\,\text{ms}}$	(9.70)	0.966	0.977	0.027	0.059	[20]
Histogram-2 (HIST2)	$\boldsymbol{\alpha = 0, D = 800\,\text{ms}}$	(9.70) (9.72)	0.977	0.987	0.004	0.021	[30]
Histogram-1 (sHIST1)	$\alpha = 0.6$, $D = 800\,\text{ms}$	(9.70)	1.650	0.858	1.025	0.311	PB
Histogram-2 (sHIST2)	$\alpha = 0.6$, $D = 800\,\text{ms}$	(9.70) (9.72)	0.920	0.855	0.043	0.210	PB
Quantile-based	$D = 800\,\text{ms}$		233.745	1.536	443.858	12.796	[23]

Note: PB, Present Book.

based on histograms of smoothed noisy speech psd (i.e., $\alpha \neq 0$ in Equation 9.70) and are labeled sHIST1 and sHIST2 algorithms.

Table 9.1 shows the performance of the noise-estimation algorithms tested. Different conclusions can be drawn regarding the performance of the various noise-estimation algorithms, depending on the measure used (MSE vs. MedSE). In terms of the MSE measure, the MS, the weighted-average methods, and the histogram-based methods (except sHIST1) performed the best, that is, yielded the smallest

MSE value. The worst performance (largest MSE) was obtained by the quantile-based algorithm [23], the likelihood ratio algorithm [13], and the spectral minimum-tracking algorithms [19]. The large MSE values obtained by the likelihood ratio and quantile methods are largely due to the presence of a few outlier frames. This is not surprising, as the MSE measure does not exclude any frames from the squared-error calculation. In that respect, the MSE measure may not always be a reliable measure, because it is extremely sensitive to outlier values. For that reason we also compare the performance of the various noise-estimation algorithms using the median of the squared-error values (MedSE).

In terms of the MedSE measure, the SNR-dependent noise-estimation method ($\beta = 0.6$), the weighted-averaging methods, and the histogram methods (sHIST1 and sHIST2) performed the best (i.e., achieved the lowest MedSE). The MedSE values obtained for each triplet set were subjected to statistical analysis (paired-samples *t*-tests [51]) to determine statistically significant differences in the performance of the various algorithms. Statistical analysis indicated that the minimal-controlled algorithms (IMCRA and MCRA-2) were found to produce significantly ($p < 0.05$) lower MedSE values than the MS algorithm. Of the three minimal-controlled algorithms, the MCRA-2 algorithm performed the best. Overall, the following three algorithms performed the best and equally well: the SNR-dependent algorithm ($\beta = 0.6$, Equations 9.26 and 9.27), the histogram algorithm (sHIST2, i.e., $\alpha = 0.6$, Equations 9.70, 9.72) and the weighted-average algorithms (Equations 9.33 and 9.34). The histogram-based algorithm achieved a low median value and the smallest IQR value. This suggests that the performance of the histogram-based algorithm is consistent across and within utterances and across the three types of noises examined. The worst performer in terms of consistency (i.e., large values of IQR) was the spectral minimal-tracking algorithm, suggesting that it does not perform well in terms of tracking the noise spectrum reliably across and within utterances.

In the foregoing discussion, we compared the performance of the various noise-estimation algorithms using normalized squared-error measures (Equation 9.77), based on either the mean or the median of the errors between the true and estimated noise power spectra. There is no evidence, however, that these measures are correlated with speech quality, and the results reported in Table 9.1 need to be interpreted with caution; that is, it is not known whether small MSE or small MedSE values are associated with better speech quality. The squared-error measure (Equation 9.77) in general has several shortcomings. For one, it treats all frames (voiced, unvoiced, and silence) identically. Second, it treats noise overestimation and underestimation errors identically. Noise overestimation errors may clip speech segments whereas noise underestimation errors may produce more residual noise; hence, these errors cannot be considered perceptually equivalent. Further research is needed to develop better objective measures for evaluating the performance of noise-estimation algorithms.

9.8 SUMMARY

This chapter presented noise-estimation algorithms. Unlike VAD algorithms, noise-estimation algorithms estimate and update the noise spectrum continuously, even during speech activity. As such, noise-estimation algorithms are more suited for speech-enhancement algorithms operating in highly nonstationary environments. Noise-estimation algorithms exploit three key observations: (a) noise does not affect the spectrum uniformly and, consequently, the effective spectral SNR can vary between different frequency bands; (b) the power of the noisy speech signal in individual frequency bands often decays to the power level of the noise, even during speech activity; and (c) histograms of energy values in individual frequency bands reveal that the most frequent value (i.e., the histogram maximum) corresponds to the noise level. Three different classes of noise-estimation algorithms were presented, each exploiting the preceding observations. Most of the noise-estimation algorithms described provide an underestimate of the noise spectrum and are not able to respond fast enough to increasing noise levels. Objective evaluation and comparison between the various noise-estimation algorithms was also presented. Although such objective evaluations are informative and provide useful insights into the performance of various noise-estimation algorithms, they need to be supplemented with subjective listening evaluations (not reported).

REFERENCES

1. Srinivasan, K. and Gersho, A. (1993), Voice activity detection for cellular networks, *Proceedings of the IEEE Speech Coding Workshop,* Sainte-Adele, QC, Canada, pp. 85–86.
2. El-Maleh, J. and Kabal, P. (1997), Comparison of voice activity detection algorithms for wireless personal communication systems, *Proceedings of the IEEE Canadian Conference on Electrical and Computer Engineering*, St. John's, NL, Canada, pp. 470–472.
3. Freeman, D., Cosier, G., Southcott, C., and Boyd, I. (1989), The voice activity detector for the Pan-European digital cellular mobile telephone service, *Proceedings of the IEEE International Conference on Acoustics, Speech, and Signal Processing,* Glasgow, U.K., pp. 369–372.
4. Haigh, J. and Mason, J. (1993), Robust voice activity detection using cepstral features, *Proceedings of the IEEE TENCON,* Beijing, China, pp. 321–324.
5. Sasaki, S. and Matsumoto, I. (1994), Voice activity detection and transmission error control for digital cordless telephone system, *IEICE Trans. Commun.*, E77B(7), 948–955.
6. Sohn, J. and Kim, N. (1999), Statistical model-based voice activity detection, *IEEE Signal Process. Lett.,* 6(1), 1–3.
7. Tanyer, S. and Ozer, H. (2000), Voice activity detection in nonstationary noise, *IEEE Trans. Speech Audio Process.,* 8(4), 478–482.
8. Tucker, R. (1992), Voice activity detection using a periodicity measure, *Proc. IEEE,* 139(4), 377–380.
9. Rabiner, L. and Sambur, M. (1977), Voiced-unvoiced-silence detection using the Itakura LPC distance measure, *Proceedings of the IEEE International Conference on Acoustics, Speech, and Signal Processing,* Hartford, CT, pp. 323–326.
10. Junqua, J. C., Reaves, B., and Mak, B. (1991), A study of endpoint detection algorithms in adverse conditions: Incidence on a DTW and HMM recognizers, *Proceedings of Eurospeech,* Genova, Italy, pp. 1371–1374.
11. Brady, P. (1965), A technique for investigating on-off patterns of speech, *Bell Syst. Tech. J.,* 44, 1–22.
12. Kondoz, A. (2004), *Digital Speech: Coding for Low Bit Rate Communication Systems,* 2nd ed., West Sussex, England: John Wiley & Sons.

13. Sohn, J. and Sung, W. (1998), A voice activity detector employing soft decision based noise spectrum adaptation, *Proceedings of the IEEE International Conference on Acoustics, Speech, and Signal Processing,* Seattle, WA, pp. 365–368.
14. Cohen, I. (2002), Noise estimation by minima controlled recursive averaging for robust speech enhancement, *IEEE Signal Process. Lett.,* 9(1), 12–15.
15. Yamauchi, J. and Shimamura, T. (2002), Noise estimation using high-frequency regions for speech enhancement in low SNR environments, *IEEE Workshop Speech Coding,* Tsukuba, Japan, pp. 59–61.
16. Lin, L., Holmes, W., and Ambikairajah, E. (2003), Subband noise estimation for speech enhancement using a perceptual Wiener filter, *Proceedings of the IEEE International Conference on Acoustics, Speech, and Signal Processing,* Vol. I, Hong Kong, pp. 80–83.
17. Sorensen, K. and Andersen, S. (2005), Speech enhancement with natural sounding residual noise based on connected time-frequency speech presence regions, *EURASIP J. Appl. Signal Process.,* 18, 2954–2964.
18. Martin, R. (2001), Noise power spectral density estimation based on optimal smoothing and minimum statistics, *IEEE Trans. Speech Audio Process.,* 9(5), 504–512.
19. Doblinger, G. (1995), Computationally efficient speech enhancement by spectral minima tracking in subbands, *Proceedings of the Eurospeech,* Madrid, Spain, Vol. 2, pp. 1513–1516.
20. Hirsch, H. and Ehrlicher, C. (1995), Noise estimation techniques for robust speech recognition, *Proceedings of the IEEE International Conference on Acoustics, Speech, and Signal Processing,* Detroit, MI, pp. 153–156.
21. McAulay, R. J. and Malpass, M. L. (1980), Speech enhancement using a soft-decision noise suppression filter, *IEEE Trans. Acoust. Speech Signal Process.,* 28, 137–145.
22. Van Compernolle, D. (1989), Noise adaptation in a Hidden Markov Model speech recognition system, *Comput. Speech Lang.,* 3, 151–167.
23. Stahl, V., Fischer, A., and Bippus, R. (2000), Quantile based noise estimation for spectral subtraction and Wiener filtering, *Proceedings of the IEEE International Conference on Acoustics, Speech, and Signal Processing*, Istanbul, Turkey, pp. 1875–1873.
24. Martin, R. (1993), An efficient algorithm to estimate the instantaneous SNR of speech signals. *Proceedings of the Eurospeech,* Berlin, Germany, pp. 1093–1096.
25. Martin, R. (1994), Spectral subtraction based on minimum statistics, *Proceedings of. European Signal Processing,* Edinburgh, U.K., pp. 1182–1185.
26. Welch, P. (1967), The use of Fast Fourier Transform for the estimation of power spectra: A method based on time averaging over short, modified periodograms, *IEEE Trans. Audio Electroacoust.,* AU-15(2), 70–73.
27. Papoulis, A. and Pillai, S. (2002), *Probability, Random Variables and Stochastic Processes*, 4th ed., New York: McGraw Hill.
28. Proakis, J. and Manolakis, D. (2001), *Digital Communications*, 4th ed., New York: McGraw-Hill.
29. Gumbel, E. (1958), *Statistics of Extremes*, New York: Columbia University Press.
30. Ris, C. and Dupont, S. (2001), Assessing local noise level estimation methods: Application to noise robust ASR, *Speech Commun.,* 34, 141–158.
31. Meyer, J., Simmer, K., and Kammeyer, K. (1997), Comparison of one- and two-channel noise estimation techniques, *Proceedings of the 5th International Workshop on Acoustics. Echo Noise Cancellation,* London, U.K., Vol. 1, pp. 137–145.
32. Rangachari, S., Loizou, P., and Hu, Y. (2004), A noise estimation algorithm with rapid adaptation for highly nonstationary environments, *Proceedings of the IEEE International Conference on Acoustics, Speech, and Signal Processing,* Vol. I, Montreal, Quebec, Canada, pp. 305–308.

33. Malah, D., Cox, R., and Accardi, A. (1999), Tracking speech-presence uncertainty to improve speech enhancement in non-stationary environments, *Proceedings of the IEEE International Conference on Acoustics, Speech, and Signal Processing,* Phoenix, AZ, pp. 789–792.
34. Lin, L., Holmes, W., and Ambikairajah, E. (2003), Adaptive noise estimation algorithm for speech enhancement, *Electron. Lett.,* 39(9), 754–755.
35. Cohen, I. (2003), Noise spectrum estimation in adverse environments: Improved minima controlled recursive averaging, *IEEE Trans. Speech Audio Process.,* 11(5), 466–475.
36. Arslan, L., McCree, A., and Viswanathan, V. (1995), New methods for adaptive noise suppression, *Proceedings of the IEEE International Conference on Acoustics, Speech, and Signal Processing,* Detroit, MI, pp. 812–815.
37. Chang, J. and Kim, N. (2001), Speech enhancement: New approaches to soft decision, *IEICE Trans. Inf. Syst.,* E84-D(9), 1231–1240.
38. Ephraim, Y. and Malah, D. (1984), Speech enhancement using a minimum mean-square error short-time spectral amplitude estimator, *IEEE Trans. Acoust. Speech Signal Process.,* 32(6), 1109–1121.
39. Cho, Y. and Kondoz, A. (2001), Analysis and improvement of a statistical model-based voice-activity detector, *IEEE Signal Process. Lett.,* 8(10), 276–278.
40. Cho, Y., Al-Naimi, K., and Kondoz, A. (2001), Mixed decision-based noise adaptation for speech enhancement, *Electron. Lett.,* 37(8), 540–542.
41. Schwab, M., Kim, H., and Noll, P. (2003), Robust noise estimation applied to different speech estimators, *Thirty-Seventh Asilomar Conference on Signals, Systems and Computers*, Vol. 2, Pacific Grove, CA, pp. 1904–1907.
42. Rangachari, S. (2004), Noise estimation algorithms for highly non-stationary environments, MS thesis, Department of Electrical Engineering, University of Texas-Dallas, Richardson, TX.
43. Rangachari, S. and Loizou, P. (2006), A noise estimation algorithm for highly nonstationary environments, *Speech Commun.,* 28, 220–231.
44. Hu, Y. and Loizou, P. (2004), Speech enhancement based on wavelet thresholding the multitaper spectrum, *IEEE Trans. Speech Audio Process.*, 12(1), 59–67.
45. Ahmed, B. and Holmes, W. (2004), A voice activity detector using the chi-square test, *Proceedings of the IEEE International Conference on Acoustics, Speech, and Signal Processing,* Vol. I, Montreal, Quebec, Canada, pp. 625–628.
46. Nemer, E., Goubran, R., and Mahmoud, S. (1999), SNR estimation of speech signals using subbands and fourth-order statistics, *IEEE Signal Process. Lett.,* 6(7), 171–174.
47. Sugiyama, A., Kato, M., and Serizawa, M. (2005), Single-microphone noise suppression for 3G handsets based on weighted noise estimation, in Benesty, J., Makino, S., and Chen, J. (Eds.), *Speech Enhancement,* Berlin, Germany: Springer.
48. Manohar, K. and Rao, P. (2006), Speech enhancement in nonstationary noise environments using noise properties, *Speech Commun.*, 48, 96–109.
49. Yamashita, K. and Shimamura, T. (2005), Nonstationary noise estimation using low-frequency regions for spectral subtraction, *IEEE Signal Process. Lett.,* 12(6), 465–468.
50. Nilsson, M., Soli, S., and Sullivan, J. (1994), Development of hearing in noise test for the measurement of speech reception thresholds in quiet and in noise, *J. Acoust. Soc. Am.,* 95(2), 1085–1099.
51. Ott, L. (1988), *An Introduction to Statistical Methods and Data Analysis*, 3rd ed., Boston, MA: PWS-Kent Publishing Company.

Part III

Evaluation

10 Evaluating Performance of Speech Enhancement Algorithms

Listening Tests

So far, we have described numerous speech enhancement algorithms, but have not discussed how to properly evaluate their performance. Performance can be assessed using either subjective listening tests or objective measures. Subjective quality evaluation, for instance, involves comparisons of original and processed speech signals by a group of listeners who are asked to rate the quality of speech along a predetermined scale. Objective evaluation involves a mathematical comparison of the original and processed speech signals. Objective measures quantify quality by measuring the numerical "distance" between the original and processed signals. Clearly, for the objective measure to be valid, it needs to correlate well with subjective listening tests, and for that reason, much research has been focused on developing objective measures that model various aspects of the auditory system. Chapter 11 focuses on objective measures, while this chapter provides an overview of the various listening tests/procedures that have been used to evaluate speech enhancement algorithms in terms of quality and intelligibility. Although historically some of these procedures have been used to evaluate speech-coding algorithms, these methods have also been used to quantify the performance of speech enhancement algorithms [1].

10.1 QUALITY VS. INTELLIGIBILITY

Quality is only one of the many attributes of the speech signal. Intelligibility is a different attribute and the two are not equivalent. Hence, different assessment methods are used to evaluate the quality and intelligibility of processed speech. Quality is highly subjective in nature and it is difficult to evaluate reliably. This is partly because individual listeners have different internal standards of what constitutes "good" or "poor" quality, resulting in large variability in rating scores among listeners. Quality measures assess "how" a speaker produces an utterance, and includes attributes such as "natural," "raspy," "hoarse," "scratchy," and so on. Quality possesses many dimensions, too many to enumerate. For practical purposes, we typically restrict ourselves to only a few dimensions of speech quality depending on the application. Intelligibility measures assess "what" the speaker said, that is, the meaning or the content of the spoken words. Unlike quality, intelligibility is not subjective and can be easily measured by presenting speech material (sentences, words, etc.) to a group of listeners and asking them to identify the words spoken. Intelligibility is quantified by counting the number of words or phonemes identified correctly.

The relationship between speech intelligibility and speech quality is not fully understood, and this is in part due to the fact that we have not yet identified the acoustic correlates of quality and intelligibility [2]. Speech can be highly intelligible, yet be of poor quality. Examples include speech synthesized using a small number (3–6) of sine waves [3,4] and speech synthesized using a small number (4) of modulated noise bands [5]. Sine wave speech, for instance, is perceived as being "tonal" and mechanical sounding, yet it is highly intelligible [3]. Conversely, speech can have good quality, yet not be completely intelligible. Consider, for example, speech transmitted over IP (VoiIP) networks and assume that a large number of packets are lost [6] in the transmission. Speech, at the receiver end, will be perceived as interrupted and perhaps less intelligible since certain words might be missing. The perceived quality of the remaining words, however, might be reasonably good. As the aforementioned examples illustrate, speech quality and speech intelligibility are not synonymous terms; hence different methods need to be used to assess the quality and intelligibility of processed (enhanced) speech.

10.2 EVALUATING INTELLIGIBILITY OF PROCESSED SPEECH

Intelligibility is an important attribute of the speech signal that needs to be preserved at all costs by speech enhancement algorithms. At the very least, we require that speech enhancement algorithm preserve the intelligibility of the input speech signal, although we would much prefer that it improves the intelligibility, particularly when speech is embedded in very low signal-to-noise (S/N) levels.

Developing and designing a reliable and valid speech intelligibility test is not as simple as it seems because several factors need to be considered. Desirable features of good intelligibility tests include the following:

1. *Good representation of all major speech phonemes:* All, or nearly all, fundamental speech sounds (phonemes) should be represented in each list of test items. Ideally, the relative frequencies of occurrence of phonemes in the test items should reflect the distribution of phonemes commonly found in normal speech. This requirement is placed to ensure that the intelligibility test will yield a score that is reflective of a real-world communicative situation. It addresses a validity issue.
2. *Equal difficulty of test lists:* For extensive testing, particularly in situations where several algorithms need to be tested in different conditions, it is preferable to have a large number of test lists. This is necessary in order to keep listeners from "learning" or memorizing somehow the speech material or the order of materials presented. A test list might comprise, say, 10 sentences or 50 monosyllabic words. Multiple test lists are needed. Test material should be grouped into a number of lists, each of which should be equally difficult to identify.

3. *Control of contextual information:* It is well known that words embedded in sentences are more intelligible than words presented in isolation [7]. This is because listeners make use of contextual information when identifying words in a sentence. That is, it is not necessary to identify all the words in a sentence in order to extract the meaning of the sentence. Human listeners utilize high-level knowledge (e.g., semantics, pragmatics, grammar) about the language and "fill in the blanks." For sentence tests, it is necessary to control the amount of contextual information present in each list so that each list is equally intelligible. As we will see later on, some chose to reduce the amount of contextual information present by varying the number of words listeners can choose from [7], others chose to eliminate it by presenting words in isolation [8], while others chose to control it [9,10].

A variety of speech tests based on different speech materials were proposed over the years (see review in [1, ch. 2]). These tests generally fall into one of the three main classes depending on the speech materials chosen: (a) recognition of syllables made up of meaningless combinations of speech sounds (e.g., "apa," "aka" [11]); (b) recognition of single meaningful words (e.g., *bar, pile* [8]) presented in isolation (i.e., out of context) or presented in a two-response format (i.e., rhyming word pairs as in *veal-feel* [12]); and (c) recognition of meaningful sentences containing all contextual information among words (e.g., [10]). Each of these tests has its advantages and disadvantages depending on the application at hand. Next, we describe some of the intelligibility tests commonly used.

10.2.1 Nonsense Syllable Tests

One of the earliest attempts to measure speech intelligibility was made by French and Steinberg [13] in the late 1920s. They suggested using a random list of 66 nonsense monosyllables in the format of consonant-vowel-consonant, abbreviated as /C-V-C/. These lists were constructed so that each initial and final consonant and each vowel were only used once. No restrictions were imposed on the initial or final consonants allowed. The number of syllables identified correctly was obtained by reading aloud the syllables to a group of listeners. This test was referred to by French and Steinberg as an *articulation* test, and similarly the intelligibility score was termed the *articulation score.*

Miller and Nicely [11] later refined the aforementioned test and reduced the total number of nonsense syllables to 16, which were presented in the format /a-C-a/, where C denotes the consonant. The following 16 consonants were chosen /p, t, k, f, th, s, sh, b, d, g, v, dh, z, zh, m, n/ as they frequently occur in fluent speech. In their study, the consonants were filtered and corrupted at varying levels of noise and then presented to a group of listeners for identification. Analysis of the confusion matrices—a matrix containing the average responses of the listeners for each stimulus presented—indicated that for the most part the confusion errors were not random. The errors could be explained in terms of five articulatory features [14] or "dimensions" that distinguish the different phonemes in terms of voicing, nasality, affrication, duration, and place of articulation. A voicing error, for instance, would suggest that listeners are not able to discriminate between /p/-/b/, or /d/-/t/ or /g/-/k/.

TABLE 10.1
Classification of Consonants into Five Articulatory Features

	Features				
Consonant	**Voicing**	**Nasality**	**Frication**	**Duration**	**Place**
/p/	0	0	0	0	0
/t/	0	0	0	0	1
/k/	0	0	0	0	2
/f/	0	0	1	0	0
/th/	0	0	1	0	1
/s/	0	0	1	1	1
/sh/	0	0	1	1	2
/b/	1	0	0	0	0
/d/	1	0	0	0	1
/g/	1	0	0	0	2
/v/	1	0	1	0	0
/dh/	1	0	1	0	1
/z/	1	0	1	1	1
/zh/	1	0	1	1	2
/m/	1	1	0	0	0
/n/	1	1	0	0	1

Source: Miller, G. and Nicely, P., *J. Acoust. Soc. Am.*, 27(2), 338, 1955.

It is called a voicing error because it is a confusion between the unvoiced stop-consonants /p, t, k/ and the voiced stop-consonants /b, d, g/. The classification of the 16 consonants in the 5 articulatory features is shown in Table 10.1.

If we apply the groupings given in Table 10.1, we can obtain five different scores, one for each of the five features. For example, we can obtain a score for the voicing feature by grouping the voiceless consonants together and all voiced consonants together and constructing a 2×2 confusion matrix (see examples in Tables 10.2 and 10.3).

Alternatively, we can use an information theoretical approach to assess the identification of the five articulatory features. More specifically, we can view the input consonant stimuli as the input to a communication channel, represented by the speech enhancement system in our case, and the listener's responses as the output of the channel. The input stimulus takes a discrete value from a finite set of M consonants and has a discrete distribution that we denote by p_i, $i = 1, 2, \ldots, M$. Similarly, the output (i.e., the listener's response) takes a discrete value from the same set of consonants, and has a discrete distribution that we denote by p_j. We can then compute the mutual information between the input stimuli $\mathbf{x}$ and the output (responses) $\mathbf{y}$ as follows:

$$I(x, y) = -\sum_{i=1}^{M}\sum_{j=1}^{M} p_{ij} \log_2 \frac{p_i p_j}{p_{ij}} \tag{10.1}$$

TABLE 10.2
Example Consonant Confusion Matrix

	/p/	/t/	/k/	/f/	/s/	/sh/	/b/	/d/	/g/	/v/	/dh/	/z/	/jh/	/l/	/m/	/n/
/p/	67						33									
/t/		33	33	33												
/k/			33						67							
/f/				100												
/s/					100											
/sh/						100										
/b/	33						33							33		
/d/		33						67								
/g/				33					67							
/v/										67						33
/dh/										33	67					
/z/					67							33				
/jh/		33											67			
/l/												33		67		
/m/											33				67	
/n/																100

Note: Mean percent correct identification was 66.67%.

where p_{ij} denotes the joint probability of occurrence of the input x_i and output y_j. The mutual information gives the average amount of information (expressed in bits per stimulus) transmitted by the system based on the input **x** and observed output **y**. In our application, the estimated mutual information $I(x, y)$ can be used to assess the amount of feature (voicing, place, affrication, duration) information transmitted by the system. The mutual information can be normalized as follows:

$$M(x,y) = \frac{I(x,y)}{H(x)} = \frac{I(x,y)}{-\sum_{i=1}^{M} p_i \log_2(p_i)} \tag{10.2}$$

where $H(x)$ denotes the *entropy* of the input. Since $H(x) \geq I(x, y) \geq 0$ [15, Chapter 3.2], the relative mutual information $M(x, y)$ takes values in the range of 0–1. In practice, the true probabilities p_i and p_{ij} are unknown and must be estimated from the relative frequencies of responses during the experiment. In place of p_i, p_j, and p_{ij}, we can use n_i/n, n_j/n, and n_{ij}/n, respectively, where n_i is the number of times the input stimulus i is presented, n_j is the number of times the output stimulus j is observed, and n_{ij} is the number of times the output j is observed when the input stimulus i is presented in a sample of n observations.

We can compute the relative information transmitted, $M(x, y)$, separately for each of the five features. For example, we can construct a 2×2 voicing confusion matrix by grouping the voiceless consonants together as one stimulus and the voiced

TABLE 10.3
Sub-Matrices of the Five Articulatory Features Extracted from the Confusion Matrix in Table 10.2

Voicing			Nasality			Frication			Duration		
	Unvoiced (%)	Voiced (%)		Non-Nasals (%)	Nasals (%)		Fricative (%)	Non-Fricative (%)		Long (%)	Short (%)
Unvoiced	83	17	Non-Nasals	97	3	Fricative	90	10	Long	100	0
Voiced	20	80	Nasals	17	83	Non-Fricative	15	85	Short	3	97

Place			
	Labial (%)	Alveolar (%)	Velar (%)
Labial	80	20	
Alveolar	9	86	5
Velar	8.5	8.5	83

Note: Numbers indicate percent correct.

consonants as the other stimulus according to Table 10.1, and tabulate the following frequencies of responses: voiceless responses to voiceless input stimuli, voiceless responses to voiced input, voiced responses to voiceless input, and voiced responses to voiced input. We can then use Equation 10.2 with $M = 2$ (voiced and unvoiced) to compute the relative information transmitted for voicing. Similarly, we can compute the relative information transmitted for nasality, affrication, duration, and place of articulation. For the place feature, we will need to construct a 3×3 place confusion matrix and use $M = 3$ in (10.2).

Table 10.2 shows an example of a confusion matrix and Table 10.3 shows the associated sub-matrices constructed for each of the five features. For this example, the percentage of information transmitted (based on Equation 10.2) for the place feature was 50.53%; for the duration feature, 85.97%; for the affrication feature, 46.51%; for the nasality feature, 58.92%; and for the voicing feature, 30.78%. The voicing score was low, suggesting that the voiced consonants were often confused with the unvoiced consonants. This in turn implies that somehow the voicing information, typically present in the low frequencies, was lost or distorted. This example illustrates that the information transmission analysis is an invaluable tool that can be used to isolate the source of confusion errors.

10.2.2 Word Tests

One problem with using nonsense syllable tests is the difficulty in constructing lists of syllables in which all items are equally difficult to recognize. Furthermore, nonsense syllable tests measure primarily the ability of the speech enhancement system to reproduce individual phonemes, and a certain degree of listener training might be required, particularly when a large list of syllables is involved.

For the aforesaid reasons, some proposed the use of single meaningful words that differed either in the leading or trailing consonant (i.e., rhyming words), while others proposed the use of words chosen to have equal phonetic decomposition.

10.2.2.1 Phonetically Balanced Word Tests

Egan [8] proposed the use of phonetically balanced monosyllable words. He constructed 20 lists, each consisting of 50 common English monosyllables (see list 1 in Table 10.4). These lists were designed to satisfy the following criteria: (a) equal average difficulty, (b) equal range of difficulty, and (c) equal phonetic content representative of normal speech. The last criterion was achieved by choosing the words in each list to have the same phonemic distribution as normal conversational speech. For that reason, the word lists are called phonetically balanced.

The requirement that the lists had an equal range of difficulty is an important one and was placed to avoid having systems always perform near zero or near 100% correct. If, for instance, the word test is too easy, then all systems will perform nearly one-hundred-percent correct and will therefore learn nothing from the test as to which system is better. This effect is referred to in the literature as the *ceiling effect*, since the system performs near the ceiling, that is, maximum performance. Similarly, if the word test is too difficult, consisting of say a large number of unfamiliar words, then all systems will perform near zero percent correct. This is referred

TABLE 10.4
Words from List 1 of the Monosyllabic Word Test

1. are	11. death	21. fuss	31. not	41. rub
2. bad	12. deed	22. grove	32. pan	42. slip
3. bar	13. dike	23. heap	33. pants	43. smile
4. bask	14. dish	24. hid	34. pest	44. strife
5. box	15. end	25. hive	35. pile	45. such
6. cane	16. feast	26. hunt	36. plush	46. then
7. cleanse	17. fern	27. is	37. rag	47. there
8. clove	18. folk	28. mange	38. rat	48. toe
9. crash	19. ford	29. no	39. ride	49. use
10. creed	20. fraud	30. nook	40. rise	50. wheat

Source: Egan, J., *Laryngoscope*, 58(9), 955, 1948.

to in the literature as the *floor effect*, since the system performs near the floor, that is, minimum performance. For these reasons, in order to avoid any floor or ceiling effects, Egan [8] designed the lists to be of equal range of difficulty.

10.2.2.2 Rhyming Word Tests

Several researchers have proposed the use of rhyming words [12,16,17], which were presented to listeners in either a single-response format, pair-response format, or in a six-response format.

In Fairbanks' test [16], all items in the test list were monosyllables of the form /C-V-C/. The trailing vowel-consonant was specified and the listener was asked to identify the leading consonant. For instance, if the word "dot" was presented, the listener would see in his response sheet "ot" and asked to fill in the blank. The test words were chosen carefully to allow a number of possible response words, with an average of about 8–9 alternative words. These words were not made available to the listener. Possible alternative (rhyming) words for the aforementioned example include *cot, got, hot, lot, not, port, rot*, and *jot*. This test effectively tests the identification of a single consonant embedded in a word using an open-set response format. Unlike the nonsense syllable test, this test is based on meaningful words familiar to the listeners.

House et al. [17] modified the aforementioned test by restricting the listener responses to a finite set of rhyming words. For each word presented, the listener response sheet contained a closed set of six alternative words to choose from. So, for instance, if the word *bean* was presented, the listener had to choose from one of the following six words written on the response sheet: *bean, beach, beat, beam, bead*, and *beak*. All words had the same leading consonant, but a different trailing consonant. This test was called the Modified Rhyme Test (MRT). Note that this test is administered in the closed-set response format with a probability of chance of 0.17 (1/6). In contrast, Fairbanks's test was administered in the open-set response format with a chance probability being considerably lower, since the listeners were not given a set of words to choose from.

Voiers [12] refined the rhyming tests mentioned earlier and developed the Diagnostic Rhyme Test (DRT), a test widely used today for evaluating the intelligibility of speech coders. He proposed a hybrid approach combining the MRT method [17] of restricting the responses to a finite set of words (two in the DRT) and the idea of Miller and Nicely [11] to divide the phonemes in terms of their distinctive features. The rhyming words in the DRT test were chosen to differ not only in the leading consonant but also in just one distinctive feature of the leading phoneme. The listener's response was restricted to two possible choices, one of which was the stimulus word. So, for instance, when the word *bond* was presented, the listener saw the following two choices on the response sheet: *bond* and *pond*. These two words differ not only in the leading consonant (/b/ vs. /p/) but also in the voicing feature, since /b/ is a voiced stop and /p/ is its unvoiced counterpart.

A total of six distinctive features were selected: voicing, nasality, sustention, sibilation, graveness, and compactness. Table 10.5 shows the list of words (total of 192) used in the DRT test, grouped by their distinctive features. Note that the features voicing and nasality were also used by Miller and Nicely [11], and the features graveness and compactness were subsets of the place feature used in [11]. Graveness is part of the grave–acute scale, where graveness describes phonemes whose spectrum is dominated by low frequencies (e.g., /p/), and acuteness describes phonemes with spectra dominated by high frequencies (e.g., /t/). The use of the word pair *peak-teak*, for instance, assesses the identification of the graveness feature. Compactness is part of the compact–diffuse scale, where compactness describes phonemes with a dominant mid-frequency peak in the spectrum (e.g., /k/,/g/) and diffuseness describes phonemes with either flat spectra (e.g., /f/) or peaks isolated in either the low or high frequencies (e.g., /d/). The use of the word pair *gill-dill*, for instance, assesses identification of the compactness feature.

The six distinctive features are scored separately by grouping the words in terms of their features (as shown in Table 10.5) and obtaining a single percent correct score for each feature. The DRT test yields in all seven scores, one for each of the six distinctive features and the mean score. All scores are corrected for chance (probability of chance is 0.5) as follows:

$$S_j = \frac{R_j - W_j}{T_j} 100 \tag{10.3}$$

where

S_j is the chance-adjusted percent correct score for feature j
R_j is the number of correct responses
W_j is the number of incorrect responses for feature j
T_j is the total number of responses

The main advantage in using the DRT test over the other rhyming tests is that it gives not only an overall intelligibility score for the speech enhancement system but also a "diagnostic" score for each of the six distinctive features. That is, much like the approach by Miller and Nicely [11], it can be used to identify any potential weakness of

TABLE 10.5
Words Used in the DRT Test

Voicing Voiced—Unvoiced	Nasality Nasal—Oral	Sustention Sustained—Interrupted
veal—feel	meat—beat	vee—bee
bean—peen	need—deed	sheet—cheat
gin—chin	mitt—bit	vill—bill
dint—tint	nip—dip	thick—tick
zoo—sue	moot—boot	foo—pooh
dune—tune	news—dues	shoes—choose
voal—foal	moan—bone	those—doze
goat—coat	note—dote	though—dough
zed—said	mend—bend	then—den
dense—tense	neck—deck	fence—pence
vast—fast	mad—bad	than—Dan
gaff—calf	nab—dab	shad—chad
vault—fault	moss—boss	thong—tong
daunt—taunt	gnaw—daw	shaw—caw
jock—chock	mom—bomb	von—bon
bond—pond	knock—dock	vox—box

Sibilation Sibilated—Un-sibilated	Graveness Grave—Acute	Compactness Compact—Diffuse
zee—thee	weed—reed	yield—wield
cheep—keep	weak—teak	key—tea
jilt—gilt	bid—did	hit—fit
sing—thing	fin—thin	gill—dill
juice—goose	moon—noon	coop—poop
chew—coo	pool—tool	you—rue
joe—go	bowl—dole	ghost—boast
sole—thole	fore—thor	show—so
jest—guest	met—net	keg—peg
chair—care	pent—tent	yen—wren
jab—dab	bank—dank	gat—bat
sank—thank	fad—thad	shag—sag
jaws—gauze	fought—thought	yawl—wall
saw—thaw	bond—dong	caught—taught
jot—got	wad—rod	hop—fop
chop—cop	pot—tot	got—dot

Note: Words are grouped by their distinctive features.

the speech system in terms of transmitting effectively the various acoustic features. If, for instance, the graveness score is found to be too low, that would suggest a deficiency in the speech system in preserving mid-frequency information. The DRT scores can therefore be used as a guide to improve the performance of a speech system.

Extensive tests showed that the DRT test is a reliable test. The standard error of the DRT total score was found to be about one percentage point when listening crews of 8–10 people were used [12]. The DRT was also found to be sensitive to various forms of signal degradations including noise masking [12]. Among all features, the graveness feature was found to be affected the most, in line with the findings by Miller and Nicely [11] on the effect of noise on the place feature. In contrast, the voicing and nasality features were found in [11] to be robust in most noise conditions and were not affected as much.

10.2.3 Sentence Tests

The use of single words eliminates contextual information, but some might argue that word tests do not adequately reflect real-world communicative situations. The validity of the test is particularly at question if the chosen test words do not occur frequently in conversational speech. For those reasons, some have proposed the use of sentence material for better or perhaps more realistic assessment of speech intelligibility.

In developing sentence tests, however, care must be taken to select speech materials in which the phonetic content is balanced (across the various lists) and reflect the distribution of speech sounds in the language. In addition, the speech materials need to be well controlled for difficulty (i.e., word predictability) in that the individual lists should be chosen so that they are equally difficult. Next, we briefly describe two such speech sentence tests in common use: the SPIN and HINT tests.

The Speech Perception in Noise (SPIN) test [9] uses sentences consisting of five-to-eight words each, and contains eight lists of 50 sentences each. To simplify the task, in terms of scoring and time, the test requires a single-word response from the listener: the last word (keyword) in the sentence. To ensure equal difficulty among lists, half of the sentences (25) in each list contain keywords of high predictability (i.e., words easier to identify given the context information) and the other half (25) contain keywords of low predictability (e.g., words difficult to identify despite context information). An example of a high-predictability sentence is *the boat sailed across the bay,* where the words *boat, sailed,* and *across* provide semantic links to the keyword *bay.* An example of a low-predictability sentence is *John was talking about the bay,* where the words *John, talking* and *about* do not provide semantic pointers to the keyword *bay.* Clearly, the identification of the keyword *bay* in the low-predictability sentence is more difficult than the identification of the same keyword in the high-predictability sentence.

Table 10.6 shows the first 10 sentences extracted from the first list. The equivalence of the lists used in the SPIN test was challenged and scrutinized in [18,19]. These studies demonstrated that there was variability in the intelligibility scores among lists, particularly in the recognition of the low-context sentences. These findings motivated the development of a new sentence test, the hearing in noise test (HINT) [10].

TABLE 10.6
Example Sentences from the SPIN Database

(H) 1. The watchdog gave a warning growl
(H) 2. She made the bed with clean sheets
(L) 3. The old man discussed the dive
(L) 4. Bob heard Paul called about the strips
(L) 5. I should have considered the map
(H) 6. The old train was powered by steam
(H) 7. He caught the fish in his net
(L) 8. Miss Brown shouldn't discuss the sand
(H) 9. Close the window to stop the draft
(H) 10. My T.V. has a 12 inch screen

Source: Kalikow, D. et al., *J. Acoust. Soc. Am.*, 61(5), 1337, 1977.
Note: The H and L at the left of each sentence indicate the keyword with high and low predictability, respectively.

The HINT test [10] contains 25 phonetically balanced lists with ten sentences per list. The sentences were originally derived from British sentence materials [20] and adapted to American English. Sentences were equalized for naturalness, length, and intelligibility. Recordings were made of the 250 sentences (at a sampling frequency of 20 kHz) using a single male professional voice actor. Unlike the SPIN test, the sentences are scored on a word-by-word basis, that is, all words are included in the scoring, and the score is reported in terms of average percent of words identified correctly. Scoring is relaxed in most sentences allowing article substitutions and differences in verb tenses. The HINT test has been particularly popular in the speech perception community and is often used to measure speech intelligibility in both normal-hearing and hearing-impaired populations [10]. Table 10.7 shows the first list (10 sentences) used in the HINT test.

The HINT test is particularly suited for measuring the speech reception threshold (SRT), which is the S/N level at which listeners obtain a 50% correct score (see the next section for more details). As we will see next, the SRT score, unlike the percent correct score, is not sensitive to floor or ceiling effects.

10.2.4 Measuring Speech Intelligibility

In most of the aforementioned tests (nonsense syllable, word, or sentence tests), speech intelligibility is quantified in terms of percentage of words (or syllables) identified correctly. Percent intelligibility is often measured at fixed speech and/or noise levels. Such intelligibility measures (i.e., percent correct scores), however, are inherently limited by floor or ceiling effects. If, for instance, we evaluate the intelligibility of speech enhanced by two different algorithms, and we obtain percent

TABLE 10.7
Example Sentences (List 1) from the HINT Database

1. (A/the) boy fell from (a/the) window
2. (A/the) wife helped her husband
3. Big dogs can be dangerous
4. Her shoes (are/were) very dirty
5. (A/The) player lost (a/the) shoe
6. Somebody stole the money
7. (A/the) first (is/was) very hot
8. She's drinking from her own cup
9. (A/the) picture came from (a/the) book
10. (A/the) car (is/was) going too fast

Source: Nilsson, M. et al., *J. Acoust. Soc. Am.*, 95(2), 1085, 1994.
Note: The variations allowed in response are shown in parentheses. The words used in the original recordings are underlined.

correct scores in the upper 90s for both algorithms, then we have no way of knowing which of the two algorithms is truly better since we are limited by ceiling effects. Therefore, in some cases, we might need a different, and perhaps more reliable, measure for assessing speech intelligibility that is not sensitive to the presentation level of speech and/or noise and is not subject to floor or ceiling effects. Next, we describe such a measure. We also present various statistical tests that can be used to examine significant differences between algorithms.

10.2.4.1 Speech Reception Threshold

The speech reception threshold (SRT) can be used as an alternative to percent correct scores for measuring speech intelligibility [21]. The SRT can be measured either in quiet or in noise. In quiet, it is defined as the presentation (or intensity) level at which listeners identify words with 50% accuracy. It can be obtained by presenting speech material (words or sentences) at different intensity levels ranging from low to high, and obtaining a performance–intensity plot, that is, a plot of percent correct scores as a function of intensity. From the performance–intensity plot, we can determine the 50% point corresponding to the SRT.

When measured in noise, the SRT is defined as the S/N level at which listeners identify words with 50% accuracy. It can be obtained by presenting speech at different S/N levels ranging from say negative S/N levels (e.g., −10 dB S/N) to positive S/N levels (e.g., 10 dB S/N), and obtaining a performance–S/N level plot, that is, a plot of percent correct scores as a function of S/N level. From this plot, we can determine the 50% point corresponding to the SRT. Clearly, performance will be poor (near zero percent correct) for small and negative values of S/N, and performance will be high (near 100% correct) for large and positive values of S/N. The performance–S/N function (also called psychometric function [10,22] in the psychophysics community) is expected to be monotonically increasing with a sigmoid-like shape (see example

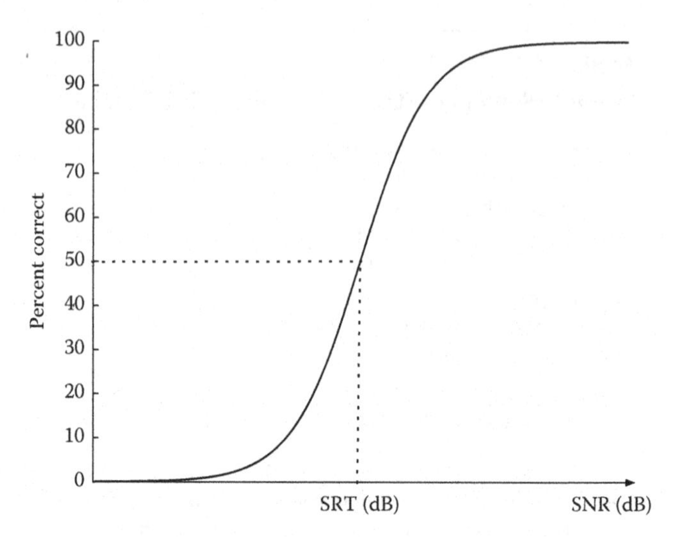

FIGURE 10.1 Typical performance–S/N function. The SRT is the S/N level corresponding to 50% correct.

in Figure 10.1). The SRT is the S/N level, in dB, at which listeners identify words with 50% accuracy. The SRT of the HINT sentences, for instance, was measured to be −2.92 dB S/N for speech-shaped noise suggesting that on the average subjects identify half of the words correctly at −2.92 dB S/N [10].

The SRT measurement requires access to the performance–intensity functions. Obtaining the performance–intensity or the performance–S/N functions, however, is time-consuming as we have to repeat the test at different intensity levels or at different S/N levels. Furthermore, it is not clear what range of S/N levels to include in order to bracket the 50% point. A more practical and efficient method is needed for obtaining the SRT. Fortunately, such a method exists and is based on adaptive psychophysical procedures [22].

The procedure is adaptive in that it systematically adjusts the S/N level (or the intensity level in quiet) depending on the listener's response. This adaptive procedure, also called the up–down procedure, works as follows. Speech materials are presented initially at a high S/N level. If the listener identifies correctly the words presented, then the S/N level is decreased by a fixed amount, say by 2 dB. This continues until the listener no longer identifies the words presented. Then, the S/N level is increased by the same amount, say by 2 dB, until the listener no longer identifies the words. This process continues for many trials while keeping track of the changes in the S/N level. The change in direction from an increase (up) to a decrease (down) in the S/N level is called a reversal as is the change in direction from a decrease to an increase in the S/N level. The first two reversals are typically ignored to reduce the bias from the initial point [22], and the midpoints of the last eight reversals are averaged to obtain the SRT. The same procedure can be used to obtain the SRT in quiet except that rather than changing the S/N level, we systematically change the sound intensity level. The increments by which the S/N level (or intensity level) is increased or decreased are known as step sizes, and need to be chosen carefully. A large step size might badly place the data relative to the 50% point, while a small step size would require a longer time for the procedure to converge. Some suggested starting with a large step size and gradually reducing it to a smaller step size [22]. A fixed step size of 2–4 dB was found to work well in [23,24].

The aforementioned up–down adaptive procedure is known to converge to the 50% point, that is, the SRT, of the performance–S/N function [22,23]. Dirks et al. [23] have shown that the up–down procedure provides the same estimate of SRT as the brute force method of extracting the 50% point from the performance–S/N level function.

10.2.4.2 Using Statistical Tests to Assess Significant Differences: Recommended Practice

After conducting speech intelligibility tests, we often want to compare the performance of various algorithms. At the very least, we are interested in knowing whether a specific speech enhancement algorithm improves speech intelligibility over the baseline condition (i.e., unprocessed noisy speech materials). Consider, for instance, the percent correct scores obtained by 10 listeners when presented with enhanced speech and with unprocessed noisy speech. The mean intelligibility score for the enhanced speech was say 90%, and the mean score for the unprocessed speech was say 85%. For this example, can we safely say with confidence that the speech enhancement algorithm improved speech intelligibility? We cannot reach such a conclusion without first performing the appropriate statistical test.

Statistical techniques [25, ch. 4] can be used to draw inferences about the means of two populations, which in our case correspond to the percent correct scores of the enhanced and unprocessed speech or more generally to scores obtained using two different algorithms. In most of these techniques, an assumption is made that the scores obtained are drawn from two Gaussian distributions with different means μ_1 and μ_2, but identical variances. Inferences about the differences between the two means can be made using hypothesis testing. More specifically, based on the available samples from the two distributions, we can test the following two hypotheses:

$$\begin{aligned} H_0 &: \mu_1 = \mu_2 \\ H_1 &: \mu_1 \neq \mu_2 \end{aligned} \tag{10.4}$$

where

H_0 is the null hypothesis that the means of the two populations are equal
H_1 is the alternate hypothesis that the means of the two populations differ

The main purpose of the hypothesis-testing technique is to establish whether experimental evidence supports the rejection (or acceptance) of the null hypothesis. A test statistic is needed to test the aforementioned hypotheses. More specifically, the said hypotheses can be tested using the t statistic, which is based on the Student's t distribution. For that reason, the associated test is known in the statistics literature as the *t-test*. The test statistic t is computed as follows:

$$t = \frac{\bar{d}}{\sigma_d}\sqrt{n} \tag{10.5}$$

where

$\bar{d}$ and σ_d are the sample mean and standard deviations, respectively, of the differences in scores between the two populations

n is the total number of samples (i.e., the number of scores in our case)

The probability distribution of t has a mound shape similar to the Gaussian distribution and it is symmetric around its mean. In fact, under certain assumptions about the distribution of $\bar{d}$, the t distribution becomes Gaussian [26, p. 358].

The computed value of t will determine if we will accept or reject the null hypotheses stated in Equation 10.4. If the value of t is found to be greater than a critical value (found in statistics tables), then we reject the null hypothesis and therefore conclude that the means of the two populations are different. For the example in Table 10.8, if t is found to be larger than the critical value, we conclude that there is a *statistically significant* difference in intelligibility and that algorithm B improved speech intelligibility. If the value of t is found to be smaller than the critical value,

TABLE 10.8
Examples of Intelligibility Scores Obtained by Four Different Algorithms

	Example 1		Example 2	
Subjects	**Alg. A**	**Alg. B**	**Alg. C**	**Alg. D**
1	87	89	97	80
2	76	76	76	70
3	84	85	80	96
4	80	81	75	85
5	76	82	76	85
6	79	85	79	86
7	83	86	83	76
8	78	80	78	81
9	80	83	75	86
10	86	89	90	91
Means	80.9	83.6	80.9	83.6
Variance	15.43	16.49	52.99	54.04

Note: The mean scores obtained for the algorithms in Examples 1 and 2 are identical, but the variances are different

then we accept the null hypothesis and conclude that the means of the two populations do not differ, that is, the performance of algorithm A is as good as the performance of algorithm B.

The critical value of t depends on the degrees of freedom, equal to $n - 1$ (i.e., one less than the total number of samples), and also on the specified criterion of significance, α. The specified criterion of significance α, which is typically set to $\alpha = 0.05$, gives the probability of rejecting H_0 erroneously. The error in rejecting H_0 when in fact H_0 is true is known as Type I error [26, p. 355]. By using $\alpha = 0.05$, for example, as the criterion of significance, we are confident, with a probability of 0.95, that our decision to reject H_0 is correct.

T-tests also yield the level of significance, denoted as p value, which provides the probability that the null hypothesis H_0 is true (i.e., the means of the two populations are the same) and should be accepted. Clearly, the smaller the p value, the more confident we are in rejecting the null hypothesis H_0. For two-tailed tests, the p value can be computed by evaluating twice the probability that t will be larger in absolute value than the computed value $\hat{t}$, that is,

$$
\begin{aligned}
p &= 2P(t > |\hat{t}\,|) \\
&= 2\int_{|\hat{t}|}^{\infty} f_t(t)dt
\end{aligned}
\tag{10.6}
$$

where

$P(\cdot)$ denotes the probability measure

$f_t(t)$ denotes the Student's probability density function

The aforementioned probability can be evaluated by computing the sum of the areas under the t distribution for which $t > \hat{t}$ or $t < -\hat{t}$ corresponding to the tails of the t distribution. Since the t distribution is symmetric, the two areas under the two tails are identical, and we only need to integrate from $|\hat{t}|$ to infinity and multiply the result by two to get the p value in (10.6).

For the examples given in Table 10.8, the t value obtained for Example 1 was $t = 4.26$, while the t value obtained for Example 2 was $t = 0.84$. The critical value ($\alpha = 0.05$) of t obtained from statistics tables for 9 (=10−1) degrees of freedom is 2.262. Since the t value obtained in Example 1 is larger than the critical value, we reject the null hypothesis and conclude that algorithm B is better than algorithm A in terms of improving speech intelligibility. The rejection areas for this example are illustrated in Figure 10.2. We say that the difference in intelligibility performance between algorithms A and B is statistically significant.

The situation in Example 2 is different. Since the t value obtained in Example 2 is smaller than the critical value, we accept the null hypothesis and conclude that algorithms C and D perform equally well. That is, we conclude that algorithm D is no better than algorithm C in terms of speech intelligibility despite the 2.7% difference in scores. The corresponding p values for Examples 1 and 2 were $p = 0.002$

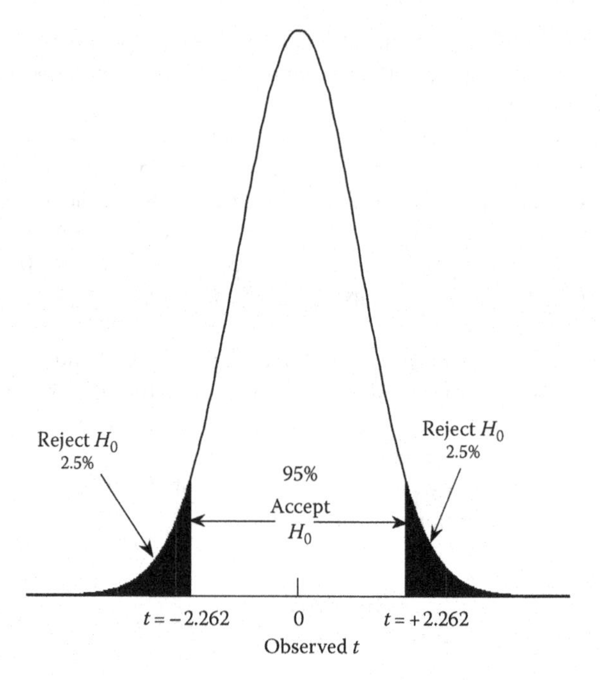

FIGURE 10.2 Acceptance and rejection regions for the example in Table 10.8.

and $p = 0.42$, respectively. The aforementioned example clearly demonstrates that providing the mean scores of the intelligibility tests is not enough as far as being able to draw reliable conclusions about the performance of various algorithms.

The t-test presented in this section is based on two assumptions. The first assumption is that the samples (percent correct scores in our case) are drawn from Gaussian distributions. Fortunately, this assumption is not unreasonable and the t-test is quite robust with regard to this assumption. As an alternative, a nonparametric test that does not require the normality assumption can be used based on Wilcoxon's rank sum test [25, p. 183]. The second assumption is that the population variances are equal. Experiments from statistics showed that the t-test is robust and still applies even when the population variances differ by as much as a factor of 3. Alternatively, the data can be transformed to a new variable to achieve uniform variance across the two populations. Some common transformations for the data y include $\sqrt{y}, \log y$ and $\arcsin \sqrt{y}$ [25, p. 417,27].

The aforementioned t-test applies only when we want to compare the means of two populations. But, what happens if we want to compare the means of M ($M > 2$) populations? This situation arises when we want to investigate, for example, the effect of varying a certain parameter of an algorithm on intelligibility. That is, suppose we vary systematically a specific parameter of the algorithm and we want to investigate whether a certain value of the parameter will improve speech intelligibility. To answer this question, we can process speech materials with each parameter value and present the processed speech materials to listeners for identification. From this test, we can obtain M sets of scores (one set per parameter value), from which we need to determine whether varying the parameter has any effect on the intelligibility, and if so, which parameter yields the largest improvement.

It is tempting to run pairwise comparisons of the population means using multiple t-tests to answer the aforementioned questions. However, the probability of falsely rejecting *at least one* of the hypotheses increases as the number of t-tests increases. That is, although we may set the probability of Type I error at the $\alpha = 0.05$ level for each individual test, the probability of falsely rejecting *at least one* of those tests might be much larger than 0.05.

For the aforementioned reason, the t-tests are not recommended for multiple pairwise comparisons. A different test, called the analysis of variance (ANOVA) test, is used in place of the t-test. The ANOVA test is based on the evaluation of the following modified hypothesis:

$$\begin{aligned} &H_0 : \mu_1 = \mu_2 = \mu_3 = \ldots. = \mu_M \\ &H_1 : \text{at least one of the population means differs from the rest} \end{aligned} \tag{10.7}$$

where
H_0 is the null hypothesis
H_1 is the alternate hypotheses

In place of the t statistic, the F statistic is used to test equality of the population means:

$$F = \frac{s_B^2}{s_W^2} \tag{10.8}$$

where
s_B^2 is the mean square between samples
s_W^2 is the mean square within samples [25, ch. 10]

The F statistic has an F distribution [26, p. 208] with (df_1, df_2) degrees of freedom, where $df_1 = M - 1$ and $df_2 = M(n - 1)$, with M being the number of populations and n the number of samples within each population (note that the number of samples within each population need not necessarily be the same). The test statistic F is compared against a critical value (which depends on df_1, df_2, and a specified α), and if it is found to be larger than the critical value, then we reject the null hypothesis and conclude that at least one of the population means differs from the rest. Likewise, if the F value is found to be smaller than the critical value, then we accept the null hypothesis and conclude that the population means are equal to each other.

Overall, the ANOVA test will tell us if any of the population means differs from the rest but it will not tell us which population means differ from each other. That is, it will not tell us, for instance, whether μ_1 differs from μ_2 or μ_4, or whether μ_2 differs from μ_4, and so on. To answer these questions, multiple comparison pairwise tests need to be conducted after performing the ANOVA test. Since these tests are performed after the ANOVA test, they are often called *post hoc* tests, and are performed *only if* the computed p value of the ANOVA test is found to be smaller than the specified level of significance, $\alpha = 0.05$. If the p value is found to be larger than $\alpha = 0.05$, then we conclude that the population means are equal to one another, that is, we say that the specified parameter had no effect on speech intelligibility.

Several *post hoc* tests can be used for multiple pairwise comparisons and include among others the Fisher's least significant difference (LSD) test, the Scheffe's test, and the Tukey's test [25, ch. 11]. The LSD test is one of the most common *post hoc* tests used to assess differences in the means between pairs of populations following the ANOVA test.

Consider the example given in Table 10.9 which examines the effect of four different values of the parameter X on speech intelligibility. Intelligibility scores were obtained for each of the four parameters using 10 listeners. We are interested in finding out whether parameter X has any significant effect on speech intelligibility, and if so, which value (A, B, C, or D) yielded the largest improvement. Based on an ANOVA test (see Table 10.10), the estimated F value was 13.68, which is larger than the critical value for $df_1 = 3$ and $df_2 = 36$ degrees of freedom and $\alpha = 0.05$ [25, p. A-8]. The associated p value was smaller than 0.005. We therefore reject the null hypotheses that the mean intelligibility scores obtained with each of the four parameters were equal, and conclude that the parameter X had a significant effect on speech intelligibility. *Post hoc* tests according to LSD indicated that the scores obtained with parameter C were significantly higher ($p < 0.05$) than the scores obtained with parameters A, B, or D. LSD tests also indicated that the scores obtained with parameters A and B were not significantly ($p = 0.556$) different from each other, and the score obtained with parameter D was significantly ($p < 0.05$) lower than all other scores.

TABLE 10.9
Intelligibility Scores for 10 Listeners as a Function of Four Different Parameters

	Parameters			
Subjects	**A**	**B**	**C**	**D**
1	56	54	68	45
2	62	60	65	55
3	59	57	68	50
4	55	53	58	48
5	65	60	65	55
6	50	52	67	40
7	56	54	59	49
8	61	65	70	60
9	60	58	63	52
10	50	48	63	53
Means	57.4	56.1	64.6	50.7

TABLE 10.10
ANOVA Results for the Example in Table 10.9

	Sum of Squares	*df*	Mean Square	*F*	*p*
Between groups	982.600	3	327.533	13.682	<.0005
Within groups	861.800	36	23.939		
Total	1844.400	39			

In this section, we described two common statistical tests that can be used to assess significant differences between algorithms, the *t*-test, and the ANOVA test. These tests are available in several software packages including Microsoft's Excel program, MATLAB® Statistics Toolbox, as well as in various statistical packages (e.g., SPSS, Inc.). Such tests are highly recommended when interested in assessing the true benefits of intelligibility of speech enhancement algorithms.

10.3 EVALUATING QUALITY OF PROCESSED SPEECH

A good speech enhancement algorithm needs to preserve or enhance not only speech intelligibility but also speech quality. This is based on the observation that it is possible for speech to be highly intelligible but be of poor quality. Also, it is not unlikely that two different algorithms may produce equal word-intelligibility scores, yet the listeners perceive the speech of one of the two algorithms as being more natural, pleasant, and acceptable than the other. There is therefore the need to measure other attributes of the speech signal besides intelligibility. Reliable evaluation of speech quality is considered to be a much more challenging task than the task of evaluating speech intelligibility. This is largely because quality assessment is highly subjective and the reliability of the subjective measurements becomes an issue.

Several methods for evaluating speech quality have been proposed in the literature [1]. These methods can be broadly classified into two categories: those that are based on relative preference tasks and those that are based on assigning a numerical value on the quality of the speech stimuli, that is, based on quality ratings. In the relative preference tests, listeners are presented with a pair of speech stimuli consisting of the test stimuli and the reference stimuli. The reference stimuli are typically constructed by degrading the original speech signal in a systematic fashion, either by filtering or by adding noise. Listeners are asked to select the stimuli they prefer the most. In the rating tests, listeners are presented with the test speech stimuli and asked to rate the quality of the stimuli on a numerical scale, typically a 5-point scale with one indicating poor quality and a five indicating excellent quality. No reference stimuli are needed in the rating tests. As we will see next, these tests have their strengths and weaknesses, and in practice, the best test might depend on the application at hand. In the following sections, we describe in more detail the relative preference and quality rating tests that can be used to assess the quality of degraded speech, which in our application is speech processed by noise suppression algorithms.

10.3.1 Relative Preference Methods

The *isopreference* test was perhaps one of the earliest paired-comparison tests used for measuring speech quality [28]. In this method, test signals, each with a different intensity level and corrupted by different levels of additive noise, were passed through a system consisting of a band-limiting filter simulating the analog characteristics of a speech transmission system. Subjects listened to pairs of test signals and asked to select the one they preferred. Test results were reported in terms of "isopreference contours" on a two-dimensional space of speech intensity level versus noise level. Any two points on the isopreference contours specified the pair of parameter values that yielded equal preference for the two test signals.

The isopreference method is quite elaborate and time-consuming due to the large number of intensity- and noise-level combinations that need to be considered. Moreover, in order to make valid comparisons between different systems, the isopreference contours need to be somehow reduced to a single number or scale. For these reasons, several modifications to the isopreference method were made.

The method proposed in [29] did not require the determination of the isopreference contours and was based on the use of five types of distorted speech as reference signals (this method was recommended by the IEEE Subcommittee on Subjective Measurements [30]). The reference stimuli used in [29] are listed in Table 10.11 and are labeled as A–E. The test involved all possible forward and reverse order comparisons between the test signal and the reference signals, and also all possible combinations among all reference signals. Listeners were presented with pairs of signals and asked to express their preference. Since each reference signal is presented exactly eight times, we can take the number of times a given reference signal is preferred and divide that by the number of listeners to get a number between 0 and 8. This number is then multiplied by 1.25, the preference rating for each of the reference signals. The reference signals were chosen so that system A would ideally have a rating of 10 as it is not distorted in any way, while systems B–E would have the ratings of 7.5, 5, 2.5, and 0, respectively [29].

The preference rating for the test signal is obtained by considering only the preference judgments obtained for the 10 comparisons involving the test signals and the reference signals. Since the test signal is presented exactly ten times to the listeners,

TABLE 10.11
Reference Conditions Used

System	Signal Description
A	High-fidelity speech (clean)
B	Speech bandpass filtered (800–3000 Hz)
C	Speech low-pass filtered (3000 Hz) and combined with low-pass filtered white noise (500 Hz). Peak SNR 10 dB
D	Speech combined with reverberant echo. Delay of first echo 150 ms
E	Speech peak clipped, then bandpass filtered (300–2000 Hz)

Source: Hecker, M. and Williams, C., *J. Acoust. Soc. Am.*, 39(5), 946, 1966.

we can compute the number of times that the test signal is preferred and divide that by the number of listeners to get a number between 0 and 10. This number, denoted as X, is entered into the formula $y = 1.25(X - 1)$ to determine the preference rating for the test signal. This formula is used to produce a numerical coincidence on the preference scale rating for the case where the test signal and the reference signal are judged to be of equal preference, that is, "isopreferent." So, by plotting the rating obtained for the test signal against the rating obtained with the reference signals, we can determine the reference signal, which is equally preferred to the test signal.

As pointed out in [30], the choice of reference signals is important in speech preference tests. At the very least, the reference signals should sound markedly different when compared to each other and they should be considerably preferred in a certain order. The reference signals listed in [29] were consistently preferred in the order of A through E. A comparison of the aforesaid preference test involving the five reference signals (Table 10.11) with a test which used as reference conditions different levels of a single type of distortion (e.g., caused by noise degradation) indicated that the preference judgments obtained with the aforesaid test exhibited a significantly smaller variance among the listeners.

Various other methods have been used to generate reference signals [31,32]. The Modulated Noise Reference Unit (MNRU) reference signal [31] in particular has been used extensively for the evaluation of speech quality (e.g., [33]). The MNRU reference signal $r(n)$ is generated as follows:

$$r(n) = x(n)\left[1 + 10^{-Q/20} d(n)\right] \tag{10.9}$$

where

$x(n)$ is the input speech signal
$d(n)$ is the random noise
Q is the desired SNR

More specifically, Q is the ratio of speech power to modulated noise power:

$$Q = \text{SNR} = 10\log_{10} \frac{E\{x^2(n)\}}{E\left\{\left[10^{-Q/20} \cdot d(n) \cdot x(n)\right]^2\right\}} \tag{10.10}$$

Note that the noise $d(n)$ is not additive but is modulated by the input speech signal. Zero-mean white noise with unit variance (i.e., $E\{d^2(n)\} = 1$) is typically used for $d(n)$. The MNRU signals produce speech distortions that are subjectively similar to those produced by companded digital codecs. Guidelines for constructing MNRU reference signals can be found in [34].

A simpler preference test suitable for evaluating high-quality voice communication systems was proposed in [35]. The test involved presentation of pairs of signals, where the first signal was the reference signal and the second signal was the test signal. Modulated noise (MNRU) was used as the reference signal. The listener's task was to rate the amount of degradation of the second signal (test signal) compared to the first

TABLE 10.12
Degradation Rating Scales

Rating	Degradation
1	Very annoying
2	Annoying
3	Slightly annoying
4	Audible but not annoying
5	Inaudible

signal (reference signal) based on a five-point rating scale shown in Table 10.12. The aforementioned method, called the Degradation Category Rating method (DCR), provides only a relative measure of degradation of the test signal and as such it is highly dependent on the specific reference signal used in the evaluation [36]. The sensitivity of the DCR method in terms of resolving small differences in quality was found to be better when evaluating wideband, high-quality systems than when evaluating narrowband systems [36].

Perhaps the simplest form of the paired-comparison test is the forced-choice paired-comparison test. In this test, listeners are presented with pairs of signals produced by systems A and B and asked to indicate which of the two signals they prefer. The same signal is processed by both systems A and B. Results are reported in terms of percent of time system A is preferred over system B. Note that unlike the previously mentioned methods, no reference signal is used. Such a method is typically used when interested in evaluating the preference of system A over other systems. The main drawback of this simple method is that it is not easy to compare the performance of system A with the performance of other systems obtained in other labs.

While the aforesaid AB preference test tells us whether system A is preferred over system B, it does not tell us by how much. That is, the magnitude of the difference in preference is not quantified. The comparison category rating (CCR) test is designed to quantify the magnitude of the preference difference on a four-point scale with the rating of 0 indicating no difference, one indicating small difference, two indicating a large difference, and three indicating a very large difference. Table 10.13 shows the category ratings [37,38]. Positive and negative numbers are used to account for both directions of preference.

10.3.2 Absolute Category Rating Methods

Preference tests typically answer the question: "How well does an average listener like a particular test signal over another signal or over a reference signal which can be easily reproduced?" Listeners must choose between two sequentially presented signals, but do not need to indicate the magnitude of their preference (except in the CCR test, Table 10.13) or the reason(s) for their decision. In some applications, however, knowing the reason why a particular signal is preferred over another is more important than the preference score itself. Another shortcoming of the preference methods is that the reference signals do not always allow for a wide range of distortions as they only capture a

TABLE 10.13
Comparison Category Ratings

Rating	Quality of Second Stimulus Compared to the First Is
3	Much better
2	Better
1	Slightly better
0	About the same
−1	Slightly worse
−2	Worse
−3	Much worse

limited scope of speech distortions that could be encountered. This could potentially result in most of the test signals being preferred (or disliked) over the reference signals, thereby introducing a bias in the quality evaluation. Lastly, most preference tests produce a *relative* measure of quality (e.g., relative to a reference signal) rather than an absolute measure. As such, it is difficult to compare preference scores obtained in different labs without having access to the same reference signals.

The aforementioned shortcomings of the preference tests can be addressed by the use of absolute judgment quality tests in which judgments of overall quality are solicited from the listeners without the need for reference comparisons. Three such tests are described next.

10.3.2.1 Mean Opinion Scores

The most widely used direct method of subjective quality evaluation is the category judgment method in which listeners rate the quality of the test signal using a five-point numerical scale (see Table 10.14), with five indicating "excellent" quality and one indicating "unsatisfactory" or "bad" quality. This method is one of the methods recommended by the IEEE Subcommittee on Subjective Methods [30] as well as by ITU [38,39]. The measured quality of the test signal is obtained by averaging the scores obtained from all listeners. This average score is commonly referred to as the Mean Opinion Score (MOS).

TABLE 10.14
MOS Rating Scale

Rating	Speech Quality	Level of Distortion
5	Excellent	Imperceptible
4	Good	Just perceptible, but not annoying
3	Fair	Perceptible and slightly annoying
2	Poor	Annoying, but not objectionable
1	Bad	Very annoying and objectionable

The MOS test is administered in two phases: training and evaluation. In the training phase, listeners hear a set of reference signals that exemplify the high (excellent), the low (bad), and the middle judgment categories. This phase, also known as the "anchoring phase," is very important as it is needed to equalize the subjective range of quality ratings of all listeners. That is, the training phase should in principle equalize the "goodness" scales of all listeners to ensure, to the extent possible, that what is perceived as "good" by one listener is perceived as "good" by the other listeners. A standard set of reference signals need to be used and described when reporting the MOS scores [30]. In the evaluation phase, subjects listen to the test signal and rate the quality of the signal in terms of the five quality categories (1–5) shown in Table 10.14.

Detailed guidelines and recommendations for administering the MOS test can be found in the ITU-R BS.562-3 standard [38] and include the following:

1. *Selection of listening crew*: Different number of listeners is recommended depending on whether the listeners had extensive experience in assessing sound quality. The minimum number of nonexpert listeners should be 20 and the minimum number of expert listeners should be 10.
2. *Test procedure and duration*: Speech material (original and degraded) should be presented in random order to subjects, and the test session should not last more than 20 min without interruption. This step is necessary to reduce listening fatigue.
3. *Choice of reproduction device*: Headphones are recommended over loudspeakers, since headphone reproduction is independent of the geometric and acoustic properties of the test room. If loudspeakers are used, the dimensions and the reverberation time of the room need to be reported.

Further guidelines pertaining to the choice of speech input levels, noise and reference conditions, etc. for proper evaluation of the quality of narrowband and wideband speech codecs can be found in the ITU standard [37] as well as in [40].

Reference signals can be used to better facilitate comparisons between MOS tests conducted at different times, different laboratories, and different languages [33]. MOS scores can be obtained, for instance, using different MNRU reference signals for various values of Q (S/N) ranging from 5 to 35 [33,37]. A plot of MOS scores as a function of Q can be constructed to transform the raw MOS scores to an equivalent Q value. The Q equivalent values can then be used to compare performance among systems in different labs.

The MOS test is based on a five-category rating of the speech quality (Table 10.14). The quality scale is in a way quantized into five discrete steps, one for each category. Listeners are therefore forced to describe the complex impressions of speech quality in terms of the five categories. It is implicitly assumed that these five steps (categories) are uniformly spaced, that is, they are equidistant from each other. This assumption, however, might not be true, in general. For these reasons, some have suggested modifying the aforementioned test to ask the listeners to evaluate the test signals in terms of real numbers from 0 to 10, where 0 indicates "bad" quality and 10 indicates "excellent" quality [41]. In this test, no quantization of the quality scale is done since the listeners are allowed to use fractions between integers, if they so desire.

10.3.2.2 Diagnostic Acceptability Measure

The absolute category judgment method (e.g., MOS test) is based on ratings of the *overall* quality of the test speech signal. These ratings, however, do not convey any information about the listeners' bases for judgment of quality. Two different listeners, for instance, may base their ratings on different attributes of the signal, and still give identical overall quality rating. Similarly, a listener might give the same rating for two signals produced by two different algorithms, but base his judgments on different attributes of each signal. In brief, the MOS score alone does not tell us which attribute of the signal affected the rating. The MOS test is therefore considered to be a single-dimensional approach to quality evaluation, and as such it cannot be used as a diagnostic tool to improve the quality of speech enhancement algorithms.

A multidimensional approach to quality evaluation was proposed by Voiers [42] based on the Diagnostic Acceptability Measure (DAM). The DAM-based test was motivated by early work done by McDermott in the late 1960s. McDermott [43] used multidimensional scaling techniques to analyze preference judgments of speech subjected to 22 different types of distortion. Her analysis suggested a three-dimensional perceptual space and labeled the three axes as: overall clarity, signal-background distortion, and subjective loudness. The DAM test incorporates elements from McDermott's analysis.

The DAM test evaluates the speech quality on three different scales classified as *parametric, metametric*, and *isometric* [1,44]. These three scales yield a total of 16 measurements on speech quality covering several attributes of the signal and background. The metametric and isometric scales represent the conventional category judgment approach where speech is rated relative to "intelligibility," "pleasantness," and "acceptability." The parametric scale provides fine-grained measurements of the signal and background distortions. Listeners are asked to rate the signal distortion on six different dimensions and the background distortion on four dimensions (see Table 10.15). Listeners are asked, for instance, to rate on a scale of 0–100 how muffled or how nasal the signal sounds are, ignoring any other signal or background distortions present. Listeners are also asked to rate separately on a scale of 0–100 the amount of hissing, buzzing, chirping, or rumbling present in the background. Table 10.15 shows the quality scales used in the DAM test. The composite acceptability (CA) measure summarizes all the information gathered from all the scales into a single number, and is computed as a weighted average of the individual scales.

The parametric portion of the DAM test relies on the listeners' ability to *detect*, perhaps more reliably, specific distortions present in the signal or in the background rather than providing preference judgments of these distortions. It therefore relies on the assumption that people tend to agree better on *what they hear* rather than on *how well they like it* [44]. To borrow an example from daily life, it is easier to get people to agree on the color of a car than how much they like it. As argued in [44], the parametric approach tends to give more accurate—more reliable—scores of speech quality as it avoids the individual listener's "taste" or preference for specific attributes of the signal from entering the subjective quality evaluation.

TABLE 10.15
Scales Used in the DAM Test

		Parametric Scales	
Name	**Abbreviation**	**Descriptor**	**Example**
Signal	SF	Fluttering, bubbling	AM speech
	SH	Distant, thin	High-pass speech
	SD	Rasping, crackling	Peak-clipped speech
	SL	Muffled, smothered	Low-pass speech
	SI	Irregular, interrupted	Interrupted speech
	SN	Nasal, whining	Bandpass speech
	TSQ	Total signal quality	
Background	BN	Hissing, rushing	Gaussian noise
	BB	Buzzing, humming	60 Hz hum
	BF	Chirping, bubbling	Narrowband noise
	BR	Rumbling, thumping	Low freq. noise
	TBQ	Total background quality	
		Metametric Scales	
	I	Intelligibility	
	P	Pleasantness	
		Isometric Scales	
	A	Acceptability	
	CA	Composite acceptability	

Compared to the MOS test, the DAM test is time-consuming and requires carefully trained listeners. Prior to each listening session, listeners are asked to rate two "anchor" and four "probe" signals. The "anchors" consist of examples of high- and low-quality speech and give the listeners a frame of reference. The "probes" are used to detect any coincidental errors that may affect the results in a particular session. In addition to the presentation of "anchors" and "probes," listeners are selected on the basis that they give consistent ratings over time and have a moderately high correlation to the listening crew's historical average rating [1]. The selected listeners are calibrated prior to the testing session so as to determine their own subjective origin or reference relative to the historical average listener's ratings.

The DAM quality scales listed in Table 10.15 consist of 12 parametric scales and 4 metametric and isometric scales. Note that a few more scales were added to the original DAM test [44, p. 143], but we will focus here only on the original set of scales. The parametric scale is separated into six ratings of signal quality and four ratings of background quality. The individual scores of the signal ratings are used to compute a total signal quality (TSQ) score as follows [1, Chapter 3]:

$$TSQ = \sum_{j=1}^{6} b_j^S S_j + c_1^S \left(\prod_{j=1}^{6} S_j \right)^{1/3} + c_2^S \left(\prod_{j=1}^{6} S_j \right)^{1/6} + c_3^S \tag{10.11}$$

where

S_j is the adjusted average (across all listeners) score of the jth signal quality scale $j = 1, 2, \ldots, 6$, with $j = 1$ corresponding to the SF (fluttering scale)

$j = 2$ corresponding to the SH (distant-thin scale), and so on

The b_j^S coefficients are weights on these scales, and the c_i^S coefficients are chosen to normalize the TSQ score relative to the acceptability scale. Note that the S_j scores are not the raw scores of signal distortion, but the scores that have been adjusted and corrected for the listener's subjective origin and scale [1, p. 79]. These scores are averaged across listeners as follows:

$$S_j = \frac{\sum_{k=1}^{N} \rho_{jk} \hat{S}_{jk}}{\sum_{k=1}^{N} \rho_{jk}}, \quad j = 1, 2, \ldots, 6 \tag{10.12}$$

where

$\hat{S}_{jk}$ is the partially adjusted score of listener k on scale j

N is the number of listeners (usually 12)

ρ_{jk} is the correlation coefficient for listener k obtained by computing the correlation of the ratings of listener k on scale j with the historical average listener's ratings on scale j

The weighted averaging is done to place the largest weight to the scores of listeners whose responses were more consistent with the ratings of the historical average listener.

Similarly, the individual scores of the background ratings are used to compute a total background quality (TBQ) score as follows:

$$TBQ = \sum_{j=1}^{4} b_j^B B_j + c_1^B \left(\prod_{j=1}^{4} B_j \right)^{1/3} + c_2^B \left(\prod_{j=1}^{4} B_j \right)^{1/6} + c_3^B \tag{10.13}$$

where B_j is the adjusted average (across all listeners, as done in Equation 10.12) score of the jth background quality scale; where $j = 1, 2, \ldots, 4$, with $j = 1$ corresponding to the BN (hissing scale); $j = 2$ corresponding to the BB (buzzing scale); and so on. The b_j's are weights on these scales, and the c_i^B are coefficients are chosen to normalize the TSQ score relative to the acceptability scale.

The acceptability score (A) is computed from the TSQ and TBQ scores as follows:

$$A = \sum_{j=1}^{6} b_j^S S_j + \sum_{j=1}^{4} b_j^B B_j + c_1^A (TSQ)(TBQ) + c_2^A \tag{10.14}$$

where c_j^A are the regression coefficients computed using scores from a set of over 200 test systems. Note that the acceptability score is a function of the product of the

TSQ and TBQ scores, suggesting that the acceptability score is high only when *both* the TSQ and TBQ scores are high. If either of the TSQ and TBQ scores is low, then the acceptability score (A) is approximately equal to the smaller of the two scores.

The metametric quality measures of intelligibility (I) and pleasantness (P) are computed as follows:

$$I = c_1^I I_R + c_2^I (I_R)^2 + c_3^I$$
$$P = c_1^P P_R + c_2^P (P_R)^2 + c_3^P \tag{10.15}$$

where

I_R and P_R are the adjusted listener's ratings of intelligibility and pleasantness, respectively

c_j^X are regression coefficients computed in a manner similar to that in Equation 10.14

The final score of CA gives the rating of the overall signal quality and is computed as follows:

$$CA = \frac{\sum_{j=1}^{6} b_j^{CA} S_j + \sum_{j=1}^{4} d_j^{CA} B_j + c_1^{CA} A + c_2^{CA} I + c_3^{CA} P}{\sum_{j=1}^{6} b_j^{CA} \sum_{j=1}^{4} d_j^{CA} \sum_{j=1}^{3} c_j^{CA}} \tag{10.16}$$

where b_j^{CA}, c_j^{CA}, and d_j^{CA} are weights proportional to the statistical reliability of the corresponding quality scores. The CA score summarizes the information from all quality scales into a single number, and it thus allows comparisons between systems. Good correlation ($\rho = 0.9$) was reported in [44] between the CA scores and the MOS scores for a large number (>200) of system conditions.

The DAM test yields a total of 16 scores, as indicated by Equations 10.11 through 10.16. Clearly, the pattern of DAM scores will depend on the type of distortion involved. Figure 10.3 shows as an example the effect of center-clipping distortion on the pattern of DAM scores [1, p. 154]. As shown, this type of distortion affected mostly the signal quality, with only a minor effect on the background. More attention needs to be paid on the pattern of the DAM scores rather than on the final score of CA. This is because different types of noise might produce the same CA score, yet have dramatically different DAM patterns [44]. This supports the idea that quality is better described as a multidimensional rather than as a single-dimensional concept.

10.3.2.3 ITU-T P.835 Standard

The aforesaid subjective listening tests (DAM and MOS) were designed primarily for the evaluation of speech coders. The speech coders, however, are evaluated mainly in quiet and generally introduce different types of distortion than those encountered in noise suppression algorithms. Speech enhancement algorithms typically degrade the speech signal component while suppressing the background

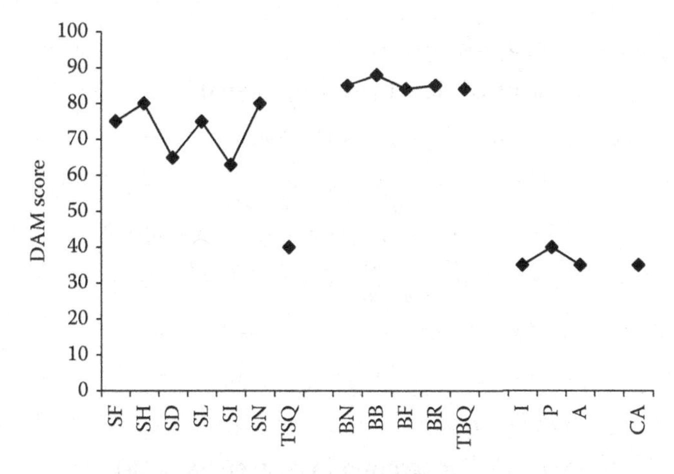

FIGURE 10.3 DAM scores obtained from the evaluation of the effect of center-clipping distortion on speech quality. (From Quackenbush, S. et al., *Objective Measures of Speech Quality*, Prentice Hall, Englewood Cliffs, NJ, 1988, p. 154.)

noise, particularly in low SNR conditions. That is, while the background noise may be suppressed, and in some cases rendered inaudible, the speech signal may get degraded in the process. This situation complicates the subjective evaluation of speech enhancement algorithms since it is not clear as to whether listeners base their overall quality judgments on the signal distortion component, noise distortion component, or both. This uncertainty regarding the different weight individual listeners place on the signal and noise distortion components introduces additional error variance in the subjects' ratings of overall quality resulting and consequently decreases the reliability of the ratings. These concerns were addressed by the ITU-T standard (P. 835) [45] that was designed to lead the listeners to integrate the effects of both signal and background distortion in making their ratings of overall quality.

The methodology proposed in [45] reduces the listener's uncertainty by requiring him/her to successively attend to and rate the waveform on: the *speech signal* alone, the *background noise* alone, and the *overall effect* of speech and noise on quality. More precisely, the ITU-T P. 835 method instructs the listener to successively attend to and rate the enhanced speech signal on

1. The speech signal alone using a five-point scale of signal distortion (SIG)—see Table 10.16.
2. The background noise alone using a five-point scale of background intrusiveness (BAK)—see Table 10.17.
3. The overall effect using the scale of the Mean Opinion Score (OVL)—[1 = bad, 2 = poor, 3 = fair, 4 = good, 5 = excellent].

Each trial contains a three-sentence sample of speech laid out in the format shown in Figure 10.4. Each sample of speech is followed by a silent period during which

TABLE 10.16
Scale of Signal Distortion (SIG)

Rating	Description
5	Very natural, no degradation
4	Fairly natural, little degradation
3	Somewhat natural, somewhat degraded
2	Fairly unnatural, fairly degraded
1	Very unnatural, very degraded

TABLE 10.17
Scale of Background Intrusiveness (BAK)

Rating	Description
5	Not noticeable
4	Somewhat noticeable
3	Noticeable but not intrusive
2	Fairly conspicuous, somewhat intrusive
1	Very conspicuous, very intrusive

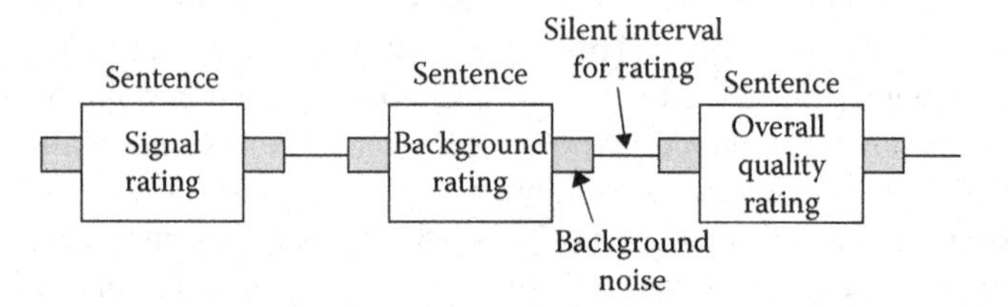

FIGURE 10.4 Stimulus presentation format for the listening tests conducted according to the ITU-T P.835 standard.

the listener rates the signal according to the SIG, BAK, or OVL scales. In the example shown in the figure, each sample of speech is approximately four seconds in duration and includes: one second of preceding background noise alone, two seconds of noisy speech (roughly the duration of a single sentence), and one second of background noise alone. Each sample of speech is followed by an appropriate silent interval for rating. For the first two samples, listeners rate either the signal or the background depending on the rating scale order specified for that trial. For the signal distortion rating, for instance, subjects are instructed to attend *only* to the speech signal and rate the speech on the five-category distortion scale shown in Table 10.16. For the background distortion rating, subjects are instructed to attend *only* to the background and rate the background on the five-category intrusiveness scale shown in Table 10.17. Finally, for the third sample in each trial, subjects are instructed to listen to the noisy speech signal and rate it on the five-category overall quality scale used in MOS tests (Table 10.14). To control for the effects of rating scale order, the order of the rating scales needs to be balanced. That is, the scale order should be "Signal, Background, Overall Effect" for half of the trials, and "Background, Signal, Overall Effect" for the other half.

The ITU-T P.835 standard was used in [46] to evaluate and compare the performance of 13 different speech enhancement algorithms (more on this in Chapter 11).

10.4 EVALUATING RELIABILITY OF QUALITY JUDGMENTS: RECOMMENDED PRACTICE

In the aforesaid subjective tests, listeners rate the quality of the processed speech on a 5-point discrete scale (MOS test) or on a 0–100 continuous scale (DAM test). For the ratings to be meaningful, however, listeners must use the scales consistently. A given listener must rate a specific speech sample the same way every time he or she hears it. That is, we would like the *intra-rater reliability* of quality judgments to be high. Listeners need, in other words, to be self-consistent in their assessment of quality. Additionally, all listeners must rate a given speech sample in a similar way. We would thus like the *inter-rater reliability* of quality judgments to be high. The measurements of *intra-* and *inter-rater* reliability are critically important as they indirectly indicate the confidence we place on the listeners' (i.e., the raters) quality judgments. High values of *inter-rater* reliability, for instance, would suggest that another sample of listeners would produce the same mean rating score for the same speech material. In other words, high inter-rater reliability implies high reproducibility of results. In contrast, a low value of *inter-rater* reliability would suggest that the listeners were not consistent in their quality judgments.

The efficacy of reliability measures has been studied extensively in behavioral sciences (see reviews in [47,48]) as well as in voice research where pathological voices are rated by clinicians in terms of breathiness or roughness [49–51]. Drawing from this body of literature, we focus next on some of the most commonly used reliability measures.

10.4.1 Intra-Rater Reliability Measures

Various statistics have been used to evaluate intra-rater reliability [48,49]. The two most common statistics are the *Pearson's correlation coefficient* between the first and second ratings, and the test–retest *percent agreement*. To obtain the Pearson's coefficient, listeners are presented with the same speech samples at two different testing sessions. The Pearson's correlation between the ratings in the first and second sessions is obtained as follows:

$$\rho_P = \frac{\sum_{j=1}^{n}(x_j - \bar{x})(y_j - \bar{y})}{n\sigma_x\sigma_y} \tag{10.17}$$

where
$\{x_i\}_{i=1}^n$ are the ratings obtained in the first session
$\{y_i\}_{i=1}^n$ are the ratings obtained in the second session
$\bar{x}$ and $\bar{y}$ are the sample means of the ratings
σ_x and σ_y are the standard deviations of the ratings
n is the total number of ratings made in each session

Note that this coefficient takes values in the range of $-1 \le \rho_P \le 1$. The value of the Pearson coefficient indicates the strength of the (assumed) linear relationship between the variables $\{x_i\}_{i=1}^n$ (first rating) and $\{y_i\}_{i=1}^n$ (second rating). A value of $\rho_P \approx 0$ indicates no linear relationship (i.e., no correlation) between $\{x_i\}_{i=1}^n$ and $\{y_i\}_{i=1}^n$ while a value of $\rho_P \approx 1$ indicates a strong positive relationship between the two variables. In the context of quality assessment, a value of $\rho_P \approx 1$ would indicate consistency in judgments between the first and second testing sessions, while a value of $\rho_P \approx 0$ would indicate inconsistency. Consider the example given in Table 10.18 where two listeners (raters) are tested in two different sessions. The estimated Pearson coefficient for Rater 1 was 0.299 while the estimated Pearson coefficient for Rater 2 was 0.913. From this, we conclude that Rater 2 was more consistent in his ratings. In this example (Table 10.18), only two raters were involved. Since most tests will involve more than two raters, it is recommended that the average (across all raters) and standard deviation of the Pearson's coefficient is reported along with the range (minimum and max) of the coefficients [49].

The values of the Pearson's correlation coefficient are used in some cases as a basis for excluding some listeners from the test. That is, we may recruit a large number of listeners but keep only those with relatively high ($\rho_P > 0.9$) intra-rater reliability [29]. When computing the average score, we may include only scores from listeners with high intra-rater reliability.

Another simple measure of intra-rater reliability is the *percent agreement* that can be computed by counting the number of ratings that agree exactly or within ± one scale value. Two different measures can thus be reported: one based on the *exact*

TABLE 10.18
Hypothetical Ratings of Degraded Speech by Two Listeners (Raters) for Two Sessions

	Rater 1		Rater 2	
Sentence Number	**First Session**	**Second Session**	**First Session**	**Second Session**
1	2	2	3	3
2	4	2	4	4
3	4	4	4	4
4	3	3	3	2
5	2	3	3	2
Means	3	2.8	3.4	3
ρ	0.299		0.913	
Agreement	60%		60%	

agreement between the ratings made in the first and second sessions, and one based on the agreement within ± one scale value. For the example given in Table 10.18, the exact agreement for Rater 1 was 60% and the exact agreement for Rater 2 was 60%. This suggests that both raters produced the same ratings in both sessions 60% of the time. Agreement within ± one scale value was 80% for Rater 1 and 100% for Rater 2.

Although the percent agreement measure is simple to compute, it needs to be interpreted with caution. This is because this measure is rarely corrected for chance and therefore is often inflated (see, for instance, the example in Table 10.18). Assuming all scale values are equally likely to occur, the chance probability of listeners responding within ± one scale value is $(3p - 2)/p^2$, where p is the number of values in the scale [49]. For a five-point ($p = 5$) scale (e.g., the MOS scale), the chance probability is equal to 0.52. So, for the example given in Table 10.18, the exact agreement is not as good as it seems, since it is in fact only 8% points above chance. The agreement scores might also be inflated if too many or too few speech samples in the test fall at the extremes of the scales. Hence, the distribution of "quality" among the test speech samples can affect the value of the percent agreement measure.

10.4.2 Inter-Rater Reliability Measures

The intra-rater reliability measures described earlier assess how self-consistent each listener is, but do not assess how consistent are the listeners with each other in making quality judgments. It is not unlikely, for instance, to have listeners who are self-consistent, but do not agree with each other. The degree of agreement among a group of listeners can be assessed using *inter-rater reliability* measures. These measures reflect the overall coherence of a group of listeners.

A number of *inter-rater reliability* measures have been used [49] and include among others the Cronbach's alpha [52], Kendall's coefficient of Concordance [53], and the intraclass correlation coefficient [54,55]. Of those measures, the intraclass coefficient is perhaps one of the most common and most recommended measures [47] used in subjective judgments.

There exist several forms of the ICC depending on the experimental design at hand, but for our application, we will focus on the one where the speech samples and the raters are treated as random effects in a two-way ANOVA (indicated as ICC(2,1) in [54] and as ICC(A,1) in [55]). That is, both the listeners and the speech samples are assumed to be randomly selected, representing the two random factors in the ANOVA. The ICC is based on the ANOVA [25, Chapter 14], and it is computed as a ratio of variances across speech samples and across raters. More specifically, the ICC is computed as [54] follows:

$$ICC = \frac{MSB - MSE}{MSB + (K-1)MSE + K(MSL - MSE)/N} \tag{10.18}$$

where

MSB is the mean square of the ratings across speech samples
MSE is the mean square of the residual
MSL is the mean square of the ratings across listeners
K is the number of speech tokens
N is the number of listeners

TABLE 10.19
Computation of the Inter-Class Rater Reliability

	Raters				
Speech Token	**1**	**2**		**N**	**Means**
1	y_{11}	y_{12}	$\cdots$	y_{1N}	$\bar{y}_1$
2	y_{21}	y_{22}	$\cdots$	y_{2N}	$\bar{y}_2$
$\vdots$	$\vdots$	$\vdots$	$\cdots$	$\vdots$	$\vdots$
K	y_{K1}	y_{K2}	$\cdots$	y_{KN}	$\bar{y}_K$
Means	$\bar{r}_1$	$\bar{r}_2$	$\cdots$	$\bar{r}_N$	

Denoting the rating of the ith speech sample by the jth rater as y_{ij} (see Table 10.19), we can compute the aforesaid mean square values as follows:

$$MSB = \frac{N}{K-1}\sum_{i=1}^{K}(\bar{y}_i - \bar{y})^2$$

$$MSL = \frac{K}{N-1}\sum_{i=1}^{N}(\bar{r}_i - \bar{y})^2$$

$$MSE = \frac{1}{(N-1)(K-1)}\left[\sum_{i=1}^{K}\sum_{j=1}^{N}(y_{ij} - \bar{y})^2 - (K-1)MSB - (N-1)MSL\right] \quad (10.19)$$

where

$\bar{y}$ is the overall sample mean

$\bar{y}_i$ is the sample mean (across listeners) rating of the ith speech token

$\bar{r}_i$ is the sample mean (across speech tokens) rating of the ith rater (see Table 10.19) Note that the MSB value measures the variability of the rating scores among the speech samples, the MSL measures the variability in ratings among the raters, and MSE measures the variability among the ratings that is not accounted for by either the selected speech samples or raters. In addition to reporting the ICC coefficient, it is also recommended that the 95% confidence intervals of the ICC estimate are reported. Formulae for estimating the 95% confidence intervals of ICC can be found in [55].

Table 10.20 shows examples of ICC estimation for two sets of listeners who were asked to rate the quality of five sentences using the MOS scale (five-point scale). The mean MOS score for the first set of three listeners was 2.86, and the mean MOS score for the second set of listeners was 2.8. The estimated ICC coefficient (according to Equation 10.18) for the first set of listeners was 0.1077 and the estimated ICC coefficient for the second set of listeners was 0.8. Clearly, the second set of listeners

TABLE 10.20
Hypothetical Ratings (Based on the MOS Scale) of Processed Speech by Two Groups of Listeners

	Listeners: Group 1			Listeners: Group 2		
Speech Tokens	**1**	**2**	**3**	**1**	**2**	**3**
1	3	4	1	3	3	3
2	2	4	3	3	2	2
3	5	5	2	2	3	3
4	4	3	1	4	4	4
5	3	2	1	2	2	2

was more consistent with each other in making quality judgments than the first set of listeners. Interestingly, the MOS scores obtained in both tests were roughly the same. However, the ICC measure suggests that we should "trust" the second set of listeners in that they are more consistent with each other.

10.5 SUMMARY

This chapter presented various listening tests and procedures that have been used to evaluate the performance of speech enhancement algorithms in terms of subjective quality and intelligibility. Several intelligibility tests were described based on the use of nonsense syllables, monosyllabic words, rhyming words, or sentences as speech materials. Several subjective listening tests were also described for evaluating the quality of enhanced speech. These tests included relative preference methods and absolute category rating methods (e.g., MOS, DAM). The ITU-T P.835 standard established for evaluating the quality of speech processed by a noise reduction algorithm was also described.

REFERENCES

1. Quackenbush, S., Barnwell, T., and Clements, M. (1988), *Objective Measures of Speech Quality*, Englewood Cliffs, NJ: Prentice Hall.
2. Voiers, W. (1980), Interdependencies among measures of speech intelligibility and speech "quality", *Proc. IEEE Int. Conf. Acoust., Speech, Signal Processing*, 5, 703–705.
3. Remez, R., Rubin, R., Pisoni, D., and Carrell, O. (1981), Speech perception without traditional cues, *Science*, 212, 947–950.
4. Loizou, P., Dorman, M., and Tu, Z. (1999), On the number of channels needed to understand speech, *J. Acoust. Soc. Am.*, 106(4), 2097–2103.
5. Shannon, R., Zeng, F.-G., Kamath, V., Wygonski, J., and Ekelid, M. (1995), Speech recognition with primarily temporal cues, *Science*, 270, 303–304.
6. James, J., Chen, B., and Garrison, L. (2004), Implementing VoIP: A voice transmission performance progress report, *IEEE Commun. Mag.*, 42(7), 36–41.

7. Miller, G., Heise, G., and Lichten, W. (1951), The intelligibility of speech as a function of the context of the test materials, *J. Exp. Psychol.*, 41, 329–335.
8. Egan, J. (1948), Articulation testing methods, *Laryngoscope*, 58(9), 955–991.
9. Kalikow, D., Stevens, K., and Elliott, L. (1977), Development of a test of speech intelligibility in noise using sentence materials with controlled word predictability, *J. Acoust. Soc. Am.*, 61(5), 1337–1351.
10. Nilsson, M., Soli, S., and Sullivan, J. (1994), Development of hearing in noise test for the measurement of speech reception thresholds in quiet and in noise, *J. Acoust. Soc. Am.*, 95(2), 1085–1099.
11. Miller, G. and Nicely, P. (1955), An analysis of perceptual confusions among some English consonants, *J. Acoust. Soc. Am.*, 27(2), 338–352.
12. Voiers, W. D. (1983), Evaluating processed speech using the Diagnostic Rhyme Test, *Speech Technol.*, January/February, 30–39.
13. Fletcher, H. and Steinberg, J. (1929), Articulation testing methods, *Bell Syst. Tech. J.*, 8, 806–854.
14. Jakobson, R., Fant, G., and Halle, M. (1967), *Preliminaries to Speech Analysis: The Distinctive Features and Their Correlates*, Cambridge, MA: MIT Press.
15. Blahut, R. (1990), *Principles and Practice of Information Theory*, Reading, MA: Addison-Wesley Publishing Company.
16. Fairbanks, G. (1958), Test of phonemic differentiation: The rhyme test, *J. Acoust. Soc. Am.*, 30(7), 596–600.
17. House, A., Williams, C., Hecker, M., and Kryter, K. (1965), Articulation-testing methods: Consonantal differentiation with a closed-response set, *J. Acoust. Soc. Am.*, 37(1), 158–166.
18. Bilger, R., Nuetzel, J., Rabinowitz, W., and Rzeczkowski, C. (1984), Standardization of a test of speech perception in noise, *J. Speech Hear. Res.*, 27, 32–48.
19. Morgan, D., Kamm, C., and Velde, T. (1981), Form equivalence of the speech perception in noise (SPIN) test, *J. Acoust. Soc. Am.*, 69(6), 1791–1798.
20. Bench, J. and Bamford, J. (1979), *Speech-Hearing Tests and the Spoken Language of Hearing-Impaired Children*, London, U.K.: Academic.
21. Plomp, R. and Mimpen, A. (1979), Speech-reception threshold for sentences as a function of age and noise level, *J. Acoust. Soc. Am.*, 66(5), 1333–1342.
22. Levitt, H. (1971), Transformed up-down methods in psychoacoustics, *J. Acoust. Soc. Am.*, 49(2), 467–477.
23. Dirks, D., Morgan, D., and Dubno, J. (1982), A procedure for quantifying the effects of noise on speech recognition, *J. Speech Hear. Disord.*, 47, 114–123.
24. Dubno, J., Dirks, D., and Morgan, D. (1984), Effects of age and mild hearing loss on speech recognition in noise, *J. Acoust. Soc. Am.*, 76(1), 87–96.
25. Ott, L. (1988), *An Introduction to Statistical Methods and Data Analysis*, 3rd ed., Boston, MA: PWS-Kent Publishing Company.
26. Papoulis, A. and Pillai, S. (2002), *Probability, Random Variables and Stochastic Processes*, 4th ed. New York: McGraw Hill, Inc.
27. Studebaker, G. A. (1985), A 'rationalized' arcsine transform, *J. Speech Hear. Res.*, 28, 455–462.
28. Munson, W. and Karlin, J. (1962), Isopreference method for evaluating speech-transmission circuits, *J. Acoust. Soc. Am.*, 34(6), 762–774.
29. Hecker, M. and Williams, C. (1966), Choice of reference conditions for speech preference tests, *J. Acoust. Soc. Am.*, 39(5), 946–952.
30. IEEE Subcommittee (1969), IEEE recommended practice for speech quality measurements, *IEEE Trans. Audio Electroacoust.*, AU-17(3), 225–246.

31. Law, H. and Seymour, R. (1962), A reference distortion system using modulated noise, *Proc. IEE*, 109B(48), 484–485.
32. Schroeder, M. (1968), Reference signal for signal quality studies, *J. Acoust. Soc. Am.*, 44(6), 1735–1736.
33. Goodman, D. and Nash, R. (1982), Subjective quality of the same speech transmission conditions in seven different countries, *IEEE Trans. Commun.*, COm-30(4), 642–654.
34. ITU-T (1996), Methods for objective and subjective assessment of quality: Modulated noise reference unit (MNRU). ITU-T Recommendation P. 810.
35. Combescure, P., Guyader, A., and Gilloire, A. (1982), Quality evaluation of 32 Kbit/s coded speech by means of degradation category ratings, *Proceeding of the IEEE International Conference on Acoustics, Speech, Signal Processing*, Paris, France, pp. 988–991.
36. Panzer, I., Sharpley, A., and Voiers, W. (1993), A comparison of subjective methods for evaluating speech quality, in Atal, B., Cuperman, V., and Gersho, A. (Eds.), *Speech and Audio Coding for Wireless and Network Applications.* Boston, MA: Kluwer Academic Publishers,
37. ITU-T (1996), Subjective performance assessment of telephone band and wideband digital codecs, ITU-T Recommendation P. 830.
38. International Telecommunication Union—Radiocommunication Sector, Recommendation BS. (1990), Subjective assessment of sound quality, pp. 562–563.
39. International Telecommunication Union—Telecommunication Sector, Recommendation (1998), Subjective performance assessment of telephone band and wideband digital codecs, p. 830.
40. Coleman, A., Gleiss, N., and Usai, P. (1988), A subjective testing methodology for evaluating medium rate codecs for digital mobile radio applications, *Speech Commun.*, 7(2), 151–166.
41. Rothauser, E., Urbanek, G., and Pachl, W. (1970), A comparison of preference measurement methods, *J. Acoust. Soc. Am.*, 49(4), 1297–1308.
42. Voiers, W. D. (1977), Diagnostic acceptability measure for speech communication systems, *Proceedings of the IEEE International Conference Acoustics, Speech, Signal Processing*, Hartford, CT, pp. 204–207.
43. McDermott, B. (1968), Multidimensional analyses of circuit quality judgments, *J. Acoust. Soc. Am.*, 45(3), 774–781.
44. Voiers, W. D., Sharpley, A., and Panzer, I. (2002), Evaluating the effects of noise on voice communication systems, in Davis, G. (Ed.), *Noise Reduction in Speech Applications,* Boca Raton, FL: CRC Press, pp. 125–152.
45. ITU-T (2003), Subjective test methodology for evaluating speech communication systems that include noise suppression algorithm, ITU-T Recommendation P. 835.
46. Hu, Y. and Loizou, P. (2006), Subjective comparison of speech enhancement algorithms, *Proc. IEEE Int. Conf. Acoust., Speech Signal Process.*, I, 153–156.
47. Tinsley, H. and Weiss, D. (1975), Interrater reliability and agreement of subjective judgments, *J. Counsel. Psychol.*, 22(4), 358–376.
48. Suen, H. (1988), Agreement, reliability, accuracy and validity: Toward a clarification, *Behav. Assess.*, 10, 343–366.
49. Kreiman, J., Kempster, G., Erman, A., and Berke, G. (1993), Perceptual evaluation of voice quality: Review, tutorial and a framework for future research, *J. Speech Hear. Res.*, 36(2), 21–40.
50. Gerratt, B., Kreiman, J., Antonanzas-Barroso, N., and Berke, G. (1993), Comparing internal and external standards in voice quality judgments, *J. Speech Hear. Res.*, 36, 14–20.

51. Kreiman, J. and Gerratt, B. (1998), Validity of rating scale measures of voice quality, *J. Acoust. Soc. Am.*, 104(3), 1598–1608.
52. Cronbach, L. (1951), Coefficient alpha and the internal structure of tests, *Psychometrika*, 16, 297–334.
53. Kendall, M. (1955), Rank correlation methods, New York: Hafner Publishing Co.
54. Shrout, P. and Fleiss, J. (1979), Intraclass correlations: Uses in assessing rater reliability, *Psychol. Bull.*, 86(2), 420–428.
55. McGraw, K. and Wong, S. (1996), Forming inferences about some intraclass correlation coefficients, *Psychological Methods*, 1(1), 30–46.

11 Objective Quality and Intelligibility Measures

Subjective listening tests provide perhaps the most reliable method for assessing speech quality or speech intelligibility. These tests, however, can be time-consuming requiring in most cases access to trained listeners. For these reasons, several researchers have investigated the possibility of devising objective, rather than subjective, measures of speech quality [1, ch. 2] and intelligibility. Ideally, the objective measure should be able to assess the quality (or intelligibility) of the enhanced speech without needing access to the original speech signal. The objective measure should incorporate knowledge from different levels of processing including low-level processing (e.g., psychoacoustics) and higher level processing such as semantics, linguistics, and pragmatics. The ideal measure should predict with high accuracy the results obtained from subjective listening tests with normal-hearing listeners. This chapter provides an overview of objective quality and intelligibility measures which have been used to assess the quality and intelligibility of speech processed by noise-reduction algorithms.

11.1 OBJECTIVE QUALITY MEASURES

Objective measures of speech quality are implemented by first segmenting the speech signal into 10–30ms frames, and then computing a distortion measure between the original and processed signals. A single, global measure of speech distortion is computed by averaging the distortion measures of each speech frame. As we will see shortly, the distortion measure computation can be done either in the time domain (e.g., signal-to-noise ratio measures) or in the frequency domain (e.g., linear predictive coding [LPC] spectral distance measures). For the frequency-domain measures, it is assumed that any distortions or differences detected in the magnitude spectra are correlated with speech quality. Note that the distortion measures are not distance measures in the strict sense, as they do not obey all properties of a distance metric. For one, these measures are not necessarily symmetric and some (e.g., log spectral distance measure) yield negative values. Psychoacoustic experiments [2] suggest that the distance measures should not be symmetric [3].

A large number of objective measures have been evaluated, particularly for speech coding applications [1]. Reviews of objective measures can be found in [4–7]. Next, we focus on a subset of those measures that have been found to correlate well, at least with speech-coder type of distortions.

11.1.1 SEGMENTAL SIGNAL-TO-NOISE RATIO MEASURES

The segmental signal-to-noise ratio can be evaluated either in the time or frequency domain. The time-domain measure is perhaps one of the simplest objective measures used to evaluate speech enhancement algorithms. For this measure to be meaningful, it is important that the original and processed signals be aligned in time and that any phase errors present be corrected. The segmental signal-to-noise (SNRseg) is defined as

$$\text{SNRseg} = \frac{10}{M}\sum_{m=0}^{M-1}\log_{10}\frac{\sum_{n=Nm}^{Nm+N-1} x^2(n)}{\sum_{n=Nm}^{Nm+N-1}(x(n)-\hat{x}(n))^2} \tag{11.1}$$

where

$x(n)$ is the original (clean) signal
$\hat{x}(n)$ is the enhanced signal
N is the frame length (typically chosen to be 15–20 ms)
M is the number of frames in the signal

Note that the SNRseg measure is based on the *geometric mean* of the signal-to-noise ratios across all frames of the speech signal.

One potential problem with the estimation of SNRseg is that the signal energy during intervals of silence in the speech signal (which are abundant in conversational speech) will be very small resulting in large negative SNRseg values, which will bias the overall measure. One way to remedy this is to exclude the silent frames from the sum in Equation 11.1 by comparing short-time energy measurements against a threshold or by flooring the SNRseg values to a small value. In [8], the SNRseg values were limited in the range of [−10, 35 dB] thereby avoiding the need for a speech/silence detector.

The aforementioned definition of the segmental SNR is based on the input (clean) and processed signals. Alternatively, we can use the signals passed through the perceptual weighting filters commonly used in CELP-type algorithms. After passing the clean and processed signals through these filters, we can compute the segmental SNR based on the outputs of these filters [9]. This perceptually weighted SNR was evaluated in [10] and found to yield a high correlation with subjective listening tests.

A different definition for the segmental SNR was proposed by Richards [11] by shifting the log function by 1, that is,

$$\text{SNRseg}_{\text{R}} = \frac{10}{M}\sum_{m=0}^{M-1}\log_{10}\left(1+\frac{\sum_{n=Nm}^{Nm+N-1} x^2(n)}{\sum_{n=Nm}^{Nm+N-1}(x(n)-\hat{x}(n))^2}\right) \tag{11.2}$$

In doing so, the possibility of getting large negative values during the silent segments of speech is avoided. Note that the smallest achievable value of SNRseg_{R} is now zero rather than negative infinity. The main advantage of the aforementioned definition for the segmental SNR is that it avoids the need for explicit marking of speech and silent segments. This measure was evaluated in [12].

The segmental SNR can be extended in the frequency domain as follows [13]:

$$\text{fwSNRseg} = \frac{10}{M}\sum_{m=0}^{M-1}\frac{\sum_{j=1}^{K} W_j \log_{10}\left[X^2(j,m)/\left(X(j,m)-\hat{X}(j,m)\right)^2\right]}{\sum_{j=1}^{K} W_j} \tag{11.3}$$

where

W_j is the weight placed on the jth frequency band
K is the number of bands
M is the total number of frames in the signal
$X(j,m)$ is the filter-bank amplitude of the clean signal in the jth frequency band at the mth frame
$\hat{X}(j,m)$ is the filter-bank amplitude of the enhanced signal in the same band

The main advantage in using the frequency-based segmental SNR over the time-domain SNRseg (Equation 11.1) is the added flexibility to place different weights for different frequency bands of the spectrum. There is also the flexibility in choosing perceptually motivated frequency spacing such as critical-band spacing.

Various forms of weighting functions W_j were suggested in [1,13]. One possibility is to choose the weights W_j based on articulation index (AI) studies [14]. Such an approach was suggested in [1] with the summation in (11.3) taken over 16 articulation bands spanning the telephone bandwidth (200–3200 Hz). Values of the weights used in [1, ch. 6.2] are given in Table 11.1. Note that the weights derived in [14] were derived assuming 1/3-octave filters, and the weights shown in Table 11.1 were interpolated to produce the equivalent weights for critical-band filter spacing.

Alternatively, the weights for each band can be obtained using regression analysis producing the so-called *frequency-variant* objective measures [1, p. 241]. This way, the weights can be chosen to give maximum correlation between the objective and subjective measures. For these measures, a total of K (one for each band) different objective measures, D_j, are computed for each file, where D_j is given by

$$D_j = \frac{1}{M}\sum_{m=1}^{M} 10\log_{10}\left[\frac{X^2(j,m)}{\left(X(j,m)-\hat{X}(j,m)\right)^2}\right] \quad j=1,2,\ldots,K \tag{11.4}$$

TABLE 11.1
Center Filter Frequencies (Hz) and Corresponding Articulation Index Weights Used for Computing the Weighted Spectral Distance Measure

Band Number	Center Freq. (Hz)	Weight	Band Number	Center Freq. (Hz)	Weight
1	50	0.003	14	1148	0.032
2	120	0.003	15	1288	0.034
3	190	0.003	16	1442	0.035
4	260	0.007	17	1610	0.037
5	330	0.010	18	1794	0.036
6	400	0.016	19	1993	0.036
7	470	0.016	20	2221	0.033
8	540	0.017	21	2446	0.030
9	617	0.017	22	2701	0.029
10	703	0.022	23	2978	0.027
11	798	0.027	24	3276	0.026
12	904	0.028	25	3597	0.026
13	1020	0.030			

Source: Quackenbush, S. et al., *Objective Measures of Speech Quality*, Prentice Hall, Englewood Cliffs, NJ, 1988, ch. 6.2.

The optimal weights for each objective measure D_j of each band are obtained using Kth-order linear regression analysis yielding the following frequency-variant objective measure

$$fwVar = a_0 + \sum_{j=1}^{K} a_j D_j \tag{11.5}$$

where
$\{a_j\}$ are the regression coefficients
D_j is given by Equation 11.4
K is the number of bands ($K = 6$ in [1, ch. 5])

Non-linear regression analysis can alternatively be used to derive the frequency-variant objective measures (more on this in Section 11.1).

11.1.2 Spectral Distance Measures Based on LPC

Several objective measures were proposed based on the dissimilarity between all-pole models of the clean and enhanced speech signals [1]. These measures assume that over short-time intervals speech can be represented by a pth order all-pole model of the form:

$$x(n) = \sum_{i=1}^{p} a_x(i)x(n-i) + G_x u(n) \tag{11.6}$$

where

$a_x(i)$ are the coefficients of the all-pole filter (determined using linear prediction techniques)

G_x is the filter gain and $u(n)$ is a unit variance white noise excitation

Perhaps two of the most common all-pole based measures used to evaluate speech-enhancement algorithms are the log-likelihood ratio (LLR) and Itakura–Saito (IS) measures. Cepstral distance measures derived from the LPC coefficients were also used.

The LLR measure is defined as

$$d_{LLR}(\mathbf{a}_x, \bar{\mathbf{a}}_{\hat{x}}) = \log \frac{\bar{\mathbf{a}}_{\hat{x}}^T \mathbf{R}_x \bar{\mathbf{a}}_{\hat{x}}}{\mathbf{a}_x^T \mathbf{R}_x \mathbf{a}_x} \tag{11.7}$$

where

$\mathbf{a}_x^T = [1, -\alpha_x(1), -\alpha_x(2), \ldots, -\alpha_x(p)]$ are the LPC coefficients of the clean signal

$\bar{\mathbf{a}}_{\hat{x}}^T = [1, -\alpha_{\hat{x}}(1), -\alpha_{\hat{x}}(2), \ldots, -\alpha_{\hat{x}}(p)]$ are the coefficients of the enhanced signal

$\mathbf{R}_x$ is the $(p + 1) \times (p + 1)$ autocorrelation matrix (Toeplitz) of the clean signal.

The aforementioned measure has an interesting interpretation in the frequency domain. Equation 11.7 can be expressed in the frequency domain as [1, p. 49]:

$$d_{LLR}(\mathbf{a}_x, \bar{\mathbf{a}}_{\hat{x}}) = \log\left(1 + \int_{-\pi}^{\pi} \left|\frac{A_x(\omega) - \bar{A}_{\hat{x}}(\omega)}{A_x(\omega)}\right|^2 d\omega\right) \tag{11.8}$$

where $A_x(\omega)$ and $\bar{A}_{\hat{x}}(\omega)$ are the spectra of $\mathbf{a}_x^T$ and $\bar{\mathbf{a}}_{\hat{x}}^T$ respectively. This equation indicates that the differences between the signal and enhanced spectra are weighted more when $1/|A_x(\omega)|^2$ is large, which is generally near the formant peaks. Hence, this measure penalizes differences in formant peak locations.

Another interpretation of the LLR measure is that it represents the ratio of the energies of the prediction residuals of the enhanced and clean signals. The numerator estimates the energy of the prediction residual of the enhanced signal when filtered by

$$A_x(z) = 1 - \sum_{i=1}^{p} a_x(i) z^{-i} \tag{11.9}$$

Similarly, the denominator estimates the energy of the prediction residual of the clean signal filtered by (11.9). Since the denominator is also the minimum (obtained over all possible prediction coefficients) residual energy, the denominator term is always smaller than the numerator, and therefore the LLR measure is always positive.

The IS measure is defined as follows:

$$d_{IS}(\mathbf{a}_x, \bar{\mathbf{a}}_{\hat{x}}) = \frac{G_x}{\bar{G}_{\hat{x}}} \frac{\bar{\mathbf{a}}_{\hat{x}}^T \mathbf{R}_x \bar{\mathbf{a}}_{\hat{x}}}{\mathbf{a}_x^T \mathbf{R}_x \mathbf{a}_x} + \log\left(\frac{\bar{G}_{\hat{x}}}{G_x}\right) - 1 \tag{11.10}$$

where G_x and $\bar{G}_{\hat{x}}$ are the all-pole gains of the clean and enhanced signals respectively. The all-pole gain G_x can be computed as follows:

$$G_x = \left(\mathbf{r}_x^T \mathbf{a}_x\right)^{1/2} \tag{11.11}$$

where $\mathbf{r}_x^T = [r_x(0), r_x(1), \ldots, r_x(p)]$ contains the auto correlations of the clean signal (it is also the first row of the auto correlation matrix $\mathbf{R}_x$). Note that unlike the LLR measure, the IS measure penalizes differences in all-pole gains, i.e., differences in overall spectral levels of the clean and enhanced signals. This can be considered as a drawback of the IS measure, since psychoacoustic studies [15] have shown that differences in spectral level have minimal effect on quality.

The LPC coefficients can also be used to derive a distance measure based on cepstrum coefficients. This distance provides an estimate of the log spectral distance between two spectra. The cepstrum coefficients can be obtained recursively from the LPC coefficients $\{a_j\}$ using the following expression [16, p. 442]:

$$c(m) = a_m + \sum_{k=1}^{m-1} \frac{k}{m} c(k) a_{m-k} \qquad 1 \leq m \leq p \tag{11.12}$$

where p is the order of the LPC analysis (Equation 11.6). A measure based on cepstrum coefficients can be computed as follows [17]:

$$d_{cep}(\mathbf{c}_x, \bar{\mathbf{c}}_{\hat{x}}) = \frac{10}{\log_e 10} \sqrt{2 \sum_{k=1}^{p} [c_x(k) - c_{\hat{x}}(k)]^2} \tag{11.13}$$

where $c_x(k)$ and $c_{\hat{x}}(k)$ are the cepstrum coefficients of the clean and enhanced signals respectively.

11.1.3 Perceptually Motivated Measures

The aforementioned objective measures are attractive in that they are simple to implement and easy to evaluate. However, their ability to predict subjective quality is limited as they do not closely emulate the signal processing involved at the auditory periphery. Much research [10,15,18–20] has been done to develop objective measures based on models of human auditory speech perception, and in this subsection we describe some of these perceptually motivated measures.

11.1.3.1 Weighted Spectral Slope Distance Measure

Psychoacoustic studies [15] indicated that when subjects were asked to rate the phonetic distance between synthetic vowels subjected to several spectral manipulations (including low-pass, high-pass filtering, level change, formant frequency differences, etc.), subjects assigned the largest distance to pairs of vowels that differed in formant frequencies. Motivated by this finding, Klatt [15] proposed a measure based on weighted differences between the spectral slopes in each band. This measure was designed to penalize heavily differences in spectral peak (formants) locations, while ignoring other differences between the spectra such as spectral tilt, overall level, etc. Those differences were found to have little effect on ratings of phonetic distance between pairs of synthetic vowels.

This measure is computed by first finding the spectral slope of each band. Let $C_x(k)$ be the original (clean) and $C_{\hat{x}}(k)$ the enhanced critical-band spectra respectively, expressed in dB. A first-order differencing operation is used to compute the spectral slopes as follows:

$$\begin{aligned} S_x(k) &= C_x(k+1) - C_x(k) \\ \bar{S}_{\hat{x}}(k) &= \bar{C}_{\hat{x}}(k+1) - \bar{C}_{\hat{x}}(k) \end{aligned} \tag{11.14}$$

where $S_x(k)$ and $\bar{S}_{\hat{x}}(k)$ denote the spectral slopes of the clean and enhanced signals respectively of the kth band. The differences in spectral slopes are then weighted according to first whether the band is near a spectral peak or valley, and second according to whether the peak is the largest peak in the spectrum. The weight for bank k, denoted as $W(k)$, is computed as follows:

$$W(k) = \frac{K_{\max}}{[K_{\max} + C_{\max} - C_x(k)]} \frac{K_{loc\max}}{[K_{loc\max} + C_{loc\max} - C_x(k)]} \tag{11.15}$$

where

$C_{\max}$ is the largest log spectral magnitude among all bands

$C_{loc\max}$ is the value of the peak nearest to band k

$K_{\max}$, $K_{loc\max}$ are constants which can be adjusted using regression analysis to maximize the correlation between the subjective listening tests and values of the objective measure

For the experiments in [15], a high correlation was found with $K_{\max} = 20$ and $K_{loc\max} = 1$.

The weighted spectral slope (WSS) distance measure is finally computed as

$$d_{WSM}(C_x, \bar{C}_x) = \sum_{k=1}^{36} W(k)\left(S_x(k) - \bar{S}_{\hat{x}}(k)\right)^2 \tag{11.16}$$

for each frame of speech. The mean WSS is computed by averaging the WSS values obtained across all frames in the sentence.

The WSS measure is attractive because it does not require explicit formant extraction. Yet, it attends to spectral peak locations and is insensitive to relative peak heights and to spectral details in the valleys. The LPC-based measures (e.g., LLR measure) are sensitive to formant frequency differences, but are also quite sensitive to changes in formant amplitude and spectral tilt changes. It was no surprise that the WSS measure yielded a higher correlation ($\rho = 0.74$) than the LPC measures with subjective quality ratings of speech degraded by speech coding distortions [1].

11.1.3.2 Bark Distortion Measures

The aforementioned measure (WSS) constituted the first step in modeling how humans perceive speech, particularly vowels. Further progress was made later on by focusing on modeling several stages of the auditory processing, based on existing knowledge from psychoacoustics about how human listeners process tones and bands of noise [21, ch. 3]. Specifically, these new measures take into account the fact that

1. The ear's frequency resolution is not uniform, i.e., the frequency analysis of acoustic signals is not based on a linear frequency scale
2. The ear's sensitivity is frequency dependent
3. Loudness is related to signal intensity in a non-linear fashion

Human hearing is modeled as a series of transformations of the acoustic signal. Both the original and processed signals undergo this series of transformations leading to the so-called loudness spectra. The Bark spectral distortion (BSD) measure, proposed in [10], uses the distance between these spectra as the subjective quality measure. Figure 11.1 shows the block diagram of the stages involved in the computation of the BSD measure. Next, we describe in detail the processing involved in the individual blocks.

11.1.3.2.1 Critical-Band Filtering

The auditory system is known to have a poorer discrimination at high frequencies than at low frequencies. This can be modeled by pre-processing the signal through a bank of bandpass filters with center frequencies and bandwidths increasing with frequency. These filters have come to be known in the psychoacoustics literature as critical-band filters and the corresponding frequency spacing as critical-band spacing. The critical-band filter spacing can be approximated by the Bark frequency scale using the following Hertz-to-Bark transformation:

$$b = 6\sinh^{-1}\left(\frac{f}{600}\right) \tag{11.17}$$

where f is specified in Hz and b in Bark units. The critical-band filtering is often done in the power spectrum domain by summing up the signal power within each Bark to obtain the so-called Bark spectrum $B(b)$, $b = 1,2, \ldots, N_b$, where N_b is the number of Barks.

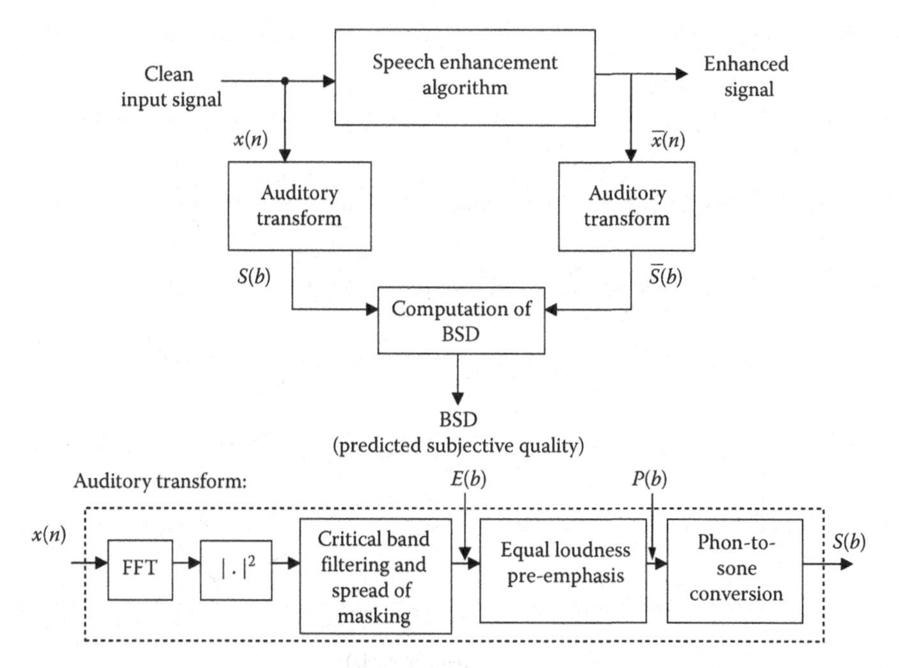

FIGURE 11.1 Block diagram of the BSD measure computation.

Following the critical-band filtering, the spread-of-masking effect is modeled by convolving the Bark spectrum $B(b)$ with a triangular-shape function of the form [22]:

$$10\log_{10}[SF(b)] = 15.81 + 7.5(b + 0.474) - 17.5\sqrt{1 + (b + 0.474)^2}\ \text{dB} \quad (11.18)$$

where b is expressed in Barks and $SF(b)$ is a triangular-shaped function. The output spectrum $E(b)$ resulting from this operation, i.e., $E(b) = B(b)^{*}SF(b)$, where * denotes convolution, is called the "excitation pattern" as it models the distribution of neuron excitation at the basilar membrane.

11.1.3.2.2 Equal Loudness Pre-Emphasis

The next stage takes into account the fact that the perceived loudness varies with frequency [23,24]. For example, a 100 Hz tone needs to be 35 dB more intense than a 1000 Hz tone for the two tones to be perceived as equally loud. This can best be explained by looking at the equal-loudness level curves (Figure 11.2) [25]. Any two points on each of those curves are perceived as equally loud. The loudness level of a tone in *phons* is defined as the intensity in dB SPL (sound-pressure level) of a 1 kHz tone which sounds equally loud.

In order to take into account the dependency of frequency on the perceived loudness, we need to convert the intensity levels in dB to loudness levels in *phons.*

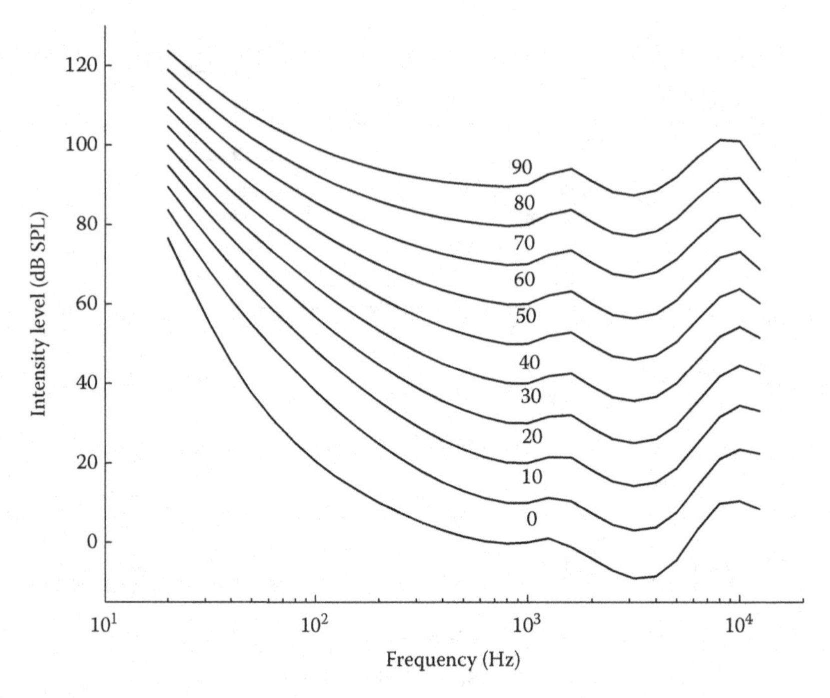

FIGURE 11.2 Equal loudness curves computed using the ISO 226 standard [25]. Numbers on each curve indicate phons.

This can be done by running the excitation spectrum through a pre-emphasis filter of the form $H(z) = (2.6 + z^{-1})/(1.6 + z^{-1})$ that boosts frequencies near and beyond the notch in the equal-loudness curves, i.e., above 1800 Hz [10]. Alternatively, the dB-to-phon conversion can be done using pre-computed equal-loudness curves (Figure 11.2) [26]. After converting the excitation spectrum $E(b)$ into *phons*, we get a new spectrum which we indicate by $P(b)$. This new spectrum $P(b)$ is expressed in loudness units of *phons* and not in dB.

11.1.3.2.3 Subjective Loudness Compensation

The last step includes yet another perceptual non-linearity: The increase in phons needed to double the subjective loudness is not a constant, but varies with the loudness level. For example, at a level of 40 phons, an extra 10 phons doubles the loudness, while near threshold the same 10 phons increase the loudness 10-fold. To incorporate this non-linearity, we need to convert the phons to *sones*. One sone is defined arbitrarily as the loudness of a 1000 Hz tone at 40 dB SPL. For instance, a 1000 Hz tone with a level of 50 dB SPL is typically judged as being twice as loud as a 40 dB tone and has therefore a loudness of two sones. Roughly a 2-fold change on loudness is produced by a 10-fold change in intensity, corresponding to a 10 dB change in level. This relationship does not hold for sound levels below 40 dB, because the loudness changes more rapidly with intensity level. The phon-to-sone conversion is modeled by the following power-law relationship:

$$S(b) = \begin{cases} 2^{(P(b)-40)/10} & \text{if } P(b) \geq 40 \\ \left[\dfrac{P(b)}{40}\right]^{2.642} & \text{if } P(b) < 40 \end{cases} \quad (11.19)$$

where $S(b)$ denotes the auditory spectrum expressed in sones. It was hypothesized in [26] that when listeners compare two signals, they respond to differences in the signals' levels expressed in *sones*, i.e., differences in the loudness spectra. The square of these differences was proposed in [26] as a viable perceptual distance for modeling judgment of vowel quality differences.

Figure 11.3 shows the different stages of the processing applied to a short-segment of the vowel/eh/. Figure 11.3a shows the signal power spectrum, Figure 11.3b shows the Bark spectrum, and Figure 11.3c shows the "excitation pattern." Note that "excitation pattern" is a smeared version of the Bark spectrum

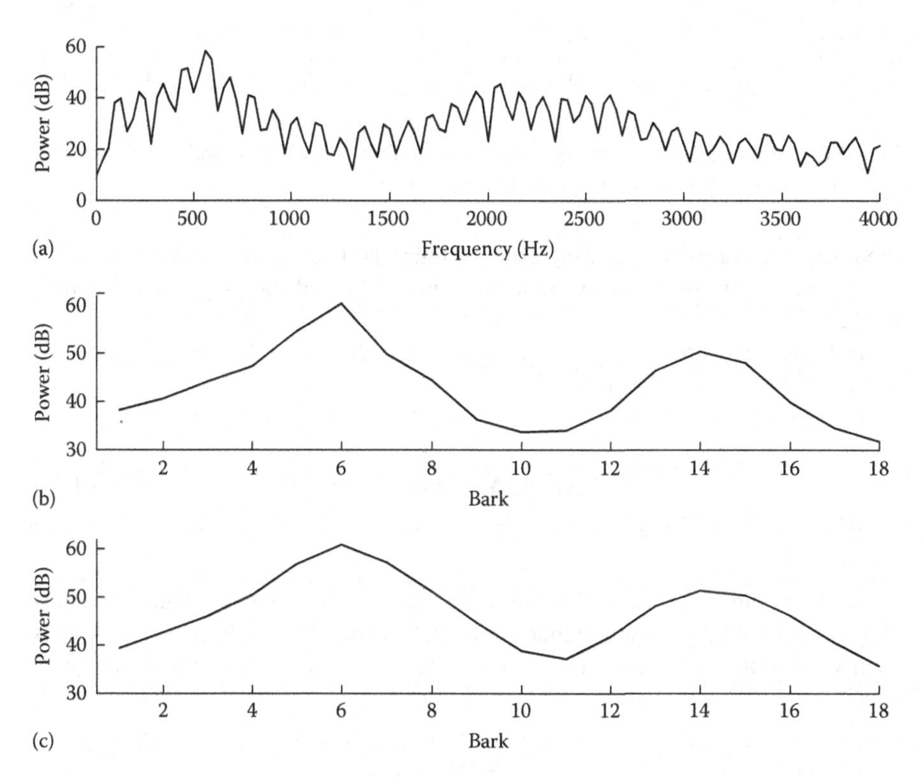

FIGURE 11.3 Panel (a) shows the power spectrum of a short segment of the vowel/eh/. Panel (b) Shows the Bark spectrum (x-axis is in Barks), and panel (c) shows the excitation spectrum obtained by convolving the Bark spectrum with a spread-masking function.

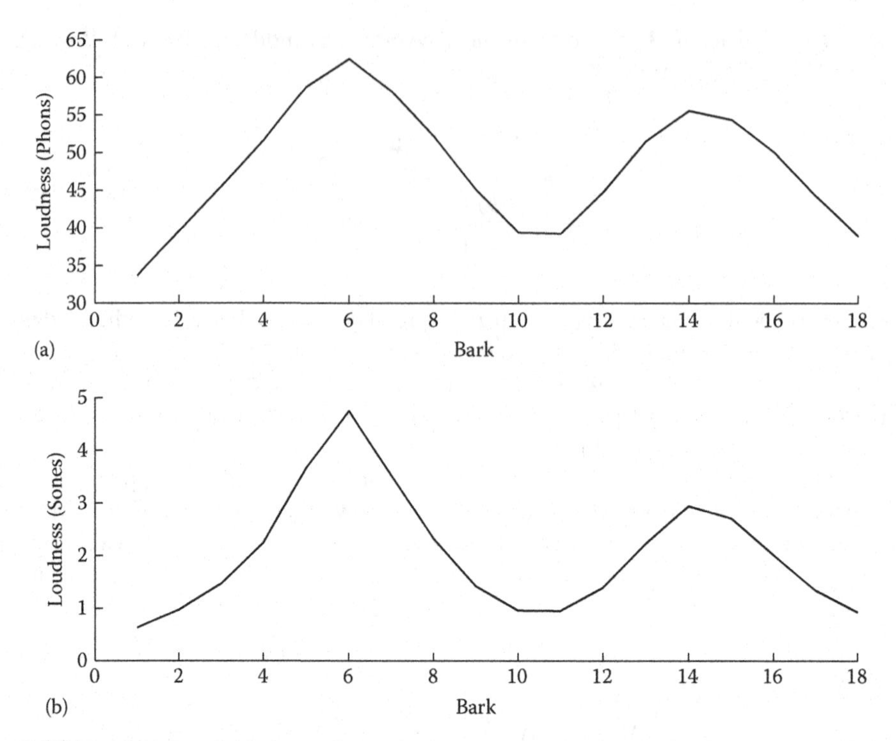

FIGURE 11.4 Panel (a) shows the excitation spectrum converted in phons and panel (b) shows the loudness spectrum expressed in units of sones.

modeling the spread-of-masking effect. Figure 11.4 shows the conversion of the excitation spectra to subjective loudness units. The auditory spectrum is shown in Figure 11.4b.

The BSD measure for frame k is based on the difference between the loudness spectra and is computed as follows:

$$BSD(k) = \sum_{b=1}^{N_b} [S_k(b) - \bar{S}_k(b)]^2 \qquad (11.20)$$

where $S_k(b)$ and $\bar{S}_k(b)$ are the loudness spectra of the clean and enhanced signals respectively and N_b is the number of critical bands. The mean BSD measure is finally computed by averaging the frame BSD measures across the sentence as follows:

$$\vec{BSD} = \frac{\sum_{k=1}^{M} BSD(k)}{\sum_{k=1}^{M}\sum_{b=1}^{N_b} [S_k(b)]^2} \qquad (11.21)$$

where M is the total number of the frames processed. The term in the denominator is used to ensure that the BSD measure is invariant under any scaling of the input signal. Experiments in [10] indicated that the BSD measure yields large values for the low-energy (unvoiced) segments of speech. This problem can be avoided by excluding the low-energy segments of speech from the BSD computation in Equation 11.21 using a voiced/unvoiced detector.

Improvements to the BSD measure were reported in [19,27,28] leading to the modified BSD measure (MBSD). The MBSD measure simply included a weighing function, $W(b)$, in the computation of the square difference of the auditory spectra as follows:

$$MBSD(k) = \sum_{b=1}^{N_b} W(b)[S_k(b) - \bar{S}_k(b)]^2 \tag{11.22}$$

where $W(b)$ was either 1 or 0 based on masking threshold calculations. In [28], $W(b)$ was set according to forward and backward masking threshold calculations, and in [19] it was set according to simultaneous masking threshold calculations. More specifically, in [19] $W(b)$ was set to 1 if the difference between the loudness spectra was above the masking threshold and set to 0 otherwise. The idea is that if the loudness difference is below the masking threshold, it will not be audible and can therefore be excluded from the MBSD computation. The weighting function $W(b)$ was determined as follows [19]:

$$W(b) = \begin{cases} 1 & |S_k(b) - \bar{S}_k(b)| \geq T(b) \\ 0 & |S_k(b) - \bar{S}_k(b)| < T(b) \end{cases} \tag{11.23}$$

where $T(b)$ is the masking threshold of the bth Bark. The masking threshold can be computed using the procedure outlined in [29]. The mean MBSD measure is computed by averaging the frame MBSD measures across the sentence as follows:

$$M\vec{B}SD = \frac{1}{M} \sum_{k=1}^{M} MBSD(k) \tag{11.24}$$

Experiments in [10,19] indicated that both BSD and MBSD measures yielded a high correlation ($\rho > 0.9$) with MOS scores. Further improvements to the MBSD measure were proposed in [27,30].

11.1.3.3 Perceptual Evaluation of Speech Quality Measure

Most of the aforementioned objective measures have been found to be suitable for assessing only a limited range of distortions which do not include distortions commonly encountered when speech goes through telecommunication networks. Packet loss, for instance, signal delays, and codec distortions would cause most objective

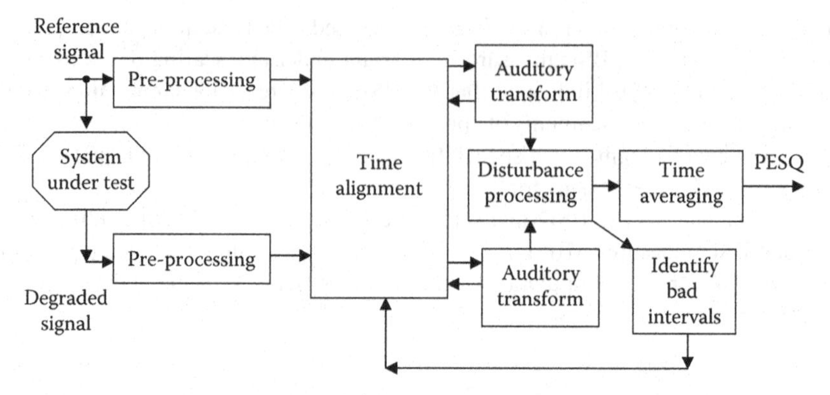

FIGURE 11.5 Block diagram of the PESQ measure computation.

measures to produce inaccurate predictions of speech quality. A number of objective measures were proposed in the 1990s focusing on this type of distortions as well as filtering effects and variable signal delays [31–33].

A competition was held in 2000 by the ITU-T study group 12 to select a new objective measure capable of performing reliably across a wide range of codec and network conditions. The perceptual evaluation of speech quality (PESQ) measure, described in [34], was selected as the ITU-T recommendation P.862 [35] replacing the old P.861 recommendation, which was based on the perceptual speech quality measure (PSQM) [32].

The structure of the PESQ measure is shown in Figure 11.5. The original (clean) and degraded signals are first level equalized to a standard listening level, and filtered by a filter with response similar to a standard telephone handset. The signals are aligned in time to correct for time delays, and then processed through an auditory transform, similar to that of BSD, to obtain the loudness spectra. The difference, termed the disturbance, between the loudness spectra is computed and averaged over time and frequency to produce the prediction of subjective MOS score. The details of the PESQ computation are given next.

11.1.3.3.1 Pre-Processing

The gain of the system under test is not known *a priori* and may vary considerably depending on the type of phone connection. Thus it is necessary to equalize the level of the original and degraded signals to a standard listening level. Gains are computed based on the rms values of bandpass-filtered (350–3250 Hz) speech. These gains are applied to the original and enhanced signals resulting in scaled versions of these signals.

Following the gain equalization, the signals are filtered by a filter with a response similar to that of a telephone handset. The intermediate reference system (IRS) receives characteristic of the telephone handset used [36, Annex D]. The IRS filtered versions of the original speech signal and degraded speech signals are computed and used in both time-alignment block and perceptual model.

11.1.3.3.2 Time Alignment

The time-alignment block provides time delay values to the perceptual model to allow corresponding signal parts of the original and degraded files to be compared. This alignment process is done in the following stages:

1. *Crude delay estimation*: Cross-correlation of the envelopes for the original and degraded signals is performed first to estimate the crude delay between them, with an approximate resolution of 4 ms. The signal envelopes are computed based on normalized frame-energy values determined by $\log(\max(E_k/ET, 1))$, where E_k is the energy in 4 ms long frame k, and ET is a threshold determined by a voice activity detector.
2. *Utterance splitting and alignment*: The estimated delays are used to divide the original signal into a number of subsections, which are referred to as utterances. Further refinement is done to determine accurate alignment of the utterances to the nearest sample and this is done in two stages:
   a. Envelope-based delay estimation of utterances. This processing only provides a crude alignment between the utterances of the original and degraded signals.
   b. Following the envelope-based alignment, frames (64 ms in duration) of the original and processed signals are Hanning-windowed and cross correlated. The index of the maximum correlation gives the delay estimate for each frame, and the maximum of the correlation, raised to the power 0.125, is used as a measure of the confidence of the alignment in each frame. These delay estimates are subsequently used in a histogram-based scheme to determine the delays to the nearest sample.

The output of the fine-time alignment procedure is a delay value and a delay confidence for each utterance. Delay changes during speech are tested by splitting and realigning time intervals in each utterance. The splitting process is repeated at several points within each utterance and the split that produces the greatest confidence is identified. Note from Figure 11.5 that after applying the perceptual model, sections that have very large disturbance (greater than a threshold value) are identified and realigned using cross-correlation.

The time-alignment section of the algorithm produces delays per time interval (d_i) along with the matched start and stop samples. This allows the delay of each frame to be identified in the perceptual model. Figure 11.6 shows an example of the alignment process.

11.1.3.3.3 Perceptual Model

The auditory transform block shown in Figure 11.5 maps the signals into a representation of perceived loudness based on a sequence of transformations similar to those used in the BSD measure [10]. The following steps are taken to compute the loudness spectra:

1. *Bark spectrum estimation*: An estimate of the power spectrum, based on the FFT, is first computed using 32 ms Hamming windows, with 50% overlap between frames. The Bark spectrum is computed by summing up the

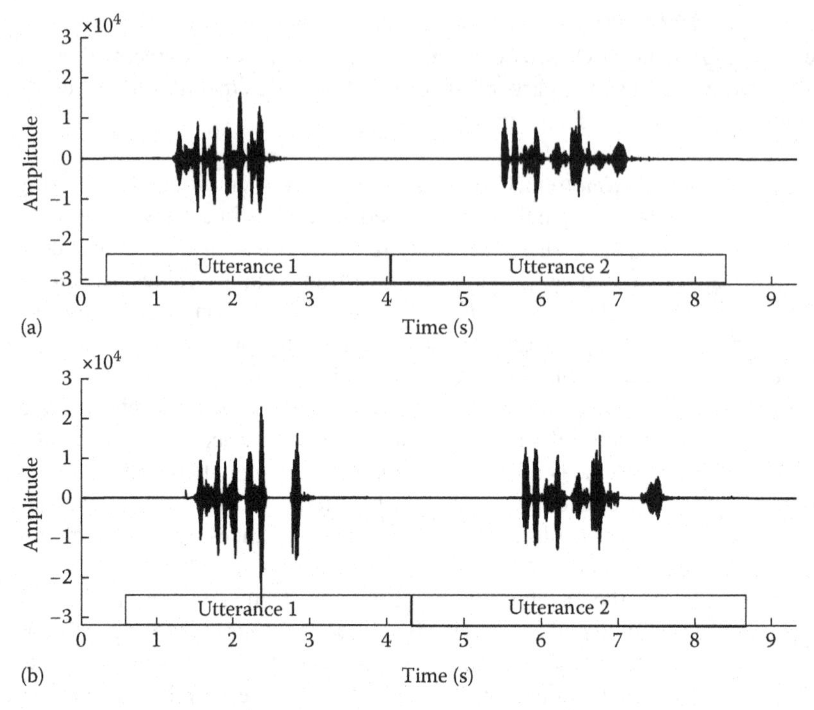

FIGURE 11.6 Comparison of two signals taken from the ITU standard [35]. The output of the time-alignment process is shown in the inserts by the x-axis. Two utterances were identified for this example by the PESQ algorithm. Note that the processed signal (b) is delayed (by 280 ms) with respect to the original signal (a), and this delay is reflected in the time marking of the two utterances. Also, the degraded signal is missing speech segments during the period of 2.6–2.9 s due to lost packets.

powers in 42 bands spaced according to a modified Bark scale (no spreading function is applied to the Bark spectrum as done in [10]). A total of 49 bands are used for signals sampled at 16 kHz.

2. *Frequency equalization*: To compensate for filtering effects, a factor is computed based on the ratio of averaged (over speech-active frames) degraded Bark spectrum to the original Bark spectrum. The original Bark spectrum is then multiplied by this factor, which is limited to the range of [−20 dB, 20 dB].
3. *Gain equalization*: To compensate for short-term gain variations, the ratio between the "audible power" of the original and degraded signals is computed. The so-called audible power is estimated in the Bark domain and includes only Bark components in the power calculation larger than the absolute hearing threshold of each band, i.e., only components that are audible. This ratio is bounded to the range $[3 \times 10^{-4}, 5]$ and is smoothed over time using a first-order low-pass filter of the form $H(z) = 0.8 + 0.2 \cdot z^{-1}$. The degraded Bark spectrum is then multiplied by this ratio.

4. *Loudness spectra computation:* After compensation of filtering and short-term gain variations, the original and degraded Bark spectra are transformed to a sone loudness scale using Zwicker's law [37]:

$$S(b) = S_l \cdot \left(\frac{P_0(b)}{0.5}\right)^{\gamma} \cdot \left[\left(0.5 + 0.5 \cdot \frac{B'_x(b)}{P_0(b)}\right)^{\gamma} - 1\right] \tag{11.25}$$

where

S_l is a loudness scaling factor

$P_0(b)$ is the absolute hearing threshold for Bark b

$B'_x(b)$ is the frequency-compensated Bark spectrum (from step 2) of the original spectrum

The power exponent γ is 0.23 for $b \geq 4$ and slightly larger for $b < 4$

Similarly, the loudness spectrum of the degraded signal, denoted as $\overline{S}(b)$, is computed from (11.25) using the gain-compensated Bark spectrum (from step 3) of the degraded signal in place of $B'_x(b)$.

Figures 11.7 through 11.11 show example speech spectra computed at different stages of the processing. The signals shown in Figure 11.6 were taken from the ITU standard [35]. Figure 11.6 shows the output of the alignment process and Figure 11.7 shows the power spectra of the original and processed signals. The IRS filtering

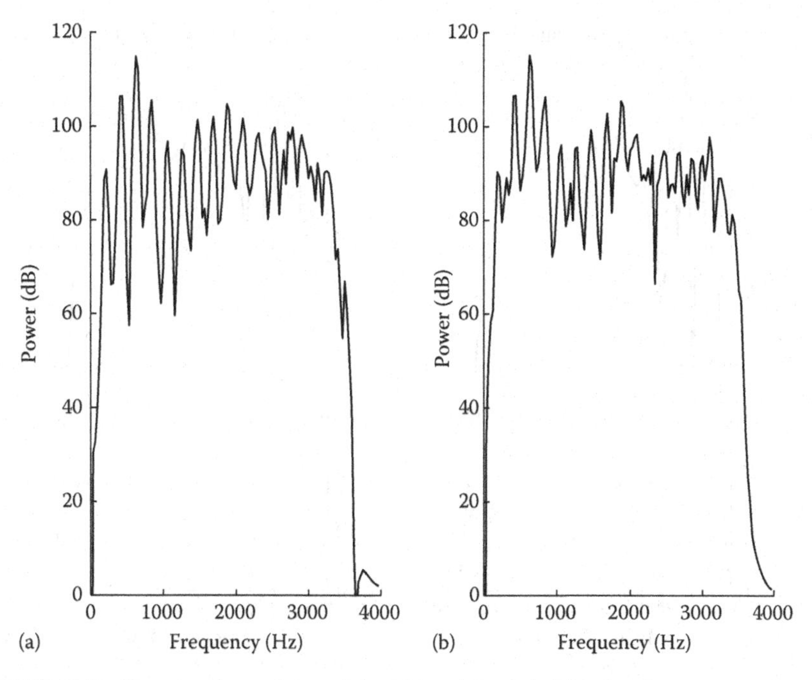

FIGURE 11.7 Power spectra of the original (a) and degraded (b) signals.

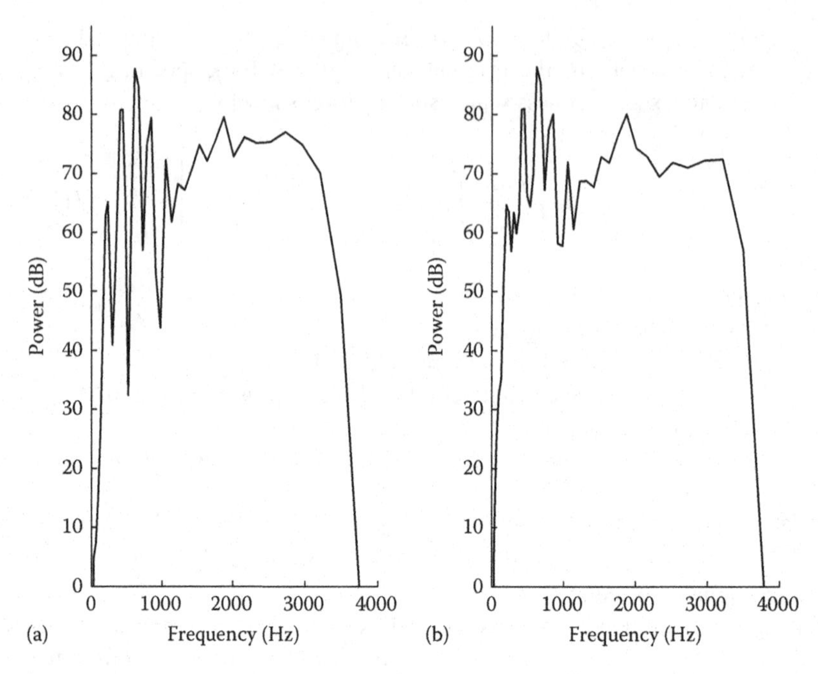

FIGURE 11.8 Bark spectra of the original (a) and processed (b) signals.

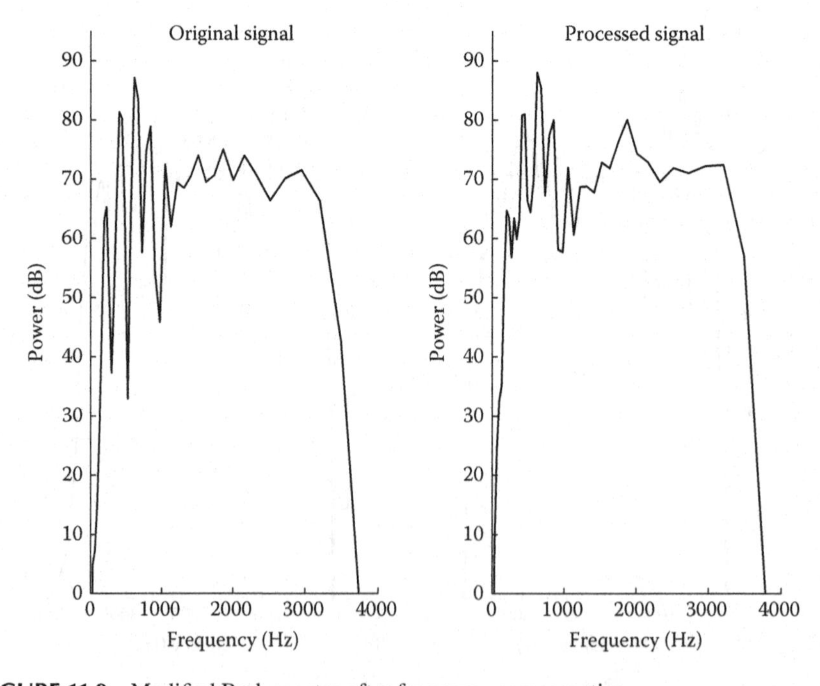

FIGURE 11.9 Modified Bark spectra after frequency compensation.

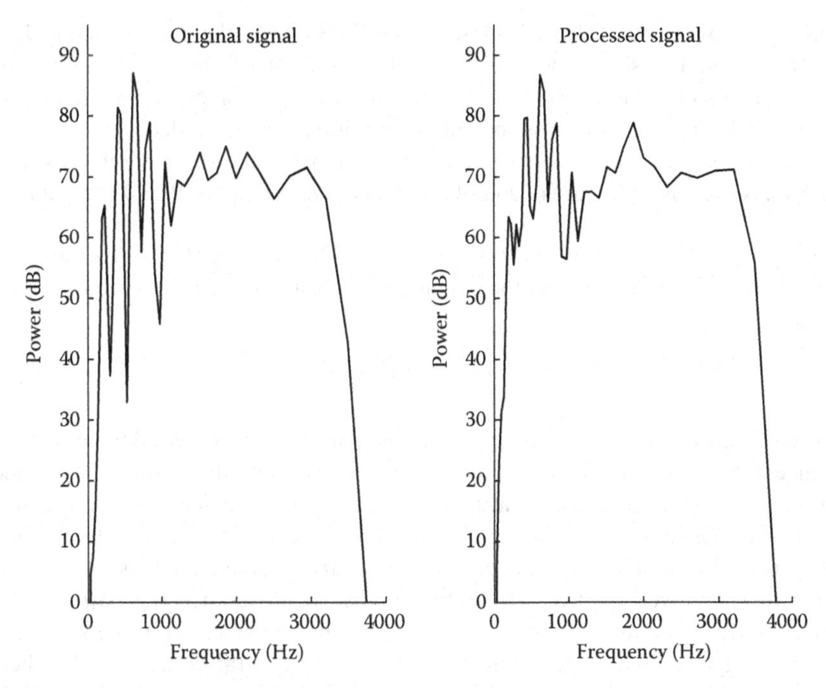

FIGURE 11.10 Modified Bark spectra after gain compensation.

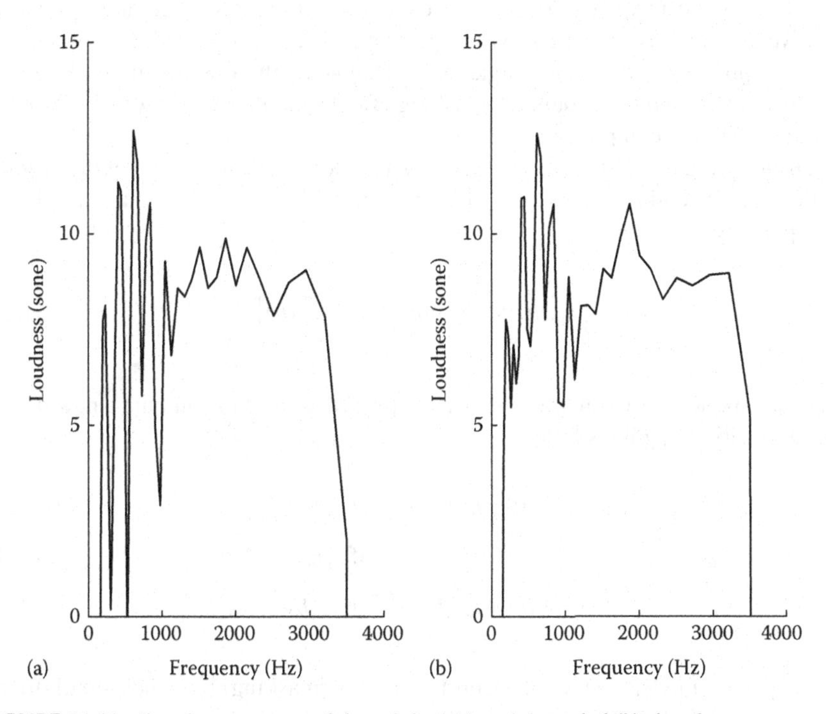

FIGURE 11.11 Loudness spectra of the original (a) and degraded (b) signals.

is evident from Figure 11.7. Likewise Figure 11.8 shows the corresponding Bark spectra, Figure 11.9 shows the modified Bark spectra after frequency compensation, Figure 11.10 shows the modified Bark spectra after gain compensation, and finally Figure 11.11 shows the loudness spectra of the original and degraded signals.

The absolute difference between the degraded, $\overline{S}(b)$, and original loudness spectra, $S(b)$, is used as a measure of audible error in the next stage of PESQ computation.

11.1.3.3.4 Disturbance Computation and Averaging Over Time and Frequency

The signed difference between the enhanced and original loudness spectra is computed as

$$r_n(b) = S_n(b) - \overline{S}_n(b) \tag{11.26}$$

where the subscript n indicates time (i.e., the frame number). We denote this difference array $\{r_n(b)\}$ as the raw disturbance density. Note that unlike most objective measures (e.g., the BSD measure), which treat positive and negative loudness differences the same (by squaring the difference), the PESQ measure treats these differences differently. This is because positive and negative loudness differences affect the perceived quality differently. A positive difference (i.e., $S(b) > \overline{S}(b)$) would indicate that a component, such as noise, has been added to the spectrum, while a negative difference would indicate that a spectral component has been omitted or heavily attenuated. Compared to additive components, the omitted components are not as easily perceived due to masking effects, leading to a less objectionable form of distortion. Consequently, different weights are applied to positive and negative differences. In addition to accounting for the asymmetrical effect of positive and negative loudness differences, the raw disturbance density $\{r_n(b)\}$ is processed to account for masking effects and non-linear weighting of the frequency (Bark) components.

The masking effect is taken into account as follows. The minimum of the original and enhanced loudness spectra is first computed for each time-frequency cell and multiplied by 0.25, that is,

$$m_n(b) = 0.25 \min\left\{S_n(b), \overline{S}_n(b)\right\} \tag{11.27}$$

The corresponding two-dimensional array, $\{m_n(b)\}$ is used to compute a new disturbance density, $\{D_n(b)\}$, as follows:

$$D_n(b) = \begin{cases} r_n(b) - m_n(b) & \text{if } r_n(b) > m_n(b) \\ 0 & \text{if } |r_n(b)| \le m_n(b) \\ r_n(b) + m_n(b) & \text{if } r_n(b) < -m_n(b) \end{cases} \tag{11.28}$$

This equation models the psychoacoustic process (masking) by which small differences are inaudible in the presence of loud signals.

The asymmetrical effect of positive and negative differences is modeled by multiplying the disturbance density $\{D_n(b)\}$ in (11.28) by an asymmetry factor $AF_n(b)$, which is estimated as follows:

$$AF_n(b) = \begin{cases} 0 & \text{if } \left\{[\bar{B}_n(b)+c]/[B_n(b)+c]\right\}^{1.2} < 3 \\ 12 & \text{if } \left\{[\bar{B}_n(b)+c]/[B_n(b)+c]\right\}^{1.2} > 12 \\ \left(\dfrac{\bar{B}_n(b)+c}{B_n(b)+c}\right)^{1.2} & \text{else} \end{cases} \quad (11.29)$$

where $B_n(b)$ and $\bar{B}_n(b)$ denote the Bark spectra of the input and processed signals respectively, and the constant c is set to $c = 50$. The aforementioned factor is then used to compute an asymmetrical disturbance density as follows:

$$DA_n(b) = AF_n(b) \cdot D_n(b) \qquad 1 \le b \le 42 \quad (11.30)$$

where $DA_n(b)$ denotes the asymmetrical disturbance density. Figure 11.12 shows the estimated frame disturbances, $D_n(b)$ and $DA_n(b)$, for the example signals shown in

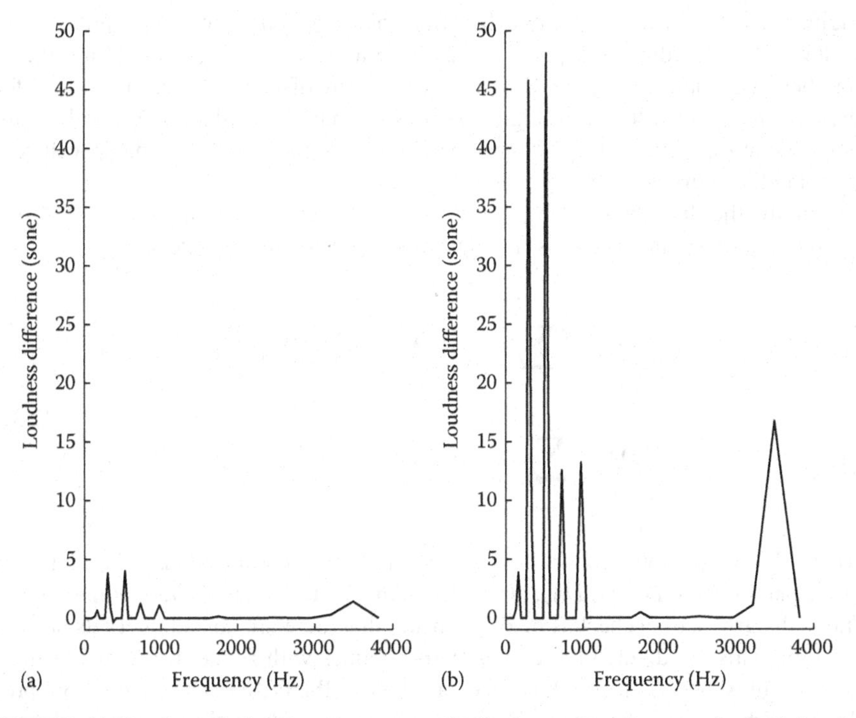

FIGURE 11.12 Symmetric (a) and asymmetric (b) frame disturbances obtained for the loudness spectra shown in Figure 11.11.

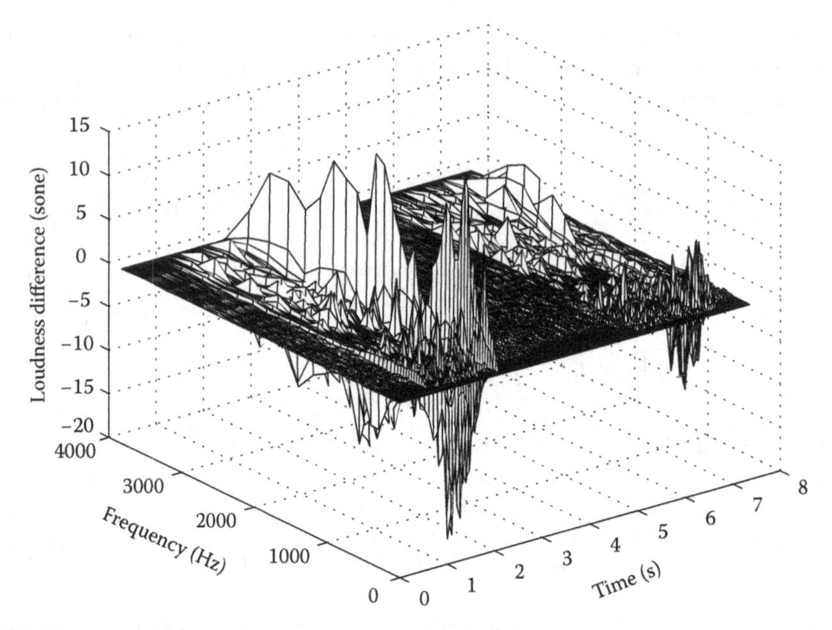

FIGURE 11.13 Disturbance density $\{D_n(b)\}$ for the pair of signals in Figure 11.6.

Figure 11.6. Note that $DA_n(b)$ has the same shape as $D_n(b)$, but it is amplified by a factor of 12 according to Equation 11.29. The asymmetric disturbances are therefore heavily penalized. Figure 11.13 shows the entire disturbance density $\{D_n(b)\}$ for the example signals shown in Figure 11.6. Note that largest disturbance values are observed at the period of 2–3 s as we would expect due to the missing speech segments in the degraded signal at that time period.

Finally, the disturbance density $\{D_n(b)\}$ and the asymmetrical density $\{DA_n(b)\}$ are integrated (summed) across frequency using two different norms:

$$D_n = \left(\sum_{b=1}^{N_b} W_b\right)^{1/2} \left(\sum_{b=1}^{N_b} [\mid D_n(b) \mid W_b]^2\right)^{1/2}$$

$$DA_n = \sum_{b=1}^{N_b} \mid DA_n(b) \mid W_b \tag{11.31}$$

where W_b are weights proportional to the width of the Bark bands. The aforesaid aggregated values, D_n and DA_n, are called frame disturbances. After computing the frame disturbances, a check is made to ensure that there are no bad intervals present (bad intervals are defined to be consecutive frames with frame disturbance values above a threshold). This check is necessary so that the PESQ measure does not predict large distortions over a small number of bad frames due to incorrect time delays. New delay values are estimated for the identified bad frames and the corresponding frame disturbances are recomputed. The recomputed frame disturbance values, denoted as D''_n and DA''_n, replace the original frame disturbances if they are found to be smaller. These frame disturbance values are scaled by the frame "audible power" (raised to the power 0.04) of the input signal and limited to a maximum of 45.

In the final stage of the PESQ measure computation, the frame disturbance values are averaged over time based on two different duration intervals and different norms. First, the frame disturbances are averaged over intervals of 20 frames (320 ms), with 50% overlap and no windowing. The averaged disturbance value for the kth 320 ms interval is computed as follows:

$$D''_k = \left(\frac{1}{20} \sum_{n=(k-1)20}^{20k-1} \left(D''_n\right)^6 \right)^{1/6}$$
$$DA''_k = \left(\frac{1}{20} \sum_{n=(k-1)20}^{20k-1} \left(DA''_n\right)^6 \right)^{1/6} \tag{11.32}$$

where the summation over n spans 320 ms. Next, the aforementioned disturbance values are averaged now over the speech-active portion of the signal using a 2-norm as follows:

$$d_{sym} = \left(\frac{\sum_k \left(D'''_k t_k\right)^2}{\sum_k (t_k)^2} \right)^{1/2}$$
$$d_{asym} = \left(\frac{\sum_k \left(DA'''_k t_k\right)^2}{\sum_k (t_k)^2} \right)^{1/2} \tag{11.33}$$

where the summation over k is performed over the speech-active intervals, and t_k are weights applied to the frame disturbances and depend on the length of the signal. For short duration signals containing less than 1000 frames, $t_k = 1$. Reduced emphasis is placed on the onset of the signal if the total duration of the signal is over 16 s, modeling the effect of short-term memory in subjective listening [38]. Note that a higher norm is used in (11.32) for averaging over 320 ms segments to give largest weight to localized distortions [39].

The final PESQ score is computed as a linear combination of the average disturbance value d_{sym} and the average asymmetrical disturbance value d_{asym} as follows:

$$PESQ = 4.5 - 0.1 \cdot d_{sym} - 0.0309 \cdot d_{asym} \tag{11.34}$$

The range of the PESQ score is −0.5 to 4.5, although for most cases the output range will be a MOS-like score, i.e., a score between 1.0 and 4.5.

High correlations (ρ > 0.92) with subjective listening tests were reported in [34] using the aforesaid PESQ measure for a large number of testing conditions taken from mobile, fixed and voice over IP (VoiIP) applications. The PESQ can be used reliably to predict the subjective speech quality of codecs (waveform and CELP-type coders) in situations where there are transmission channel errors, packet loss or varying delays in the signal. It should be noted that the PESQ measure does not provide a comprehensive evaluation of telephone transmission quality, as it only reflects the effects of one-way speech or noise distortion perceived by the end-user. Effects such as loudness loss, sidetone, and talker echo are not reflected in the PESQ scores.

11.1.4 Wideband PESQ

A number of changes were made to PESQ (ITU-T P.862) to accommodate binaural or monaural wideband headphone presentation with a frequency response that is either flat or equalized to be flat (as opposed to using a telephone handset). The recommendations for wideband extension to PESQ were documented in ITU P.862.2 [40] and included two small changes to the PESQ implementation. First, the IRS filter used originally for modeling the response of telephone headsets was removed. Instead, an infinite impulse response (IIR) filter with a flat response above 100 Hz was used. Second, the PESQ raw output values were mapped using a logistic-type function to better fit the subjective mean opinion score (MOS)

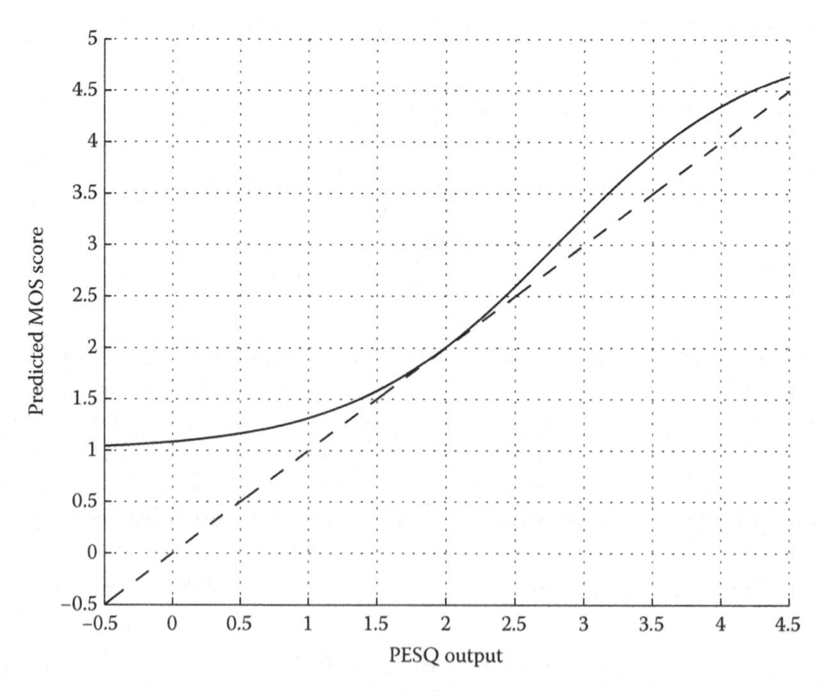

FIGURE 11.14 Output mapping functions to MOS scores as used for the narrowband PESQ (dashed lines) and wideband PESQ (solid lines) implementations.

scores (see Figure 11.14). As mentioned in the previous section, the basic ITU P.862 model provides raw scores in the range −0.5 to 4.5. The wideband extension to ITU-T P.862 includes a mapping function that allows linear comparisons with MOS values produced from subjective experiments that include wideband speech conditions with an audio bandwidth of 50–7000 Hz. The output mapping function used in the wideband extension had the following form:

$$y = 0.999 + \frac{4.999 - 0.999}{1 + e^{-1.3669 \cdot x + 3.8224}} \tag{11.35}$$

where x is the raw PESQ output (ITU P.862). The mapping function was derived from data from a number of subjective listening experiments involving some wideband speech conditions as well as a mixture of narrow-band, wideband, and intermediate bandwidth speech. The difference in output mapping functions between the original PESQ (ITU P.862) and the wideband PESQ (ITU P.862.2) is illustrated in Figure 11.14. Raw PESQ values smaller than 1 are now mapped to values close to 1, a step found necessary since the subject's MOS scores are never smaller than 1.

The aforementioned mapping function was designed and tested with wideband speech. A different mapping function was developed for transforming the raw PESQ scores (ITU P.862) of narrowband speech to MOS scores, and this was documented in ITU P.862.1 [41]. The output mapping function used for narrowband speech had the following form:

$$y = 0.999 + \frac{4.999 - 0.999}{1 + e^{-1.4945 \cdot x + 4.6607}} \tag{11.36}$$

where x is the raw PESQ output (ITU P.862). The aforementioned function was evaluated, in terms of correlation, using speech material from nine languages (including Japanese) processed in a large number of conditions that included voice over internet protocol (VoIP) and wireless applications. The resulting correlation with human subjective quality ratings was found to be slightly higher than when using the raw PESQ scores [41].

11.1.5 Composite Measures

In addition to the aforementioned measures, one can form the so-called *composite measures* [1, Chapter 9] by combining multiple objective measures. The rationale behind the use of composite measures is that different objective measures capture different characteristics of the distorted signal, and therefore combining them in a linear or non-linear fashion can potentially yield significant gains in correlations. Regression analysis can be used to compute the optimum combination of objective measures for maximum correlation. One possibility is to use the following linear regression model:

$$
\begin{aligned}
y_i &= f(\mathbf{x}) + \varepsilon_i \\
&= \alpha_0 + \sum_{j=1}^{P} \alpha_j x_{ij} + \varepsilon_i
\end{aligned} \tag{11.37}
$$

where

$f(\mathbf{x})$ is the mapping function presumed to be linear
P is the number of objective measures involved
$\{y_i\}_{i=1}^{N}$ are the dependent variables corresponding to the subjective ratings of N samples of degraded speech
x_{ij} is the independent (predictor) variable corresponding to the jth objective measure computed for the ith observation (degraded file)
ε_i is a random error associated with each observation

The regression coefficients α_i can be estimated to provide the best fit with the data using a least-squares approach [1, p. 184]. The P objective measures considered in (11.37) may include, among other measures, the LPC-based measures (e.g., IS, LLR), segmental SNR measures (e.g., SNRseg) or the PESQ measure. The selection of objective measures to include in the composite measure is not straightforward and in some cases it is based solely on experimental evidence (trial and error) and intuition. Ideally, we would like to include objective measures that capture complementary information about the underlying distortions present in the degraded signal.

The frequency-variant fwSNRseg measure described earlier (see Equation 11.5) is a composite measure obtained by linearly combining K frequency-domain segmental SNRs (Equation 11.4). Note that in the computation of the frequency-variant fwSNRseg measure, $P = K$ in (11.37) corresponding to the segmental SNR values in the K frequency bands. The composite measures were found in [1, ch. 9] and [42] to yield the highest correlations with subjective quality. High correlations ($\rho = 0.82 - 0.84$) were obtained in [1, ch. 9] with composite measures composed of 21–35 variables.

A linear function $f(\mathbf{x})$ was assumed in (11.37) for mapping P objective measures to the observed subjective ratings, $\{y_i\}_{i=1}^{N}$. Such a model is accurate only when the true form of the underlying function is linear. If it is not, then the modeling error will likely be large and the fit will be poor. Non-parametric models which make no assumptions about the form of the mapping function can alternatively be used. More specifically, models based on multivariate adaptive regression splines (MARS) have been found to yield better performance for arbitrary data sets [43]. Unlike linear and polynomial regression analysis, the MARS modeling technique is data driven and derives the functional form from the data. The basic idea of the MARS modeling technique is to recursively partition the domain into smaller sub-regions and use spline functions to locally fit the data in each region. The number of splines used in each sub-region is automatically determined from the data. The MARS model has the following form:

$$y_i = \alpha_0 + \sum_{j=1}^{M} \alpha_j B_j(\mathbf{x}) + \varepsilon_i \tag{11.38}$$

where $B_j(\mathbf{x})$ are the basis functions and M is the number of basis functions which are automatically determined from the data (note that M could be larger than the number of objective measures, $\boldsymbol{P}$). Spline basis functions of the following form were proposed in [43]:

$$B_j(\mathbf{x}) = \prod_{k=1}^{K_j} s_{kj} \cdot \max(0, x_{kj} - t_{kj}) \tag{11.39}$$

where

x_{kj} are the predictor variables (values of the objective measures)

t_{kj} are the split points (knots) determined from a recursive algorithm that partitions the domain into smaller sub-regions

K_j is the number of splits involved in the computation of the jth basis function and $s_{kj} = \pm 1$

One of the most powerful features of the MARS modeling is that it allows for possible interactions between the predictor (independent) variables so that a better fit can be found for the target (dependent) variable. Composite measures derived from the aforementioned MARS regression model are evaluated (see Section 11.2) with subjective ratings of enhanced speech.

In addition to the measures described so far, several other distortion measures have been proposed in the literature for speech recognition and speech coding applications. The interested reader can find more information about these measures in [5,44,45].

11.1.6 Non-Intrusive Objective Quality Measures

The aforementioned objective measures for evaluating speech quality are "intrusive" in nature as they require access to the input (clean) signal. These measures predict speech quality by estimating the "distortion" between the input (clean) and output (processed) signals and then mapping the estimated "distortion" value to a quality metric. In some applications, however, the input (clean) signal is not readily available and therefore the said objective measures are not practical or useful. In VoIP applications, for instance, where we are interested in monitoring continuously the performance of telecommunication networks (in terms of speech quality), we only have access to the output signal. In such cases, a non-intrusive objective measure of speech quality would be highly desirable for continuous monitoring of quality of speech delivered to a customer or a particular point in the network. Based on such quality assessment, network traffic can be routed, for instance, through less congested parts of the network and therefore improve the quality of service.

A fundamentally different approach is required to analyze a processed signal when the clean (reference) input signal is not available, and several *non-intrusive* measures have been proposed in the literature [46–51]. Some methods are based on comparing the output signal to an artificial reference signal derived from an appropriate codebook [49,50]. Other methods use vocal-tract models to identify distortions [47]. This latter method [47] first extracts a set of vocal-tract shape parameters (e.g., area functions, cavity size) from the signal, and then evaluates these parameters for physical production violations, i.e., whether the parameters could have been generated by the human speech-production system. Distortions are identified when the vocal-tract parameters yield implausible shape and cavity sizes. A variant of the vocal-tract method was adopted as the ITU-T P.563 [52] standard for non-intrusive evaluation of speech quality. More information on non-intrusive methods can be found in [46,53].

11.1.7 Figures of Merit of Objective Measures

So far we described numerous objective measures, but have not yet discussed what makes a certain objective measure better than other. Some objective measures are "optimized" for a particular type of distortion and may not be meaningful for another type of distortion. The task of evaluating the validity of objective measures over a wide range of distortions is immense [1]. A suggested process to follow is to create a large database of speech distorted in various ways and evaluate the objective measure for each file in the database and for each type of distortion [1, ch. 1]. At the same time, the distorted database needs to be evaluated by human listeners using one of the subjective listening tests (e.g., MOS test) described earlier. Statistical analysis needs to be used to assess the correlation between subjective scores and the values of the objective measures. For the objective measure to be valid and useful, it needs to correlate well with subjective listening tests.

The correlation between subjective listening scores and objective measures can be obtained using Pearson's correlation coefficient (see Equation 10.17). This correlation coefficient ρ can be used to predict the subjective results based on the values of the objective measures as follows:

$$P_k = \bar{P} + \rho \frac{\sigma_P}{\sigma_O}(O_k - \bar{O}) \tag{11.40}$$

where

O_k denotes the value of the objective measure obtained for the kth speech file in the database

P_k denotes the predicted subjective listening score

σ_P and σ_O denote the standard deviations of the subjective and objective scores respectively

$\bar{P}$ and $\bar{O}$ denote the mean values of the subjective and objective scores respectively

Note that Equation 11.40 is based on first-order linear regression analysis assuming a single objective measurement. Higher order polynomial regression analysis could also be used if the objective measure is composed of multiple measurements [1, ch. 4.5].

A second figure-of-merit is an estimate of the standard deviation of the error obtained by using the objective measures to predict the subjective listening scores. This figure-of-merit is computed as

$$\sigma_e = \sigma_P \sqrt{1-\rho^2} \tag{11.41}$$

where σ_e is the *standard error of the estimate.* The standard error of the estimate of the subjective scores provides a measure of variability of the subjective scores about the regression line, averaged over all objective scores. For good predictability of the subjective scores, we would like the objective measure to yield a small value of σ_e. Both figures of merit, i.e., correlation coefficient and standard error of the estimate σ_e, need to be reported when evaluating objective measures.

An alternative figure-of-merit to σ_e is the root-mean-square error (RMSE) between the per-condition averaged objective measure and subjective ratings computed over all conditions:

$$RMSE = \sqrt{\frac{\sum_{i=1}^{M} (\bar{S}_i - \bar{O}_i)^2}{M}} \tag{11.42}$$

where

$\bar{S}_i$ indicates the averaged subjective score in the ith condition
$\bar{O}_i$ indicates the averaged objective score in the ith condition
M is the total number of conditions

Figure 11.15 shows two hypothetical examples obtained by two different objective measures. The estimated correlation coefficients and error estimate for the example shown in Figure 11.15a are $\rho = -0.76$ and $\sigma_e = 0.5$ respectively, and for the example in Figure 11.15b are $\rho = -0.94$ and $\sigma_e = 0.23$. Clearly, for this example, the second objective measure is a better predictor of the speech quality. Note that estimated correlation coefficients are negative since large distortion values suggest poor quality, i.e., low MOS scores.

As shown in Figure 11.14, the experimental data (objective scores) are fitted with a straight line to the subjective scores. Hence, the aforementioned analysis assumes that the objective and subjective scores are *linearly* related (see Equation 11.40). This is not always the case, however, and in practice, it is not easy to uncover the best-fitting function or the true relationship between the objective and subjective measurements. Some found a better fit with a quadratic relationship [10,17] while others found a good fit with a logistic function [39]. Kitawaki et al. [17], for instance,

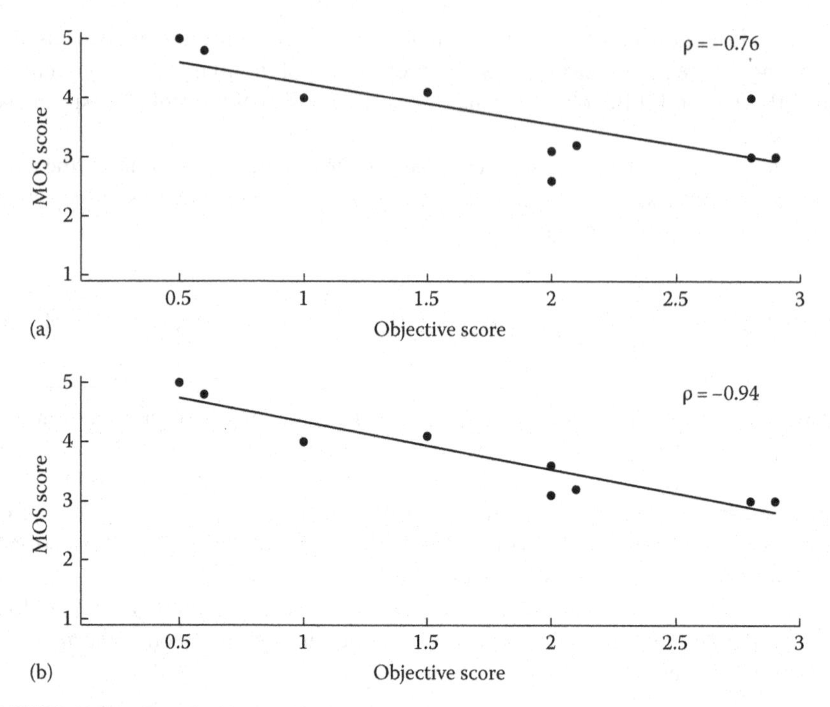

FIGURE 11.15 Panels (a) and (b) show two hypothetical scatter plots of objective measure values and MOS scores. The regression (best fit) line is shown with the corresponding correlation coefficients.

derived the following quadratic expression for predicting MOS scores from cepstral distance measures for Japanese speech:

$$\text{MOS} = 0.04(d_{cep})^2 - 0.8 \cdot d_{cep} + 3.56 \tag{11.43}$$

where d_{CD} denotes the cepstral distortion distance (see Equation 11.13). Nonparametric regression techniques, such as the MARS technique described in Section 11.1, can alternatively be used to uncover the mapping function between (multiple) objective measures and subjective ratings.

A large number of studies [1, ch. 1, 5, 54–56] reported correlations of objective measures with subjective listening tests. The majority of these studies, however, estimated these correlations based on subjective evaluations of degraded speech containing distortions produced by speech coders and not distortions produced by noise suppression algorithms. Next, we report in more detail on the evaluation of objective quality measures for speech processed by noise suppression algorithms [42,57].

11.2 EVALUATION OF OBJECTIVE QUALITY MEASURES

Although a large number of objective speech quality measures have been proposed in the past [1] to predict the subjective quality of speech, the majority of those measures were developed for the purpose of evaluating the distortions introduced by speech coders and/or communication channels [58]. Only a few, if any, of these measures have been formally evaluated with speech enhanced by noise suppression algorithms. Next, we make use of the subjective test results collected in [59] (and discussed in more detail in Chapter 12) to evaluate the correlation of several widely used objective measures [42,57]. The objective measures considered a wide range of distortions introduced by four types of real-world noise at two SNR levels by 13 speech enhancement algorithms encompassing four classes of speech enhancement algorithms: spectral-subtractive, subspace, statistical-model based, and Wiener algorithms. The subjective quality ratings were obtained using the ITU-T P.835 methodology designed to evaluate the quality of enhanced speech along three dimensions: signal distortion (SIG), noise distortion (BAK), and overall quality (OVL).

Several widely used objective speech quality measures were evaluated: the segmental SNR (segSNR) measure, the weighted spectral slope (WSS) distance [15], the perceptual evaluation of speech quality (PESQ) measure [34], the log likelihood ratio (LLR) measure, the Itakura–Saito (IS), the cepstrum distance (CEP) measure [1], the frequency-weighted segmental SNR [13], and the frequency-variant spectral distance measures [1, p. 241]. Composite measures, combining a subset of the aforesaid measures, as well as modifications to the PESQ and WSS measures were also evaluated.

The LLR and IS measures were computed using Equations 10.26 and 10.29, respectively [1]. The IS values were limited to the range of [0, 100]. This was necessary in order to limit the number of outliers, known to influence linear regression analysis. For the same reason, the LLR values were limited to the range of [0, 2]. The segSNR measure was computed as per [8]. Only frames with segmental SNR in the range of [−10 dB, 35 dB] were considered in the average. The CEP was computed using Equation 10.32 and was limited in the range of [0, 10]. To further minimize the number of outliers, only 95% of the frames with the lowest distance were considered in the computation of the average of the LLR, IS, and CEP measures.

The frequency-weighted segmental SNR (fwSNRseg) was computed as per Equation 10.22 using different weighting functions and different numbers of frequency bands ($K = 25$ and $K = 13$). The following form of the fwSNRseg measure was considered:

$$\text{fwSNRseg} = \frac{10}{M}\sum_{m=0}^{M-1}\frac{\sum_{j=1}^{K} W(j,m)\log_{10}\dfrac{|X(j,m)|^2}{\left(|X(j,m)|-|\hat{X}(j,m)|\right)^2}}{\sum_{j=1}^{K} W(j,m)} \tag{11.44}$$

where

$W(j, m)$ is the weight placed on the jth frequency band
K is the number of bands
M is the total number of frames in the signal
$|X(j, m)|$ is the filter-bank magnitude of the clean signal in the jth frequency band at the mth frame
$|\hat{X}(j, m)|$ is the filter-bank magnitude of the enhanced signal in the same band

The computed SNR of the jth frequency band in (11.44) was limited in the range of [−10 dB, 35 dB].

Two types of weighting functions, $W(j, m)$, were considered in (11.44). The first weighting function was the spectrum of the clean signal in each band raised to a power, that is,

$$W(j,m) = |X(j,m)|^{\gamma} \tag{11.45}$$

where $|X(j, m)|$ is the filter-bank magnitude of the clean signal in the jth band at frame m and γ is the power exponent, which can be varied for maximum correlation. In our experiments, we varied γ from 0.1 to 2 and obtained maximum correlation with $\gamma = 0.2$. The second weighting function considered were the AI weights given in Table 11.1, i.e.,

$$W(j,m) = A(j) \tag{11.46}$$

where $A(j)$ is the articulation index weight of the jth band. Note that these weights, unlike those given in (11.45), remain fixed for all frames.

The filter-bank spectra in (11.44) were obtained as follows. The signal bandwidth was first divided into K frequency bands ($K = 25$ or $K = 13$) spaced in proportion to the ear's critical bands (see Table 11.1). The 13 bands were formed by merging adjacent critical bands. The filter-bank spectra, $|X(j, m)|$, used in (11.44) and (11.45) were computed after multiplying the FFT magnitude spectra by the Gaussian-shaped windows shown in Figure 11.16, and summing up the weighted spectra within

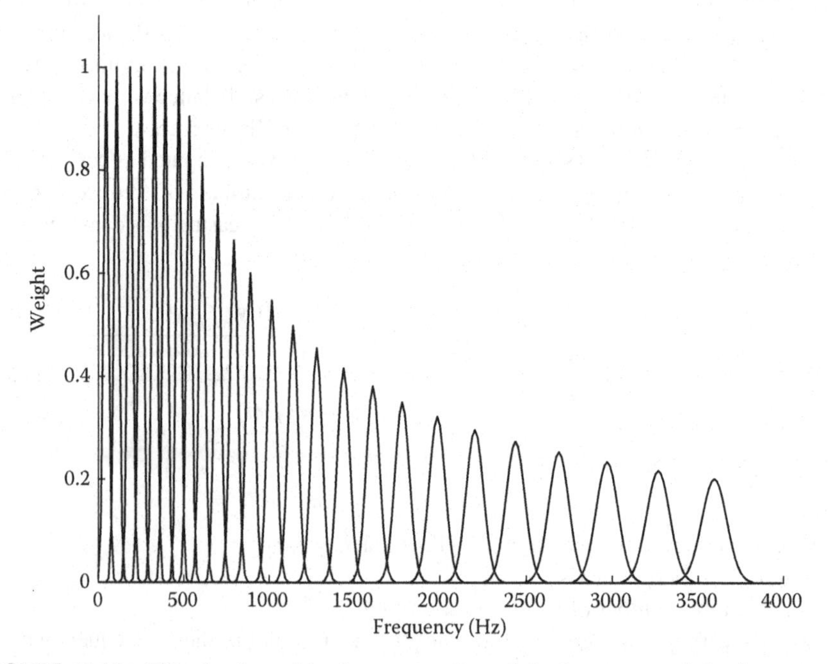

FIGURE 11.16 Filter bank used in the computation of the frequency-weighted segmental SNR measure (fwSNRseg).

each band. Prior to the distance computation in (11.44) and multiplication by the Gaussian-shaped windows, the clean and enhanced FFT magnitude spectra were normalized to have an area equal to 1. In addition to using $K = 25$ and $K = 13$ bands in the computation of the fwSNRseg measure, we also considered using $K = 256$, i.e., half the size of the FFT length, for comparative purposes. In this case, the FFT magnitude spectra were not multiplied by Gaussian-shaped windows (Figure 11.16).

The WSS measure [15] was also considered:

$$d_{WSS} = \frac{1}{M} \sum_{m=0}^{M-1} \frac{\sum_{j=1}^{K-1} W(j,m)\left[S(j,m) - \hat{S}(j,m)\right]^2}{\sum_{j=1}^{K-1} W(j,m)} \tag{11.47}$$

where $W(j, m)$ are the weights computed as per Equation 10.34 [15], $K = 25$, and $S(j, m)$, $\hat{S}(j, m)$ are the spectral slopes of the jth frequency band at frame m of the clean and enhanced speech signals, respectively.

A modified version of the PESQ measure was also considered. As described in Section 11.1.3.3, the final PESQ score is obtained by linear combining the average disturbance value D_{ind} with the average asymmetrical disturbance values A_{ind} as follows [35]:

$$PESQ = a_0 - a_1 D_{ind} - a_2 A_{ind} \tag{11.48}$$

where $a_0 = 4.5$, $a_1 = 0.1$, and $a_2 = 0.0309$. The parameters a_0, a_1, and a_2 in Equation (11.48) were optimized for speech processed through networks and not for speech enhanced by noise suppression algorithms. As we cannot expect the PESQ measure to correlate highly with all three quality rating scales (speech distortion, noise distortion, and overall quality), we considered optimizing the PESQ measure for each of the three rating scales by choosing a different set of parameters (a_0, a_1, a_2) for each scale. The modified PESQ measures were obtained by treating a_0, a_1, and a_2 in Equation 11.48 as the parameters that need to be optimized for each of the three rating scales: speech distortion, noise distortion, and overall quality. Multiple linear regression analysis was used to determine the values of the a_0, a_1, and a_2 parameters. The values of D_{ind} and A_{ind} in Equation 11.48 were treated as independent variables in the regression analysis. The actual subjective scores for the three scales were used in the regression analysis. This analysis yielded the following three different measures for signal distortion ($PESQ_S$), noise distortion ($PESQ_N$), and overall speech quality ($PESQ_O$):

$$\begin{aligned} PESQ_S &= 5.736 \;\; -0.250 \;\; D_{ind} + 0.003 A_{ind} \\ PESQ_N &= 5.758 \;\; -0.121 \;\; D_{ind} - 0.057 A_{ind} \\ PESQ_O &= 5.413 \;\; -0.205 \;\; D_{ind} - 0.016 A_{ind} \end{aligned} \tag{11.49}$$

We refer to modified PESQ measures as mPESQ measures.

Aiming to improve further the correlation coefficients, composite measures based on linear and non-linear (non-parametric) regression analysis were considered. Composite objective measures can be obtained by linearly combining existing objective measures to form a new measure [1] (see Section 11.1.5). The weights applied to each objective measure can be obtained optimally by utilizing linear and non-linear (non-parametric) regression analysis techniques such as MARS [43], or by using other non-linear techniques (e.g., [60]). Multiple linear regression analysis was used to derive three composite measures, one for each quality rating scale. The derived composite measures for signal distortion (C_S), noise distortion (C_N), and overall quality (C_O) were as follows:

$$\begin{aligned} C_S &= -0.261 + 1.562 \cdot IS - 0.02 \cdot PESQ \\ C_N &= 1.893 + 0.007 \cdot IS + 0.8 \cdot PESQ - 0.468 \cdot CEP \\ &\quad + 0.291 \cdot LLR - 0.008 \cdot WSS \\ C_O &= -0.736 - 0.012 \cdot IS + 1.50 \cdot PESQ \end{aligned} \tag{11.50}$$

The said regression coefficients were computed following cross-validation of the data [57]. Only 50% of the data were used to derive the aforesaid regression coefficients, with the remaining data used to evaluate the prediction power of the composite measures.

Aside from the PESQ measures, all other measures were computed by segmenting the sentences using 30 ms duration Hanning windows with 75% overlap between adjacent frames. A tenth-order LPC analysis was used in the computation of the LPC-based objective measures (CEP, IS, LLR). MATLAB® implementations of the aforementioned objective measures are provided in the accompanying DVD-ROM of this book (see Appendix C).

Correlations were run between the aforesaid objective measures and each of the three subjective rating scores (SIG, BAK, OVL) [57]. A total of 1792 processed speech samples were included in the correlations encompassing two SNR levels, four different types of background noise and speech/noise distortions introduced by 13 different speech enhancement algorithms. Ratings collected for each scale were averaged across subjects. Similarly, the objective scores were averaged across all sentences involved in each condition. Correlation analysis involved the use of mean objective scores and ratings computed across a total of 112 conditions (14 algorithms × SNR levels × noise types).

11.2.1 Correlations of Objective Measures with Quality and Signal/Background Distortions

Pearson's correlation coefficients (Pearson's correlation—see Equation 10.17) and standard deviation of the error, $\hat{\sigma}_e$ (see Equation 10.50) were used to assess the prediction power of the objective measures. The correlation coefficients obtained

TABLE 11.2
Correlation Coefficients, $|\rho|$, of Objective Measures with Overall Quality, Signal Distortion, and Background Noise Distortion

Objective Measure	Overall Quality	Signal Distortion	Background Distortion
SegSNR	0.36	0.22	0.56
Weighted spectral slope (WSS)	0.64	0.59	0.62
PESQ	0.89	0.81	0.76
Log-likelihood ratio (LLR)	0.85	0.88	0.51
Itakura–Saito distance (IS)	0.60	0.73	0.09
Cepstrum distance (CEP)	0.79	0.84	0.41
fwSNRseg (K = 13 bands)	0.85	0.87	0.59
fwSNRseg (K = 25 bands)	0.84	0.84	0.62
Modified PESQ (Equation 11.49)	0.92	0.89	0.76
Composite measure (Equation 11.50)	0.91	0.89	0.82

with each of the three subjective rating scales (SIG, BAK, OVL) were computed and tabulated separately (Table 11.2). Table 11.2 shows the resulting correlation coefficients (values of the prediction error $\hat{\sigma}_e$ can be found in [57]).

From Table 11.2, we can see that of the seven basic objective measures tested, the PESQ measure yielded the highest correlation ($r = 0.89$) with overall quality, followed by the fwSNRseg measure ($r = 0.85$) and the LLR measure ($r = 0.85$). Compared to the PESQ measure, the LLR and fwSNRseg measures are computationally simpler to implement, and yield approximately the same correlation coefficient. The lowest correlation ($r = 0.36$) was obtained with the SNRseg measure. The correlations with signal distortion were of the same magnitude as those of overall quality. This suggests that the same basic objective measure predicts equally well signal distortion and overall quality. This finding is consistent with a previous finding [59] suggesting that listeners are more sensitive to signal distortion than background distortion when making judgments on overall quality. The correlations, however, with noise distortion were generally poorer suggesting that the basic objective measures are inadequate in predicting background distortion. Note that measures that predict musical-noise type of distortion were proposed in [61], but have not been validated or evaluated with other types of background distortion, such as those encountered in [57]. A significant improvement in correlation with background distortion was obtained in [57] with the use of composite measures (see Equation 11.50). Significant improvements were also obtained in correlations with overall quality and signal distortion. Highest correlation ($r = 0.92$) with overall quality was obtained with the modified PESQ measure ($PESQ_O$, Equation 11.49), and highest correlation ($r = 0.82$) with background distortion was obtained with the composite measure C_N (see Equation 11.50).

11.2.2 Summary of Findings

Based on the correlation analysis reported earlier, we can draw the following conclusions:

1. Of the seven basic objective measures tested, the PESQ measure yielded the highest correlation ($r = 0.89$) with overall quality and signal distortion. The LLR and fwSNRseg measures performed nearly as well at a fraction of the computational cost.
2. The segSNR measure, which is widely used for evaluating the performance (quality) of speech enhancement algorithms, yielded the lowest correlation coefficient ($r = 0.36$) with overall quality. This makes the segSNR measure highly unsuitable for evaluating the quality of speech processed via enhancement algorithms.
3. The majority of the basic objective measures predict equally well signal distortion and overall quality, but not background distortion. This was not surprising given that most measures take into account both speech-active and speech-absent segments in their computation. Measures that would place more emphasis on the speech-absent segments would be more appropriate and likely more successful in predicting noise distortion (BAK).

11.3 QUALITY MEASURES: SUMMARY OF FINDINGS AND FUTURE DIRECTIONS

Presently, there is no single objective measure that correlates well with subjective listening evaluations for a wide range of speech distortions. Most measures have been validated for a specific type of distortion. Some measures correlate well with distortions introduced by speech coders while others (e.g., PESQ measure) correlate well with distortions introduced by telecommunication networks. Of all the measures examined and evaluated, the PESQ measure is currently the most reliable measure for assessment of overall quality of speech processed by noise-reduction algorithms. The PESQ measure, however, fails to predict reliably the effects of noise distortion (see Table 11.2). Further research is warranted to design measures that can predict noise distortion effects.

Ideally, the objective quality measure should predict the quality of speech independent of the type of distortions introduced by the system whether be a network, a speech coder or a speech enhancement algorithm. This is extremely challenging and would require a deeper understanding of the human perceptual processes involved in quality assessment. For one, little is known as to how we should best integrate or somehow combine the frame computed distance measures to a single global distortion value. The simplest approach used in most objective measures is to compute the arithmetic mean of the distortions computed in each frame, i.e.,

$$D = \frac{1}{M} \sum_{k=0}^{M-1} d(\mathbf{x}_k, \overline{\mathbf{x}}_k) \tag{11.51}$$

where

M is the total number of frames

D denotes the global (aggregate) distortion

$d(\mathbf{x}_k, \overline{\mathbf{x}}_k)$ denotes the distance between the clean and processed signals in the kth frame

This distance measure could take, for instance, the form of either (11.7), (11.10), or (11.20). The averaging in Equation 11.51 implicitly assumes that all frames (voiced, unvoiced, and silence) should be weighted equally, but this is not necessarily consistent with quality judgments. For one, the aforementioned averaging does not take into account temporal masking effects.

Alternatively, we can consider using a time-weighted averaging approach to estimate the global distortion, i.e.,

$$D_W = \frac{\sum_{k=0}^{M-1} w(k) d(\mathbf{x}_k, \overline{\mathbf{x}}_k)}{\sum_{k=0}^{M-1} w(k)} \tag{11.52}$$

where $w(k)$ represents the weighting applied to the kth frame. Computing the frame weights, $w(k)$, however, is not straightforward and no optimal methods (at least in the perceptual sense) exist to do that.

Accurate computation of $w(k)$ would require a deeper understanding of the factors influencing quality judgments at least at two conceptual levels: the supra segmental (spanning syllables or sentences) and the segmental (spanning a single phoneme) levels. At the supra segmental level we need to know how humans integrate information across time, considering at the very least temporal (non-simultaneous) masking effects such as forward and backward masking. Forward masking is an auditory phenomenon which occurs when large energy stimuli (maskers) precede in time, and suppress (i.e., mask) later arriving and lower energy stimuli from detection. In the context of speech enhancement, this means that the distortion introduced by the noise-reduction algorithm may be detectable beyond the time window in which the signal and distortion are simultaneously present. Masking may also occur before the masker onset and the corresponding effect is called backward masking [62, ch. 4]. Backward masking effects are relatively short (less than 20 ms), but forward masking effects can last longer than 100 ms [62, ch. 4.4] and its effects are more dominant. Attempts to model forward masking effects were reported in [1, p. 265, 18,28].

At the segmental (phoneme) level, we need to know which spectral characteristics (e.g., formants, spectral tilt, etc.) of the signal affect quality judgments the most. We know much about the effect of spectral manipulations on perceived vowel quality but comparatively little on consonant quality [15,26]. Klatt [15] demonstrated that of all spectral manipulations (e.g., low-pass filtering, notch filtering, spectral tilt) applied to vowels, the formant frequency changes had the largest effect on quality judgments. His findings, however, were only applicable to vowels and not necessarily to stop consonants or any other sound class. For one, Klatt concluded that spectral tilt is unimportant in vowel perception [15], but that is not the case however in stop-consonant perception. We know from the speech perception literature that spectral tilt is a major cue to stop place of articulation [63, ch. 6, 64]. The labial stops (/b, p/) are characterized by a positive (rising) spectral tilt, the alveolar stops (/d, t/) by a negative (falling) spectral tilt and the velar stops (/g, k/) by a compact (with a peak in mid-frequencies) spectrum. Some [64] explored the idea of constructing a spectral template that could be associated with each place of stop articulation, and used those templates to classify stops. In brief, the stop consonants, and possibly the other consonants, need to be treated differently than vowels, since different cues are used to perceive consonants.

There has been a limited number of proposals in the literature on how to estimate the weights $w(k)$ in (11.52) or how to best combine the local distortions to a single global distortion value [1, ch. 7, 18, 39, 65, 66]. Perhaps the most successful approach is to segment the utterance into low, mid and high-level segments according to their RMS level. Such an approach was used in coherence-based measures with great success (more on this in Section 11.4.3).

11.4 SPEECH INTELLIGIBILITY MEASURES

Most intelligibility measures are based on the assumption that intelligibility depends on the audibility of the signal in each frequency band. Audibility is often expressed in terms of SNR with bands having positive SNR more likely to contribute to intelligibility while bands with un-favorable SNR not contributing to intelligibility. Speech intelligibility is predicted based on a linear combination of band SNRs appropriately weighted by some functions, known as band-importance functions (BIFs). Thus, the majority of the intelligibility measures bear the following form:

$$SI = \sum_{k=1}^{K} W_k \cdot SNR_k \tag{11.53}$$

where

K is the number of bands (K is often equal to 20)

W_k denotes the BIF in band k $\left(\text{normalized such that } \sum_k W_k = 1\right)$

SI denotes the *objective* speech intelligibility (SI) value

A mapping (transfer) function is subsequently needed to transform the objective SI value into the predicted SI score. The computation of the SNR in each band differs across the various measures proposed and depends on the background (e.g., reverberation, additive noise) and type of processing (e.g., noise reduction, filtering, etc.) applied to the corrupted speech signal. Depending on the method used to compute the SNR, different intelligibility measures were developed, and these are described next.

11.4.1 Articulation Index

Much of the work done in the 1920s by Fletcher et al. at AT&T Bell Labs led to the development of the AI theory (see review in [67]). Of interest at the time was finding ways to quantify the transmission of information through telephone channels. Another important question was: What was the minimum bandwidth required to transmit speech over telephone while maintaining SI? The answer to this question required an extensive series of listening experiments wherein speech was low-pass or high-pass filtered at various cut-off frequencies and intelligibility scores were collected for each cut-off frequency. Acknowledging the influence of context on SI, all tests involved primarily non-sense syllables consisting of a mixture of CVCs, CVs, and VCs. To distinguish between recognition of meaningful sentences and recognition of vowels/consonants in non-sense syllables, the word *articulation* was used to indicate the latter. This term is rather misleading as it implies a speech production mechanism or task. Nonetheless, the term persisted till today. While the theoretical foundations were first laid out by Fletcher et al. in the 1920s, the AI index as a predictive measure was first published in the 1940s by French and Steinberg [68]. The AI measure itself underwent a number of changes leading to the ANSI 1969 standard [69] and later on the ANSI 1997 standard [70], where its name was finally changed to speech intelligibility index (SII).

11.4.1.1 Theory

The series of listening experiments performed by Fletcher and Galt [71] were designed to establish a relationship between the intelligibility of speech filtered into various bands. For instance, if the intelligibility of speech low-pass filtered at 1000 Hz is s_L and the intelligibility of speech high-pass filtered at 1000 Hz (i.e., complementary filtered) is s_H, what can we deduce about the relationship between s_L, s_H, and s, where s is the intelligibility score of full-bandwidth (non-filtered) speech? Fletcher sought for a non-linear transformation $f(.)$ that would satisfy the following relationship: $f(s) = f(s_L) + f(s_H)$. He succeeded in finding such a transformation after making the assumption that the band articulation errors are independent. Assume that $e_L = 1 - s_L$ is the articulation error (AE) obtained when speech is low-pass filtered at f_L Hz and $e_H = 1 - s_H$ is the AE obtained when speech is high-pass filtered at f_H Hz. Then, the AE made when listeners are presented with full-bandwidth speech is given by

$$e = e_L \cdot e_H \tag{11.54}$$

suggesting that the AEs (which may be interpreted as probabilities of error) made in the two bands are independent. That is, the probability of making an error in one band is not influenced by the probability of making an error in another band. Suppose that listeners are presented with 100 words. When these words are low-pass filtered at 1100 Hz, suppose that listeners make 30 errors in word identification, i.e., $e_L = 0.3$. When the words are high-pass filtered at 1100 Hz, listeners make 12 word errors, i.e., $e_H = 0.12$. Then, based on the aforesaid independence model, when the listeners are presented with full-bandwidth (i.e., with no filtering) words, the overall error ought to be

$$e = 0.3 \times 0.12 = 0.036 \tag{11.55}$$

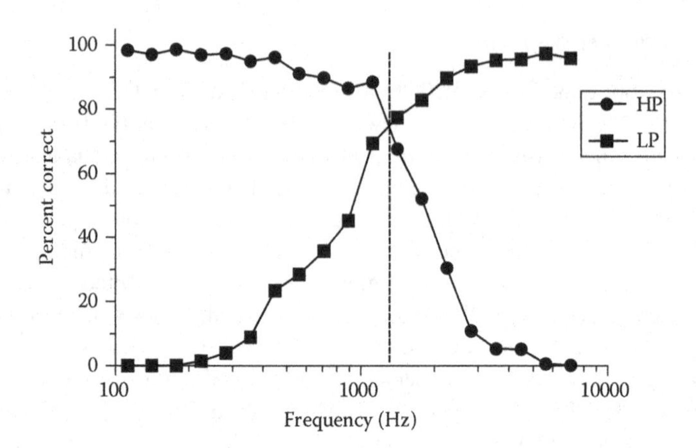

FIGURE 11.17 Monosyllabic word recognition as a function of low-pass and high-pass cut-off frequency. (From Studebaker, G. and Sherbecoe, R., *J. Speech Hear. Res.*, 34, 427, 1991.)

That is, nearly four errors (=96.4% correct) should be made when listening to full-bandwidth speech.

But, how accurate is the said independence model? A number of studies have verified that it is relatively accurate, at least for single words or non-sense syllables and for speech corrupted with steady (stationary) noise. Figure 11.17 shows the intelligibility scores obtained by low-pass/high-pass filtering monosyllabic (and meaningful) words in various noise conditions ranging from SNR = −10 to SNR = 8 dB [72]. Clearly, high intelligibility scores are obtained as the low-pass cut-off frequency f_L increases (since more information is presented to the listener) and low intelligibility scores are obtained as the high-pass cut-off frequency f_H increases (since low-frequency information is eliminated). The two curves intersect at approximately f = 1.4 kHz, a frequency known as cross-over frequency. The cross-over frequency divides equally the spectrum into two equal-intelligibility regions since the intelligibility is the same regardless whether speech is low-pass filtered or high-pass filtered at that particular frequency. To verify whether Equation 11.54 holds, one could compute the model error as

$$ME = e - e_L \cdot e_H \tag{11.56}$$

where ME denotes the model error made for each pair of low-pass and high-pass cut-off frequencies. The absolute value of ME is plotted (in percentage) in Figure 11.18 as a function of frequency (based on 1/3-octave frequency spacing) using the data taken from [72]. For this particular condition (SNR = 8 dB) shown in Figure 11.18, e = 0.016 for the recognition of full-bandwidth words. As can be seen, the model error is for the most part less than 7%. Error is largest near the cross-over frequency region. This has also been verified in other studies with consonants embedded in vowel-consonant-vowel (VCV) context [73–75].

The two-band independence model mentioned earlier can also be extended into K bands. Let e_1 be the AE obtained when only the first band is presented to the listener, e_2 the error when only the second band is presented to the listener, and so forth.

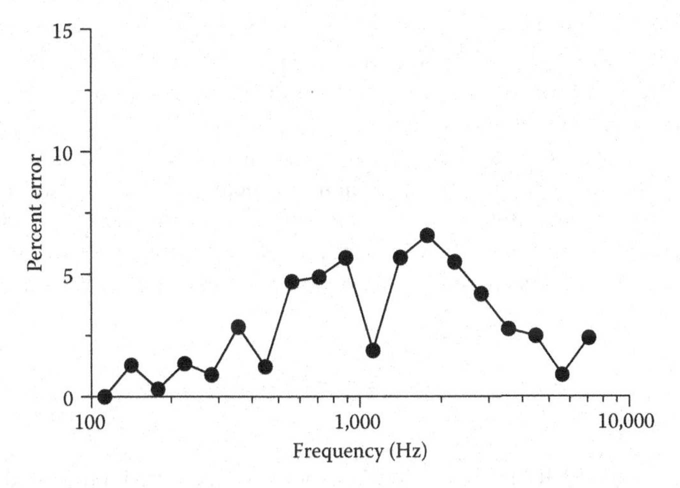

FIGURE 11.18 Overall band error, in percent, for the data shown in Figure 11.17.

When all the bands are presented to the listener (i.e., full signal bandwidth), the total error is given by the following product:

$$e = e_1 e_2 \cdots e_j \cdots e_K \tag{11.57}$$

Note that the said equation assumes that the K bands are independent and as such contribute to K independent channels of information. Let s denote the percent correct score obtained when all bands are used, and s_k the percent correct score when only the kth band is used. Hence, from Equation 11.57, we have

$$1 - s = (1 - s_1)\cdot(1 - s_2)\ldots(1 - s_K) \tag{11.58}$$

Taking the logarithm of both sides, we get

$$\log(1 - s) = \sum_{j=1}^{K} \log(1 - s_j) = \sum_{j=1}^{K} \log(e_j) \tag{11.59}$$

Next, let us assume that the overall AE is proportional to log (1 − s), i.e.,

$$AE = \frac{Q}{P}\log(1 - s) \tag{11.60}$$

where Q and P are free parameters that can be adjusted for different speech materials. After solving for s in the aforesaid equation and using Equation 11.59, we get

$$\begin{aligned} s &= 1 - 10^{\frac{P}{Q}AE} \\ &= 1 - 10^{\frac{P}{Q}\sum_j \log(e_j)} \end{aligned} \tag{11.61}$$

This equation relates the overall SI score s with the intelligibility score (i.e., $1 - e_j$) of each band alone, i.e., the intelligibility of speech that is filtered through each band and presented to the listener. Note that for the aforesaid to be true, the band independence assumption (i.e., Equation 11.57) needs to hold. The band AEs e_j can be obtained from laborious listening tests (as shown in Figure 11.17), but those are time-consuming making the said equation impractical. If we could instead relate the band AEs e_j with something we can measure from the signals (target and masker), we can relate that to the overall (wideband) SI, thus avoiding the need for listening tests. Let us assume that the band AE e_j decreases exponentially with increasing band SNR [68], i.e.,

$$e_j = 10^{-SNR_j} \tag{11.62}$$

where SNR_j is the SNR in band j, which can be easily measured if provided access to the target and masker signals prior to mixing. Equation 11.62 constitutes a reasonable assumption given that the lower the SNR is in a given band, the lower the amount of useful information transmitted to the listener by that band. To one extreme, the band may be completely masked by background noise rendering the band useless. Substituting the aforementioned expression for e_j into Equation 11.61, we get an expression for the intelligibility score as a function of the band SNRs:

$$\begin{aligned} s &= 1 - 10^{-\frac{P}{Q}\left(\sum_j SNR_j\right)} \\ &= 1 - 10^{-\frac{P}{Q}AI} \end{aligned} \tag{11.63}$$

where $AI = \sum_k \text{SNR}_k$ is defined to be the AI. Since the aforementioned function is monotonically increasing, the higher the AI value is the higher the predicted intelligibility score. Consequently, the higher the SNRs are in each band, the higher the intelligibility. In practice, the SNR_k values are normalized between 0 and 1 (see Section 11.4.1.4), and subsequently AI takes values between 0 and 1. Note that the AI equation bears the same form as the original expression given in Equation 11.53 assuming $W_k = 1$ for all bands. It is clear from the previous equation that AI is the objective intelligibility index and s is the predicted intelligibility score obtained by the sigmoidal-shaped mapping function of the form ($1–10^{-c \cdot AI}$). That is, $s = f(\text{AI})$, where $f(.)$ is the AI-to-intelligibility mapping function, which is also known in the literature as the *transfer function*. It is clear from Equation 11.63 that as $AI \rightarrow 0$ we have $s \rightarrow 0$ (predicted intelligibility is low), and as $AI \rightarrow 1$ we have $s \rightarrow 1$ (predicted intelligibility is high). In general, the shape of the transfer function differs depending on the speech materials (e.g., sentences, words, non-sense syllables) and can be obtained by fitting the data (AI values) to the intelligibility scores obtained from listening tests or by low-pass and high-pass filtering the signal at various cut-off frequencies [71].

11.4.1.2 Transfer Function

By changing the parameters P and Q in Equation 11.60, one can derive different sigmoidal-like transfer functions. For the most part and in most cases, $P = 1$. The parameter P is often referred to as the proficiency factor reflecting different speaker characteristics, practice effects, etc. When P is greater or smaller than 1, performance is accounted for by factors other than audibility and effective SNR alone. The parameter Q varies depending on the speech materials used and in particular whether these materials contain contextual information (e.g., sentences) or not (e.g., non-sense syllables, single words). Figure 11.19 shows the transfer functions for sentences [71,76] and monosyllabic words [72]. As shown in Figure 11.19, the choice of transfer function is critical for prediction of SI and it reflects the influence of context on speech recognition [77]. Note that the same value of AI may predict a different intelligibility score for different speech materials. A value of AI = 0.5 for instance, would predict a 74% score on monosyllabic word recognition and a 99% score on sentence recognition. A more general expression of the transfer function bears the form

$$s = \left(1 - 10^{-\frac{P}{Q}AI}\right)^N \tag{11.64}$$

where N is an additional fitting constant. The parameter values for the transfer functions shown in Figure 11.19 are $P = 2.3$, $Q = 0.428$, and $N = 2.729$ for sentence

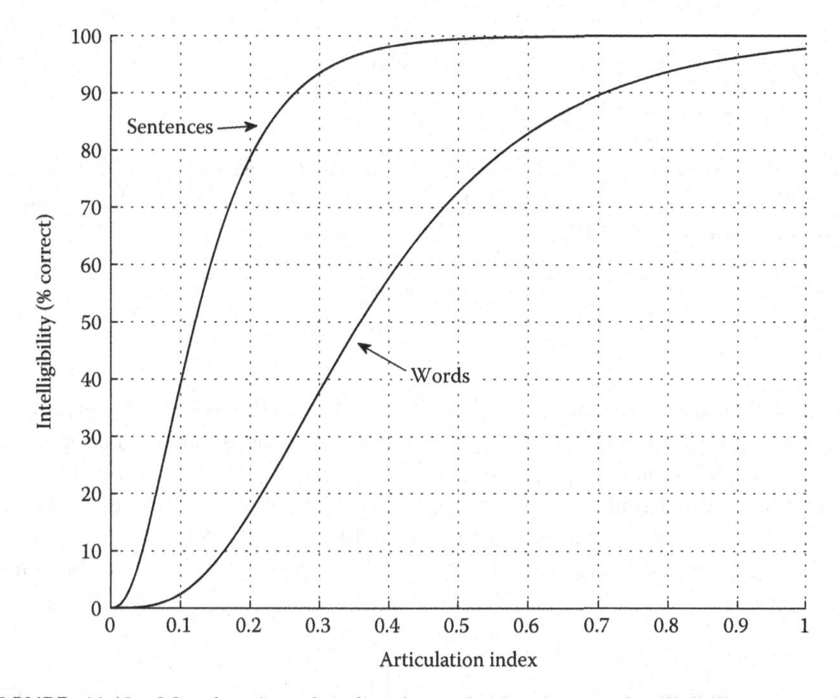

FIGURE 11.19 Mapping (transfer) functions of AI values to intelligibility scores for sentences and words.

intelligibility prediction and $P = 1$, $Q = 0.445$, and $N = 4.077$ for word intelligibility prediction. Transfer functions for other speech materials can be found in [76].

11.4.1.3 Derivation of Band-Importance Functions

The BIFs, denoted as W_k, in Equation 11.53, represent the relative contribution of different frequency bands to SI. It is a laborious task to estimate them as it involves low-pass and high-pass filtering the speech stimuli using a large number of cut-off frequencies and SNR levels. The derivation of the BIFs for monosyllabic words [72], for instance, required a total of 301 listening conditions. As one might expect, the relative importance of each frequency band varies across different speech materials (i.e., words versus sentences).

To derive the BIF, we first need to consider the continuous version of Equation 11.53, i.e.,

$$AI = \int_0^{Fc} W(f)SNR(f)df \tag{11.65}$$

where F_c denotes the signal bandwidth. For a low-pass filter system with cut-off frequency f, and assuming that the speech band is delivered at optimum intensity levels (SNR >> 1) such that is audible, the aforementioned equation reduces to

$$AI(f) = \int_0^{f} W(f)df \tag{11.66}$$

where $AI(f)$ indicates the AI obtained assuming the listener has only access to the spectral information present in the low-pass region of [0–f] Hz. From the said equation, we can compute the BIF as

$$W(f) = \frac{dAI(f)}{df} \tag{11.67}$$

where $dAI(f)$ denotes the amount of AI carried by the small frequency band df spanning the region between f and $f + df$ when the speech band is delivered at optimum levels. The derivation of $W(f)$ suggests a two-step process. First, the AI needs to be determined for different low-pass and high-pass filter cut-off frequencies. Note that the low-pass/high-pass filtering tests involving different cut-off frequencies provide intelligibility scores rather than AI values. These scores, however, can be transformed into AI values by solving Equation 11.64 for AI:

$$AI(f_B) = -\frac{Q}{P}\log\left(1 - s_{f_B}^{\frac{1}{N}}\right) \tag{11.68}$$

where s_{f_B} denotes the intelligibility score for a specific low-/high-pass filtering condition with cut-off frequency f_B and $AI(f_B)$ denotes the corresponding AI value. Following the aforementioned conversion to AI values, a function is fit through all data points involving the various low/pass filtering conditions and SNR levels to obtain $AI(f)$, i.e., the AI as a function of frequency. Second, the derivative of $AI(f)$ is computed with respect to frequency as per Equation 11.67, yielding the BIF $W(f)$. The BIF is finally normalized so that its sum (or area) over all frequencies is equal to 1. The said procedure has been used in [71] to compute the BIF of non-sense syllables (parameters in Equation 11.68 were set to $P = 1$, $Q = 0.55$ and $N = 1$).

A simplified method was used in [72] to compute the BIF for a specific band by approximating $W(f)$ in Equation 11.67 as follows:

$$W(f_{L-H}) \approx AI(f_H) - AI(f_L) \tag{11.69}$$

where the band spans the frequency range of f_L–f_H Hz, with $AI(f_L)$ and $AI(f_H)$ indicating the corresponding AI values (transformed from the corresponding intelligibility scores according to Equation 11.68) of the lower and higher cut-off frequencies of the band respectively.

BIFs for different speech materials are shown in Figure 11.20. BIFs for other speech materials are tabulated in [70, Table B.2]. As can be seen from Figure 11.20, most BIFs place more emphasis in the region near the F2 formant. As described earlier, the derivation of BIFs requires extensive listening tests and are speech-material specific.

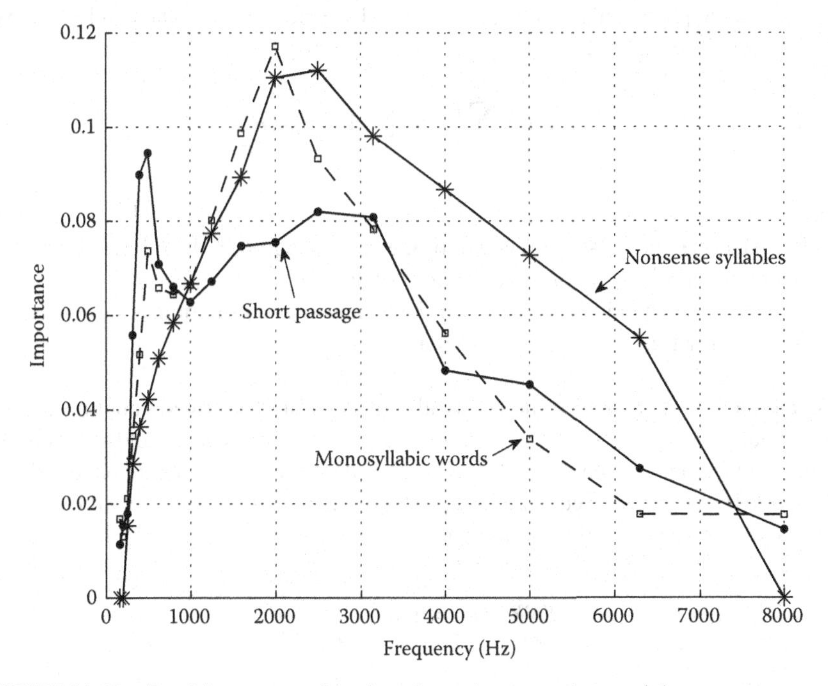

FIGURE 11.20 Band-importance functions for various speech materials.

They are appropriate for the prediction of intelligibility of monosyllabic words or consonants (e.g., in VCV context) corrupted by steady background noise. These BIFs are not appropriate, however, for predicting the intelligibility of speech corrupted by fluctuating maskers (e.g., competing talker). It is also not appropriate to use them in intelligibility measures operating on short-term intervals since the spectral characteristics of the speech signal vary over time. Signal and phonetic-segment dependent BIFs were proposed in [78]. These BIFs are derived directly from the target signal and change accordingly from segment to segment. More specifically, the critical-band spectrum, computed in short-term intervals and raised to a power can be used as BIF [78]. That is, the target signal spectrum can serve as its own BIF. The power exponent controls the emphasis placed on spectral peaks and valleys and can be varied for maximum correlation with the data. Improved correlations were obtained in [78] with the signal-dependent BIFs when compared to the fixed BIFs shown in Figure 11.20.

11.4.1.4 Articulation Index Measure

The basic form of the AI measure is described in the following [14,79]:

Step 1: Computation of SNR in each band

Prior to mixing the speech and noise (masker) signals, the long-term average spectra of speech and noise are computed. This can be done, for instance, using Welch's periodogram technique [80] with a 125 ms integration window. This window size is used in the literature since it has been found that the corresponding distribution of the speech root-mean-square (rms) values is approximately linear over a 30 dB dynamic range [14,81]. The spectrum is divided into 1/3-octave bands and the power in each band is computed as [70]

$$P_X(f_k) = \sum_m |S(m)|^2 - 10\log_{10}(B_k) \tag{11.70}$$

where

- $P_x(f_k)$ denotes the 1/3-octave power of the speech signal in the kth band
- $|S(m)|^2$ denotes FFT magnitude-squared spectrum
- B_k denotes the bandwidth of the kth band and the summation is done over all frequency bins spanning the kth band

The subtraction of the log of the bandwidth in the aforementioned equation is done for normalization purposes to account for the progressively wider bandwidths in the higher frequencies. A total of 18 1/3-octave bands spanning the signal bandwidth of 150–8000 Hz are often used. The said procedure is repeated for noise, and the SNR in the kth 1/3-octave band is computed as

$$SNR_{dB}(f_k) = 10\log_{10}\frac{P_X(f_k)}{P_N(f_k)} \tag{11.71}$$

where $PN(f_k)$ denotes the 1/3-octave level of the noise in the kth band.

Step 2: Mapping of the band SNRs in the range of [0,1]

The dynamic range of SNR values computed as per Equation 11.71 is extremely large and may vary from −60 to +60dB. The effective speech dynamic range, however, is approximately 30dB [81]. For that reason, the SNRdB values are limited within a 30dB dynamic range, and more specifically within −15 and +15dB. The limiting is done as follows:

$$SNR''_{dB} = \begin{cases} -15 & \text{if } SNR_{dB} < -15 \\ SNR_{dB} & -15 \le SNR_{dB} \le 15 \\ 15 & \text{if } SNR_{dB} > 15 \end{cases} \tag{11.72}$$

where SNR''_{dB} denote the limited SNR_{dB} values. The SNR''_{dB} values are next linearly mapped to the range of 0–1 as follows:

$$SNR_M(f_k) = \frac{SNR''_{dB}(f_k) + 15}{30} \tag{11.73}$$

where the normalized SNR_M takes values in the range of 0 and 1 (see Figure 11.21).

Step 3: Computation of AI

The AI is finally computed using Equation 11.53 as

$$AI = \sum_{k=1}^{K} W_k \cdot SNR_M(f_k) \tag{11.74}$$

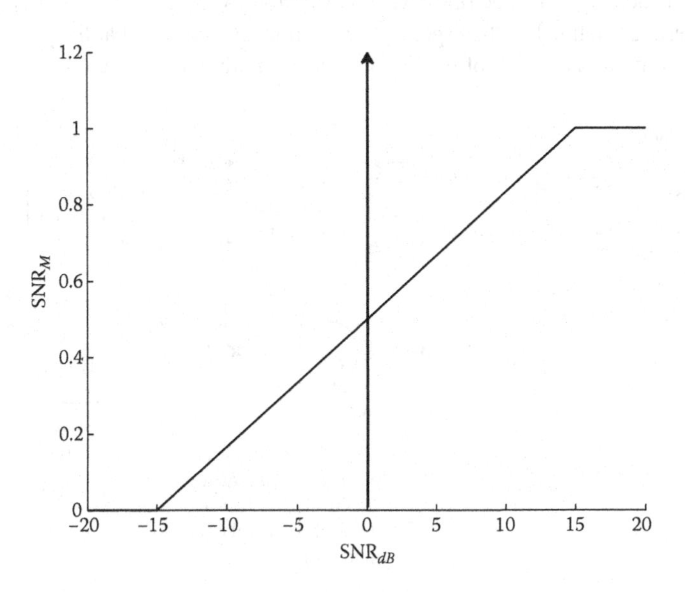

FIGURE 11.21 Function used for mapping the SNR to the range of 0–1.

where W_k denotes the BIF function of band k. The BIF is normalized such that $\sum_k W_k = 1$. Note that the AI measure yields values between 0 and 1, with values near 1 suggesting high intelligibility and values near 0 suggesting poor intelligibility.

Finally, to get the predicted intelligibility score, the appropriate transfer (mapping) function needs to be used (see transfer functions in Figure 11.19) that takes as input the AI value and produces the intelligibility score.

11.4.1.5 Speech Intelligibility Index (ANSI 1997 Standard)

A series of studies [82] were published validating the AI culminating with the creation of the ANSI S3.5-1969 standard [69]. These studies investigated among other things the impact of low-pass, high-pass, and bandpass filtering of speech in various noise masking conditions [82]. The standard was later revised in 1997. In the ANSI S3.5-1997 standard [70], the name of the measure changed from AI to SII. The computation of the audibility function (SNR) was modified to take into account the effects of spread of masking and vocal effort. Masking becomes an issue when higher energy vowels make lower energy consonants inaudible. The revised standard takes into consideration the fact that SI can decrease at extremely high sound pressure levels, something known as "roll-over" effect [68,83]. In the presence of high background noise levels, a talker is likely to raise the voice level (vocal effort) due to the Lombard effect. Increased vocal effort is associated with variation in the amplitude spectrum causing possible changes to intelligibility. The audibility function was also modified in the revised standard to accommodate individuals with conductive hearing loss. Hearing threshold levels may be used as additional input to the SII computation.

The block diagram showing the computation of the SII is given in Figure 11.22. The inputs to the SII model are as follows:

1. Equivalent speech spectrum levels (in dB) for 18 1/3-octave frequency bands. These are defined as the "speech spectrum levels measured at the point corresponding to the center of the listener's head (midpoint between the ears), with

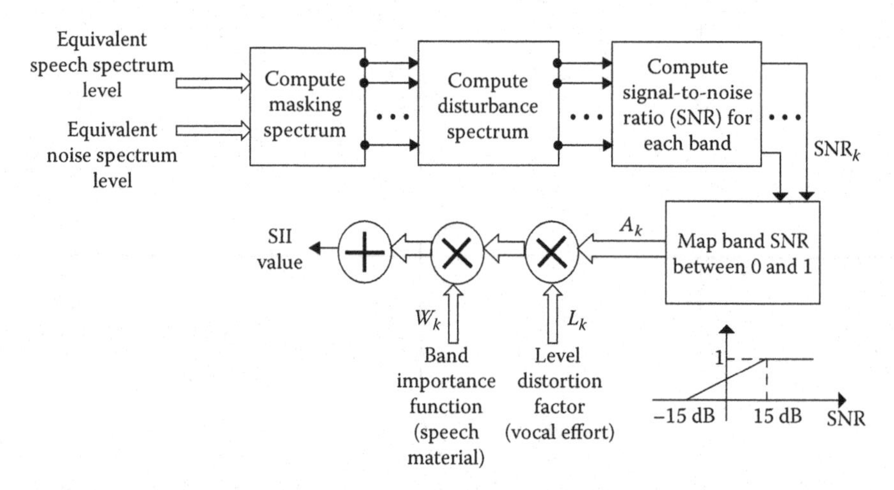

FIGURE 11.22 Block diagram showing the computation of the SII.

the listener absent" [70, p. 6]. If these levels are not available, the free-field-to-eardrum transfer function can be used (see Table 11.3). This function can be used to compute the difference between the pure-tone SPL at the eardrum and the pure-tone SPL at the center of the listener's head. If for instance, the SPL at the eardrum of the listener is 50 dB at 1000 Hz, then after using the free-field-to-eardrum transfer function at 1000 Hz (see Table 11.3), we can compute the equivalent speech spectrum level by subtracting the two, i.e., 50 − 2.6 = 47.4 dB. We denote the equivalent speech spectrum level (in dB) in band k as S_k.

2. Equivalent noise spectrum levels (in dB) for 18 1/3-octave frequency bands measured the same way as already discussed. We denote the noise spectrum level (in dB) in band k as N_k.
3. Equivalent hearing threshold levels, denoted as T_k, for 18 1/3-octave frequency bands.

TABLE 11.3
Table Showing 1/3-Octave Center Frequencies, Internal Noise Spectrum Levels, Speech Spectrum Levels for Different Vocal Efforts and Free-Field to Eardrum Transfer Function

Band No.	Center Frequency (Hz)	Reference Internal Noise Spectrum Level (dB)	Speech Spectrum Level for Stated Vocal Effort (dB)				Free-Field to Eardrum Transfer Function (dB)
			Normal	Raised	Loud	Shout	
1	160	0.6	32.41	33.81	35.29	30.77	0.00
2	200	−1.7	34.48	33.92	37.76	36.65	0.50
3	250	−3.9	34.75	38.98	41.55	42.5	1.00
4	315	−6.1	33.98	38.57	43.78	46.51	1.40
5	400	−8.2	34.59	39.11	43.3	47.4	1.50
6	500	−9.7	34.27	40.15	44.85	49.24	1.80
7	630	−10.8	32.06	38.78	45.55	51.21	2.40
8	800	−11.9	28.30	36.37	44.05	51.44	3.10
9	1000	−12.5	25.01	33.86	42.16	51.31	2.60
10	1250	−13.5	23.00	31.89	40.53	49.63	3.00
11	1600	−15.4	20.15	28.58	37.7	47.65	6.10
12	2000	−17.7	17.32	25.32	34.39	44.32	12.00
13	2500	−21.2	13.18	22.35	30.98	40.8	16.80
14	3150	−24.2	11.55	20.15	28.21	38.13	15.00
15	4000	−25.9	9.33	16.78	25.41	34.41	14.30
16	5000	−23.6	5.31	11.47	18.35	28.24	10.70
17	6300	−15.8	2.59	7.67	13.87	23.45	6.40
18	8000	−7.1	1.13	5.07	11.39	20.72	1.80
	Overall SPL, dB		62.35	68.34	74.85	82.3	

Source: ANSI S3-5, Methods for calculation of the speech intelligibility index, American National Standards Institute, 1997.

In the following we outline the steps involved in the computation of the SII, assuming 1/3-octave frequency spacing:

Step 1: Compute the equivalent masking spectra

For each band, compute the self-masking spectrum V_k as

$$V_k = S_k - 24 \tag{11.75}$$

and

$$B_k = \max(V_k, N_k) \tag{11.76}$$

Compute the slope per 1/3-octave band of spread of masking as follows:

$$C_k = -80 + 0.6[B_k + 10\log_{10} F_k - 6.353] \tag{11.77}$$

where F_k are the center-frequencies of the 1/3-octave bands as listed in Table 11.3. For all bands, except the first one, compute the equivalent masking spectrum as follows:

$$Z_k = 10\log_{10}\left\{10^{0.1N_k} + \sum_{m=1}^{k-1} 10^{0.1[B_m + 3.32C_m \log_{10}(0.89F_k/F_m)]}\right\} \tag{11.78}$$

Step 2: Compute the disturbance spectrum levels

Compute the equivalent internal noise spectrum as

$$X_k = R_k + T_k \tag{11.79}$$

where

R_k is the reference internal noise spectrum listed in Table 11.3
T_k the hearing threshold levels

The reference internal noise spectrum is the spectrum of a fictitious internal noise in the ear of the listener computed such that if it were an external masker, it would produce the pure-tone threshold in quiet [68,79]. Compute

$$D_k = \max(Z_k, X_k) \tag{11.80}$$

where D_k denotes the disturbance spectrum level.

Step 3: Compute the level distortion factors

Calculate the level distortion factor, L_k, as [68]

$$L_k = 1 - \frac{S_k - U_k - 10}{160} \tag{11.81}$$

where U_k is the standard speech spectrum level at normal vocal effort (listed in Table 11.3). Values of U_k for other vocal efforts including raised, loud, and shout and are tabulated in Table 11.3. The level distortion factor, L_k, is limited to 1, i.e., $L''_k = \min(L_k,1)$.

Step 4: Compute the effective band SNR (audibility function)

Compute the SNR in band k as

$$SNR_k = \frac{S_k - D_k + 15}{30} \quad (11.82)$$

Note that this equation is the same as in Equation 11.73 except that the noise spectrum is replaced with the disturbance spectrum (Equation 11.80). The SNR_k values are limited within the range of 0–1, and are adjusted to account for the speech level distortion factor L_k:

$$SNR''_k = L''_k \cdot SNR_k \quad (11.83)$$

Step 5: Compute the speech intelligibility index

Calculate the speech intelligibility index (SII) as

$$SII = \sum_{k=1}^{18} W_k \cdot SNR''_k \quad (11.84)$$

where W_k is the band-importance function.

Figure 11.23 shows an example computation of the SII for an IEEE sentence corrupted by SSN at 0 dB. Figure 11.23a shows the long-term average spectra (1/3-octave levels) of the masker and target signals (prior to mixing) computed using a 125 ms integration window. Figure 11.23b shows the SNR in each band computed simply by subtracting the target from the masker spectra (note that the spectra are given in dB). The equivalent masking spectrum, computed using Step 2, is shown in Figure 11.23c along with the original masker spectrum. Finally, Figure 11.23d shows the normalized SNR given by Equation 11.83. For this example, the vocal effort was normal and the level distortion factor was computed to be 1 for all bands. The band SNR was extremely low near 1000 Hz yielding normalized SNR values close to 0 (Figure 11.23d). For the remaining frequencies, the band SNR was near 0 dB, and the corresponding normalized SNR was near 0.5 according to the linear mapping function shown in Figure 11.21. Following the computation of the SII, as per Equation 11.84, using short passage BIFs, the resultant SII value is 0.37. Based on the transfer function shown in Figure 11.20 for sentences, the predicted intelligibility score for this sentence should be nearly 95% correct.

11.4.1.6 Limitations of AI

The AI measure has been successful in predicting intelligibility of speech in additive noise or speech that has been filtered [82]. It has, however, a number of limitations. First, it has been validated for the most part only for steady (stationary) masking noise since

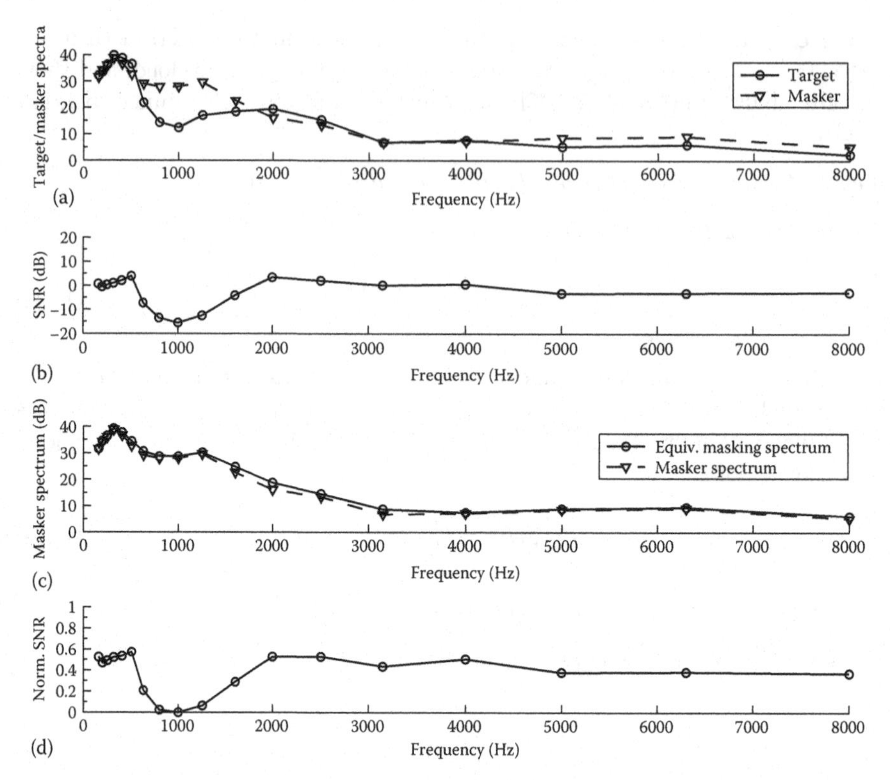

FIGURE 11.23 Example computation of the SII for an IEEE sentence corrupted by speech-shaped noise at 0 dB SNR. (a) Long-term average spectra (1/3 octave levels) of masker and target signals prior to mixing; (b) SNR in each band; (c) equivalent masking spectrum and the original masker spectrum; (d) normalized SNR computed from equation 11.83.

it is based on the long-term average spectra of the speech and masker signals. As such, it cannot be applied to situations in which speech is embedded in fluctuating maskers (e.g., competing talkers). Several attempts have been made to extend the AI measure to assess SI in fluctuating maskers [84,85] and these are briefly discussed in the next section. Second, according to the ANSI (1997) standard [70], the SII measure cannot be used in conditions that include multiple sharply filtered bands of speech or sharply filtered noises. Incidentally, sharply filtered bands of speech can be produced when speech is processed via spectral-subtractive algorithms due to the non-linear thresholding of the speech envelopes. Third, it cannot be applied in situations where non-linear operations (e.g., non-linear gain functions used in speech enhancement) are involved and additive noise is present. This is because the definitions of the target and masker signals are no longer clear following non-linear processing, as both the target and masker signals are affected. Consequently, the definition of the true output SNR, namely the effective SNR following non-linear processing, poses a great challenge. In contrast, in situations wherein speech is subjected to linear filtering operations (e.g., low-pass filter), the SNR can be determined based on the target and masker signals prior to mixing. In the following sections, we provide a brief description of some of the methods proposed to address the said limitations.

11.4.1.6.1 Addressing Fluctuating Maskers

The existing SII model does not take into account any fluctuations (or modulations) in the masking noise, since the SII is computed from the long-term averaged speech and noise spectra. This refers to situations where speech is embedded in say train noise or interruptive (e.g., on/off) type of noise. This also includes situations where a competing-talker(s) is present. Numerous studies have reported on experiments assessing SI in fluctuating or modulated noise [86–88], and the general conclusion is that normal-hearing listeners perform better in conditions where fluctuating (modulated) noise is present compared to conditions where stationary noise (e.g., white noise, speech-shaped noise) of the same SNR level is present (see also discussion in Section 4.1.1). This was attributed to the listeners exploiting the "dips" in the temporal envelope or "glimpsing" the target during the silent, and higher-SNR, gaps in the waveform (see Section 4.3.2)

The SII model (Section 11.4.1.5) does not predict SI accurately in fluctuating noise maskers (e.g., [86]). To account for the perceptual effect of fluctuating maskers, Rhebergen et al. [84] adapted the SII model such that the SII value was calculated within short duration frames, after which the short-term SII values were averaged. The approach taken to determine the SII within small time frames is to first window the speech and noise signal in short-time frames, compute the spectrum using say the Fourier transform, and derive the SII from the resulting short-term speech and noise spectra. In order to be able to track the perceptually relevant fluctuations over time, the window length was chosen in accordance with the temporal resolution of normal-hearing listeners, as determined using gap-detection experiments [89]. It is known, for instance, that the temporal resolution of the auditory system is frequency dependent with time constants (i.e., integration times) for the lower frequency bands being larger than those of the higher bands [21,89]. Rhebergen et al. [84] filtered the signal into 21 critical bands, and extracted the envelope of the target and masker signals in each band using the Hilbert transform. The envelopes were windowed (rectangular window) and the window length was chosen to be relatively short in the higher bands and relatively long in the lower bands. More precisely, window lengths ranging from 35 ms in the lower band (150 Hz) to 9.4 ms in the highest band (8000 Hz) were considered. The envelopes of the target and masker signals, along with the thresholds of hearing were input to the SII model to derive instantaneous values of SII for each time frame. The final SII value was computed by averaging across all instantaneous SII values. The modified SII model was tested using various fluctuating maskers including noise with speech-like modulation spectrum, interrupted (gated) noise with 50% duty cycle, sinusoidally modulated noise, and competing-talker modulated noise. Good correlation was reported between the predicted SRT and observed SRT values in the various conditions. The said SII model was later modified and extended in [85] to account for forward masking.

11.4.1.6.2 Addressing Non-Linear Operations

Most (if not all) noise-suppression algorithms discussed in this book involve a gain reduction stage, in which the noisy (mixture) spectrum is multiplied by a gain function G_k (taking typically values ranging from 0 to 1) with the intent of suppressing background noise, if present. The noisy speech spectrum is non-linear processed by a gain function to produce the enhanced spectrum $\hat{X}_k$ for frequency bin k. In the power spectral-subtractive algorithm [38], for instance, the gain function takes the form

$$G_k = \max\left(0, 1 - \frac{\hat{N}_k^2}{Y_k^2}\right) \tag{11.85}$$

where

$\hat{N}_k^2$ denotes the magnitude-squared spectrum of the estimated (e.g., using a noise-estimation algorithm) masker

Y_k denotes the corrupted magnitude spectrum (the max operator is used to ensure that the gain function is always positive)

The non-linear processing of the noisy speech spectra poses certain challenges in terms of defining the effective output band SNR based on $\hat{X}_k$. This is so because the non-linear function (e.g., gain G_k) affects both the target and masker signals and thus we can no longer assume that the enhanced spectrum $\hat{X}_k$ always corresponds to the modified (e.g., attenuated, etc.) target signal. To see this, we can express the magnitude-squared spectrum of the enhanced signal, i.e., $\hat{X}_k^2$, as follows:

$$\begin{aligned} \hat{X}_k^2 &= G_k^2 Y_k^2 = G_k^2\left(X_k^2 + N_k^2\right) \\ &= G_k^2 X_k^2 + G_k^2 N_k^2 \\ &= S_T^2 + S_M^2 \end{aligned} \tag{11.86}$$

where

X_k denotes the clean signal magnitude spectrum

N_k indicates the masker spectrum

S_T^2 denotes the power of the modified (by non-linear processing) target component

S_M^2 (the subscript k was omitted for clarity) denotes the power of the modified masker component of $\hat{X}_k^2$

Knowing whether the target component (i.e., S_T^2) of the enhanced spectrum is dominant is important in as far as defining the effective or output SNR.

11.4.1.6.2.1 Defining the Output Band SNR Consider the corrupted (mixture) spectrum Y_k in frequency bin k being processed by a noise-reduction algorithm specified by the gain function G_k. Since the masker is additive, the gain function is applied to both the target spectrum X_k and the masker spectrum N_k (see Equation 11.86). Consequently the output SNR in bin k, denoted as $SNR_{\text{out}}(k)$, can be computed as follows:

$$SNR_{\text{out}}(k) = \frac{S_T^2}{S_M^2} = \frac{(G_k X_k)^2}{(G_k N_k)^2} = \frac{X_k^2}{N_k^2} = SNR_k \tag{11.87}$$

where

$(G_k X_k)^2$ denotes the power of the modified (by G_k) target signal in bin k
$(G_k N_k)^2$ indicates the power of the modified masker signal
SNR_k denotes the input band SNR as determined prior to mixing

According to the aforesaid equation, the *output band SNR cannot be improved by any choice of G_k beyond the value of the input band SNR_k*. This observation partially explains the lack of intelligibility with existing noise-reduction algorithms by NH listeners [90] and hearing-impaired listeners [91], at least for algorithms that make use of gain functions to suppress the background noise. It is worth mentioning that while noise-reduction algorithms do not improve the SNR in a specific band, they *can* improve the *overall* SNR accumulated (and appropriately weighted) across all bands (for more detailed discussion see Chapter 13). Note that the overall SNR (computed across all bands) and the output band SNR (computed for a specific band as per Equation 11.87) are different. One strategy for improving the overall SNR (defined as the weighted sum of SNRs across all bands) is to discard bands with unfavorable (extremely low) SNRs while retaining bands with favorable SNR (see proof in [92]). Such an approach was taken in [93] and has been shown to improve SI by normal-hearing listeners (see Chapter 13).

Clearly, the definition here of output band SNR is not useful as it does not involve the enhanced spectrum $\hat{S}$. Alternatively, the output band SNR can be defined as follows [78]:

$$\overline{SNR_k} = \frac{\hat{X}_k^2}{N_k^2} \tag{11.88}$$

where $\overline{SNR_k}$ denotes the new definition of the output SNR in bin k. Similar to the AI computation, the said SNR was limited, mapped to [0, 1] and weighted by BIFs in the study by Ma et al. [78]. The aforementioned measure, however, yielded a poor correlation ($r < 0.4$) with intelligibility scores [78]. This was attributed to the inherent ambiguity associated with non-linear processing when the G_k suppression function is applied to the noisy speech envelopes. More specifically, when the noisy signal is processed by a noise-reduction algorithm (via the application of the gain function G_k), it is not clear whether the resulting spectrum $\hat{X}$ corresponds predominantly to, say, the modified (e.g., attenuated) target spectrum or the modified masker spectrum (see Equation 11.86). Consequently, we cannot easily define the "true" output band SNR as we do not know beforehand whether $\hat{X}$ reflects primarily the modified masker envelope or the modified target envelope.

It is clear from the discussion here that a distinction needs to be made in Equation 11.88 to reflect the scenarios in which the non-linear processing affects primarily (or predominantly) the target spectrum rather than the masker spectrum. If the target magnitude spectrum is dominantly larger than the masker spectrum (i.e., SNR >> 0 dB) then the enhanced spectrum $\hat{X}$ will most likely reflect the modified target spectrum (since the masker component will be extremely small), whereas if the masker spectrum is dominantly larger than the target spectrum (i.e., SNR << 0 dB) then the enhanced spectrum $\hat{X}$ will most likely reflect the modified masker spectrum (since the target component will be extremely small). Determining, however, the appropriate SNR threshold to discriminate between these two scenarios is not straightforward given that the non-linear processing affects both the target and masker envelopes; hence an alternative strategy for making the distinction is needed.

There are two possible scenarios to consider. In the first scenario $\hat{X} < X$, suggesting attenuation of the target signal and in the second scenario $\hat{X} > X$, suggesting amplification of the target signal. As $\hat{X}$ gets significantly larger than X (i.e., overestimation occurs), the corresponding masker magnitude spectrum also gets larger and at some point the input band SNR will become negative. In fact, it can be proven [94] that for a certain range of gain values, the input band SNR is always negative when $\hat{X} > X$. Furthermore, it can also be proven analytically [94] that when $\hat{X} \geq 2 \cdot X$, the corresponding input band SNR is always negative. Consequently, bands for which $\hat{X} \geq 2 \cdot X$ is true should not be included since the speech information is masked. Hence, for the most part, when $\hat{X} > X$ the enhanced spectrum $\hat{X}$ will likely reflect the modified masker spectrum and thus should not be used in the definition of the output SNR in Equation 11.88. Put differently, when $\hat{X} > X$ the masker component of $\hat{X}$ will for the most part be larger than the target component (i.e., $S_M > S_T$ in Equation 11.86), and thus $\hat{X}$ should not be used in Equation 11.88.

11.4.1.6.2.2 Modifying the AI Measure In brief, as shown in Equation 11.87 the output band SNR cannot exceed the input band SNR. Second, the limitations discussed in using Equation 11.88 to compute the output band SNR can be circumvented to some extent if we identify the situations where X better reflects the effects of non-linear processing (e.g., noise reduction) on the target spectrum rather than on the masker spectrum. As discussed earlier, the processed spectrum $\hat{X}$ reflects more reliably the effect of suppression on the target spectrum when $\hat{X} < X$ than when $\hat{X} > X$. It seems reasonable then to restrict X in Equation 11.88 to be always smaller than X, and thus consider in the computation of the proposed measure only bands in which $\widehat{X < X}$. The implicit hypothesis is that those bands will contribute more to intelligibility and should thus be included. This was confirmed in listening studies [93] in which normal-hearing listeners were presented with speech synthesized to contain either target attenuation distortions alone (i.e., bands with $\hat{X} < X$) or target amplification distortions alone (i.e., bands with $\hat{X} > X$). Speech synthesized to contain only target attenuation was always more intelligible, and in fact, it was found to be more intelligible than either the un-processed (noise corrupted) or processed (via the noise-reduction algorithm) speech.

After taking the discussed facts into account, a new measure can be derived, which computes the fraction or proportion of the input SNR transmitted as follows [94]:

$$fSNR_k = \begin{cases} \dfrac{\min\left(\overline{SNR}_k, SNR_k\right)}{SNR_k} & \text{if } SNR_k \geq SNR_L \\ 0 & \text{else} \end{cases} \tag{11.89}$$

where

$fSNR_k$ denotes the fraction (or proportion) of the input SNR transmitted (by the noise-reduction algorithm)

$\overline{SNR_k}$ is given by Equation 11.88

SNR_k is the true SNR and SNR_L denotes the smallest SNR value allowed

It is clear that $fSNR_k$ is bounded by 1, i.e., $0 \leq fSNR_k \leq 1$, and thus denotes the fraction (or proportion) of the input SNR preserved (or transmitted) by the noise-reduction algorithm in a specific band. The maximum value of 1 is attained by $fSNR_k$ when: (1) no non-linear processing (i.e., $G_k = 1$) is applied to the noisy spectrum, and/or (2) when $\hat{X} \approx X$, i.e., when the noise-reduction algorithm produces an accurate estimate of the clean target spectrum. The use of minimum operation in Equation 11.89 ensures that only frequency bins for which $\hat{X} < X$ are included. Furthermore, only bins with SNR falling above a certain value (e.g., $SNR_L > 0\,\text{dB}$) are considered. This is necessary for two reasons. First, the condition $\hat{X} < X$ does not guarantee that the input SNR will always be positive. Second, use of $SNR_L > 0\,\text{dB}$ always guarantees that the target component of the output spectrum will always be larger than the masker component (see Equation 11.86). Following Equation 11.89 the new measure is weighted and accumulated across all bands to produce the fractional AI (fAI) index:

$$fAI = \frac{1}{\sum_{k=1}^{M} W_k} \sum_{k=1}^{M} W_k \cdot fSNR_k \tag{11.90}$$

where

W_k denotes the band-importance function applied to band k

M is the total number of bands used

Experiments reported in [94] indicated that the fAI measure was clearly influenced by the choice of BIF and SNR_L value. The data used in the evaluation of the fAI measure were taken from the intelligibility assessment of noise-corrupted speech processed through eight different noise suppression algorithms [90]. High correlation ($r = 0.9$) was obtained with the fAI measure with $SNR_L = 11\,\text{dB}$. It is interesting to note that the average fAI values did not exceed the value of 0.4, at least for the SNR levels tested (0 and 5 dB). The individual short-term values of fAI, however, exceeded sometimes the value of 0.4, but the average was biased toward lower values due to the extremely low fAI values obtained during unvoiced segments, which also happened to be the low SNR segments. This implies that on the average only 10%–40% of the input SNR was transmitted by most noise-reduction algorithms, at least for algorithms operating at the two SNR levels examined (0 and 5 dB).

The aforementioned measure made use of the fact that the output band SNR following noise reduction cannot exceed the input band SNR. This observation motivated another objective measure that quantified the amount of SNR loss incurred by noise suppression [95]. More specifically, the SNR loss in band j was defined as follows:

$$
\begin{aligned}
L(j) &= SNR_{dB}(j) - \overline{SNR}_{dB}(j) \\
&= 10 \cdot \log_{10} \frac{X_j^2}{N_j^2} - 10 \cdot \log_{10} \frac{\hat{X}_j^2}{N_j^2} \\
&= 10 \cdot \log_{10} \frac{X_j^2}{\hat{X}_j^2}
\end{aligned}
\tag{11.91}
$$

where

$L(j)$ is the SNR loss in band j
$SNR(j)$ is the input SNR in band j
$\overline{SNR}(j)$ is the effective SNR of the enhanced signal (same as in Equation 11.88)
$\hat{X}_j$ is the excitation spectrum of the enhanced signal (note that this measure operates in the excitation spectrum domain)

The first SNR term in Equation 11.91 provides the original SNR in band j before processing the input signal, while the second SNR term provides the SNR of the processed (enhanced) signal as defined in Equation 11.88. The term $L(j)$ in Equation 11.91 thus defines the loss in SNR, termed SNR_{LOSS}, incurred when the corrupted signal goes through a noise-suppression algorithm. Clearly, when $\hat{X}(j) = X(j)$, the SNR_{LOSS} is zero.

Following the computation of the SNR loss in Equation 11.91, the $L(j)$ term is limited within the SNR range of $[-\text{SNR}_{\text{Lim}}, \text{SNR}_{\text{Lim}}]$ dB as follows:

$$
\hat{L}(j) = \min\left(\max(L(j), -\text{SNR}_{\text{Lim}}), \text{SNR}_{\text{Lim}}\right) \tag{11.92}
$$

and subsequently mapped to the range of [0, 1] using the following equation:

$$
\text{SNR}_{\text{LOSS}}(j) = \begin{cases} -\dfrac{C_-}{\text{SNR}_{\text{Lim}}} \hat{L}(j) & \text{if } \hat{L}(j) < 0 \\[2ex] \dfrac{C_+}{\text{SNR}_{\text{Lim}}} \hat{L}(j) & \text{if } \hat{L}(j) \geq 0 \end{cases} \tag{11.93}
$$

where C_+ and C_- are parameters (defined in the range of [0, 1]) controlling the slopes of the mapping function. This equation normalizes the SNR_{LOSS} measure to the range of $0 \le \text{SNR}_{\text{LOSS}}(j) \le 1$ since $0 \le C_+, C_- \le 1$. The average (across all bands) SNR_{LOSS} for a given frame is denoted as $\text{fSNR}_{\text{LOSS}}$ and is computed as follows:

$$\text{fSNR}_{\text{LOSS}} = \frac{\sum_{j=1}^{K} W(j) \cdot \text{SNR}_{\text{LOSS}}(j)}{\sum_{j=1}^{K} W(j)} \tag{11.94}$$

where $W(j)$ is the band-importance function. Finally, the average SNR_{LOSS} across the utterance is computed by averaging the $\text{fSNR}_{\text{LOSS}}$ values across all frames in the signal.

From Equations 11.92 and 11.93, it is clear that the SNR_{LOSS} measure depends on the SNR_{Lim} and the parameters C_+ and C_-, both of which control the slope of the mapping function in Equation 11.93. The parameters C_+ and C_- are quite important, as they can tell us about the individual contribution of the spectral attenuation (occurring when $X > \hat{X}$) and spectral amplification (occurring when $X < \hat{X}$) distortions introduced by noise-suppression algorithms to SI. By setting $C_+ = 1$ and $C_- = 0$, for instance, we can assess whether we can better predict SI when accounting only for spectral attenuation distortions while ignoring spectral amplification distortions. Similarly, by setting $C_+ = 1$ and $C_- = 1$, we can assess whether both distortions (spectral amplification and attenuation) should be weighted equally. In brief, the parameters C_+ and C_- can help us assess the perceptual impact of the spectral distortions introduced by noise-suppression algorithms. The influence of the parameters SNR_{Lim}, C_+ and C_- was investigated in [95]. Optimum values for the parameters C_+ and C_-, in terms of highest correlation with SI scores, were found to be 1 and 1 respectively. Furthermore, results indicated that only spectral distortions falling within a 6 dB range (i.e., within [−3, 3] dB) should be included in the computation of the SNR_{LOSS} measure. Modestly high correlation was obtained when $\text{SNR}_{\text{Lim}} = 3\,\text{dB}$.

Other extensions to the AI index that were designed for handling non-linear processing were based on a different definition of the SNR. Such measures were proposed by Kates and Arehart [96] to predict the intelligibility of peak-clipping and center-clipping distortions, such as those introduced by hearing aids. The modified index, called the CSII index, used the base form of the SII procedure, but with the signal-to-noise ratio estimate replaced by the signal-to-distortion ratio, which was computed using the coherence function between the input and processed signals. This measure will be described in more detail later in Section 11.4.3.

11.4.2 Speech Transmission Index

The speech-transmission index (STI), developed by Houtgast and Steeneken in the early 1970s [97], is based on an acoustic transmissions or systems approach. More precisely, it is based on the concept of modulation transfer function (MTF) which has been used as a design tool for auditorium acoustics. The MTF has been used as a measure for assessing the effects of a room (e.g., reverberation, etc.) on SI. For instance, given the volume (size) of the room, the reverberation time, ambient noise level, the talker's vocal level, and talker-to-listener distance, one can derive analytically the MTF function and use that to derive a SII, called the speech transmission index [98]. As will be shown in the next sections, this index borrows some of the principles used in the AI but uses an *indirect* method for deriving the SNR in each band [98–100].

11.4.2.1 Theory

The derivation of the MTF is rooted in a linear systems and channel estimation theory, where the channel denotes here the transmission path from the speaker to the listener. The enclosure (or room) is considered to the linear system that might be subjected to reverberation or ambient noise. The input to this system is the speaker's signal and the output of this system is the signal received at the listener's ears. Clearly, in the absence of room reflections (reverberation) or additive noise, the signal received (and perceived) by the listener is identical to the signal produced by the speaker. In realistic scenarios, however, it is of interest to know the effect of this linear system (room) on the output (received by the listener) signal. In traditional DSP theory, this effect is characterized by the transfer function of the system and in the context of the STI, the transfer function is defined in the envelope modulation domain.

The question now is how to measure this MTF for a given room. This can be done by exciting the system using an input signal with a simple and well-defined envelope and observing the envelope of the received (output) signal. Consider the following sinewave-modulated signal fed as input to the system:

$$I(t) = I_{INP} \cdot (1 + \cos 2\pi F t) \tag{11.95}$$

where F denotes the modulation frequency (Hz). At the receiving end, the output signal becomes

$$I_o(t) = I_{OUT} \cdot (1 + m \cdot \cos 2\pi F t) \tag{11.96}$$

where m denotes the modulation depth, which is also called modulation index. The input and output signals are also known as *probe* and *response* signals, respectively. The value of m takes values in the range of 0–1 and denotes the reduction in modulation caused by the transmission channel. Small values of m suggest large degradations of the input envelope (note that at the input, $m = 1$) in that the peak-to-dip ratio (temporal envelope contrast) is greatly reduced. Figure 11.24 shows examples of input and output signals produced with different values of m. As can be seen, as the value of m gets smaller, the signal envelope gets flatter, i.e., the peaks and dips in the signal come closer to each other.

Although simplistic, the aforementioned probe and response envelope signals reflect the true effects of reverberation and noise. Reverberation is known to smear the signal envelope, and the degree of smearing is reflected in the value of m. The smaller the value of m is, the more severe the smearing is and the more echoic (reverberant) the signal sounds.

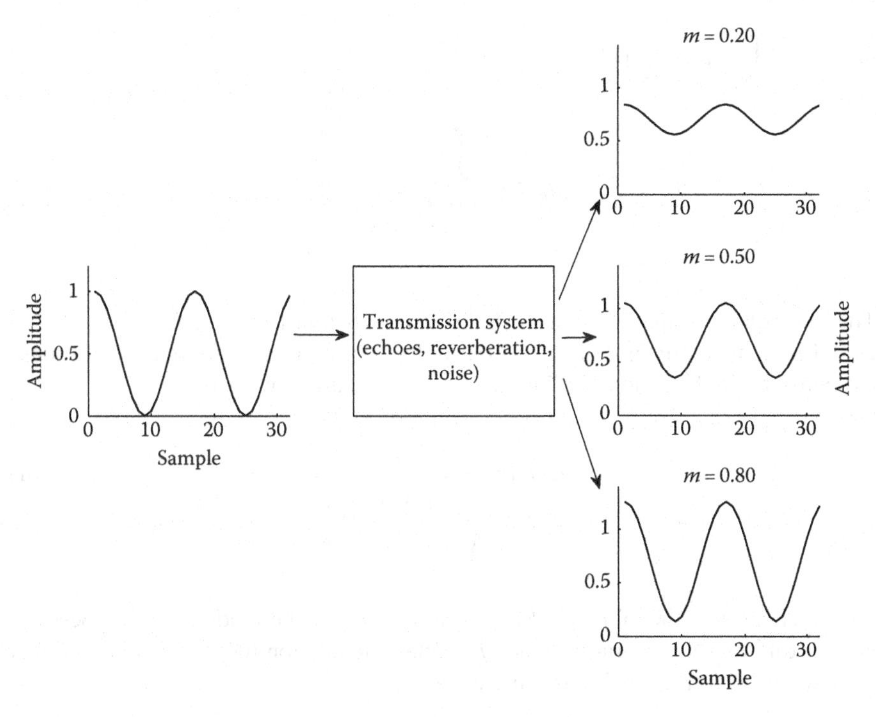

FIGURE 11.24 Example input and output sinusoidal-modulated signals for different values of *m*.

Equations 11.95 and 11.96 provide the input and output (received) envelopes at a specific modulation frequency *F*. After taking a sweep of modulation frequencies *F* and observing the output modulation index for each *F*, we can determine the function *m*(*F*), namely, the *modulation transfer function* (MTF). This function provides the reduction in modulations (i.e., *m*) in the output envelopes for each value of modulation frequency *F*.

In reverberation and/or noise, the MTF can be derived analytically. In reverberant conditions, after disregarding the impact of the direct sound and assuming that the room impulse response is given by the following decaying exponential

$$r(t) = C \cdot e^{-13.8 \cdot t/T} \tag{11.97}$$

where *C* is a constant and *T* is the reverberation time (i.e., T_{60} value), we can compute the output envelope as the convolution of the input envelope (Equation 11.95) with *r*(*t*):

$$I_o(t) = \int_0^{\infty} I(t-\tau) \cdot r(\tau)\, d\tau \tag{11.98}$$

After some manipulation, $I_o(t)$ can be written as

$$I_o(t) = I_{INP} \cdot b(1 + m_R(F) \cdot \cos 2\pi Ft) \tag{11.99}$$

where $b = \int_0^\infty r(t)dt$ and

$$m_R(F) = \frac{\left| \int_0^\infty r(t) e^{j2\pi Ft} dt \right|}{\int_0^\infty r(t)dt} \tag{11.100}$$

The said equation suggests that the MTF of reverberant rooms can be computed in closed form using the (normalized) Fourier transform of the room impulse response $r(t)$. Substituting Equation 11.97 in the previous equation, we get

$$m_R(F) = \frac{1}{\sqrt{1 + \left(\frac{2\pi F \cdot T}{13.8} \right)^2}} \tag{11.101}$$

Figure 11.25 plots the aforesaid MTF as a function of the modulation frequency F and for different reverberation times T. Higher modulation reduction is observed at high modulation frequencies as T increases.

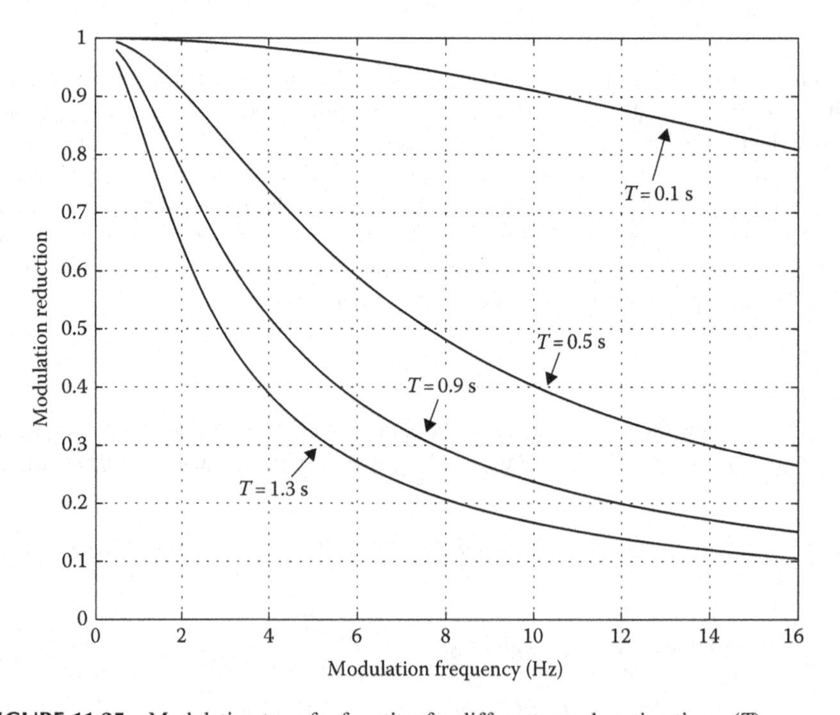

FIGURE 11.25 Modulation transfer function for different reverberation times (T).

In the case of (steady) additive noise with a constant mean envelope I_N, the noise-corrupted envelope can be written as

$$\begin{aligned} I_{NSY}(t) &= I(t) + I_N \\ &= I_{INP} \cdot (1 + \cos 2\pi Ft) + I_N \\ &= (I_{INP} + I_N) \cdot \left(1 + \underbrace{\frac{I_{INP}}{I_{INP} + I_N}}_{m_N} \cos 2\pi Ft \right) \end{aligned} \tag{11.102}$$

From this equation, we can write the MTF for additive noise as

$$\begin{aligned} m_N &= \frac{I_{INP}}{I_{INP} + I_N} = \frac{I_{INP}/I_N}{I_{INP}/I_N + 1} = \frac{SNR}{SNR + 1} \\ &= \frac{1}{1 + 10^{-SNR_{dB}/10}} \end{aligned} \tag{11.103}$$

where $SNR \triangleq I_{INP}/I_N$ and $SNR_{dB} = 10\log_{10}(SNR)$. Note that the MTF for additive noise (Equation 11.103) is independent of the modulation frequency. Solving for SNR_{dB} in the previous equation, we get

$$SNR_{dB} = 10\log_{10}\left(\frac{m_N}{1 - m_N} \right) \tag{11.104}$$

This equation suggests that if we are provided with the modulation reduction factor m_N, we can compute the corresponding SNR that produced this reduction in modulation. Equation 11.104 is the key equation used in the computation of the STI.

Figure 11.26 plots m_N (Equation 11.103) as a function of SNR. As expected, a greater modulation reduction is observed as the SNR level decreases. This is also evident in speech envelopes extracted at a specific band following corruption by noise. Figure 11.27 shows example speech envelopes extracted (using the Hilbert transform) from a band centered at f = 800 Hz in quiet (Figure 11.27a) and in speech-weighted noise at SNR = −5 and 0 dB (Figure 11.27b and c). For this example (SNR = 0 dB), the peaks and valleys of the envelopes are clearly evident. At SNR = −5 dB, however, the noise floor (indicated with arrow on right and shown with a horizontal dashed line) is raised considerably and the peak-to-valley contrast is reduced. Alternatively, we say that the modulation depth (or modulation index) is markedly reduced. For the example shown in Figure 11.27 we can derive m_N using Equation 11.103. The mean envelope amplitude of the input signal in quiet is 176, i.e., I_{INP} = 176. For the example in Figure 11.27b (SNR = 0 dB), the mean amplitude of the noisy envelope is 407, i.e., $I_{INP} + I_N$ = 407, and the resulting modulation index is 0.44.

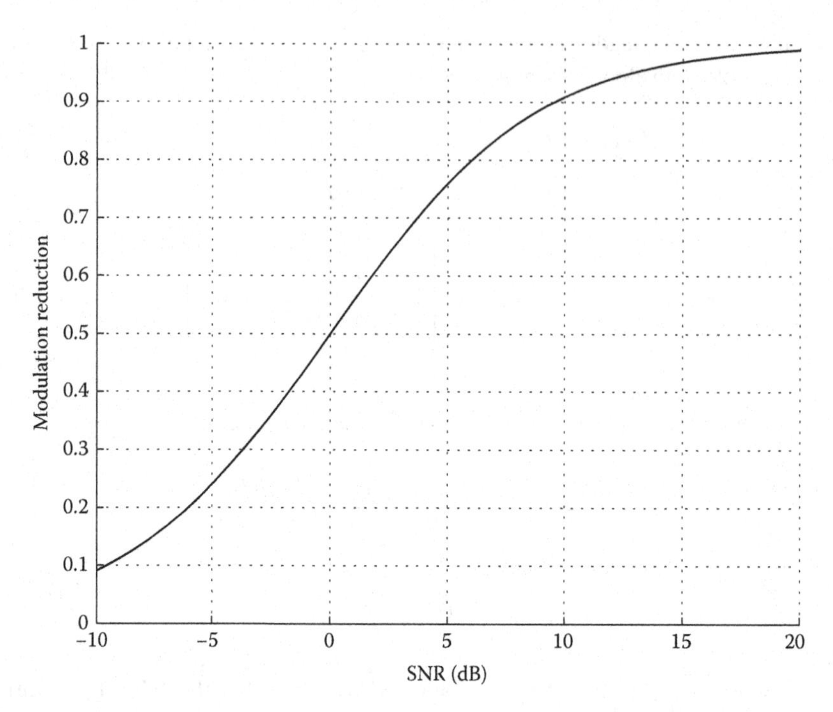

FIGURE 11.26 Modulation transfer function for additive noise conditions.

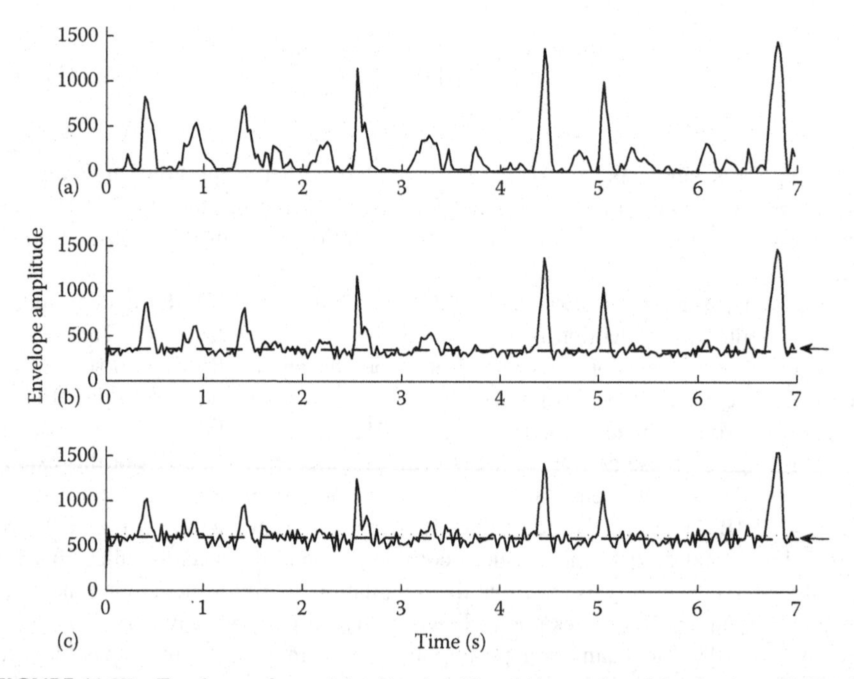

FIGURE 11.27 Envelopes of speech in: (a) quiet, (b) and (c) speech-weighted noise at SNR = 0 and −5 dB, respectively. Arrows point to the mean envelopes of the background noise.

Using Equation 11.104, we can infer the SNR level that produced the corresponding reduction in modulation. In doing so, we get $SNR_{dB} = -1.1$ dB, which is close to the true SNR of 0 dB (i.e., the true SNR at which the envelopes were created). Similarly, for the example in (SNR = −5 dB) Figure 11.27c, we have $I_{INP} + I_N = 632$, yielding a modulation index of 0.28. The inferred SNR (based on Equation 11.103) that produced this reduction in modulation is −4 dB. The earlier example demonstrated that the reduction in modulations, as quantified by the MTF, can tell us a great deal about the underlying SNR.

Additive noise is not the only external factor that could reduce modulations. Reverberation, if chosen appropriately, could also yield the same modulation index value m. That is, by solving for T in Equation 11.101, we can find the reverberation time (T) required to yield the equivalent reduction in modulation (m) for a given modulation frequency F. For instance, the reverberant condition wherein the modulation frequency is $F = 2.5$ Hz and the reverberation time is $T = 1.5$ s is just as detrimental (in terms of predicted intelligibility) as additive noise at SNR = 0 dB. This is so because both listening scenarios result in $m = 0.5$. Put differently, using Equations 11.101 and 11.104, one could find the reverberation time T that would yield the same intelligibility as that with speech corrupted by additive noise at an SNR level determined by Equation 11.104. In general, the m value obtained in any condition involving reverberation, noise or combination of the two, can be used to infer the *apparent* SNR, namely the SNR that would have resulted in that very same m value. This transformation of m values to SNR is a key step in the STI implementation.

11.4.2.2 Speech Modulation Spectrum

So far, we talked about typical modulation frequencies involved in the computation of the MTF, but have not elaborated on the range of frequencies to consider. A number of intelligibility studies determined the range of modulation frequencies important for SI [101–103]. Drullman et al. [101] assessed the effect of smearing the temporal envelope, via low-pass filtering, on speech recognition in noise. Speech was bandpass filtered into a number of bands (width of ½ to 1 octave) and the envelope of each band was low-pass filtered at several different cut-off frequencies ranging from 0.5 to 64 Hz. Severe reduction in intelligibility was observed when the envelopes were low-pass filtered at $f < 2$ Hz. Preserving modulation frequencies above 16 Hz did not improve further the intelligibility of speech in noise compared to the intelligibility of un-processed noisy speech. Overall, this study showed that modulation frequencies in the range of 2–16 Hz are important for SI and should be maintained by noise-reduction algorithms. Follow-up studies [102] assessed the effect of high-pass filtering the envelopes and intelligibility data showed that at 8–10 Hz the modulation spectrum can be divided into two equally intelligible parts. That is, analogous to the AI low-pass/high-pass filtering studies (see Section 11.4.1.1), the cross-over frequency of the modulation spectrum is at 8–10 Hz. Consistent with the outcome in [102], the study in [103] showed that high-pass filtering the envelopes at 12 Hz resulted in significant reduction in intelligibility.

Figure 11.28 shows the modulation spectrum of speech in quiet for a specific frequency band. This spectrum was computed as follows. Speech was filtered

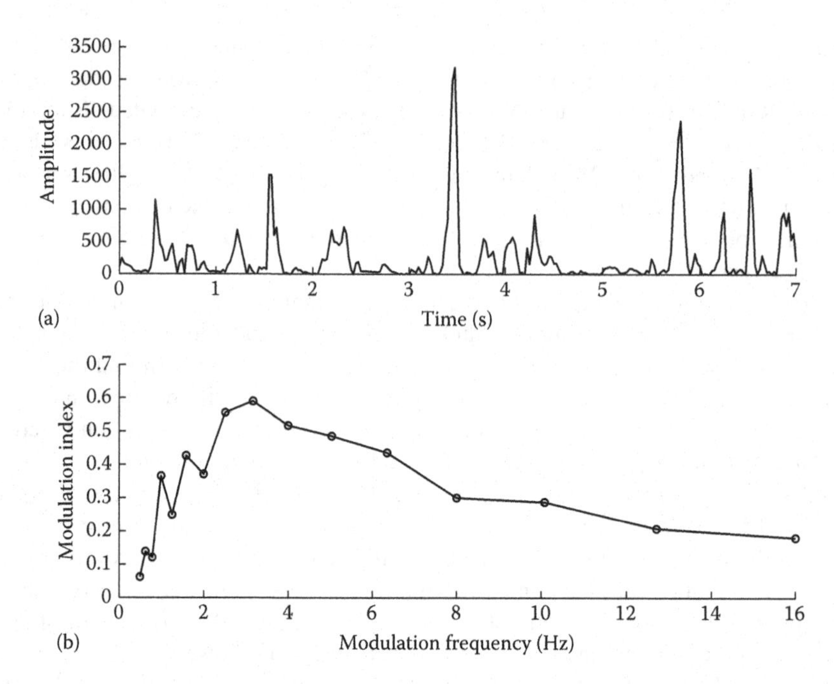

FIGURE 11.28 Panel (a) shows the speech envelope (in quiet) extracted at a band centered at 1300 Hz. Panel (b) shows the corresponding modulation spectrum.

into seven bands and the envelope of each band (see Figure 11.28a) was computed using the Hilbert transform (alternatively, the envelope could be computed by full-wave rectification and low-pass filtering). The envelope was down-sampled at 40 Hz and then filtered into 16 1/3-octave bands spanning the modulation frequency range of 0.5–16 Hz. The energy within each of the 16 bands was computed and normalized by the mean energy of the acoustic frequency band. Figure 11.28b shows the normalized modulation energies computed in each band, which taken together constitute the modulation spectrum. Note that there is a distinct peak at 3–4 Hz reflecting the rate at which syllables are produced in spoken English. Figure 11.29 shows the modulation spectra of speech-weighted noise. As can be seen, the modulation spectrum of the noise lacks the peak at 4 Hz. Higher modulation frequencies ($f > 10$ Hz) are also evident and that is not surprising given the high frequency fluctuations present in the envelope (see Figure 11.29a). Overall, the speech modulation spectrum is quite distinct from non-speech maskers. Figures 11.30 and 11.31 show, for comparative purposes, the modulation spectra of multi-talker babble and train respectively. In general, the shape of the modulation spectrum differs for different types of maskers. In fact, some hearing aids make use of this fact to discriminate between speech and non-speech sounds [104].

In brief, as shown by intelligibility studies, modulation frequencies in the range of 2–16 Hz play an important role on SI and this range is considered in the computation of the STI measure.

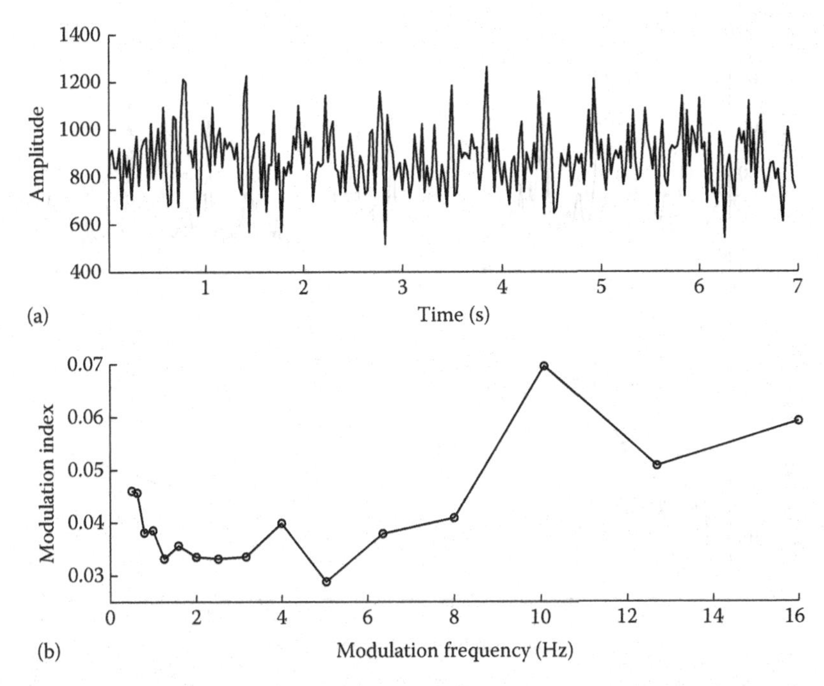

FIGURE 11.29 Panel (a) shows the envelope of speech-shaped noise extracted at a band centered at 1300 Hz. Panel (b) shows the corresponding modulation spectrum.

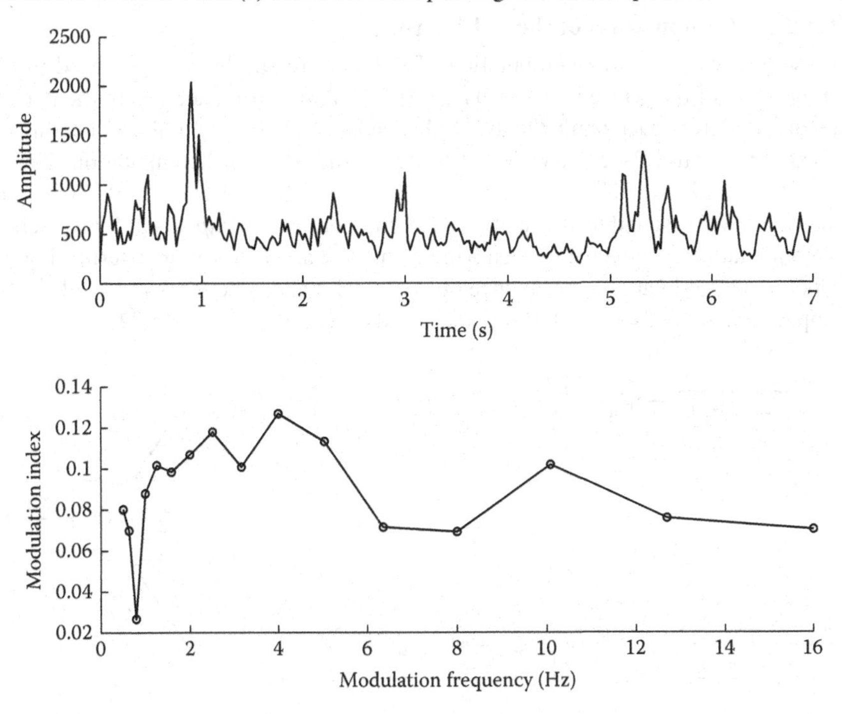

FIGURE 11.30 Envelope and modulation spectrum of babble.

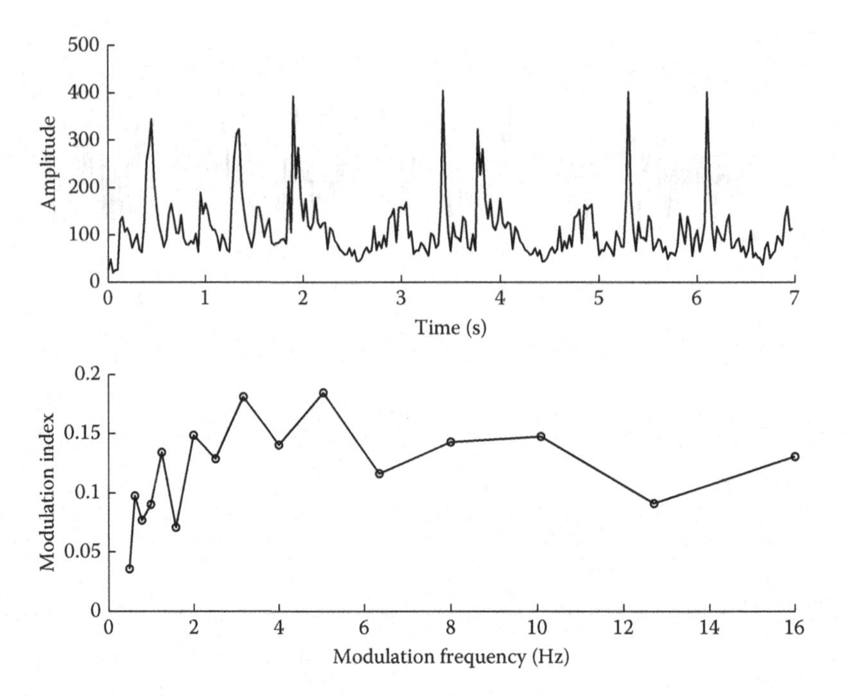

FIGURE 11.31 Envelope and modulation spectrum of train noise.

11.4.2.3 Computation of the STI Measure

The steps involved in the computation of the STI are similar to those used in the computation of the AI (see Section 11.4.1.4). The main difference lies in the derivation of the SNR in each band. Octave-wide bands are often used in the STI computation as opposed to 1/3-octave wide bands used in the AI (or SII) computation. The AI derives explicitly the SNR in each band as per Equation 11.71 whereas the STI computes the MTF first and uses Equation 11.104 to compute the *apparent* SNR. Hence, the computation of the SNR in each band is indirect and is based on determining the reduction of modulations in the envelopes of each band. The steps involved in STI computation are outlined as follows and are also shown in Figure 11.32.

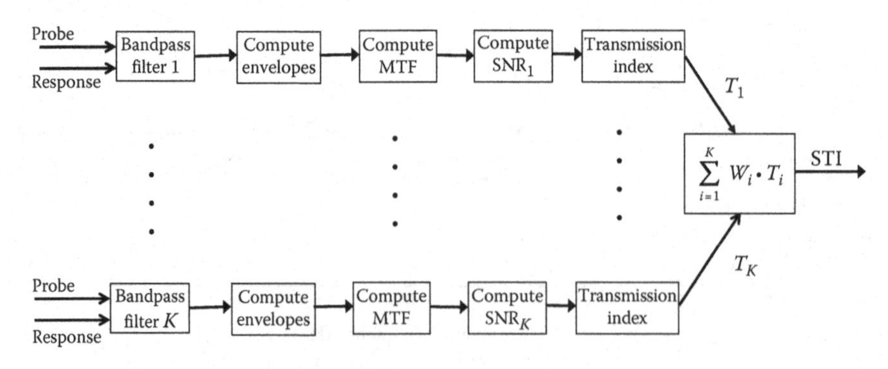

FIGURE 11.32 Steps used in the computation of the STI measure.

Step 1: Computation of band envelopes

The input (probe) and output (response) signals are first bandpass-filtered into a number of bands. (Note that in the original form of the STI [100], sinewave-modulated signals—see Equation 11.95—rather than speech signals were used as input signals.) Octave bands are often used with center frequencies spanning the range of 125–8000 Hz. The envelope of each acoustic frequency band is computed using either the Hilbert transform or via full-wave rectification and low-pass filtering. The cut-off of the low-pass filter is often set to encompass the range of modulation frequencies of interest (<16 Hz). In some studies, the envelopes are alternatively down-sampled to reduce the bandwidth and make it easier to design the modulation filters (in [105], the envelopes were down-sampled to 200 Hz while in [78] the envelopes were down-sampled to 25 Hz).

Step 2: Computation of MTF

The MTF is defined as the ratio of the modulation spectra of the input and output envelopes. The MTF can be viewed as the transfer function (in the modulation domain) of the transmission channel and can be computed as [102]

$$MTF(f) = \alpha\sqrt{\frac{P_{yy}(f)}{P_{xx}(f)}} \tag{11.105}$$

where

$\alpha = \mu_x/\mu_y$, μ_x and μ_y are the means of the input and output envelope signals respectively
$P_{xx}(f)$ and $P_{yy}(f)$ are the modulation spectra of the input and output envelopes, respectively [102]

The MTF is typically evaluated for modulation frequencies (f) ranging from $f = 0.63$ Hz to $f = 12.7$ Hz using 1/3-octave filter spacing. Note that a number of other methods have been proposed for deriving the MTF (see review and evaluation in [105]).

Step 3: Computation of SNR

The SNR in band i is computed for each modulation frequency f according to Equation 11.104, i.e.,

$$SNR_i(f) = 10\log_{10}\left(\frac{\text{MTF}(f)}{1-\text{MTF}(f)}\right) \tag{11.106}$$

Similar to Equation 11.72 used in the AI measure computation, the SNR is limited within the range of −15 to 15 dB, and then averaged across all modulation frequencies to produce the mean SNR in the ith band, denoted as $\overline{SNR_i}$.

Step 4: Computation of transmission index

The average SNR in each band is limited between 0 and 1 as follows:

$$\text{TI}_i = \frac{\overline{SNR_i} + 15}{30} \tag{11.107}$$

where TI denotes the transmission index.

Step 5: Computation of STI

Finally, the overall STI is computed as the weighted average of the TI values:

$$\text{STI} = \sum_{k=1}^{K} W_k \cdot TI_k \tag{11.108}$$

where

W_k are the band-importance weights (normalized so that their sum is 1)
K is the total number of bands

In [100], seven octave-wide bands (spanning 125–8000 Hz) were used with $W_k = [0.13, 0.14, 0.11, 0.12, 0.19, 0.17, 0.14]$.

The STI has been evaluated in a large number of conditions involving reverberation, noise, reverberation + noise, bandpass filtering, peak-clipping, and automatic gain control operations [99]. High correlations with intelligibility scores were obtained in all conditions (prediction error reported was smaller than 6%).

Equation 11.108 makes the implicit assumption that the K bands are independent. Modifications to the STI that relaxed this assumption were proposed in [106]. The STI term was computed as follows:

$$\text{STI} = \sum_{k=1}^{K} \alpha_k \cdot \text{TI}_k - \sum_{k=1}^{K-1} \beta_k \sqrt{\text{TI}_k \cdot \text{TI}_{k+1}} \tag{11.109}$$

where $K = 7$, α_k and β_k are coefficients determined from fitting the experimental data and satisfying the following relationship:

$$\sum_{k=1}^{K} \alpha_k - \sum_{k=1}^{K-1} \beta_k = 1 \tag{11.110}$$

The β_k coefficients are called the inter-band "redundancy correction factors" as they are designed to compensate for the fact that the information present in two adjacent bands might be redundant. Consequently, adding the corresponding transmission indices (TI) of the two bands might overestimate the true amount of information present, and for that reason, their contribution is subtracted. Better correlation with intelligibility was observed in [106] when the inter-band correction factors were included.

The STI, in its basic form, analyzes envelope modulations along the time dimension, derives from these temporal modulations the apparent SNR in each band and integrates the SNR information across the spectrum. A measure that analyzes temporal envelope and spectral modulations jointly, rather than separately, was proposed in [107]. This measure was grounded on neurophysiological data [108] and has been shown to be comparable to the traditional STI for additive noise and reverberation. The measure was found to perform better than the STI, for non-linear distortions (e.g., phase jitter and phase shifts) that are inseparable across the temporal and spectral dimensions.

Note that in the traditional STI method [99], the probe signal (Figure 11.32) is speech-shaped noise that has been bandpass filtered and intensity modulated at a particular modulation frequency. The probe signal is passed through the system to be evaluated and the change in modulation depth between the probe and response envelopes is measured for that particular modulation frequency. This process is repeated for other modulation frequencies to determine the complete MTF for a given frequency band. Alternatively, the artificial probe signals can be replaced with speech [102,109]. A number of studies [109,110] have shown, however, that when speech is used as the probe stimulus, artifacts are observed in the modulation spectra, particularly at the higher modulation frequencies. In the low-frequency octave bands of noisy and/or reverberant speech, the computed modulated spectra were found to be distorted at the higher modulation frequencies (>10 Hz) as reflected by elevated modulation values. These increases in modulation values were inconsistent with the theoretical values (Equations 11.101 and 11.103) and could thus affect the computation of the MTF, and subsequently the STI. Methods to reduce these artifacts were proposed in [109], and were based on identifying (using the coherence metric) the set of modulation frequencies to include in the STI computation. For the aforementioned reasons, some STI-based measures avoid the computation of the MTF altogether, and one such a measure is described next.

11.4.2.4 Normalized-Covariance Measure

The normalized-covariance measure (NCM) [111] is one of several speech-based STI measures reviewed and compared in [105]. It is called a speech-based STI measure because it uses speech as a probe signal rather than the sinewave-modulated signal given in Equation 11.95. As mentioned earlier, it does not use the MTF to compute the SNR in each band, but rather uses the covariance between the input (probe) and output (response) envelope signals, i.e.,

$$r_i = \frac{\sum_t (x_i(t) - \mu_i) \cdot (y_i(t) - \nu_i)}{\sqrt{\sum_t (x_i(t) - \mu_i)^2} \cdot \sqrt{\sum_t (y_i(t) - \nu_i)^2}} \tag{11.111}$$

where μ_i and ν_i are the mean values of the input ($x_i(t)$) and output ($y_i(t)$) envelopes respectively in the ith band. The values of r_i fall within the range of $-1 \le r_i \le 1$. The apparent SNR in each band is computed as

$$\overline{SNR_i} = 10 \log_{10} \left(\frac{r_i^2}{1 - r_i^2} \right) \tag{11.112}$$

and limited between −15 and 15 dB. Following the SNR computation, the STI is computed as discussed before using Equations 11.107 and 11.108. That is, the transmission index (TI) in each band is computed by linearly mapping the limited (within −15 to 15 dB) $\overline{SNR_i}$ values between 0 and 1 using the following equation:

$$\text{TI}_i = \frac{\overline{SNR_i} + 15}{30} \tag{11.113}$$

Finally, the transmission indices are averaged across all frequency bands to produce the NCM index:

$$\text{NCM} = \frac{1}{\sum_{i=1}^{K} W_i} \sum_{i=1}^{K} W_i \cdot \text{TI}_i \tag{11.114}$$

where W_i are the band-importance weights applied to each of the K bands. Comparing Equation 11.112 with the equation used in the STI computation (Equation 11.106), we observe that the two equations bear the same form. It is clear from Equation 11.112, that the higher the correlation (covariance) is between the clean and processed (or noisy) envelopes, the higher the SNR. Note that the correlation is performed using envelopes containing limited modulations (<16 Hz) known to be important for SI.

The covariance equation (Equation 11.111) is no other than the equation of the Pearson's correlation coefficient between two data vectors. The Pearson's correlation coefficient has many attractive properties that can be exploited for the analysis and derivation of optimal and sub-optimal gain functions [112,113]. It can be used, for instance, to quantify speech and noise distortions based on its relationship with the input SNR. Assume that the observed time-domain noisy signal, $y(n)$, is given by

$$y(n) = x(n) + d(n) \tag{11.115}$$

where

$x(n)$ is the clean speech signal
$d(n)$ is the additive noise, both of which are zero mean

The Pearson's square correlation between vectors $\mathbf{x}$ and $\mathbf{y}$, denoted as $r^2(\mathbf{x}, \mathbf{y})$, is given by

$$\begin{aligned} r^2(\mathbf{x},\mathbf{y}) &= \frac{E^2(\mathbf{x}^T\mathbf{y})}{E(\mathbf{x}^T\mathbf{x})E(\mathbf{y}^T\mathbf{y})} \\ &= \frac{E^2[\mathbf{x}^T(\mathbf{x}+\mathbf{d})]}{E(\mathbf{x}^T\mathbf{x})E(\mathbf{y}^T\mathbf{y})} \\ &= \frac{\sigma_x^2}{\sigma_y^2} = \frac{\sigma_x^2}{\sigma_x^2 + \sigma_d^2} \\ &= \frac{SNR}{SNR+1} \end{aligned} \tag{11.116}$$

where $\sigma_x^2 = E(\mathbf{x}^T\mathbf{x})$ and $SNR \triangleq \sigma_x^2 / \sigma_d^2$. In the aforesaid equation, we made use of the fact that the input speech signal (**x**) and noise (**d**) are uncorrelated (and zero mean). Solving for the SNR term in Equation 11.116 yields Equation 11.112, which is used in the NCM measure. Note that the envelopes in Equation 11.111 are always positive and have non-zero mean, but became zero mean after subtracting their mean. The said relationship (Equation 11.116) is very important as it tells us that one can use the degree of correlation between two signals (which are related according to Equation 11.115) to infer the underlying SNR (note that Equation 11.116 denotes the SNR in the time-domain and not in the frequency domain). The relationship discussed here also holds in the frequency domain and is derived later in Section 11.4.3 when describing the coherence measure.

The NCM has been evaluated extensively in a number of studies [114–118]. It has been shown to correlate highly with the intelligibility of vocoded speech [116] (used to simulate speech processed via a cochlear implant) as well as the intelligibility of Mandarin Chinese [117]. A low-frequency version of the NCM which encompasses only bands in the low frequency region (<1000 Hz) was shown in [78] to yield nearly the same correlation as the NCM implementation that used all bands. In fact, high correlation was maintained even when only one band (e.g., band 1) was used in the implementation of NCM [115]. Plotting the NCM correlations obtained when a single band (out of a total of 20 bands) is used at a time in the computation of the NCM measure reveals a masker-specific pattern, referred to as the *r*-pattern [115]. Figure 11.33 shows

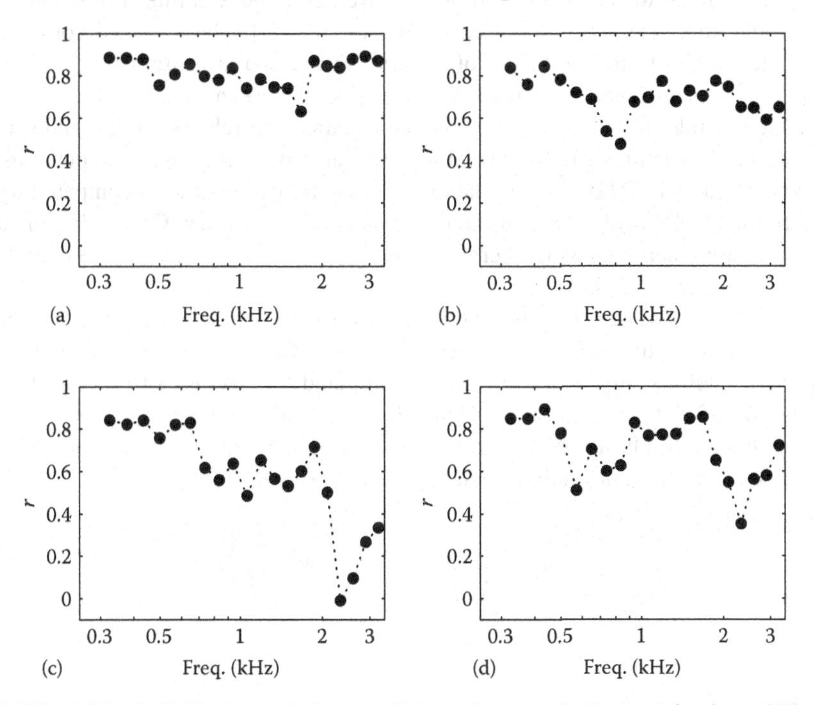

FIGURE 11.33 Individual correlation coefficients (*r-pattern*) obtained for four different maskers tested using a modified NCM measure when only one band is used a time. (a) Babble, (b) car, (c) street, and (d) train. (From Chen, F. and Loizou, P., *J. Acoust. Soc. Am.*, 128(6), 3715, 2010. With permission.)

the r-patterns for the four maskers tested in [115]. The frequency location of the dips in the r-pattern identifies inconsistencies (or perhaps differences) in the way the noise suppression algorithm(s) affects (e.g., distorts) different bands (regions) of the spectrum. These inconsistencies are caused by the fact that some bands are severely distorted while other bands are effectively "cleaned" by the noise-suppression algorithm. In the r-pattern shown in Figure 11.33, bands with high correlation indicate consistent performance with overall intelligibility scores, and one can view those bands as being representative of overall performance. As such, when the TI, or equivalently the effective SNR, is high in those bands, intelligibility is high, and when the TI is low in those bands, intelligibility is low. In contrast, bands with low correlation are likely affected differently by the noise-suppression algorithm (compared to the other bands), and in a way that is inconsistent with the overall intelligibility score. For instance, the dip in the r-pattern (band 8) of car noise suggests that the corresponding band (8) has been severely distorted by car noise and reflects the inability of the enhancement algorithm in suppressing the noise at that band (see [115, Fig. 4f]). Hence, the r-pattern can be used as a diagnostic tool for assessing algorithms in as far as determining the degree at which they can effectively suppress noise in certain regions of the spectrum.

The NCM uses the whole utterance to compute the correlation between the clean and processed envelopes in each band. Measures, similar to NCM, which compute the correlation between clean and processed envelopes in relatively shorter intervals (ranging from 20 to 384 ms in duration) and averaging the resulting correlations over the whole utterance, were proposed in [95,114,118–121]. The averaged correlation, computed across frames or blocks of frames, is used as a measure for predicting SI. In [95,121], for instance, the (squared) correlation of 20-band excitation spectra was computed using 20 ms frames. In [119], the (squared) correlation of 32-band excitation spectra, which have been normalized by their rms energy, was computed using 25.6 ms frames. In [114], the correlations of excitation spectra were computed using 192-frame blocks, with 32 ms duration frames and 75% overlap. Combining the correlation-based measures with other measures has proven to improve the correlation of a composite measure [95,114].

In [118], a measure was proposed that used 384 ms long blocks containing excitation spectra of the clean and processed signals. This measure, called short-time objective intelligibility measure (STOI), computed the average of the correlations across all 1/3-octave bands and 384 ms blocks and used the average correlation to predict the intelligibility scores. Prior to the computation of the correlation, the processed envelope was normalized and clipped as follows:

$$\bar{\mathbf{y}} = \min\left(\frac{\|\mathbf{x}\|_2}{\|\mathbf{y}\|_2}\mathbf{y}, (1-10^{-\beta/20})\cdot\mathbf{x}\right) \tag{11.117}$$

where

$\beta = -15\,\text{dB}$

$\mathbf{x}$ denotes the clean envelope vector (accumulated over 384 ms frames)

$\mathbf{y}$ denotes the processed envelope vector

$\|\cdot\|_2$ denotes the 2-norm of the vector

The clipping operation (as controlled by the parameter β) is effective primarily in noise-only regions and is thus used to de-emphasize the importance or impact of those regions on SI. The STOI measure yielded high correlations with intelligibility data, particularly with speech processed by the ideal binary mask algorithm (see description in Chapter 13).

11.4.2.5 Limitations of STI Measures

When speech is subjected to non-linear processes such as those introduced by speech-enhancement algorithms or dynamic envelope compression (or expansion) in hearing aids, the STI measure fails to successfully predict SI since the processing itself might introduce additional modulations which the STI measure interprets as increased SNR [105,122,123]. The STI measure, for instance, has failed to predict the lack of intelligibility benefit with spectral-subtractive algorithms. Ludvigsen et al. [123] have shown that in spite of the increased speech modulations and increase in STI values, the intelligibility of signals processed via the spectral-subtractive algorithm is not better than that of unprocessed signals. The lack of intelligibility improvement with spectral-subtractive algorithms has also been confirmed by numerous other studies (e.g., [90])—see Chapter 12.

For illustration purposes, Figure 11.34c shows the envelopes of speech processed by the spectral subtraction (SS) algorithm. For this example, speech (consisting of three concatenated IEEE sentences) was corrupted at 5 dB SNR with speech-shaped noise and

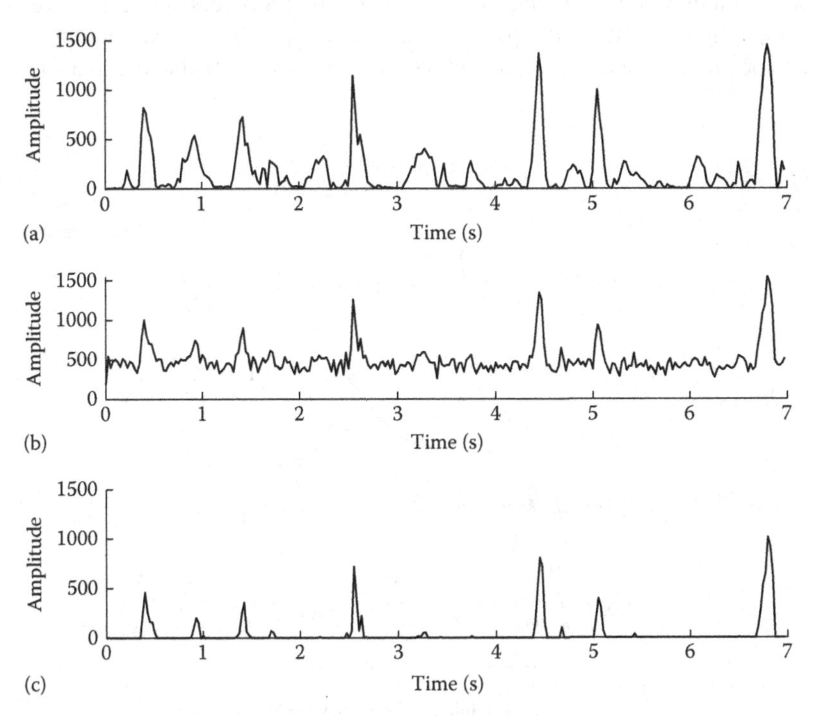

FIGURE 11.34 Panel (a) shows the envelopes (at $f = 800$ Hz) of speech in quiet. Panel (b) shows the envelopes of speech in SSN at 5 dB SNR. Panel (c) shows the envelopes obtained after spectral subtraction.

bandpass filtered into a number of bands. Figure 11.34 shows the envelopes of the clean signal envelope (Figure 11.34a), noisy envelope (Figure 11.34b), and SS-processed envelope (Figure 11.34c), computed using the Hilbert transform, for a band centered at 800 Hz. The spectral subtraction was implemented using the following envelope gain function:

$$G_k = \max\left(0, 1 - k \cdot \frac{\overline{N}_k^2}{Y_k^2}\right) \tag{11.118}$$

where

k is the over-subtraction factor ($k = 1.1$ for this example)
$\overline{N}_k$ is the mean intensity of the noise floor ($\overline{N}_k = 500$ for example in Figure 11.34) in band k
Y_k is the noisy envelope in band k

The subtraction operation removes for the most part the mean intensity (DC) of the background noise and shifts the overall envelope amplitude down to 0. The dominant envelope peaks are preserved (e.g., see peaks at $t = 2.5$, 4.5, and 6.8 s), but the smaller peaks (e.g., see peaks at $t = 2.2$, 3.2, and 6 s) are eliminated. Compared to the reduced modulations present in the noisy envelope (Figure 11.34b), the modulations present in the SS-processed envelope seem to be increased. Put differently, the peak-to-trough ratio greatly improves following the SS processing. This is verified by computing the modulation spectra of these envelopes. The corresponding modulation spectra are shown in Figure 11.35. As can be seen the modulation index of

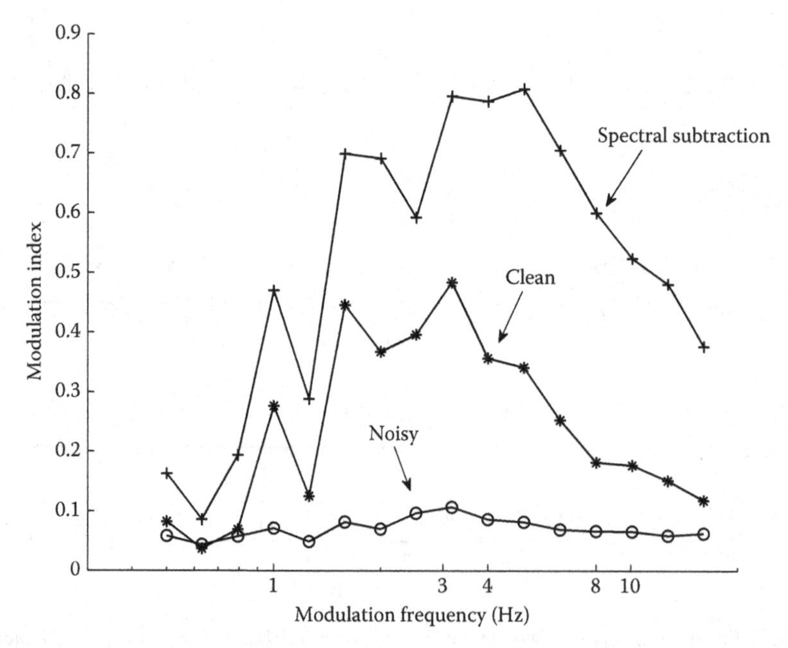

FIGURE 11.35 Modulation spectra of clean speech, noisy speech, and speech processed via spectral subtraction.

the SS-processed envelopes increases. In fact, it is larger than the modulation index of the clean envelopes. According to STI theory, the intelligibility of SS-processed speech ought to improve, since a higher modulation index implies a higher SNR and consequently a higher STI value. In reality, however, the SS processing does not improve intelligibility and this has been confirmed by a number of studies (see Chapter 12). In summary, the STI measure cannot predict the intelligibility of speech that has been subjected to non-linear processing, such as that of spectral subtraction (see Equation 11.118). The reason for that is the non-linear processing itself introduces additional modulations which the STI measure interprets as increased SNR.

A number of techniques [78,105,124,125] have been proposed to circumvent the earlier limitation. Dubbelboer and Houtgast [124] proposed a method for measuring the SNR in the modulation domain using a new test (probe) signal. The new test signal comprised of speech with a "hole" in the modulation spectrum at 4 Hz. The new signal, called "peephole" speech, was generated by band-stop filtering the temporal envelope at 4 Hz. The modulation spectrum of this signal is similar to that of clean speech except for one band (centered at 4 Hz), which is completely suppressed. When noise is added to this signal, each band in the modulation spectrum shows a reduction of speech modulations as expected (see for example Figure 11.27). The peephole band (4 Hz), however, shows an increase in modulations with increasing noise level. The modulations in the peephole band were referred to as the modulation floor reflecting the spurious modulations introduced after mixing noise and speech signals. These spurious modulations contain noise modulations and modulations originating from the interaction of the speech and noise envelopes, analogous to the interaction terms produced when adding the magnitude spectra of speech and noise (see Equation 5.20). When spectral subtraction is applied to the noisy speech envelopes, the speech modulations increase along with the modulation floor in the peephole band (4 Hz). This suggests that the ratio of speech modulations to spurious modulations remains unchanged, a favorable outcome consistent with the lack of intelligibility improvement with spectral subtraction. For that reason, the signal-to-noise ratio in the modulation domain, denoted as $(\mathrm{S/N})_{\mathrm{mod}}$, was defined in [124] as the ratio of the strength of speech modulations to spurious modulations. The term $(\mathrm{S/N})_{\mathrm{mod}}$ was proposed as a substitute of the SNR term in the STI measure. Estimating or delineating the spurious modulations from noisy envelopes is, however, difficult in practice. The modified STI, based on $(\mathrm{S/N})_{\mathrm{mod}}$, was not tested or validated with intelligibility scores, hence it remains to be seen whether the modified STI measure would predict the intelligibility of SS-processed speech.

A different method was proposed in [125] for computing the SNR in the modulation domain. This was done by computing the envelope power of noisy speech (P_{S+N}) and that of the noise alone (P_N) for each modulation band and then forming the modulation SNR ratio ($\mathrm{SNR}_{\mathrm{mod}}$) as

$$\mathrm{SNR}_{\mathrm{mod}} = \frac{P_{S+N} - P_N}{P_N} \tag{11.119}$$

Unlike [124], the interaction modulations are not included in the computation as they are assumed to have a negligible influence on intelligibility. The $\mathrm{SNR}_{\mathrm{mod}}$ is summed across all modulation bands and acoustic frequency bands resulting in the overall $\overline{SNR}_{\mathrm{mod}}$. This in turn is converted to a sensitivity index, d', using the relation

$$d' = k \cdot \left(\overline{SNR}_{\mathrm{mod}}\right)^{q} \tag{11.120}$$

where k and q are constants determined experimentally. Finally, the value of d' is converted to percent correct responses using an m-alternative forced choice (mAFC) model [126] ("ideal observer model") as follows:

$$P_{\mathrm{correct}}(d') = \Phi\left(\frac{d' - \mu_N}{\sqrt{\sigma_S^2 + \sigma_N^2}}\right) \tag{11.121}$$

where

P_{correct} is the predicted intelligibility score

Φ is the cumulative Gaussian distribution

μ_N and σ_N are determined by the response-set size (m) of the speech material

σ_S is a free parameter accounting for the redundancy of speech material (e.g., meaningful sentences have high redundancy while monosyllabic words have low redundancy)

Note that the shape of the cumulative Gaussian distribution is sigmoidal (see [127, Fig. 1]), and similar to the transfer functions shown in Figure 11.19 for mapping AI values to percent correct scores. In the mAFC model [126,128, p. 69], the ideal observer is assumed to compare the input speech item against m stored alternatives and select the one with the highest similarity to the input speech pattern (the $m - 1$ remaining items are assumed to contain noise). A similar mAFC model was also used in [127]. The aforementioned intelligibility measure was tested with speech in noise and reverberation as well as speech subjected to spectral subtraction [125]. High correlations ($r > 0.98$) with human intelligibility scores were obtained in nearly all conditions, including SS-processed speech.

The measure proposed in [125] was only tested with noisy speech processed by a basic spectral subtraction algorithm. The non-linear distortions introduced by various speech enhancement algorithms, however, differ across various algorithms. The study by Ma et al. [78] evaluated the performance of the NCM measure using speech processed via eight different speech enhancement algorithms, which included spectral-subtractive algorithms, subspace algorithms, and statistical-model based (e.g., MMSE) algorithms. High correlation ($r = 0.89$) with intelligibility scores was obtained with the NCM when signal-dependent BIFs were used in Equation 11.108 in place of the ANSI BIFs.

11.4.3 Coherence-Based Index

The STI measures utilize the reduction in envelope modulations to derive the apparent SNR in each band (e.g., see Equation 11.106). In contrast, the coherence-based measures make use of the coherence between the clean and noisy (or processed) signals to derive the SNR in each band.

11.4.3.1 Theory

Consider the noisy spectrum $Y(\omega)$ defined as

$$Y(\omega) = X(\omega) + N(\omega) \tag{11.122}$$

where $X(\omega)$ and $N(\omega)$ denote the (complex) spectra of the clean and noise signals respectively. The magnitude-squared coherence (MSC) between $Y(\omega)$ and $X(\omega)$ is given by

$$|\gamma_{XY}(\omega)|^2 = \frac{|P_{XY}(\omega)|^2}{P_{XX}(\omega)P_{YY}(\omega)} \tag{11.123}$$

where $P_{XY}(\omega) = E[X(\omega)Y^*(\omega)]$ is the cross power spectrum density between the zero-mean stationary signals $x(n)$ and $y(n)$ with power spectrum densities $P_{XY}(\omega)$ and $P_{YY}(\omega)$, respectively. The MSC has the following properties [129]:

1. The MSC is real and takes values between 0 and 1.
2. The MSC between two signals is not affected when processing these signals through a linear system. That is, if $Y_1(\omega) = H_1(\omega)Y(\omega)$ and $X_1(\omega) = H_2(\omega)X(\omega)$, for some linear systems described by $H_1(\omega)$ and $H_2(\omega)$, then we have $|\gamma_{X_1Y_1}(\omega)|^2 = |\gamma_{XY}(\omega)|^2$.
3. The MSC of two signals which are scaled with respect to one another is unity. That is, if $Y(\omega) = c\,X(\omega)$, for some constant c, then $|\gamma_{XY}(\omega)|^2 = 1$.

Yet, another property of the MSC is its relationship with the SNR and this is proven next. Following the derivation of the Wiener filter in Equation 6.36 and after assuming that the speech signal and noise are uncorrelated, it is easy to show that $P_{XY}(\omega) = P_{XX}(\omega)$ (Equation 6.34) and $P_{YY}(\omega) = P_{XX}(\omega) + P_{NN}(\omega)$ (Equation 6.35). Substituting the latter expressions into Equation 11.123, we get

$$\begin{aligned} |\gamma_{XY}(\omega)|^2 &= \frac{P_{XX}(\omega)^2}{P_{XX}(\omega)[P_{XX}(\omega) + P_{NN}(\omega)]} \\ &= \frac{P_{XX}(\omega)}{P_{XX}(\omega) + P_{NN}(\omega)} \\ &= \frac{SNR(\omega)}{SNR(\omega) + 1} \end{aligned} \tag{11.124}$$

where $SNR(\omega) = P_{XX}(\omega)/P_{NN}(\omega)$. After solving for $SNR(\omega)$ in the said equation, we get

$$SNR(\omega) = \frac{|\gamma_{XY}(\omega)|^2}{1 - |\gamma_{XY}(\omega)|^2} \tag{11.125}$$

This equation clearly shows how one can use the coherence function to estimate the SNR at each frequency bin.

The relationship (Equation 11.125) between SNR and coherence holds exactly assuming that the noisy speech signal has not been processed by a speech enhancement algorithm. As such, the said equation is not useful when the corrupted speech is not processed as it does not reflect the effects of noise-reduction on SI (note that the enhanced spectrum is not included in the equation). Suppose now that the noisy speech spectrum $Y(\omega)$ is processed by a speech-enhancement algorithm producing the enhanced (complex) spectrum $\hat{X}(\omega)$. Let us express the enhanced spectrum $\hat{X}(\omega)$ as

$$\hat{X}(\omega) = X(\omega) + R(\omega) \tag{11.126}$$

where $R(\omega)$ denotes the residual spectrum reflecting inaccuracies in the estimation of the clean signal spectrum. Let us compute the MSC between $X(\omega)$ and $\hat{X}(\omega)$. Assuming that $X(\omega)$ and $R(\omega)$ are uncorrelated (and zero mean), we get [95]

$$\begin{aligned} |\gamma_{X \cdot \hat{X}}(\omega)|^2 &= \frac{P_{XX}(\omega)^2}{P_{XX}(\omega)[P_{XX}(\omega) + P_{RR}(\omega)]} \\ &= \frac{P_{XX}(\omega)}{P_{XX}(\omega) + P_{RR}(\omega)} \\ &= \frac{SNR_{ESI}(\omega)}{SNR_{ESI}(\omega) + 1} \end{aligned} \tag{11.127}$$

where $SNR_{ESI}(\omega) \triangleq P_{XX}(\omega)/P_{RR}(\omega)$ denotes the SigNal-to-RESIdual (SNR_{ESI}) spectrum ratio, which can be explicitly written as

$$SNR_{ESI}(\omega) = \frac{E\left[|X(\omega)|^2\right]}{E\left[|R(\omega)|^2\right]} \frac{E\left[|X(\omega)|^2\right]}{E\left[|X(\omega) - \hat{X}(\omega)|^2\right]} \tag{11.128}$$

Solving for SNR_{ESI} in Equation 11.127, we get

$$SNR_{ESI}(\omega) = \frac{|\gamma_{X \cdot \hat{X}}(\omega)|^2}{1 - |\gamma_{X \cdot \hat{X}}(\omega)|^2} \tag{11.129}$$

Hence, the MSC between the processed (enhanced) signal and the clean speech signal is related to the SNR_{ESI} rather than the SNR. It is the SNR_{ESI} term that is used in the computation of the coherence-based index [96]. Note that the short-term version of SNR_{ESI} is the frequency-weighted segmental SNR (fwSNRseg) measure described in Equation 11.44. The SNR_{ESI} term is referred to as the signal-to-distortion ratio in [96] since the denominator in Equation 11.128 quantifies to some extent the distortion incurred by the processing algorithm. Note that the denominator does not differentiate between positive and negative distortions since it is squared (see discussion in [92,114]). An effective intelligibility measure that decouples the positive and negative distortions was proposed in [114].

It is interesting to note that if the corrupted speech signal is not processed via a noise suppression algorithm, we have $SNR_{ESI}(\omega) = \text{SNR}(\omega)$. This can be easily proven by letting $\hat{X}(\omega) = Y(\omega)$ in Equation 11.128. Alternatively, if the corrupted signal is processed by a gain function such that $\hat{X}(\omega) = G(\omega) \cdot Y(\omega)$ and $G(\omega) = 1$ (for most algorithms, $G(\omega) = 1$ in high-SNR segments), then we also have $SNR_{ESI}(\omega) = \text{SNR}(\omega)$. More generally, when $0 \leq G(\omega) < 1$ (the region where most enhancement algorithms operate), $SNR_{ESI}(\omega)$ is related to $\text{SNR}(\omega)$ as follows [130]:

$$SNR_{ESI}(\omega) = \frac{SNR(\omega)}{[1 - G(\omega)]^2 \; SNR(\omega) + G^2(\omega)} \tag{11.130}$$

Figure 11.36 plots $SNR_{ESI}(\omega)$ as a function of $\text{SNR}(\omega)$ for fixed values of $G(\omega)$. As can be seen, SNR_{ESI} provides a biased estimate of SNR (except when $G(\omega) = 1$).

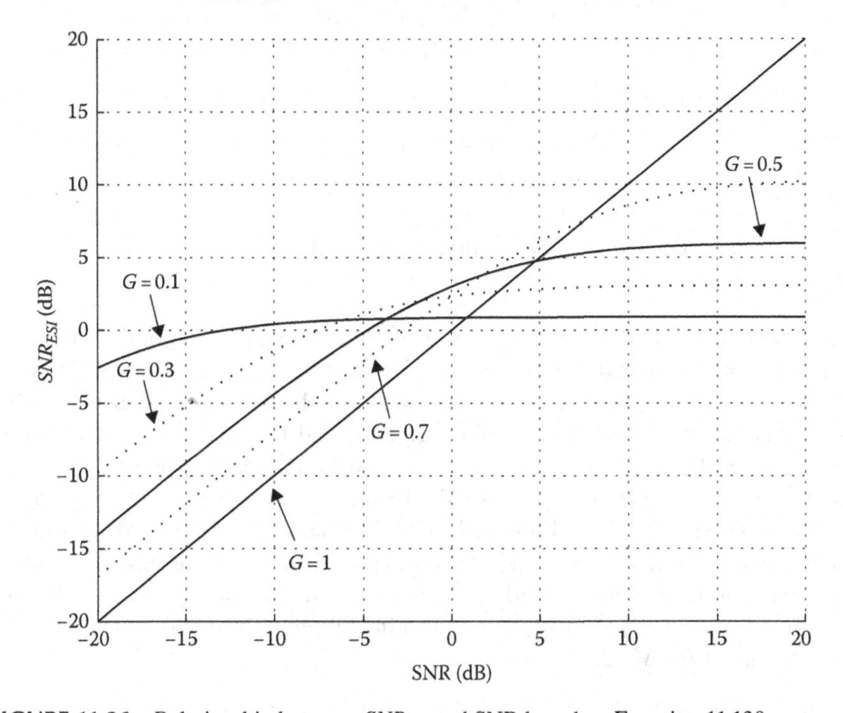

FIGURE 11.36 Relationship between SNR_{ESI} and SNR based on Equation 11.130.

The amount of bias depends largely on the value of the gain function $G(\omega)$. Larger bias is obtained as $G(\omega) \to 0$ and the bias gets progressively smaller as $G(\omega) \to 1$. The $SNR_{ESI}(\omega)$ has been shown in [92] to provide useful insights regarding spectral distortions induced by noise-suppressive gain functions (for more thorough discussion, see Chapter 13).

In summary, the MSC between the clean and processed spectra depends on SNR_{ESI} (see Equation 11.127), which is in turn related to SNR (see Equation 11.130) assuming that the processed spectra can be written as $\hat{X}(\omega) = G(\omega) \cdot Y(\omega)$.

11.4.3.2 Implementation of MSC

Implementation of MSC in Equation 11.123 requires the application of expectation operations and assumes stationary signals. In practice, the MSC can be computed by dividing the input (clean) and output (processed) signals in a number (M) of windowed segments (that may be overlapping), computing the cross power spectrum for each segment using the FFT, and then averaging across all segments. For M data segments (frames), the MSC at frequency bin ω is given by

$$|\gamma_{XY}(\omega)|^2 = \widehat{MSC}(\omega) = \frac{\left|\sum_{m=1}^{M} X_m(\omega)\, Y_m^*(\omega)\right|^2}{\sum_{m=1}^{M} |X_m(\omega)|^2 \cdot \sum_{m=1}^{M} |Y_m(\omega)|^2} \tag{11.131}$$

where

$\widehat{MSC}(\omega)$ denotes the estimated MSC
$X_m(\omega)$ and $Y_m(\omega)$ denote the FFT spectra of the clean ($x(t)$) and corrupted ($y(t)$) signals respectively computed in the mth frame

Note that if $M = 1$ in the said equation, $\widehat{MSC}(\omega) = 1$ independent of the true value of MSC, suggesting that the estimate is biased. A thorough analysis of the MSC estimate was carried out in [129] and revealed that the bias and variance of $\widehat{MSC}$ are a function of M (number of data segments) and the true MSC values. More precisely, the bias and variance were found to be inversely proportional to the number of available data segments (M). Increasing the overlap between frames increases the value of M and thus reduces the variance and bias of MSC. In [78], for instance, the $\widehat{MSC}$ was computed by segmenting the sentences using 30 ms duration Hamming windows with 75% overlap between adjacent frames. The use of a large frame overlap (>50%) was shown in [129] to reduce bias and variance in the estimate of the MSC.

Another form of bias in the estimate of the MSC is the time-delay or misalignment between the two signals. Methods for compensating the time-delay induced bias in MSC were proposed in [131].

11.4.3.3 Computation of the CSII Measure

The MSC, computed using the procedure described earlier, was incorporated in a measure for assessing the effects of hearing-aid distortions (e.g., peak clipping) on SI by normal-hearing and hearing-impaired subjects [96]. The new measure, called coherence SII (CSII), used the SII index as the base measure, and replaced the SNR term with the SNR_{ESI} (or signal-to-distortion ratio) term, i.e., Equation 11.129. That is, the SNR term in Equation 11.71 was replaced with the following expression:

$$SNR_{ESI}(j,m) = 10 \cdot \log_{10} \frac{\sum_{k=1}^{N} G_j(\omega_k) \cdot \widehat{MSC}(\omega_k) \cdot |Y_m(\omega_k)|^2}{\sum_{k=1}^{N} G_j(\omega_k) \cdot \left[1 - \widehat{MSC}(\omega_k)\right] \cdot |Y_m(\omega_k)|^2} \tag{11.132}$$

where

$G_j(\omega)$ denotes the ro-ex filter [132] centered around the jth critical band

$\widehat{MSC}(\omega)$ is given by Equation 11.131

$Y_m(\omega_k)$ is the FFT spectrum of the enhanced (or noisy) signal in the mth frame

N is the FFT size

Note that the main difference between the aforementioned equation and Equation 11.129 is that the latter equation computes the SNR_{ESI} for every frequency bin whereas Equation 11.132 computes the SNR_{ESI} for every critical band (the operation $\sum_k G_j(\omega_k) \cdot |Y_m(\omega_k)|^2$ simply integrates the power within the jth band). The ro-ex filters provide approximations to the auditory filters and can be computed using the following equation [132]:

$$G_j(f) = (1 + p_j\, g)e^{-p_j g} \tag{11.133}$$

where

$p_j = 4000 \cdot q_j/b_j$

$g = |1 - f/q_j|$

b_j is the bandwidth

q_j is the center frequency of the jth band

Figure 11.37 shows the frequency response of ro-ex filters assuming mel-frequency spacing and 16 bands.

The SNR_{ESI} term (Equation 11.132) is limited to [−15, 15] dB and is mapped linearly between 0 and 1 (similar to Figure 11.21) to produce a new term denoted

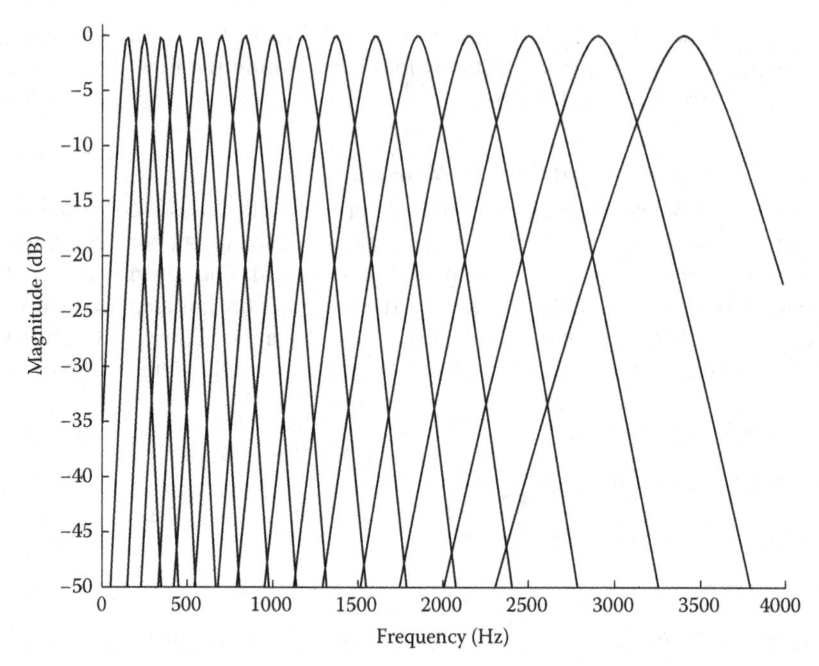

FIGURE 11.37 Frequency response of ro-ex filters.

as $T_{CSII}(j, m)$. The latter term is finally used in the computation of the CSII value as follows:

$$\text{CSII} = \frac{1}{M}\sum_{m=0}^{M-1}\frac{\sum_{j=1}^{K} W(j)\cdot T_{CSII}(j,m)}{\sum_{j=1}^{K} W(j)} \tag{11.134}$$

where

K is the number of bands spanning the signal bandwidth
$W(j)$ is the band-importance function

The aforesaid CSII measure is computed using all M frames of the utterance placing equal emphasis on all segments including vowels, consonants and vowel/consonant transitions. Computing separately the CSII measure for different phonetic segments (i.e., vowels vs. weak consonants) was found to increase the correlation of CSII with intelligibility scores [96].

11.4.3.4 Computation of the Three-Level CSII

Three CSII-based measures were derived in [96] by first dividing the M speech segments into three level regions, and computing separately the CSII measure for each region. Let us denote the overall root-mean-square (rms) level (in dB) of the whole utterance as RMS. The high-level region consisted of segments at

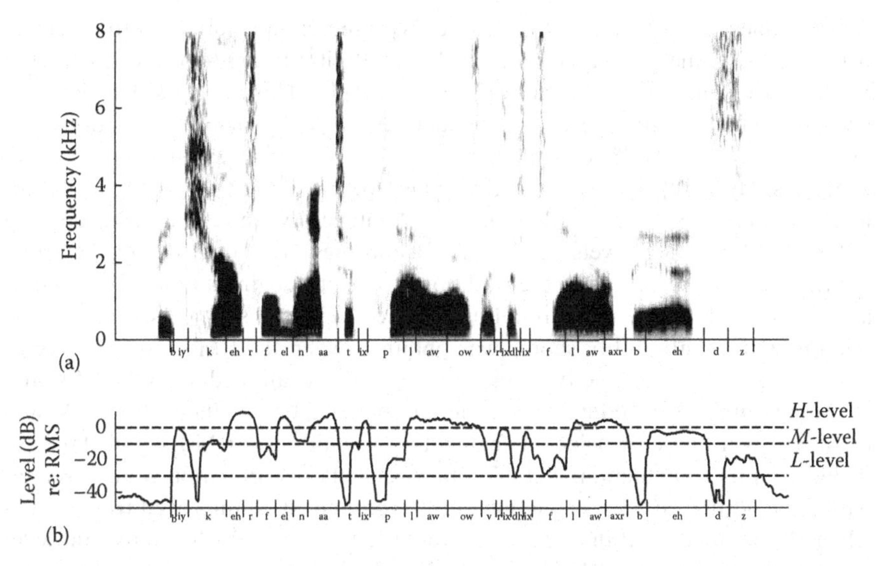

FIGURE 11.38 Panel (a) shows the spectrogram of the TIMIT sentence "Be careful not to plow over the flower beds." Panel (b) shows the segmentation of the sentence based on RMS levels.

or above the overall rms level of the whole utterance, i.e., RMS, and included for the most part sonorant segments (vowels, semivowels, and nasals). The mid-level region consisted of segments ranging from the RMS level to 10 dB below, and the low-level region consisted of segments ranging from RMS-10 dB to RMS-30 dB. Figure 11.38 shows an example segmentation of a sentence into high, medium, and low-level segments. High-level (H-level) segments contain primarily vowels, mid-level (M-level) segments contain vowel/consonant transitions, and low-level (L-level) segments contain weak consonants (e.g., /f/,/z/). Segmentation similar to that shown in Figure 11.38 was recommended in [133] for assessment of the effect of distortions on the performance of noise-reduction algorithms. Segmentation was done relative to active speech levels rather than overall RMS levels [133].

The three-level CSII measures obtained for the low-, mid-, and high-level segments were denoted as CSII_{Low}, CSII_{Mid}, and $\text{CSII}_{\text{High}}$ respectively. A linear combination of the three CSII values followed by a logistic function transformation was subsequently used to model the intelligibility scores, and the resulting intelligibility measure was called I3 [96]. The optimal weights applied to each of the three CSII measure were determined using regression analysis and as such these weights are data specific (different weights were used for predicting subjective quality [134]). For the data used in [96], the optimal combination leading to I_3 was computed as follows:

$$c = -3.47 + 1.84 \cdot CSII_{Low} + 9.99 \cdot CSII_{Mid} + 0.0 \cdot CSII_{High}$$

$$I_3 = \frac{1}{1 + e^{-c}} \tag{11.135}$$

The I_3 values were subsequently used for the prediction of intelligibility scores. It is clear from the said equation, that the intelligibility prediction is dominated by the $CSII_{Mid}$ measure carrying the largest weight. This suggests that the mid-level segments containing weak consonants and vowel/consonant transitions (see example in Figure 11.38) contribute the most to SI. This was also confirmed in another study [135] that assessed the impact of three different methods of segmenting sentences on the prediction of SI. Sentences were segmented according to low-mid-high RMS levels (as in CSII), according to the cochlea-scaled entropy (CSE) [136] and according to the traditional phonetic segmentation of obstruents and sonorants, corresponding roughly to voiced/unvoiced segments. Highest correlation with intelligibility scores was obtained when the RMS-level segmentation method was used. The two objective measures examined were the CSII and NCM measures. To account for the different segmentation methods, the NCM was modified such that only selected segments (e.g., mid-level RMS segments) were included in its computation. Notable improvements in correlation were observed with the modified NCM. Correlation of the modified NCM improved from $r = 0.8$ when all segments (within a sentence) were used to $r = 0.89$ when only mid-level segments were included. While the CSE method makes no distinction between spectral changes occurring within vowels/consonants, the RMS-level segmentation method places more emphasis on the vowel-consonant boundaries wherein the spectral change is often most prominent, and perhaps most robust, in the presence of noise. Higher correlation with intelligibility scores was obtained when including sentence segments containing a large number of consonant-vowel boundaries than when including segments with highest entropy or segments based on obstruent/sonorant classification.

Note that the data used in [96] involved HINT sentences corrupted by additive noise and subjected to symmetric peak-clipping and center-clipping distortions. This was done to mimic some of the non-linear distortions encountered in hearing aids. Further evaluation of the *I*3 measure was reported in [78] using corrupted sentences processed by different speech enhancement algorithms.

11.5 EVALUATION OF INTELLIGIBILITY MEASURES

For the objective intelligibility measure to be useful and meaningful, it has to correlate highly with human intelligibility scores. A number of studies reported on the evaluation and comparison of correlations of intelligibility measures with the intelligibility of speech processed by low-rate codecs [137], speech processed by the ideal binary mask [118–120]), and speech processed by noise-reduction algorithms [78,114,118]. The conditions under which the intelligibility measures were tested in these studies differed in terms of SNR level, speech material, and type of processing applied to the corrupted stimuli. The measures examined in [118], for instance, were evaluated at extremely low SNR levels (–3 to −10 dB) while the measures examined in [78] were evaluated at relatively more favorable conditions (0 and 5 dB). Hence, caution needs to be exercised not to presume that a high correlation obtained by a specific intelligibility measure in certain conditions (e.g., speech processed by low-rate codecs) will be maintained in other conditions (e.g., speech processed by noise-reduction algorithms).

Next, we make use of the intelligibility data collected in [90] (and discussed in more detail in Chapter 12) with normal-hearing listeners to evaluate the correlation of a number of intelligibility (and quality) measures [78] described in this chapter. The intelligibility study [90] produced a total of 72 noisy conditions including the noise-corrupted (unprocessed) conditions. The 72 conditions included distortions introduced by eight different noise-suppression algorithms operating at two SNR levels (0 and 5 dB) in four types of real-world environments (babble, car, street, and train). The intelligibility scores obtained in the 72 conditions by normal-hearing listeners were used to evaluate the predictive power of intelligibility measures as well as measures (e.g., PESQ) that were originally designed for quality assessment.

Much focus was placed in [78] on the design of band-importance weighting functions which can be used in objective measures operating on short-time intervals (e.g., 20 ms). That is, unlike the BIFs used in the STI and SII measures which are fixed for the whole utterance, these BIFs change from frame to frame depending on the spectral content of the target signal. More precisely, the following band-importance weighting functions were investigated for the coherence-based (see Equation 11.134) and fwSNRseg measures (see Equation 11.3):

$$W(j,m) = X(j,m)^p \tag{11.136}$$

where

p is a power exponent

$X(j,m)$ is the critical-band excitation spectrum of the clean target signal in jth band and frame m

The power exponent p can be optimized to fit the data and has been found in [78] to differ across speech materials (consonants vs. sentences). For the NCM measure, the following weighting function was used in Equation 11.114:

$$W_j = \left(\sum_t x_j^2(t) \right)^p \tag{11.137}$$

where $x_j(t)$ denotes the envelope of the target signal in the jth band.

11.5.1 Correlation of Intelligibility Measures with Human Intelligibility Scores

Table 11.4 shows the resulting correlations along with prediction errors for the quality and intelligibility measures examined in [78]. Of the seven measures designed

TABLE 11.4
Correlation Coefficients, *r*, and Standard Deviations of the Error, σ_e, between Sentence Intelligibility Scores and Various Objective Intelligibility Measures

Objective Measure	Band-Importance Function	*r*	σ_e
PESQ		0.79	0.11
LLR		−0.56	0.15
SNRseg		0.46	0.15
WSS		−0.27	0.17
Itakura–Saito (IS)		−0.22	0.17
Cepstrum (CEP)		−0.49	0.15
Coherence (MSC)		0.71	0.12
CSII		0.82	0.10
$CSII_{High}$		0.85	0.09
$CSII_{Mid}$		0.91	0.07
$CSII_{Low}$		0.86	0.09
I3		0.92	0.07
CSII	$p = 4$, Equation 11.136	0.86	0.09
$CSII_{High}$	$p = 2$, Equation 11.136	0.88	0.08
$CSII_{Mid}$	$p = 1$, Equation 11.136	0.94	0.06
$CSII_{Low}$	W_4, $p = 0.5$, Equation 11.136	0.86	0.09
fwSNRseg	ANSI (Table 1)	0.78	0.11
fwSNRseg	$p = 1$, Equation 11.136	0.81	0.10
NCM	ANSI (Table 2)	0.82	0.10
NCM	$p = 1.5$, Equation 11.137	0.89	0.07
SNR_{Loss} [95]		0.82	0.10
fAI [94]	$p = 2$, Equation 11.136	0.90	0.08
STOI [118]		0.85	0.09
CSII + NDR [114]		0.91	0.07

for subjective quality assessment, the PESQ and fwSNRseg measures performed the best. The fwSNRseg measure, based on the weighting function given in Equation 11.136, performed better than the PESQ measure and yielded a correlation of $r = 0.81$, compared to $r = 0.79$ obtained with the PESQ measure. The LLR measure, which was found in [57] to yield a correlation coefficient that was nearly as good as that of the PESQ measure (see Table 11.2), performed comparatively worse than the PESQ measure. The conventional segmental SNR measure, which is widely used for assessing performance of noise-suppression algorithms, performed poorly ($r = 0.46$). In summary, of all the measures tested [57] for subjective quality prediction (see Table 11.2), the fwSNRseg and PESQ measures seem to predict modestly well both speech quality and speech intelligibility, at least for the two SNR levels tested (0 and 5 dB). It should be noted, however, that the performance of the PESQ measure seems to depend highly on the input SNR level. For instance, high correlation between PESQ and speech processed via low-rate coders was reported in [137] for high SNR conditions, but low correlation ($r = 0.4$) was reported in [119] for extremely low SNR (<0 dB) conditions. Hence, the PESQ measure is not reliable for predicting SI.

Of all the intelligibility measures considered, the coherence-based (CSII) and NCM measures performed the best. The I_3 measure [96] (Equation 11.135), in particular, produced the highest correlation ($r = 0.92$). High correlation was maintained for all noise types, including modulated (e.g., train) and non-modulated (e.g., car) maskers. The correlations ranged from $r = 0.88$ with train noise to $r = 0.98$ with babble. Among the three-level CSII measures, the mid-level CSII ($CSII_{Mid}$) measure yielded the highest correlation, consistent with the outcome reported in [96]. The $CSII_{Mid}$ measure captures information about envelope transients and spectral transitions, critical for the transmission of information regarding place of articulation. Further improvements in correlation were obtained with the three-level CSII measures for the sentence materials after applying the signal-dependent BIF given in Equation 11.136. The correlation of the modified $CSII_{Mid}$ measure improved from $r = 0.92$ (7% prediction error) with ANSI weights to $r = 0.94$ (6% prediction error) with the BIF given in Equation 11.136. The resulting correlation was the highest correlation obtained in [78].

The next highest correlations were obtained with the modified NCM measure that used the signal-dependent BIF given in Equation 11.137. The resulting correlation coefficient improved from $r = 0.82$ (with ANSI weights) to $r = 0.89$ (7% prediction error). A high correlation was maintained for all noise types, including modulated (e.g., train) and non-modulated (e.g., car) maskers. The correlations ranged from $r = 0.85$ with car noise to $r = 0.94$ with babble. In the implementation of the NCM measure, the number of bands was fixed to 20, the speech dynamic range to [−15, 15] dB, and the range of modulation frequencies to 0–12.5 Hz. Additional experiments were run to assess the influence of the number of bands, range of modulation frequencies, and speech dynamic range on the prediction of SI in noise. Results indicated no significant improvements in correlation when the SNR dynamic range, range of modulation frequencies, and/or number of bands increased.

The last few rows in Table 11.4 show correlations obtained with measures reported in other studies [94,95,114] when evaluated on the same corpus and conditions. The STOI measure [118] (discussed in Section 11.4.2.4) yielded a correlation of $r = 0.85$, while the CSII measure when combined with the NDR measure, proposed in [114], yielded a correlation of $r = 0.91$ [114]. The NDR measure is a variant of the fwSNRseg measure in that it treats positive and negative distortions differently.

11.5.2 Summary of Findings

The following conclusions can be drawn from the study in [78] regarding the intelligibility measures evaluated with speech processed by enhancement algorithms:

1. Of all the intelligibility measures considered in [78], the coherence-based (CSII) and NCM measures performed the best.
2. Most measures (e.g., CSII, AI, STI) utilize a 30 dB speech dynamic range that is mapped linearly in the range of 0–1. Extending the 30 dB speech dynamic range did not seem to influence the correlation with intelligibility scores.

3. The number of bands utilized in the spectral representation did not seem to influence the correlation.
4. Of all parameters examined in [78], the BIFs influenced the performance of the STI-based (NCM) and coherence-based (CSII) measures the most (see Table 11.4). The signal (and phonetic-segment) dependent BIFs (Equations 11.19 through 11.22) are suitable for predicting the intelligibility of speech in fluctuating maskers. Additional flexibility is built in the proposed BIFs for emphasizing spectral peaks and/or spectral valleys by varying the power exponents in Equations 11.136 and 11.137.

11.6 INTELLIGIBILITY MEASURES: SUMMARY OF FINDINGS AND FUTURE DIRECTIONS

Presently, there is no single measure that correlates well with intelligibility scores for a wide range of conditions involving different types of maskers and/or speech distortions. Most measures have been validated for a specific type of distortion (e.g., such as those introduced by speech-enhancement algorithms) or type of background interference (e.g., noise, reverberation). Table 11.5 summarizes the characteristics of conventional, well-established, and well-tested measures for various types of interference and processing. With the exception of the work done in [84,85], no measure correlates highly with the intelligibility of speech embedded in modulated maskers (e.g., competing talker). This challenge is due to the fact that most measures are ineffective in modeling the human's ability to "listen in the dips" or "glimpse" the target during favorable SNR segments (see Chapter 4). The strengths and limitations of each family of measures described previously are summarized as follows.

Articulation index measures: The AI measures have been shown to predict well the intelligibility of monosyllabic words and non-sense syllables in steady noise and in conditions involving low-pass and high-pass filtering. They were not designed to predict intelligibility of sentences as the AI measures are based on long-term average spectra. They cannot be used to predict intelligibility of speech processed by enhancement algorithms as the SNR definition becomes vague following the application of the noise-suppressive gain function (see Section 11.4.1.6). Techniques such as those proposed in [94] can be used, however, to extend the capability of AI measures to handle non-linear distortions. The SII measure requires as input the SPL level of the target speech and masker at the eardrum, something that might be readily available in clinical applications (i.e., in audiological settings [76]) but not in practical applications. The AI has been criticized for its assumption of channel independence, but in reality *all* measures (with the exception of [106,127]) utilize this assumption. Channel independence has been shown to hold in a number of studies involving isolated words or non-sense syllables (e.g., [73–75]). It might arguably not hold for sentences, but nonetheless high correlation with intelligibility scores is obtained with existing intelligibility measures despite the lack of independence between adjacent channels.

TABLE 11.5
Characteristics of Established Intelligibility Measures in Terms of Limitations and Capabilities

		Type of Interference			Processing	
Intelligibility Measure	**Speech Material**	**Steady Noise**	**Modulated (e.g., Competing Talker)**	**Reverberation**	**Filtering (e.g., Low-Pass, High-Pass)**	**Non-Linear Distortions, Noise Reduction**
Articulation Index and SII	Words, non-sense syllables (e.g., /aCa/)	✓			✓	
Speech Transmission Index (STI)	Words, sentences	✓		✓	✓	
Speech-based STI	Words, sentences	✓		✓	✓	✓
Coherence	Words, sentences	✓			✓	✓

Note: Empty cells indicate the background environment or signal manipulation in which the corresponding measure does not predict reliably SI. Cells marked with a check symbol indicate the background environment in which the corresponding measure is known to predict reliably SI.

STI measures: In the absence of non-linear distortions, the conventional STI measure is the best, and simplest, measure for predicting the effects of steady noise, reverberation, or the combined effects of reverberation and noise on SI. High correlations with intelligibility scores were found even with the use of artificial signals (sinewave-modulated signals) as probe signals. Furthermore, the STI is the ideal measure to use when designing rooms and auditoria, and when there exists the need to account (or compensate) for room reflections. As discussed in Section 11.4.2.5, distortions such as those produced by spectral subtraction, introduce additional modulations that are interpreted as increased SNR by the STI (see Figure 11.35). Consequently, the STI measure fails to predict the intelligibility of non-linearly processed speech and is thus not appropriate for assessment of the intelligibility of speech enhanced by noise-reduction algorithms and particularly spectral-subtractive algorithms.

Speech-based STI measures and correlation-based measures: The STI measures use the reduction in envelope modulation depth as an indirect measure of SNR (see Equation 11.104). Measures, such as the NCM, do not explicitly assess the reduction in modulation but rather compute the covariance between the processed and clean envelopes, and from that an apparent SNR. The correlation is computed in the modulation domain taking into account envelope modulations limited to up to 16 Hz. High correlation was reported with the NCM measure when evaluated with the intelligibility of speech processed by various speech enhancement algorithms, including spectral subtraction [78]. The NCM has also been shown to correlate highly with the intelligibility of reverberant speech [138], vocoded speech [116], and Mandarin Chinese [117]. Correlation-based measures, such as those proposed in [95,114,118,119], have been found to perform well in the prediction of ideal-binary masked speech [118] and noise-suppressed speech [95,114]. The two main differences between the correlation-based measures and NCM is that: (1) the NCM operates on the whole utterance while the correlation-based measures operate in relatively shorter intervals (30–400 ms), (2) the NCM operates in the modulation domain and utilizes primarily information present in low-frequency (<16 Hz) envelope modulations.

Coherence-based measures: These measures have been validated for the most part with non-linearly processed speech and have been found to correlate highly with speech processed by noise-reduction algorithms [78] and with speech subjected to non-linear distortions (e.g., clipping) such as those encountered in hearing aids [96]. Much of the benefit provided by these measures lies in the novel segmentation of sentences into low, mid, and high RMS levels (see Figure 11.38). The coherence measures based on mid-level segments have been shown to correlate the highest with the intelligibility of English speech [78]. Coherence measures based on high-level segments have been shown to correlate the highest with the intelligibility of Mandarin Chinese [117], and this was attributed to the fact that the high-RMS levels contain primarily vowels and semivowels, which carry important F0 information for tonal language recognition.

Of the four families of intelligibility measures (Table 11.5), the speech-based STI and coherence-based measures are the most appropriate (and most reliable) for evaluating the intelligibility of noise-suppressed (via enhancement algorithms) speech. Caution needs to be exercised when evaluating the intelligibility of enhancement algorithms in background environments other than the ones in which the measure has been validated.

Table 11.5 can serve as a guide for choosing a measure for different listening environments. It is clear from this table that future work is warranted in developing objective measures that can predict reliably intelligibility in competing-talker(s) scenarios.

11.7 SUMMARY

This chapter provided a description of common objective quality and intelligibility measures. Quality measures included segmental SNR measures, spectral distance measures based on LPC (e.g., Itakura–Saito measure), and perceptually motivated measures (e.g., Bark distortion measure). The PESQ measure was also described in detail. Correlations of the objective quality measures with subjective quality ratings collected with human listeners were provided. The second part of this chapter covered common intelligibility measures. This included the AI measure, which later became an ANSI standard (SII measure), the STI measure, speech-based STI measures, and coherence-based measures. The limitations of these measures were also discussed. Correlations of the intelligibility measures with human listener's intelligibility scores were provided. This chapter focused primarily on providing an overview of the various objective measures used for quality and intelligibility assessment. A thorough evaluation of the performance of representative speech enhancement algorithms described in this book is given next in Chapter 12.

REFERENCES

1. Quackenbush, S., Barnwell, T., and Clements, M. (1988), *Objective measures of Speech Quality*, Englewood Cliffs, NJ: Prentice Hall.
2. Flanagan, J. (1955), A difference limen for vowel formant frequency, *J. Acoust. Soc. Am.*, 27, 613–617.
3. Viswanathan, R., Makhoul, J., and Russell, W. (1976), Towards perceptually consistent measures of spectral distance, *Proceedings of the IEEE International Conference on Acoustics, Speech, and Signal Processing*, Vol. 1, Philadelphia, PA, pp. 485–488.
4. Dimolitsas, S. (1989), Objective speech distortion measures and their relevance to speech quality assessments, *IEE Proc.—Vision, Image Signal Process.*, 136(5), 317–324.
5. Kubichek, R., Atkinson, D., and Webster, A. (1991), Advances in objective voice quality assessment, *Global Telecommunications Conference*, Phoenix, AZ, Vol. 3, pp. 1765–1770.
6. Kitawaki, N. (1991), Quality assessment of coded speech, in Furui, S. and Sondhi, M. (Eds.), *Advances in Speech Signal Processing*, New York: Marcel Dekker, pp. 357–385.
7. Barnwell, T. (1979), Objective measures for speech quality testing, *J. Acoust. Soc. Am.*, 66(6), 1658–1663.
8. Hansen, J. and Pellom, B. (1998), An effective quality evaluation protocol for speech enhancement algorithms, *Proceedings of International Conference on Spoken Language Processing*, Sydney, NSW, Australia, Vol. 7, pp. 2819–2822.
9. Be'ery, Y., Shpiro, Z., Simchony, T., Shatz, L., and Piasetzky, J. (1990), An efficient variable-bit-rate low-delay (VBR-LD-CELP) coder, in Atal, B. et al. (Eds.), *Advances in Speech Coding,* New York: Marcel Dekker, pp. 37–46.

10. Wang, S., Sekey, A., and Gersho, A. (1992), An objective measure for predicting subjective quality of speech coders, *IEEE J. Select. Areas Commun.*, 10(5), 819–829.
11. Richards, D. (1965), Speech transmission performance of PCM systems, *Electron. Lett.*, 1, 40–41.
12. Mermelstein, P. (1979), Evaluation of segmental SNR measure as an indicator of the quality of ADPCM coded speech, *J. Acoust. Soc. Am.*, 66(6), 1664–1667.
13. Tribolet, J., Noll, P., McDermott, B., and Crochiere, R. E. (1978), A study of complexity and quality of speech waveform coders, *Proceedings of the IEEE International Conference on Acoustics, Speech, and Signal Processing*, Tulsa, OK, pp. 586–590.
14. Kryter, K. (1962), Methods for calculation and use of the articulation index, *J. Acoust. Soc. Am.*, 34(11), 1689–1697.
15. Klatt, D. (1982), Prediction of perceived phonetic distance from critical band spectra, *Proceedings of the IEEE International Conference on Acoustics, Speech, and Signal Processing*, Vol. 7, pp. 1278–1281.
16. Rabiner, L. and Schafer, R. (1978), *Digital Processing of Speech Signals*, Englewood Cliffs, NJ: Prentice Hall.
17. Kitawaki, N., Nagabuchi, H., and Itoh, K. (1988), Objective quality evaluation for low bit-rate speech coding systems, *IEEE J. Select. Areas Commun.*, 6(2), 262–273.
18. Karjalainen, M. (1985), A new auditory model for the evaluation of sound quality of audio system, *Proceedings of the IEEE International Conference on Acoustics, Speech, and Signal Processing*, Vol. 10, Tampa, FL, pp. 608–611.
19. Yang, W., Benbouchta, M., and Yantorno, R. (1998), Performance of the modified Bark spectral distortion as an objective speech quality measure, *Proceedings of the IEEE International Conference on Acoustics, Speech, and Signal Processing*, Seattle, WA, pp. 541–544.
20. Karjalainen, M. (1984), Sound quality measurements of audio systems based on models of auditory perception, *Proceedings of the IEEE International Conference on Acoustics, Speech, and Signal Processing*, Vol. 9, San Diego, CA, pp. 132–135.
21. Moore, B. (2003), *An Introduction to the Psychology of Hearing*, 5th ed., London, U.K.: Academic Press.
22. Schroeder, M., Atal, B., and Hall, J. (1979), Optimizing digital speech coders by exploiting masking properties of the human ear, *J. Acoust. Soc. Am.*, 66(6), 1647–1651.
23. Fletcher, H. and Munson, W. (1933), Loudness, its definition, measurement and calculation, *J. Acoust. Soc. Am.*, 5, 82–108.
24. Robinson, D. and Dadson, R. (1956), A re-determination of the equal-loudness relations for pure tones, *Br. J. Appl. Phys.*, 7, 166–181.
25. ISO 226. (1987), Acoustics—Normal equal-loudness level contours, Geneva, Switzerland: International Organization for Standardization (ISO).
26. Bladon, R. and Lindblom, B. (1981), Modeling the judgment of vowel quality differences, *J. Acoust. Soc. Am.*, 69(5), 1414–1422.
27. Yang, W. (1999), Enhanced modified Bark spectral distortion (EMBSD): An objective speech quality measure based on audible distortion and cognition model, PhD dissertation, Temple University, Philadelphia, PA.
28. Novorita, B. (1999), Incorporation of temporal masking effects into bark spectral distortion measure, *Proceedings of the IEEE International Conference on Acoustics, Speech, and Signal Processing*, Vol. 2, Phoenix, AZ, pp. 665–668.
29. Johnston, J. (1988), Transform coding of audio signals using perceptual noise criteria, *IEEE J. Select. Areas Commun.*, 6, 314–323.
30. Yang, W. and Yantorno, R. (1999), Improvement of MBSD by scaling noise masking threshold and correlation analysis with MOS difference instead of MOS, *Proceedings of the IEEE International Conference on Acoustics, Speech, and Signal Processing*, Vol. 2, Phoenix, AZ, pp. 673–676.

31. Rix, A. and Hollier, M. (2000), The perceptual analysis measurement for robust end-to-end speech quality assessment, *Proceedings of the IEEE International Conference on Acoustics, Speech, and Signal Processing*, Vol. 3, Istanbul, Turkey, pp. 1515–1518.
32. Beerends, J. and Stemerdink, J. (1994), A perceptual speech-quality measure based on a psychoacoustic sound representation, *J. Audio Eng. Soc.*, 42(3), 115–123.
33. Voran, S. (1999), Objective estimation of perceived speech quality—Part I: Development of the measuring normalizing block technique, *IEEE Trans. Speech Audio Process.*, 7(4), 371–382.
34. Rix, A., Beerends, J., Hollier, M., and Hekstra, A. (2001), Perceptual evaluation of speech quality (PESQ)—A new method for speech quality assessment of telephone networks and codecs, *Proceedings of the IEEE International Conference on Acoustics, Speech, and Signal Processing*, Vol. 2, Salt Lake City, UT, pp. 749–752.
35. ITU. (2000), Perceptual evaluation of speech quality (PESQ), and objective method for end-to-end speech quality assessment of narrowband telephone networks and speech codecs, ITU-T Recommendation P. 862.
36. ITU-T. (1996), Subjective performance assessment of telephone band and wideband digital codecs, ITU-T Recommendation P. 830.
37. Zwicker, E. and Feldtkeller, R. (1967), *Das Ohr als Nachrichtenempfanger*, Stuttgart, Germany: S. Hirzel Verlag.
38. Boll, S. F. (1979), Suppression of acoustic noise in speech using spectral subtraction, *IEEE Trans. Acoust., Speech, Signal Process.*, ASSP-27(2), 113–120.
39. Hollier, M., Hawksford, M., and Guard, D. (1994), Error activity and error entropy as a measure of psychoacoustic significance in the perceptual domain, *IEE Proc.—Vision, Image Signal Process.*, 141(3), 203–208.
40. ITU. (2007), Wideband extension to Recommendation P.862 for the assessment of wideband telephone networks and speech codecs, ITU-T Recommendation P. 862. 2.
41. ITU. (2003), Mapping function for transforming P.862 raw result scores to MOS-LQO, ITU-T Recommendation P. 862. 1.
42. Hu, Y. and Loizou, P. (2006), Evaluation of objective measures for speech enhancement, *Proceedings of Interspeech*, Pittsburg, PA, pp. 1447–1450.
43. Friedman, J. (1991), Multivariate adaptive regression splines, *Ann. Stat.*, 19(1), 1–67.
44. Gray, R., Buzo, A., Gray, A., and Matsuyama, Y. (1980), Distortion measures for speech processing, *IEEE Trans. Acoust., Speech, Signal Process.*, 28(4), 367–376.
45. Gray, A. and Markel, J. (1976), Distance measures for speech processing, *IEEE Trans. Acoust., Speech, Signal Process.*, ASSP-24(5), 380–391.
46. Rix, A. (2004), Perceptual speech quality assessment—A review, *Proceedings of the IEEE International Conference on Acoustics, Speech, and Signal Processing*, Montreal, Quebec, Canada, Vol. 3, pp. 1056–1059.
47. Gray, P., Hollier, M., and Massara, R. (2000), Non-intrusive speech quality assessment using vocal-tract models, *IEE Proc.—Vision, Image Signal Process.*, 147(6), 493–501.
48. Chen, G. and Parsa, V. (2005), Nonintrusive speech quality evaluation using an adaptive neurofuzzy inference system, *IEEE Signal Process. Lett.*, 12(5), 403–406.
49. Jin, C. and Kubichek, R. (1996), Vector quantization techniques for output-based objective speech quality, *Proceedings of the IEEE International Conference on Acoustics, Speech, and Signal Processing*, Atlanta, GA, pp. 491–494.
50. Picovici, D. and Madhi, A. (2003), Output-based objective speech quality measure using self-organizing map, *Proceedings of the IEEE International Conference on Acoustics, Speech, and Signal Processing*, Hong Kong, China, pp. 476–479.

51. Kim, D. and Tarraf, A. (2004), Perceptual model for nonintrusive speech quality assessment, *Proceedings of the IEEE International Conference on Acoustics, Speech, and Signal Processing*, Montreal, Quebec, Canada, Vol. 3, pp. 1060–1063.
52. ITU. (2004), Single ended method for objective speech quality assessment in narrowband telephony applications, ITU-T Recommendation P. 563.
53. Moller, S., Chan, W., Cote, N., Falk, T., Raake, A., and Waltermann, M. (2011), Speech quality testing, *IEEE Signal Process. Mag.*, 28(6), 18–28.
54. Kitawaki, N., Itoh, K., Honda, N., and Kakehi, K. (1982), Comparison of objective speech quality measure for voiceband codecs, *Proceedings of the IEEE International Conference on Acoustics, Speech, and Signal Processing*, Paris, France, pp. 1000–1003.
55. Barnwell, T. (1980), Correlation analysis of subjective and objective measures of speech quality, *Proceedings of the IEEE International Conference on Acoustics, Speech, and Signal Processing*, Denver, CO, pp. 706–709.
56. Kubichek, R. (1991), Standards and technology issues in objective quality assessment, *Digit. Signal Process.*, I, 38–44.
57. Hu, Y. and Loizou, P. (2008), Evaluation of objective quality measures for speech enhancement, *IEEE Trans. Speech Audio Process.*, 16(1), 229–238.
58. Thorpe, L. and Yang, W. (1999), Performance of current perceptual objective speech quality measures, *Proceedings of IEEE Speech Coding Workshop*, Provo, Finland, pp. 144–146.
59. Hu, Y. and Loizou, P. (2007), Subjective evaluation and comparison of speech enhancement algorithms, *Speech Commun.*, 49, 588–601.
60. Grundlehner, B., Lecocq, J., Balan, R., and Rosca, J. (2005), Performance assessment method for speech enhancement systems, *Proceedings of First Annual IEEE BENELUX/DSP Valley Signal Processing Symposium*, Antwerp, Belgium.
61. Derakhshan, N., Rahmani, M., Akbari, A., and Ayatollahi, A. (2009), An objective measure for the musical noise assessment in noise reduction systems, *Proceedings of the IEEE International Conference on Acoustics, Speech, and Signal Processing*, Taipei, Taiwan, China, pp. 4429–4432.
62. Zwicker, E. and Fastl, H. (1999), *Pschoacoustics: Facts and Models*, 2nd ed., Berlin, Germany: Springer-Verlag.
63. Kent, R. and Read, C. (1992), *The Acoustic Analysis of Speech*, San Diego, CA: Singular Publishing Group.
64. Stevens, K. and Blumstein, S. (1978), Invariant cues for the place of articulation in stop consonants, *J. Acoust. Soc. Am.*, 64, 1358–1368.
65. Breitkopf, P. and Barnwell, T. (1981), Segmental preclassification for improved objective speech quality measures, *Proceedings of the IEEE International Conference on Acoustics, Speech, and Signal Processing*, Atlanta, GA, pp. 1101–1104.
66. Kubichek, R., Quincy, E., and Kiser, K. (1989), Speech quality assessment using expert pattern recognition techniques, *IEEE Pacific Rim Conference on Communication, Computers, and Signal Processing*, Victoria, British Columbia, Canada, 208–211.
67. Allen, J. (2005), Articulation and intelligibility, LaPorte, IN: Morgan & Claypool Publishers.
68. French, N. and Steinberg, J. (1947), Factors governing the intelligibility of speech sounds, *J. Acoust. Soc. Am.*, 19, 90–119.
69. ANSI S3-5. (1969), Methods for the calculation of the articulation index. Washington, DC: American National Standards Institute.
70. ANSI S3-5. (1997), Methods for calculation of the speech intelligibility index. Washington, DC: American National Standards Institute.
71. Fletcher, H. and Galt, R. H. (1950), The perception of speech and its relation to telephony, *J. Acoust. Soc. Am.*, 22, 89–150.
72. Studebaker, G. and Sherbecoe, R. (1991), Frequency-importance and transfer functions for recorded CID W-22 word lists, *J. Speech Hear. Res.*, 34, 427–438.

73. Li, F. and Allen, J. (2009), Multiband product rule and consonant identification, *J. Acoust. Soc. Am.*, 126, 347–353.
74. Whitmal, N. and DeRoy, K. (2011), Adaptive bandwidth measurements of importance functions for speech intelligibility prediction, *J. Acoust. Soc. Am.*, 130(6), 4032–4043.
75. Apoux, F. and Healy, E. (2009), On the number of auditory filter outputs needed to understand speech: Further evidence for auditory channel independence, *Hearing Res.*, 255, 99–108.
76. Amlani, A., Punch, J., and Ching, T. (2002), Methods and applications of the audibility index in hearing aid selection and fitting, *Trends Amplif.*, 6(3), 81–129.
77. Miller, G., Heise, G., and Lichten, W. (1951), The intelligibility of speech as a function of the context of the test materials, *J. Exp. Psychol.*, 41, 329–335.
78. Ma, J., Hu, Y., and Loizou, P. (2009), Objective measures for predicting speech intelligibility in noisy conditions based on new band-importance functions, *J. Acoust. Soc. Am.*, 125(5), 3387–3405.
79. Pavlovic, C. (1987), Derivation of primary parameters and procedures for use in speech intelligibility prediction, *J. Acoust. Soc. Am.*, 82(2), 413–422.
80. Welch, P. (1967), The use of fast Fourier transform for estimation of power spectra: A method based on time averaging over short, modified periodograms, *IEEE Trans. Audio Electroacoust.*, AU15, 70–73.
81. Dunn, H. and White, S. (1940), Statistical measurements on conversational speech, *J. Acoust. Soc. Am.*, 11, 278–288.
82. Kryter, K. (1962), Validation of the articulation index, *J. Acoust. Soc. Am.*, 34(11), 1698–1702.
83. Studebaker, G., Sherbecoe, R., McDaniel, M., and Gwaltney, C. (1999), Monosyllabic word recognition at higher-than-normal speech and noise levels, *J. Acoust. Soc. Am.*, 105, 2431–2444.
84. Rhebergen, K. S. and Versfeld, N. J. (2005), A speech intelligibility index based approach to predict the speech reception threshold for sentences in fluctuating noise for normal-hearing listeners, *J. Acoust. Soc. Am.*, 117, 2181–2192.
85. Rhebergen, K. S., Versfeld, N. J., and Dreschler, W. (2006), Extended speech intelligibility index for the prediction of the speech reception threshold in fluctuating noise, *J. Acoust. Soc. Am.*, 120, 3988–3997.
86. Festen, J. and Plomp, R. (1990), Effects of fluctuating noise and interfering speech on the speech-reception threshold for impaired and normal hearing, *J. Acoust. Soc. Am.*, 88, 1725–1736.
87. Miller, G. (1947), The masking of speech, *Psychol. Bull.*, 44(2), 105–129.
88. Brungart, D. (2001), Informational and energetic masking effects in the perception of two simultaneous talkers, *J. Acoust. Soc. Am.*, 109(3), 1101–1109.
89. Shailer, M. J. and Moore, B. C. (1983), Gap detection as a function of frequency, bandwidth, and level, *J. Acoust. Soc. Am.*, 74, 467–473.
90. Hu, Y. and Loizou, P. (2007), A comparative intelligibility study of single-microphone noise reduction algorithms, *J. Acoust. Soc. Am.*, 122(3), 1777–1786.
91. Bentler, R., Wu, H., Kettel, J., and Hurtig, R. (2008), Digital noise reduction: Outcomes from laboratory and field studies, *Int. J. Audiol.*, 47(8), 447–460.
92. Loizou, P. and Kim, G. (2011), Reasons why current speech-enhancement algorithms do not improve speech intelligibility and suggested solutions, *IEEE Trans. Audio Speech Lang. Process.*, 19(1), 47–56.
93. Kim, G., Lu, Y., Hu, Y., and Loizou, P. (2009), An algorithm that improves speech intelligibility in noise for normal-hearing listeners, *J. Acoust. Soc. Am.*, 126(3), 1486–1494.
94. Loizou, P. and Ma, J. (2011), Extending the articulation index to account for non-linear distortions introduced by noise suppression algorithms, *J. Acoust. Soc. Am.*, 130(2), 986–995.

95. Ma, J. and Loizou, P. (2011), SNR loss: A new objective measure for predicting the intelligibility of noise-suppressed speech, *Speech Commun.*, 53(3), 340–354.
96. Kates, J. and Arehart, K. (2005), Coherence and the speech intelligibility index, *J. Acoust. Soc. Am.*, 117(4), 2224–2237.
97. Houtgast, T. and Steeneken, H. (1973), The modulation transfer function in room acoustics as a predictor of speech intelligibility, *Acustica*, 28, 66–73.
98. Houtgast, T., Steeneken, H., and Plomp, R. (1980), Predicting speech intelligibility in rooms from the modulation transfer function, *Acustica*, 46, 60–72.
99. Steeneken, H. and Houtgast, T. (1980), A physical method for measuring speech transmission quality, *J. Acoust. Soc. Am.*, 67(1), 318–326.
100. Houtgast, T. and Steeneken, H. (1985), A review of the MTF concept in room acoustics and its use for estimating speech intelligibility in auditoria, *J. Acoust. Soc. Am.*, 77(3), 1069–1077.
101. Drullman, R., Festen, J., and Plomp, R. (1994), Effect of temporal envelope smearing on speech reception, *J. Acoust. Soc. Am.*, 95(2), 1053–1064.
102. Drullman, R., Festen, J., and Plomp, R. (1994), Effect of reducing slow temporal modulations on speech reception, *J. Acoust. Soc. Am.*, 95(5), 2670–2680.
103. Elliott, T. and Theunissen, F. (2009), The modulation transfer function for speech intelligibility, *PLos Comput. Biol.*, 5, 1–14.
104. Bentler, R. and Chiou, L. (2006), Digital noise reduction: An overview, *Trends Amplif.*, 10(2), 67–82.
105. Goldsworthy, R. and Greenberg, J. (2004), Analysis of speech-based speech transmission index methods with implications for nonlinear operations, *J. Acoust. Soc. Am.*, 116, 3679–3689.
106. Steeneken, H. and Houtgast, T. (1999), Mutual dependence of the octave-band weights in predicting speech intelligibility, *Speech Commun.*, 28, 109–123.
107. Elhilali, M., Chi, T., and Shamma, S. (2003), A spectro-temporal modulation index (STMI) for assessment of speech intelligibility, *Speech Commun.*, 41, 331–348.
108. Chi, T., Gao, M., Guyton, M., Ru, P., and Shamma, S. (1999), Spectro-temporal modulation transfer functions and speech intelligibility, *J. Acoust. Soc. Am.*, 106(5), 2719–2732.
109. Payton, K. and Braida, L. (1999), A method to determine the speech transmission index from speech waveforms, *J. Acoust. Soc. Am.*, 106(6), 3637–3648.
110. Payton, K., Uchanski, R., and Braida, L. (1993), Computation of modulation spectra for the Speech Transmission Index using real speech, *Proceedings of the IEEE Workshop on Applications of Signal Processing to Audio and Acoustics*, paper 5.4
111. Holube, I. and Kollmeier, B. (1996), Speech intelligibility prediction in hearing-impaired listeners based on a psychoacoustically motivated perception model, *J. Acoust. Soc. Am.*, 100, 1703–1715.
112. Benesty, J., Chen, J., and Huang, Y. (2008), On the importance of the Pearson correlation coefficient in noise reduction, *IEEE Trans. Audio Speech Lang. Process.*, 16(4), 757–765.
113. Benesty, J., Chen, J., Huang, Y., and Cohen, I. (2009), Noise reduction in speech processing. Heidelberg, Germany: Springer-Verlag.
114. Gomez, A., Schwerin, B., and Paliwal, K. (2012), Improving objective intelligibility prediction by combining correlation and coherence based methods with a measure based on the negative distortion ratio, *Speech Commun.*, 54, 503–515.
115. Chen, F. and Loizou, P. (2010), Analysis of a simplified normalized covariance measure based on binary weighting functions for predicting the intelligibility of noise-suppressed speech, *J. Acoust. Soc. Am.*, 128(6), 3715–3723.
116. Chen, F. and Loizou, P. (2011), Predicting the intelligibility of vocoded speech, *Ear Hear.*, 32(3), 331–338.
117. Chen, F. and Loizou, P. (2011), Predicting the intelligibility of vocoded and wideband Mandarin Chinese, *J. Acoust. Soc. Am.*, 129, 3281–3290.

118. Taal, C., Hendricks, R., Heusdens, R., and Jensen, J. (2011), An algorithm for intelligibility prediction of time–frequency weighted noisy speech, *IEEE Trans. Audio Speech Lang. Process.*, 19(7), 2125–2136.
119. Taal, C., Hendricks, R., Heusdens, R., and Jensen, J. (2011), An evaluation of objective measures for intelligibility prediction of time-frequency weighted noisy speech, *J. Acoust. Soc. Am.*, 130(5), 3013–3027.
120. Boldt, J. and Ellis, D. (2009), A simple correlation-based model of intelligibility for nonlinear speech enhancement and separation, *Proceedings of EUSIPCO*, Glasgow, U.K., 1849–1853.
121. Christiansen, C., Pedersen, M., and Dau, T. (2010), Prediction of speech intelligibility based on an auditory preprocessing model, *Speech Commun.*, 52, 678–692.
122. Hohmann, V. and Kollmeier, B. (1995), The effect of multichannel dynamic compression on speech intelligibility, *J. Acoust. Soc. Am.*, 97, 1191–1195.
123. Ludvigsen, C., Elberling, C., and Keidser, G. (1993), Evaluation of a noise reduction method—Comparison of observed scores and scores predicted from STI, *Scand. Audiol.*, 38, 50–55.
124. Dubbelboer, F. and Houtgast, T. (2008), The concept of signal-to-noise ratio in the modulation domain and speech intelligibility, *J. Acoust. Soc. Am.*, 124(6), 3937–3946.
125. Jorgensen, S. and Dau, T. (2011), Predicting speech intelligibility based on the signal-to-noise envelope power ratio after modulation-frequency selective processing, *J. Acoust. Soc. Am.*, 130(3), 1475–1487.
126. Green, D. and Birdsall, T. (1964), The effect of vocabulary size, in Swets, J. (Ed.), *Signal Detection and Recognition by Human Observers*, New York: Willey, pp. 609–619.
127. Musch, H. and Buus, S. (2001), Using statistical decision theory to predict speech intelligibility. I. Model structure, *J. Acoust. Soc. Am.*, 109(6), 2896–2909.
128. Green, D. and Swets, J. (1988), *Signal Detection Theory and Psychophysics*, Los Altos Hills, CA: Peninsula Publishing.
129. Carter, G., Knapp, C., and Nuttall, A. (1973), Estimation of the magnitude-squared coherence function via overlapped fast Fourier transform processing, *IEEE Trans. Audio Electroacoust.*, 21, 337–344.
130. Lu, Y. and Loizou, P. (2010), Speech enhancement by combining statistical estimators of speech and noise, *Proc. IEEE International Conference on Acoustics, Speech, and Signal Processing*, Dallas, TX, pp. 4754–4757.
131. Kates, J. M. (1992), On using coherence to measure distortion in hearing aids, *J. Acoust. Soc. Am.*, 91(4), 2236–2244.
132. Moore, B. and Glasberg, B. (1983), Suggested formulae for calculating auditory-filter bandwidths and excitation patterns, *J. Acoust. Soc. Am.*, 74(3), 750–753.
133. ETSI. (2010), Minimum performance requirements for noise suppresser application to the Adaptive Multi-Rate (AMR) speech encoder, *ETSI TS* 126 077, v. 9, Release 9.
134. Arehart, K., Kates, J., Anderson, M., and Harvey, L. (2007), Effects of noise and distortion on speech quality judgments in normal-hearing and hearing-impaired listeners, *J. Acoust. Soc. Am.*, 122, 1150–1164.
135. Chen, F. and Loizou, P. (2012), Contributions of cochlea-scaled entropy and consonant-vowel boundaries to prediction of speech intelligibility in noise, *J. Acoust. Soc. Am.*, 131(5), 4104–4113.
136. Stilp, C. and Kluender, K. (2010), Cochlea-scaled entropy, not consonants, vowels or time, best predicts speech intelligibility, *Proc. Natl. Acad. Sci. USA*, 107, 12387–12392.
137. Liu, W., Jellyman, K., Mason, J., and Evans, N. (2006), Assessment of objective quality measures for speech intelligibility estimation, *Proceedings of the IEEE International Conference on Acoustics, Speech, and Signal Processing*, Vol. I, Toulouse, France, 1225–1228.
138. Hazrati, O. and Loizou, P. (2012), Tackling the combined effects of reverberation and masking noise using ideal channel selection, *J. Speech Lang. Hear. Res.*, 55, 500–510.

12 Comparison of Speech Enhancement Algorithms

In the previous chapters, we described a number of speech enhancement algorithms that have been proposed to improve the performance of modern communication devices in noisy environments. We also reported on the subjective and objective evaluation of these algorithms using various types of noise. The scope of those evaluations was, however, limited to the individual algorithms tested in each study. We mentioned little about speech intelligibility, as most studies did not report intelligibility scores for the algorithms tested. It therefore remains unclear as to which speech enhancement algorithm performs the best, in terms of quality and/or intelligibility, in real-world listening situations where the background noise level and characteristics are constantly changing. Reliable and fair comparison between algorithms has been elusive for several reasons, including lack of common speech database for evaluation of new algorithms, differences in the types of noise used, and differences in the testing methodology. Without having access to a common speech database, it is nearly impossible for researchers to compare at the very least the objective performance of their algorithms with that of others.

In this chapter, we report on the quality and intelligibility evaluation of a number of speech enhancement algorithms described in this book. The speech enhancement algorithms were chosen to encompass four different classes of noise reduction methods: spectral subtractive, subspace, statistical-model-based, and Wiener-type algorithms. The subjective quality evaluations were done using a noisy speech corpus (NOIZEUS) developed in our lab [1]. This corpus was designed to facilitate comparisons of speech enhancement algorithms among research labs. The enhanced speech files were sent to Dynastat, Inc. (Austin, TX) for subjective quality evaluation based on the ITU-T P.835 methodology (see Chapter 10). The subjective ratings were subsequently used to evaluate the correlation of several widely used objective measures with speech quality. The intelligibility evaluations were done using the IEEE sentence corpus. Noisy sentences enhanced by the various algorithms were presented to normal-hearing listeners and asked to identify the words spoken. The results of the intelligibility studies are summarized in this chapter.

12.1 NOIZEUS: A NOISY SPEECH CORPUS FOR QUALITY EVALUATION OF SPEECH ENHANCEMENT ALGORITHMS

NOIZEUS is a noisy speech corpus recorded in our lab to facilitate comparison of speech enhancement algorithms among research groups. The noisy database contains 30 IEEE sentences [2,3] produced by three male and three female speakers and was corrupted by eight different real-world noises at different SNRs.

The noise was taken from the AURORA database [4] and includes suburban train noise, multitalker babble, car, exhibition hall, restaurant, street, airport, and train-station noise.

Thirty sentences from the IEEE sentence database were recorded in a sound-proof booth using Tucker Davis Technologies recording equipment. The sentences were produced by three male and three female speakers (five sentences/speaker). The IEEE database was selected because it contains phonetically balanced sentences with relatively low word-context predictability. Thirty sentences were selected from the IEEE database so as to include all phonemes in the American English language. The sentences were originally sampled at 25 kHz and downsampled to 8 kHz. A subset of the sentences recorded is given in Table 12.1.

To simulate the receiving frequency characteristics of telephone handsets, the speech and noise signals were filtered by the modified Intermediate Reference System (IRS) filters used in ITU-T P.862 [5] for evaluation of the PESQ measure. Noise was artificially added to the speech signal as follows. The IRS filter was independently applied to the clean and noise signals. The active speech level of the filtered clean speech signal was first determined using method B of ITU-T P.56 [6]. A noise segment of the same length as the speech signal was randomly cut out of the noise recordings, appropriately scaled to reach the desired SNR level and finally added to the filtered clean speech signal.

Noise signals were taken from the AURORA database [4] and included the following recordings from different places: babble (crowd of people), car, exhibition hall, restaurant, street, airport, train station, and train. The noise signals were added to

TABLE 12.1
Subset of Sentences from the NOIZEUS Speech Corpus Used in the Subjective Quality Evaluation

Filename	Speaker	Gender	Sentence Text
sp01.wav	CH	M	The birch canoe slid on the smooth planks
sp02.wav	CH	M	He knew the skill of the great young actress
sp03.wav	CH	M	Her purse was full of useless trash
sp04.wav	CH	M	Read verse out loud for pleasure
sp06.wav	DE	M	Men strive but seldom get rich
sp07.wav	DE	M	We find joy in the simplest things
sp08.wav	DE	M	Hedge apples may stain your hands green
sp09.wav	DE	M	Hurdle the pit with the aid of a long pole
sp11.wav	JE	F	He wrote down a long list of items
sp12.wav	JE	F	The drip of the rain made a pleasant sound
sp13.wav	JE	F	Smoke poured out of every crack
sp14.wav	JE	F	Hats are worn to tea and not to dinner
sp16.wav	KI	F	The stray cat gave birth to kittens
sp17.wav	KI	F	The lazy cow lay in the cool grass
sp18.wav	KI	F	The friendly gang left the drug store
sp19.wav	KI	F	We talked of the sideshow in the circus

the speech signals at SNRs of 0, 5, 10, and 15 dB. The NOIZEUS speech corpus was used in the subjective quality evaluation of several speech enhancement algorithms. This evaluation is described next.

12.2 COMPARISON OF ENHANCEMENT ALGORITHMS: SPEECH QUALITY

A total of 13 different speech enhancement methods were evaluated (see list in Table 12.2) [3]. Representative algorithms from four different classes of enhancement algorithms described in this book were chosen: three spectral subtractive algorithms, two subspace algorithms, three Wiener-type algorithms, and five statistical-model-based algorithms. The Wiener-type algorithms were grouped separately since these algorithms estimate the complex spectrum in the mean-square sense while the statistical-model algorithms estimate the magnitude spectrum. A subset of those algorithms was evaluated with and without noise estimation algorithms (denoted in Table 12.2 with the suffix -ne). The parameters used in the implementation of these algorithms were the same as those published unless stated otherwise. No adjustments were made for the algorithms (e.g., [7]) originally designed for a sampling rate of 16 kHz.

A statistical-model-based voice activity detector (VAD) [8] was used in all algorithms to update the noise spectrum during speech-absent periods. The following VAD decision rule was used:

$$\frac{1}{N}\sum_{k=1}^{N-1}\log\Lambda_k \underset{H_0}{\overset{H_1}{\gtrless}} \delta \tag{12.1}$$

TABLE 12.2
List of the 13 Speech Enhancement Algorithms Evaluated

Algorithm	Equation/Parameters	Reference	Chapter/Section (This Book)
KLT	Equations 14,48	[12]	Section 8.7.4.1
pKLT	Equation 34	[13]	Section 8.9.2
MMSE-SPU	Equations 7,51, $q = 0.3$	[9]	Section 7.13.2
logMMSE	Equation 20	[25]	Section 7.7
logMMSE-ne	Equation 20	[25,27]	Sections 7.7 and 9.4.3.2.2
logMMSE-SPU	Equations 2,8,10,16	[7]	Section 7.13.3
pMMSE	Equation 12	[28]	Section 7.12.2
RDC	Equations 6,7,10,14,15	[17]	Section 5.9
RDC-ne	Equations 6,7,10,14,15	[17,27]	Sections 5.9 and 9.4.3.2.2
MB	Equations 4 through 7	[15,16]	Section 5.6
WT	Equations 11, 25	[19]	Section 6.10
Wiener-as	Equations 3 through 7	[18]	Section 6.10
AudSup	Equations 26, 38, $\nu = 1, 2$ iterations	[22]	Section 6.13

SPU, speech presence uncertainty; ne, noise estimation.

where

$$\Lambda_k = \frac{1}{1+\xi_k} \exp\left\{ \frac{\gamma_k \xi_k}{1+\xi_k} \right\} \quad (12.2)$$

where
γ_k and ξ_k are the posterior and *a priori* SNRs, respectively [9]
ξ_k is computed using the decision-directed approach with $a = 0.98$
N is the size of the FFT
H_1 denotes the hypothesis of speech presence
H_0 denotes the hypothesis of speech absence
δ is a fixed threshold, which was set to $\delta = 0.15$ in [1]

When speech absence was detected, the noise power spectrum was updated according to:

$$D_k(i) = (1-\beta) \cdot Y_k^2(i) + \beta D_k(i-1) \quad (12.3)$$

where
$\beta = 0.98$
$D_k(i)$ is the noise power spectrum in frame i (for frequency bin k)
$Y_k^2(i)$ is the noisy speech power spectrum

The subspace methods used a different VAD method [10] with the threshold value set to 1.2.

12.2.1 Quality Evaluation: Procedure

To reduce the length and cost of the subjective evaluations, only a subset of the NOIZEUS corpus was processed by the 13 algorithms and submitted to Dynastat, Inc. for formal subjective evaluation. A total of 16 sentences (see Table 12.1) corrupted in four background noise environments (car, street, babble, and train) at two levels of SNR (5 and 10 dB) were processed. These sentences were produced by two male speakers and two female speakers.

The subjective listening tests were conducted by Dynastat, Inc. (Austin, TX) according to the ITU-Trecommendation P.835 [11]. As mentioned in Chapter 10, the P.835 methodology was designed to reduce the listener's uncertainty in a subjective test as to which component(s) of a noisy speech signal, that is, the speech signal, the background noise, or both, should form the basis of their ratings of overall quality. This method instructs the listener to successively attend to and rate the enhanced speech signal on the following:

1. The speech signal alone using a five-point scale of signal distortion (SIG)—see Table 10.16
2. The background noise alone using a five-point scale of background intrusiveness (BAK)—see Table 10.17
3. The overall effect using the scale of the mean opinion score (OVL)—[1 = bad, 2 = poor, 3 = fair, 4 = good, 5 = excellent]

The total number of test conditions was too large to present in a single P.835 test. Therefore, the test conditions were partitioned into two subsets, which were evaluated in two separate P.835 tests. A total of 32 listeners were recruited by Dynastat, Inc. for the listening tests. Listeners were native speakers of North American English and were between the ages of 18 and 50 years. No listener had participated in a listening test in the previous 3 months.

12.2.2 Subjective Quality Evaluation: Results

Figures 12.1 through 12.4 show the mean scores for the SIG, BAK, and OVL scales for speech processed by 13 different speech enhancement algorithms evaluated in four types of background noise and at two SNR levels (5 and 10 dB). The mean scores for the noisy speech (unprocessed) sentence are also shown for reference.

Comparative analysis is presented next at three levels. At the first level, we compare the performance of the algorithms within each of the four classes (subspace, statistical-model, subtractive, and Wiener-type). This comparison was meant to examine significant differences between algorithms within each class. At the second level, we compare the performance of the various algorithms across all classes aiming to find the algorithm(s) that performed the best across all noise conditions. Lastly, at the third level, we compare the performance of all algorithms in reference to the noisy speech (unprocessed). This latter comparison will provide valuable information as to which algorithm(s) improves (or not) significantly the quality of noisy speech.

In order to assess significant differences between the ratings obtained with each algorithm, we subjected the ratings of the 32 listeners to statistical analysis. Multiple comparison statistical tests according to Tukey's HSD test were conducted to assess significant differences between algorithms. Differences between scores were deemed significant if the obtained p value (level of significance) was smaller than 0.05.

12.2.3 Within-Class Algorithm Comparisons

In terms of overall quality, the two subspace algorithms examined performed equally well for most SNR conditions and four types of noise, except at +5 dB car noise. The generalized subspace (KLT) approach [12] performed significantly ($p = 0.006$) better than the pKLT approach [13] in +5 dbB car noise. Lower noise distortion (i.e., higher BAK scores) was observed with the pKLT method in most conditions; however, the difference in scores was not found to be statistically significant. Significantly ($p = 0.017$), lower noise distortion (i.e., higher BAK scores) was observed with the pKLT method only in +5 dB train noise. Lower signal distortion was generally observed with the generalized subspace method in most conditions with significant differences in +5 dB train noise and in both car noise conditions (5 and 10 dB). In brief, of the two subspace methods, the generalized subspace approach performed slightly better in terms of overall quality and lower signal distortion. The pKLT approach was more successful in suppressing background noise at the expense of introducing signal distortion.

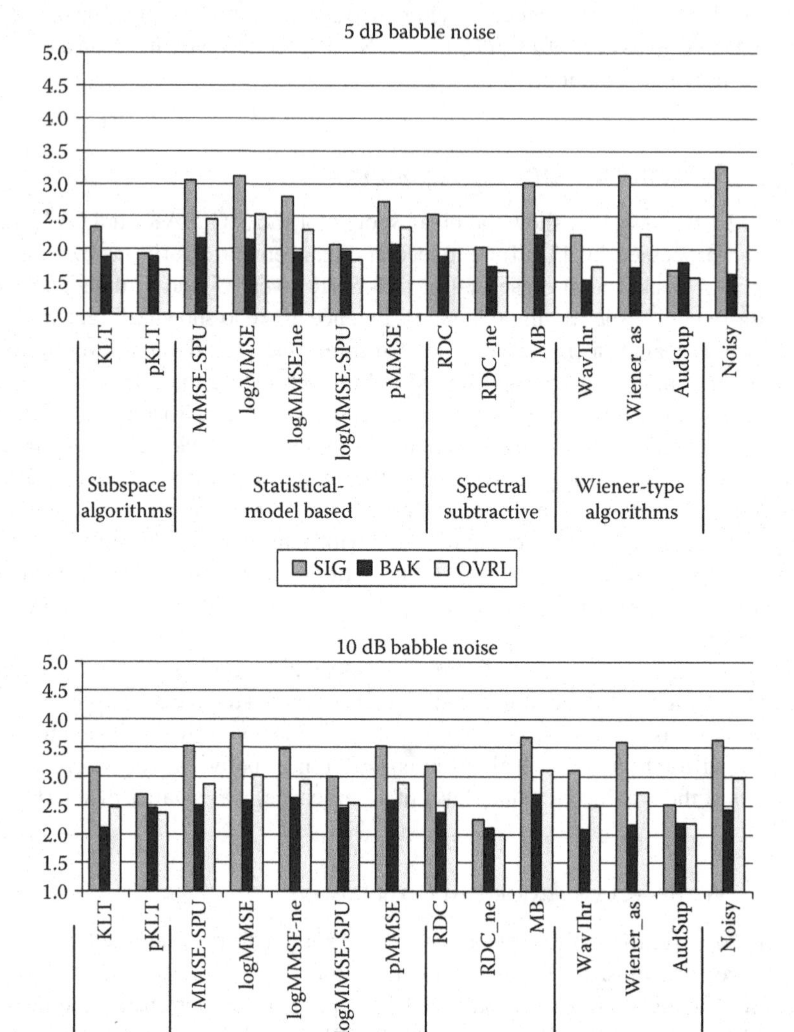

FIGURE 12.1 The mean scores for SIG, BAK, and OVL scales for the 13 methods evaluated in babble background and for SNR levels of 5 and 10 dB.

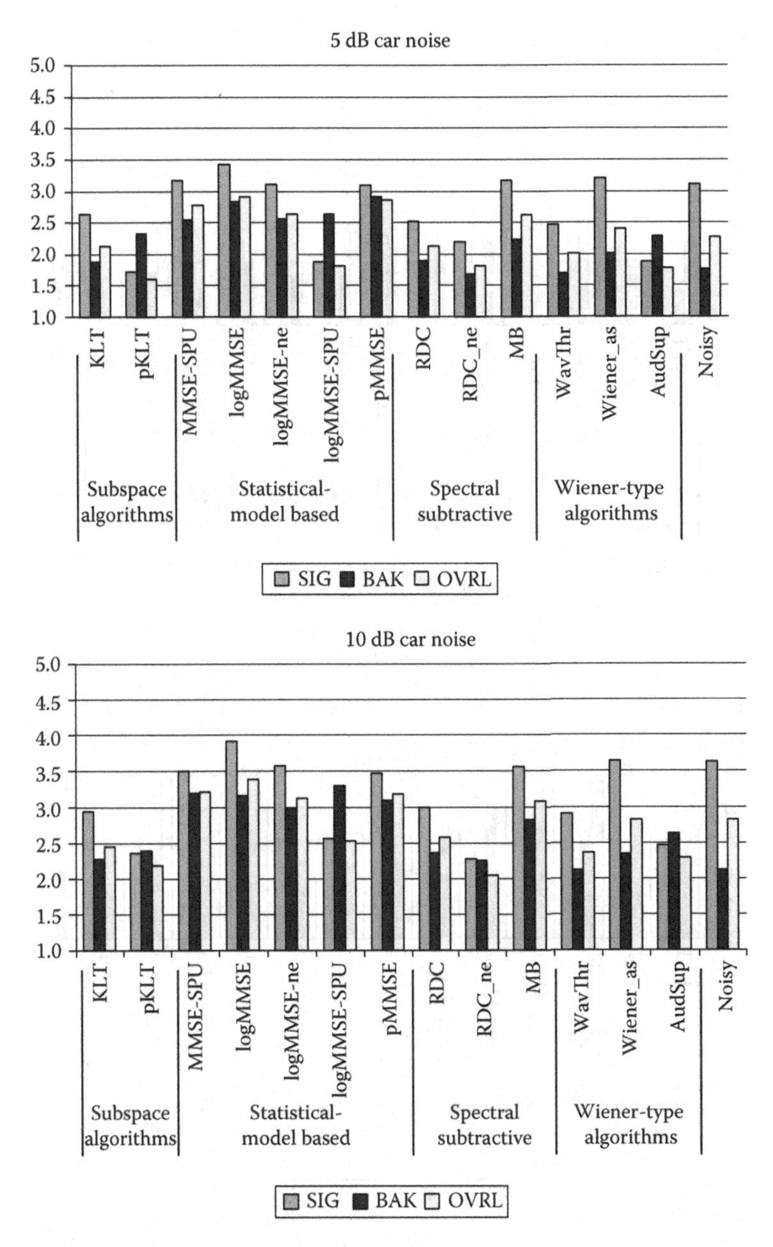

FIGURE 12.2 The mean scores for SIG, BAK, and OVL scales for the 13 methods evaluated in car noise and for SNR levels of 5 and 10 dB.

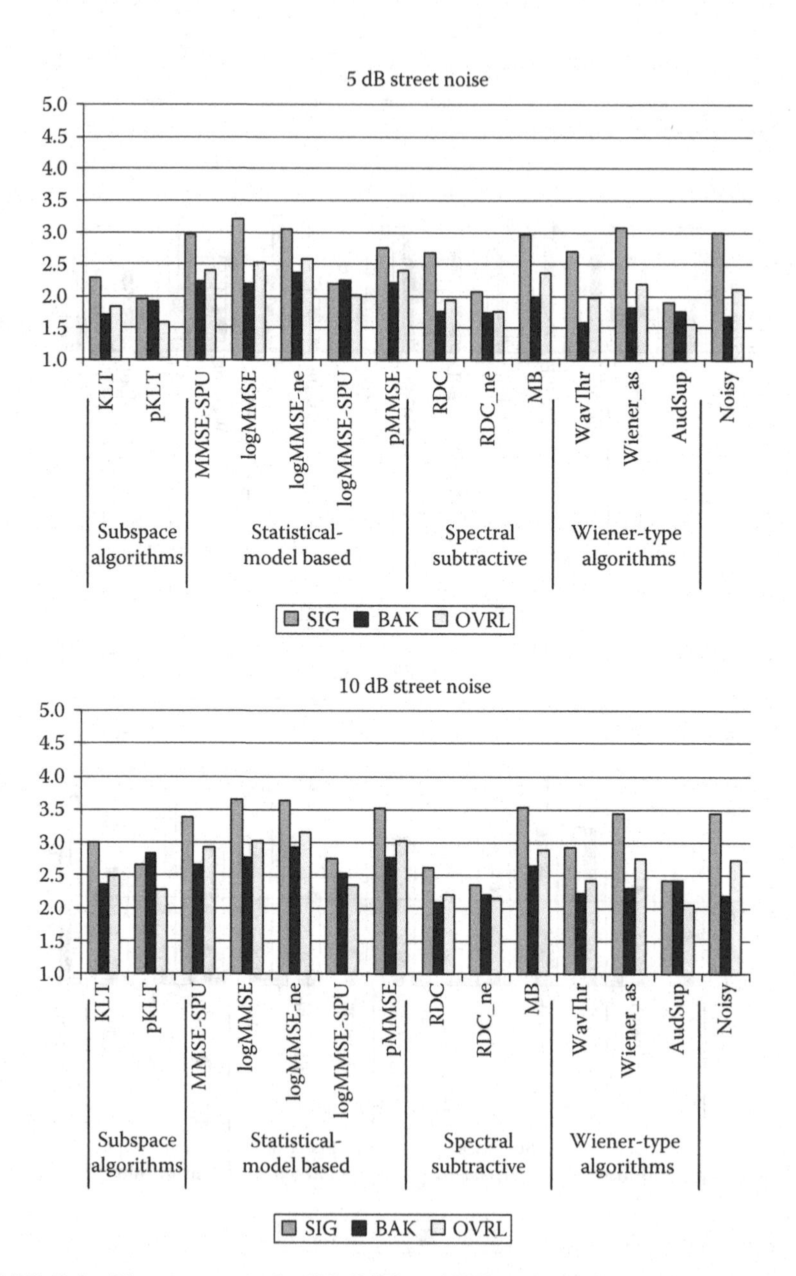

FIGURE 12.3 The mean scores for SIG, BAK, and OVL scales for the 13 methods evaluated in street noise and for SNR levels of 5 and 10 dB.

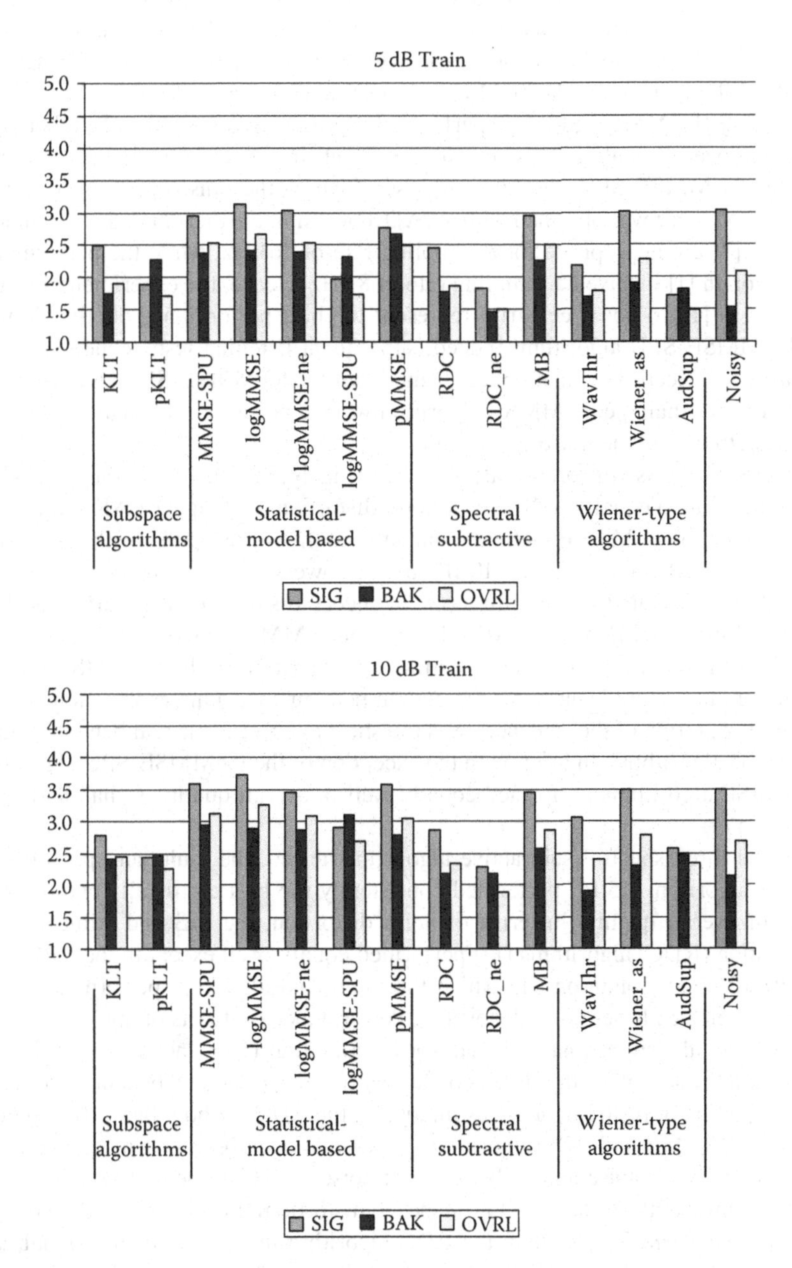

FIGURE 12.4 The mean scores for SIG, BAK, and OVL scales for the 13 methods evaluated in train noise and for SNR levels of 5 and 10dB.

The majority of the statistical-model-based algorithms examined performed equally well in terms of overall quality. There was no statistically significant difference in the overall quality between the MMSE-SPU, the log minimum mean square error (logMMSE), the logMMSE with noise estimation (logMMSE-ne), and the pMMSE algorithms. The logMMSE algorithm that incorporated signal-presence uncertainty (logMMSE-SPU) [7] performed significantly worse than the other algorithms in overall quality. This was surprising at first, but close analysis indicated that the logMMSE-SPU algorithm was sensitive to the noise spectrum estimate, which in our case was obtained with a VAD algorithm. Furthermore, the parameters given in [7] are appropriate for a sampling rate of 16 kHz, while the performance evaluation in [1] involved a sampling rate of 8 kHz. Hence, the experimental results reported in [1] do not necessarily represent the best performance obtainable with the logMMSE-SPU algorithm. Indeed, subsequent listening tests (conducted after Dynastat's subjective evaluation) confirmed that the logMMSE-SPU algorithm performed better than the logMMSE algorithm when a noise estimation algorithm [14] was used to update the noise spectrum.

In terms of noise distortion, all algorithms, including the logMMSE-SPU algorithm, performed equally well. Lower noise distortion (i.e., higher BAK scores) was obtained with the pMMSE method (compared to the MMSE-SPU method) in some conditions (5 dB train, 5 dB car, 10 dB street); however, the difference was not statistically significant ($p > 0.05$). In terms of speech distortion, nearly all algorithms (MMSE-SPU, logMMSE, logMMSE-ne, and pMMSE algorithms) performed equally well. Incorporating a noise estimation algorithm in the logMMSE method did not produce significant improvements in performance. One explanation for that is that the duration of the sentences was too short to observe the real benefit of noise estimation algorithms. In brief, with the exception of the logMMSE-SPU algorithm, the MMSE algorithms performed equally well in overall quality, signal, and noise distortion.

Of the three spectral subtractive algorithms tested, the multibandspectral subtraction algorithm [15,16] performed consistently the best across all conditions, in terms of overall quality. In terms of noise distortion, the MB and reduced-delay convolution (RDC) algorithms [17] performed equally well except in the 5 dB train and 10 dB street conditions, in which the multiband algorithm performed significantly better (i.e., lower noise distortion). Performance (in terms of noise distortion) of the RDC algorithm that included noise estimation (RDC-ne) was significantly lower than the MB algorithm in all conditions. There was no real benefit, in terms of overall quality, of including noise estimation in the RDC method. In terms of speech distortion, the MB and RDC algorithms performed equally well in most conditions except in 5 dB car noise and in 10 dB street noise, in which the MB algorithm performed significantly better (i.e., lower speech distortion). In brief, the MB algorithm generally performed better than the RDC algorithm in overall quality, signal, and noise distortion. It should be noted that the MB algorithm has an unfair advantage over the RDC algorithm in that it uses noncausal filtering (Equation 5.58) to smooth out the noisy speech spectra. That is, it assumes access to information from two future frames of speech.

Finally, of the three Wiener-filtering-type algorithms examined, the Wiener-as [18] and wavelet-thresholded (WT) algorithms [19] performed the best. In terms of overall quality, the Wiener-as method performed better than the WT method in three conditions: 5dB train, 10dB car, and 5dB babble noise. In the remaining five conditions, the Wiener-as method performed as well as the WT method. The Wiener-as method also produced consistently lower signal distortion for most conditions, except in 10dB train, 10dB babble, and street conditions, in which it performed equally well with the WT method. All three Wiener-type algorithms produced the same level of noise distortion in all conditions. In brief, the Wiener-as method performed, for the most part, better than the other Wiener-type algorithms in terms of overall quality and low signal distortion.

12.2.4 Across-Class Algorithm Comparisons

The aforementioned comparisons assessed differences between algorithms within each of the four classes of speech enhancement methods, but did not provide the answer as to which algorithm(s) performed the best overall across all noise conditions. Such comparisons are reported next.

Multiple-paired comparisons (Tukey's HSD) were conducted between the algorithm with the highest score against all other algorithms. Tables 12.3 through 12.5 report the results for the overall quality, signal distortion, and noise distortion comparisons, respectively.

Table 12.3 shows the results obtained from the statistical analysis for overall quality. Asterisks in the table indicate the absence of statistically significant difference (i.e., $p > 0.05$) between the algorithm with the highest score and the denoted algorithm. That is, the algorithms denoted by asterisks in Table 12.3 performed equally well. It is clear from Table 12.3 that there is no single best algorithm, but rather that several algorithms performed equally well across most conditions. In terms of overall quality, the following algorithms performed equally well across all conditions: MMSE-SPU, logMMSE, logMMSE-ne, pMMSE, and MB. The Wiener-as method also performed well in five of the eight conditions.

Table 12.4 shows the results obtained from the statistical analysis for signal distortion. The following algorithms performed the best, in terms of yielding the lowest speech distortion, across all conditions: MMSE-SPU, logMMSE, logMMSE-ne, pMMSE, MB, and Wiener-as. The KLT, RDC, and WT algorithms also performed well in a few isolated conditions.

Finally, Table 12.5 shows the results obtained from the statistical analysis for noise distortion. The following algorithms performed the best, in terms of yielding the lowest noise distortion across nearly all conditions: MMSE-SPU, logMMSE, logMMSE-ne, pMMSE, and MB. The pKLT method also performed well in five of the eight conditions. The KLT, RDC, RDC-ne, Wiener-as, and AudSup algorithms performed well in a few isolated conditions.

Comparing the results in Tables 12.3 through 12.5, we observe that the algorithms that yielded the lowest noise distortion (i.e., lowest noise residual) were not necessarily the algorithms that yielded the highest overall quality. The pKLT algorithm, for instance, performed well in terms of noise distortion, but performed poorly in

TABLE 12.3
Results Obtained from Comparative Statistical Analysis of Overall Quality (OVL) Scores

Noise	SNR	Subspace		Statistical-Model-Based					Spectral Subtractive			Wiener-Type		
Type	(dB)	KLT	pKLT	MMSE-SPU	logMMSE	logMMSE-ne	logMMSE-SPU	pMMSE	RDC	RDC-ne	MB	WT	Wiener-as	AudSup
Car	5			*	*	*		*			*			
	10			*	*	*		*			*			
Babble	5			*	*	*		*			*		*	
	10			*	*	*		*			*		*	
Street	5			*	*	*		*			*		*	
	10			*	*	*		*			*		*	
Train	5			*	*	*		*			*		*	
	10			*	*	*		*			*			

Algorithms indicated by asterisks performed equally well.
Algorithms with no asterisks performed poorly.

TABLE 12.4
Results Obtained from Comparative Statistical Analysis of Speech Distortion (SIG) Scores

Noise	SNR	Subspace		Statistical-Model-Based					Spectral Subtractive			Wiener-Type		
Type	(dB)	KLT	pKLT	MMSE-SPU	logMMSE	logMMSE-ne	logMMSE-SPU	pMMSE	RDC	RDC-ne	MB	WT	Wiener-as	AudSup
Car	5			*	*	*		*			*		*	
	10			*	*	*		*			*		*	
Babble	5			*	*	*		*			*		*	
	10	*		*	*	*		*	*		*		*	
Street	5			*	*	*		*	*		*	*	*	
	10			*	*	*		*			*		*	
Train	5			*	*	*		*			*		*	
	10			*	*	*		*			*		*	

Algorithms indicated by asterisks performed equally well.
Algorithms with no asterisks performed poorly.

TABLE 12.5
Results Obtained from Comparative Statistical Analysis of Noise Distortion (BAK) Scores

Noise	SNR	Subspace		Statistical-Model-Based					Spectral Subtractive			Wiener-Type		
Type	(dB)	KLT	pKLT	MMSE-SPU	logMMSE	logMMSE-ne	logMMSE-SPU	pMMSE	RDC	RDC-ne	MB	WT	Wiener-as	AudSup
Car	5			*	*	*	*	*						
	10			*	*	*	*	*			*		*	*
Babble	5	*	*	*	*	*	*	*	*	*	*			*
	10		*	*	*	*	*	*	*		*			
Street	5		*	*	*	*	*	*			*			
	10		*	*	*	*	*	*			*			
Train	5		*	*	*	*	*	*			*			
	10			*	*	*	*	*						

Algorithms indicated by asterisks performed equally well.
Algorithms with no asterisks performed poorly.

terms of overall quality and speech distortion. In contrast, the algorithms that performed the best in terms of speech distortion were also the algorithms with the highest overall quality. This suggests that listeners are influenced more by the distortion imparted on the speech signal than on the background noise when making judgments of overall quality (more on this in later section). That is, listeners seem to place more emphasis on the speech rather than on the noise distortion when judging the quality of speech enhanced by a noise suppression algorithm.

12.2.5 Comparisons in Reference to Noisy Speech

Lastly, we report on the comparisons between the enhanced speech and the noisy (unprocessed) speech. Such comparisons are important as they tell us about the possible benefits (or lack thereof) of using speech enhancement algorithms.

Multiple-paired comparisons (Tukey's HSD) were conducted between the ratings obtained with noisy speech (unprocessed) samples and the ratings obtained with speech enhanced by the various algorithms. The results are reported in Tables 12.6 through 12.8 for overall quality, signal distortion, and noise distortion comparisons, respectively. In these tables, asterisks indicate significant differences (i.e., significant benefits) between the ratings of noisy speech and enhanced speech. Table entries indicated as "ns" denote nonsignificant differences between the ratings of noisy speech and enhanced speech, that is, noisy and enhanced speech were rated equally. Blank entries in the tables indicate inferior ratings (i.e., significantly poorer ratings) for the enhanced speech compared to the ratings of noisy (unprocessed) speech samples.

Table 12.6 shows the comparisons of the ratings of overall quality of noisy (unprocessed) speech and enhanced speech. The striking finding is that only a subset of the algorithms tested provided significant benefit to overall quality and only in a few conditions (car, street, and train). The algorithms MMSE-SPU, logMMSE, logMMSE-ne, and pMMSE improved significantly the overall speech quality but only in a few isolated conditions. The majority of the algorithms (indicated with 'ns' in Table 12.6) did not provide significant improvement in overall quality when compared to the noisy (unprocessed) speech.

Table 12.7 shows the comparisons of the ratings of signal distortion of noisy speech and enhanced speech. For this comparison, we do not expect to see any asterisks in the table. That is, good performance is now indicated with "ns," suggesting that the enhanced speech did not contain any notable speech distortion. The algorithms MMSE-SPU, logMMSE, logMMSE-ne, pMMSE, MB, and Wiener-as performed the best (i.e., no notable speech distortion was introduced) in all conditions. The algorithms WT, RDC, and KLT also performed well in a few isolated conditions.

Finally, Table 12.8 shows the comparisons of the ratings of noise distortion of noisy speech and enhanced speech. The algorithms MMSE-SPU, logMMSE, logMMSE-ne, logMMSE-SPU, and pMMSE lowered significantly noise distortion for most conditions. The MB, pKLT, and AudSup also lowered noise distortion in a few (2–3) conditions. The remaining algorithms (indicated with "ns" in Table 12.8) did not lower significantly noise distortion compared to that of noisy (unprocessed) speech. That is, the background noise level was not perceived to be significantly lower in the enhanced speech than the noisy speech.

TABLE 12.6
Statistical Comparisons between the Ratings of Overall Quality of Noisy (Unprocessed) Speech and Enhanced Speech

Noise	SNR	Subspace		Statistical-Model-Based					Spectral Subtractive			Wiener-Type		
Type	(dB)	KLT	pKLT	MMSE-SPU	logMMSE	logMMSE-ne	logMMSE-SPU	pMMSE	RDC	RDC-ne	MB	WT	Wiener-as	AudSup
Car	5	ns		*	*	ns		*	ns		ns	ns	ns	
	10	ns		ns	*	ns	ns	ns	ns		ns		ns	
Babble	5	ns		ns	ns	ns		ns	ns		ns		ns	
	10			ns	ns	ns	ns	ns	ns		ns		ns	
Street	5	ns		ns	ns	*	ns	ns	ns	ns	ns	ns	ns	
	10	ns	ns	ns	ns	ns	ns	ns			ns	ns	ns	
Train	5	ns	ns	*	*		ns	ns	ns		ns	ns	ns	
	10	ns	ns	ns	*	ns	ns	ns	ns		ns	ns	ns	ns

Algorithms denoted with asterisks improved significantly the overall quality of noisy speech. That is, the quality of the enhanced speech was judged to be significantly better than that of noisy speech. In contrast, algorithms denoted with "ns" did not improve the overall quality of noisy speech.

TABLE 12.7
Statistical Comparisons between the Ratings of Speech Distortion (SIG) of Noisy (Unprocessed) Speech and Enhanced Speech

Noise	SNR	Subspace		Statistical-Model-Based					Spectral Subtractive			Wiener-Type		
Type	(dB)	KLT	pKLT	MMSE-SPU	logMMSE	logMMSE-ne	logMMSE-SPU	pMMSE	RDC	RDC-ne	MB	WT	Wiener-as	AudSup
Car	5	ns		ns	ns	ns		ns	ns		ns		ns	
	10			ns	ns	ns		ns			ns		ns	
Babble	5			ns	ns	ns		ns			ns		ns	
	10	ns		ns	ns	ns		ns	ns		ns	ns	ns	
Street	5			ns	ns	ns		ns	ns		ns	ns	ns	
	10	ns		ns	ns	ns		ns			ns	ns	ns	
Train	5	ns		ns	ns	ns		ns			ns		ns	
	10			ns	ns	ns	ns	ns			ns		ns	ns

Algorithms denoted with "ns" did not introduce notable speech distortion. In contrast, algorithms with blank table entries introduced notable speech distortion when compared to the noisy (unprocessed) speech.

TABLE 12.8
Statistical Comparisons between the Ratings of Noise Distortion (BAK) of Noisy (Unprocessed) Speech and Enhanced Speech

Noise	SNR	Subspace		Statistical-Model-Based					Spectral Subtractive			Wiener-Type		
Type	(dB)	KLT	pKLT	MMSE-SPU	logMMSE	logMMSE-ne	logMMSE-SPU	pMMSE	RDC	RDC-ne	MB	WT	Wiener-as	AudSup
Car	5	ns	*	*	*	*	*	*	ns	ns	ns	ns	ns	*
	10	ns	ns	*	*	*	*	*	ns	ns	*	ns	ns	*
Babble	5	ns	ns	*	*	ns	ns	ns	ns	ns	*	ns	ns	ns
	10	ns	ns	ns	ns	ns	ns	ns	ns	ns	ns	ns	ns	ns
Street	5	ns	ns	*	*	*	*	*	ns	ns	ns	ns	ns	ns
	10	ns	*	ns	*	*	ns	*	ns	ns	ns	ns	ns	ns
Train	5	ns	*	*	*	*	*	*	ns	ns	*	ns	ns	ns
	10	ns	ns	*	*	*	*	*	ns	ns	ns	ns	ns	ns

Algorithms denoted with asterisks significantly lowered noise distortion compared to that of unprocessed noisy speech. In contrast, algorithms denoted with “ns” did not lower noise distortion.

12.2.6 Contribution of Speech and Noise Distortion to Judgment of Overall Quality

As mentioned earlier, the P.835 process of rating the signal and background of noisy speech was designed to lead the listener to integrate the effects of the signal and the background in making their ratings of overall quality. Of great interest is understanding the individual contribution of speech and noise distortion to judgment of overall quality. Previous data (Tables 12.3 and 12.4) led us to believe that listeners were influenced more by speech distortion when making quality judgments. To further substantiate this, we performed multiple linear regression analysis on the ratings obtained for overall quality, speech, and noise distortion. We treated the overall quality score as the dependent variable and the speech and noise distortion scores as the independent variables. Regression analysis revealed the following relationship between the three rating scales:

$$R_{OVL} = -0.0783 + 0.571 R_{SIG} + 0.366 R_{BAK} \tag{12.4}$$

where

R_{OVL} is the predicted overall (OVL) rating score
R_{SIG} is the SIG rating
R_{BAK} is the BAK rating

The resulting correlation coefficient was ρ = 0.927, and the standard deviation of the error was 0.22. Figure 12.5 shows the scatter plot of the listener's overall quality ratings against the predicted ratings obtained with Equation 12.4. The aforementioned

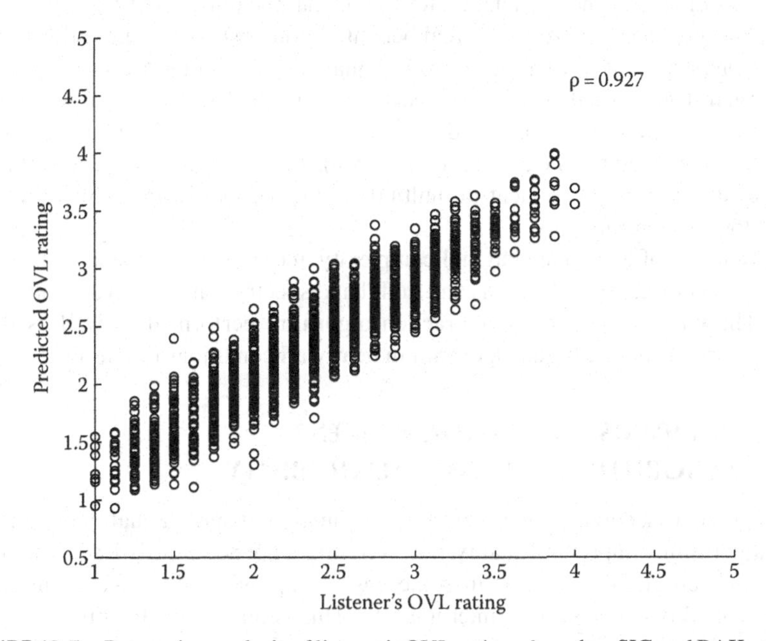

FIGURE 12.5 Regression analysis of listener's OVL ratings, based on SIG and BAK ratings.

equation confirms that listeners were indeed integrating the effects of both signal and background distortion when making their ratings. Different emphasis was placed, however, on the two types of distortion. Consistent with our previous observation, listeners seem to place more emphasis on the distortion imparted on the speech signal itself rather than on the background noise, when making judgments of overall quality.

12.2.7 Summary of Findings

Based on the statistical analysis of the listener's ratings of the enhanced speech, in terms of overall quality, speech, and noise distortion, we can draw the following conclusions:

- In terms of overall quality, the following algorithms performed the best: MMSE-SPU, logMMSE, logMMSE-ne, pMMSE, and MB. These algorithms also yielded the lowest speech distortion. The Wiener-as algorithm also performed well in some conditions. The subspace algorithms performed poorly.
- The algorithms that performed the best in terms of yielding the lowest speech distortion were also the algorithms that yielded the highest overall quality. This suggests that listeners were influenced for the most part by the distortion imparted on the speech signal than on the background noise when making judgments of overall quality. This was also confirmed by regression analysis (Equation 12.4).
- Incorporating noise estimation algorithms in place of VAD algorithms for updating the noise spectrum did not produce significant improvements in performance. One explanation for that is that the duration of the sentences was too short to observe the real benefit of noise estimation algorithms.
- Comparisons of ratings of the overall quality of noisy (unprocessed) speech against that of enhanced (processed) speech revealed that only a subset of the algorithms tested provided significant benefit to overall quality and only in a few conditions (car, street, and train). No algorithm produced significant quality improvement in multitalker babble, that is, in highly nonstationary environments.
- In terms of low computational complexity and good performance, the two winners were the Wiener-as and multiband spectral subtraction algorithms. The multiband spectral subtraction algorithm performed as well as the statistical-model-based algorithm in nearly all conditions (Table 12.3).

12.3 COMPARISON OF ENHANCEMENT ALGORITHMS: SPEECH INTELLIGIBILITY

In the previous section, we focused on the evaluation of speech quality of enhancement algorithms. Improving quality, however, might not necessarily lead to improvement in intelligibility. In fact, in some cases, improvement in quality might be accompanied by a decrease in intelligibility. This is due to the distortion imparted on the clean speech signal resulting in the process of suppressing the acoustic noise.

In some applications, the main goal of speech enhancement algorithms is to improve speech quality and preserve, at the very least, speech intelligibility. Hence, much of the focus of most speech enhancement algorithms has been to improve speech quality. Only a small number of algorithms have been evaluated using formal intelligibility tests [20–23], and in those studies, only a single speech enhancement algorithm was evaluated and in a limited number of noise conditions. It therefore remains unclear as to which of the many speech enhancement algorithms proposed in the literature performs well in terms of speech intelligibility. At the very least, we would like to know which algorithm(s) preserve or maintain speech intelligibility in reference to the noisy (unprocessed) speech, and which algorithm(s) impair speech intelligibility, particularly in extremely low-SNR conditions.

In this section, we report on the intelligibility evaluation of eight speech enhancement methods encompassing four classes of algorithms: spectral subtractive, subspace, statistical-model-based, and Wiener-type algorithms [24]. A subset of the algorithms used in the subjective quality evaluation (Section 12.2) was used. The enhanced speech files were presented to normal-hearing subjects in a double-walled sound-proof booth and asked to identify the words in the spoken sentences. Next, we present the summary of these intelligibility tests.

12.3.1 Listening Tests: Procedure

IEEE sentences [2] were used in the listening tests. The IEEE database was selected as it contains phonetically balanced sentences with relatively low word-context predictability. The IEEE sentences were recorded in a sound-proof booth using Tucker Davis Technologies recording equipment. The sentences, produced by one male speaker, were originally sampled at 25 kHz and downsampled to 8 kHz. Noise was artificially added to the sentences the same way as done with the sentences used in the NOIZEUS corpus (see Section 12.1). The noise signals were taken from the AURORA database [4] and included the following recordings from different places: babble (crowd of people), car, street, and train. The noise signals were added to the speech signals at SNRs of 0 and 5 dB.

The noise-corrupted sentences were processed by eight different speech enhancement algorithms, which included the generalized subspace (KLT) approach [12], the perceptual KLT approach (pKLT) [13], the logMMSE algorithm [25], the logMMSE algorithm implemented with speech presence uncertainty (logMMSE-SPU) [7], the spectral subtraction algorithm based on RDC [17], the multiband spectral subtraction algorithm (MB) [15], the Wiener-filtering algorithm based on WT multitaper spectra [19], and the Wiener algorithm based on *a priori* SNR estimation (Wiener-as) [18]. The parameters used in the implementation of the aforementioned algorithms were the same as those used in the subjective quality evaluation (Section 12.2) and are given in Table 12.2.

A total of 24 listeners (all native speakers of American English) were recruited for the listening tests. The subjects were paid for their participation. The 24 listeners were divided into 4 panels with each panel consisting of 6 listeners. Each panel of listeners listened to sentences corrupted by a different type of noise. This was done to ensure that no subject listened to the same sentence twice. Each subject participated in a total of 19 listening conditions (= 2 SNR levels × 8 algorithms + 2 noisy references + 1 quiet). Two sentence lists (10 sentences per list) were used for each condition. The presentation order of the listening conditions was randomized among subjects. The processed speech files, along with the clean and noisy speech files, were presented to the listeners in a double-walled sound-proof booth via Sennheiser's (HD250 Linear II) circumaural headphones at a comfortable level. Tests were conducted in multiple sessions with each session lasting no more than 2h. The subjects were allowed to take break during the listening session to reduce fatigue.

12.3.2 Intelligibility Evaluation: Results

Listening tasks involved recognition of sentences in noise. Speech intelligibility was assessed in terms of percentage of words identified correctly. All words were considered in the scoring. Figures 12.6 and 12.7 show the mean intelligibility scores for

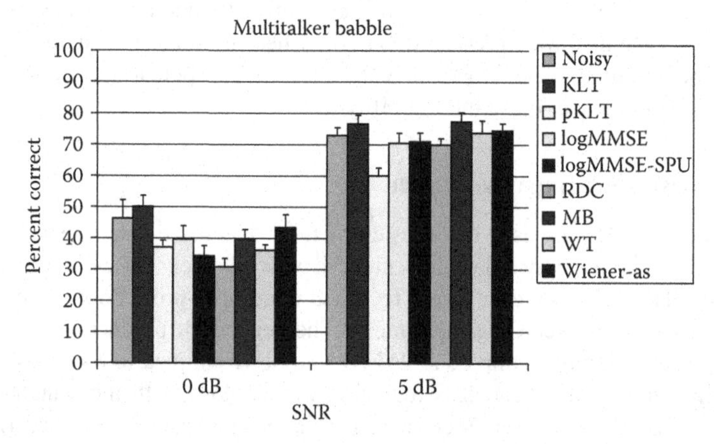

FIGURE 12.6 Mean intelligibility scores of eight speech enhancement algorithms for the sentences corrupted in multitalker babble (0 and 5dB).

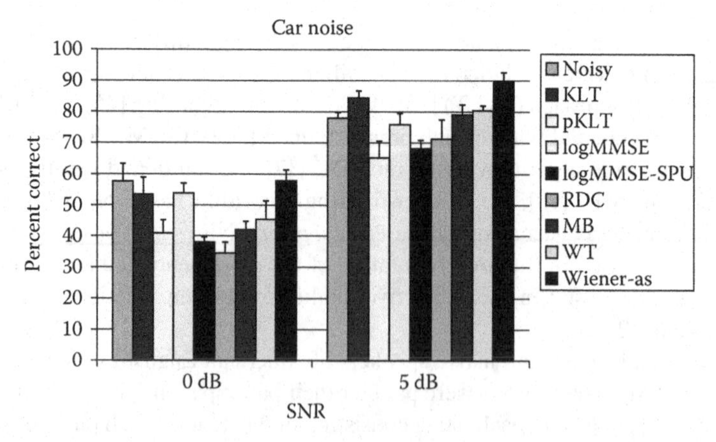

FIGURE 12.7 Mean intelligibility scores of eight speech enhancement algorithms for the sentences corrupted in car noise (0 and 5dB).

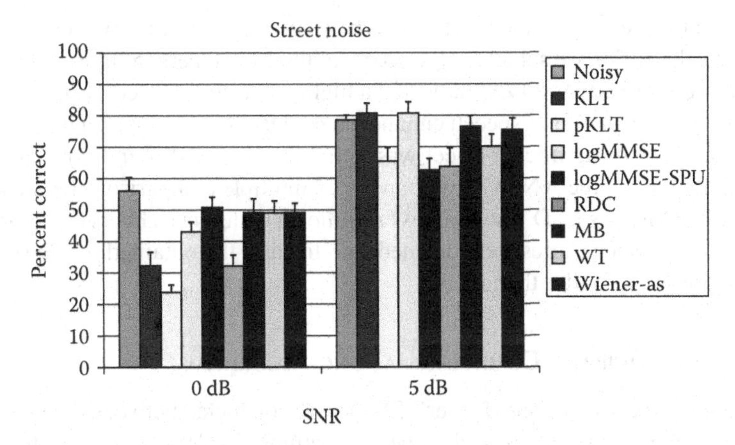

FIGURE 12.8 Mean intelligibility scores of eight speech enhancement algorithms for the sentences corrupted in street noise (0 and 5 dB).

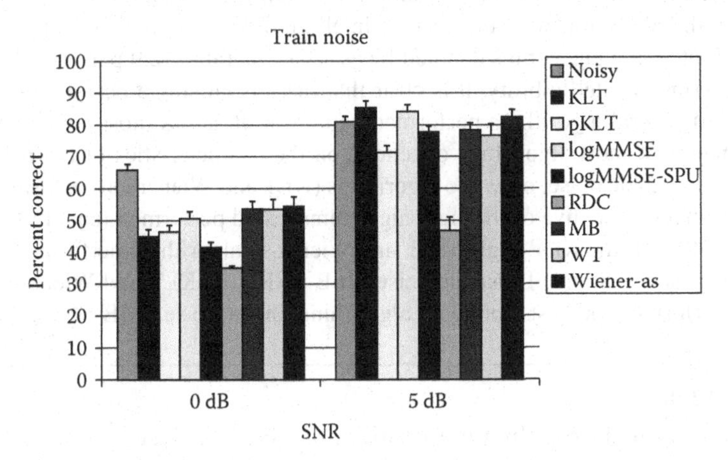

FIGURE 12.9 Mean intelligibility scores of eight speech enhancement algorithms for the sentences corrupted in train noise (0 and 5 dB).

multitalker babble and car noise, respectively. Figures 12.8 and 12.9 show the mean scores for street and train noise, respectively. The error bars in the figures give the standard errors of the mean. The intelligibility scores of noisy (unprocessed) speech are also given for comparative purposes.

We present comparative analysis of speech intelligibility at two levels [24]. At the first level, we compare the performance of the various algorithms across all classes aiming to find the algorithm(s) that performed the best across all noise conditions. At the second level, we compare the performance of all algorithms in reference to the noisy speech (unprocessed). This latter comparison will provide valuable information as to which, if any, algorithm(s) improve significantly the intelligibility of noisy speech. If no improvement is obtained, we will find out at the very least which algorithm(s) maintain speech intelligibility and which algorithm(s) diminish speech intelligibility.

In order to assess significant differences between the intelligibility scores obtained from each algorithm, we subjected the scores of the 24 listeners to statistical analysis. Analysis of variance (ANOVA) indicated a highly significant effect (e.g., for babble, $F(8,40) = 3.8$, $p < 0.005$) of speech enhancement algorithms on speech intelligibility. Similarly, a highly significant effect was found in other SNR conditions and types of noise. Following the ANOVA, we conducted multiple comparison statistical tests according to Fisher's LSD test to assess significant differences between algorithms. Differences between scores were deemed significant if the obtained p value (level of significance) was smaller than 0.05.

12.3.3 Intelligibility Comparison among Algorithms

Multiple-paired comparisons (Fisher's LSD) were conducted between the algorithms with the highest score against all other algorithms. Table 12.9 shows the results obtained from the comparative statistical analysis of intelligibility scores. Asterisks in the table indicate the absence of statistically significant difference (i.e., $p > 0.05$) between the algorithm with the highest intelligibility score and the denoted algorithm. That is, the algorithms denoted by asterisks in Table 12.9 performed equally well in terms of intelligibility. It is clear that there is no single best algorithm, but rather that several algorithms performed equally well across most conditions. The performance of most algorithms depended on the characteristics of the noise. For instance, in babble noise, only two algorithms (KLT and Wiener-as) performed well, while in street noise, five of the eight algorithms tested performed (equally) well.

At 0 dB SNR, the KLT, logMMSE, and Wiener-as algorithms performed equally well for most conditions. In babble noise (0 dB SNR), the KLT and Wiener-as algorithms performed the best among all algorithms. In car noise (0 dB SNR), the KLT,

TABLE 12.9
Results Obtained from the Comparative Statistical Analysis of Intelligibility Scores

Noise	SNR	Subspace		Statistical Model		Spectral Subtractive		Wiener-Type	
Type	(dB)	KLT	pKLT	logMMSE	logMMSE-SPU	RDC	MB	WT	Wiener-as
Car	0	*		*					*
Babble		*							*
Street				*	*		*	*	*
Train				*				*	*
Car	5	*						*	*
Babble		*		*	*		*	*	*
Street		*		*			*	*	*
Train		*		*			*		*

Algorithms indicated by asterisks performed equally well, in terms of speech intelligibility. Algorithms with no asterisks performed poorly.

logMMSE, and Wiener-as algorithms performed equally well and significantly better than the other algorithms. At 5 dB SNR, five algorithms (KLT, logMMSE, MB, WT, and Wiener-as) performed equally well in most conditions. Lowest performance was obtained by the pKLT and RDC algorithms in all conditions. Considering all SNR × (noise type) conditions, the Wiener-as algorithm performed consistently well in all eight conditions, followed by the KLT and logMMSE algorithms, which performed well in six of the eight noise conditions, followed by the WT and MB algorithms, which performed well in five and four conditions, respectively.

12.3.4 Intelligibility Comparison against Noisy Speech

Further analysis was performed to find out whether intelligibility was improved or at least maintained (i.e., speech was equally intelligible) in reference to noisy (unprocessed) speech. Multiple-paired comparisons (Fisher's LSD) were conducted between the intelligibility scores obtained with noisy speech (unprocessed) samples and the scores obtained with speech enhanced by the various algorithms. The results from the statistical analysis are given in Table 12.10. In this table, algorithms indicated with "E" yielded equal intelligibility to noisy speech, algorithms indicated with "L" yielded lower intelligibility, and algorithms indicated with "B" yielded higher intelligibility. The pattern of results for the two SNR levels (0 and 5 dB) is different. At 5 dB SNR, the majority of the algorithms maintained speech intelligibility, that is, enhanced speech was as intelligible as noisy (unprocessed) speech. At 0 dB SNR, a fair number of algorithms (about half) yielded significantly lower intelligibility scores compared to the noisy speech. Overall, the majority of the algorithms (KLT, logMMSE, MB, WT, and Wiener-as) maintained speech intelligibility in six of the eight noise conditions tested.

TABLE 12.10
Statistical Comparisons between the Intelligibility of Noisy (Unprocessed) Speech and Enhanced Speech

Noise	SNR	Subspace		Statistical Model		Spectral Subtractive		Wiener-Type	
Type	(dB)	KLT	pKLT	logMMSE	logMMSE-SPU	RDC	MB	WT	Wiener-as
Car	0	E	L	E	L	L	L	L	E
Babble		E	E	E	L	L	E	E	E
Street		L	L	L	E	L	E	E	E
Train		L	L	L	L	L	L	L	L
Car	5	E	L	E	E	E	E	E	B
Babble		E	L	E	E	E	E	E	E
Street		E	L	E	L	L	E	E	E
Train		E	L	E	E	L	E	E	E

Algorithms indicated with "E" were found to be equally intelligible to noisy speech.
Algorithms indicated with "L" obtained lower intelligibility scores and algorithms indicated with "B" obtained significantly better intelligibility scores than noisy speech.

That is, enhanced speech was found to be as intelligible as noisy (unprocessed) speech. The Wiener-as algorithm improved the intelligibility in one noise condition (car noise, 5 dB SNR). The improvement was small (roughly 10%) but statistically significant. All algorithms produced a decrement in intelligibility in the 0 dB train condition. The pKLT and RDC algorithms reduced significantly the intelligibility in most conditions.

12.3.5 Summary of Findings

Based on the earlier statistical analysis of the intelligibility scores, we can draw the following conclusions:

1. With the exception of a single noise condition (car noise at 5 dB SNR), no algorithm produced significant improvements in speech intelligibility. The majority of the algorithms (KLT, logMMSE, MB, WT, Wiener-as) tested were able to maintain intelligibility at the same level as that of noisy speech.
2. Comparing the performance of the various algorithms, we find that the Wiener-as algorithm performed consistently well in nearly all conditions. The KLT (subspace) and logMMSE algorithms performed equally well, followed by the WT and MB algorithms. In babble noise (0 dB SNR), the KLT and Wiener-as algorithms performed the best among all algorithms.
3. The algorithms that were found in the previous section (Section 12.2) to perform the best in terms of overall quality were not the same algorithms that performed the best in terms of speech intelligibility. The KLT (subspace) algorithm was found to perform the worst in terms of overall quality, but performed well in terms of preserving speech intelligibility. In fact, in babble noise (0 dB SNR), the KLT algorithm performed significantly better than the logMMSE algorithm, which was found previously (see Section 12.2) to be among the algorithms with the highest overall speech quality [1].
4. The Wiener-as algorithm [18] performed the best in terms of preserving speech intelligibility (it even improved intelligibility in one noise condition). We believe that this is due to the fact that it applies the least amount of attenuation to the noisy signal. Consequently, it introduces negligible speech distortion. This is done, however, at the expense of introducing a great deal of noise distortion (residual noise). At the other extreme, the pKLT approach reduces significantly the noise distortion but introduces a great deal of speech distortion, which in turn impairs speech intelligibility. In between the two extremes of speech and noise distortion lie the KLT and logMMSE algorithms.
5. The performance of speech enhancement algorithms seems to be dependent on the temporal/spectral characteristics of the noise, and this dependence is more evident in the low-SNR conditions (0 dB). In the 0 dB train condition, for instance, none of the tested speech enhancement algorithms preserved speech intelligibility. Yet, the same algorithms preserved speech intelligibility in other noise conditions at the same SNR level.

Finally, it is important to point out that the disappointing conclusion drawn from the earlier intelligibility study that enhancement algorithms do not improve speech intelligibility is only applicable to normal-hearing listeners and not necessarily to hearing-impaired listeners wearing hearings aids [23] or cochlear implants. The KLT algorithm, for instance, was found in [26] to produce significant improvements in speech intelligibility in cochlear implant users. Further research is therefore needed to investigate the performance of speech enhancement algorithms, such as those described in this book, in hearing-impaired listeners.

12.5 SUMMARY

This chapter provided a comprehensive evaluation and comparison of major speech enhancement algorithms in terms of quality and intelligibility. The subjective evaluation was done by Dynastat, Inc. using the ITU-T P.830 methodology. Results indicated that the statistical-model-based algorithms performed consistently the best (i.e., yielded the highest quality) across all conditions. Only a few algorithms improved significantly the overall quality of enhanced speech in comparison to the noisy (unprocessed) speech. No algorithm provided significant quality improvement in the restaurant noise condition. The intelligibility evaluation of the speech enhancement algorithms indicated that no algorithm provided significant improvements in intelligibility in reference to the noisy (unprocessed) speech. The majority of the algorithms tested preserved speech intelligibility. Three algorithms performed consistently the best in most noise conditions: the KLT (subspace), logMMSE, and Wiener-as algorithms. The algorithms that were found to perform the best in terms of overall quality were not the same algorithms that performed the best in terms of speech intelligibility. The generalized subspace (KLT) algorithm was poor in terms of speech quality, but performed very well in terms of speech intelligibility. Algorithms that hold promise in improving speech intelligibility in noise are presented in the next chapter. These algorithms do not belong to the four classes of algorithms evaluated in this chapter and are therefore presented separately.

REFERENCES

1. Hu, Y. and Loizou, P. (2006), Subjective comparison of speech enhancement algorithms, *Proceedings of the IEEE International Conference on Acoustics, Speech, and Signal Processing*, Toulouse, France, Vol. I, pp. 153–156.
2. IEEE Subcommittee (1969), IEEE recommended practice for speech quality measurements, *IEEE Trans. Audio Electroacoust.*, AU-17(3), 225–246.
3. Hu, Y. and Loizou, P. (2007), Subjective evaluation and comparison of speech enhancement algorithms, *Speech Commun.*, 49, 588–601.
4. Hirsch, H. and Pearce, D. (2000), The AURORA experimental framework for the performance evaluation of speech recognition systems under noisy conditions, *Proceedings of ISCA ITRW ASR2000*, Paris, France.
5. ITU (2000), Perceptual evaluation of speech quality (PESQ), and objective method for end-to-end speech quality assessment of narrowband telephone networks and speech codecs, ITU-T Recommendation P. 862.
6. ITU-T (1993), Objective measurement of active speech level, ITU-T Recommendation P. 56.
7. Cohen, I. (2002), Optimal speech enhancement under signal presence uncertainty using log-spectra amplitude estimator, *IEEE Signal Process. Lett.*, 9(4), 113–116.

8. Sohn, J. and Kim, N. (1999), Statistical model-based voice activity detection, *IEEE Signal Process. Lett.*, 6(1), 1–3.
9. Ephraim, Y. and Malah, D. (1984), Speech enhancement using a minimum mean-square error short-time spectral amplitude estimator, *IEEE Trans. Acoust., Speech, Signal Process.*, ASSP-32(6), 1109–1121.
10. Mittal, U. and Phamdo, N. (2000), Signal/noise KLT based approach for enhancing speech degraded by noise, *IEEE Trans. Speech Audio Process.*, 8(2), 159–167.
11. ITU-T (2003), Subjective test methodology for evaluating speech communication systems that include noise suppression algorithm, ITU-T Recommendation P. 835.
12. Hu, Y. and Loizou, P. (2003), A generalized subspace approach for enhancing speech corrupted by colored noise, *IEEE Trans. Speech Audio Process.*, 11, 334–341.
13. Jabloun, F. and Champagne, B. (2003), Incorporating the human hearing properties in the signal subspace approach for speech enhancement, *IEEE Trans. Speech Audio Process.*, 11(6), 700–708.
14. Cohen, I. (2003), Noise spectrum estimation in adverse environments: Improved minima controlled recursive averaging, *IEEE Trans. Speech Audio Process.*, 11(5), 466–475.
15. Kamath, S. and Loizou, P. (2002). A multi-band spectral subtraction method for enhancing speech corrupted by colored noise. *Proceedings of the IEEE International Conference on Acoustics, Speech, and Signal Processing*, Orlando, FL.
16. Kamath, S. (2001). A multi-band spectral subtraction method for speech enhancement, Master's Thesis, University of Texas-Dallas, Department of Electrical Engineering, Richardson, TX.
17. Gustafsson, H., Nordholm, S., and Claesson, I. (2001), Spectral subtraction using reduced delay convolution and adaptive averaging, *IEEE Trans. Speech Audio Process.*, 9(8), 799–807.
18. Scalart, P. and Filho, J. (1996), Speech enhancement based on a priori signal to noise estimation, *Proceedings of the IEEE International Conference on Acoustics, Speech, and Signal Processing*, Atlanta, GA, pp. 629–632.
19. Hu, Y. and Loizou, P. (2004). Speech enhancement based on wavelet thresholding the multitaper spectrum, *IEEE Trans. Speech Audio Process.*, 12(1), 59–67.
20. Boll, S.F. (1979), Suppression of acoustic noise in speech using spectral subtraction, *IEEE Trans. Acoust. Speech Signal Process.*, ASSP-27(2), 113–120.
21. Lim, J. (1978), Evaluation of a correlation subtraction method for enhancing speech degraded by additive noise, *IEEE Trans. Acoust. Speech Signal Process.*, 37(6), 471–472.
22. Tsoukalas, D.E., Mourjopoulos, J.N., and Kokkinakis, G. (1997), Speech enhancement based on audible noise suppression, *IEEE Trans. Speech Audio Process.*, 5(6), 497–514.
23. Arehart, K., Hansen, J., Gallant, S., and Kalstein, L. (2003), Evaluation of an auditory masked threshold noise suppression algorithm in normal-hearing and hearing-impaired listeners, *Speech Commun.*, 40, 575–592.
24. Hu, Y. and Loizou, P. (2007), A comparative intelligibility study of single-microphone noise reduction algorithms, *J. Acoust. Soc. Am.*, 122(3), 1777–1786.
25. Ephraim, Y. and Malah, D. (1985), Speech enhancement using a minimum mean-square error log-spectral amplitude estimator, *IEEE Trans. Acoust. Speech Signal Process.*, ASSP-23(2), 443–445.
26. Loizou, P., Lobo, A., and Hu, Y. (2005), Subspace algorithms for noise reduction in cochlear implants, *J. Acoust. Soc. Am.*, 118(5), 2791–2793.
27. Rangachari, S. and Loizou, P. (2006), A noise estimation algorithm for highly nonstationary environments, *Speech Commun.*, 28, 220–231.
28. Loizou, P. (2005), Speech enhancement based on perceptually motivated Bayesian estimators of the speech magnitude spectrum, *IEEE Trans. Speech Audio Process.*, 13(5), 857–869.

Part IV

Future Steps

13 Algorithms That Can Improve Speech Intelligibility

As discussed in Chapter 12, the speech enhancement algorithms described in this book can improve speech quality but not speech intelligibility. Similarly, (single-microphone) noise-reduction algorithms implemented in wearable hearing aids revealed no significant intelligibility benefit [1,2], although they have been found to improve speech quality and ease of listening in hearing-impaired (HI) listeners (e.g., [2,3]). In brief, the ultimate goal of developing (and implementing) an algorithm that would improve substantially speech intelligibility for normal-hearing (NH) and/or HI listeners has been elusive for nearly three decades. The present chapter describes a family of algorithms that are capable of improving speech intelligibility. Many of these algorithms are motivated by articulation index (AI) theory. Unlike the conventional algorithms that use (soft) smooth gain functions, the algorithms discussed in this chapter use binary gain functions.

13.1 REASONS FOR THE ABSENCE OF INTELLIGIBILITY IMPROVEMENT WITH EXISTING NOISE-REDUCTION ALGORITHMS

Our knowledge surrounding the factors contributing to the lack of intelligibility benefit with existing single-microphone noise-reduction algorithms is limited [1,4,5]. In most cases, we do not know how, and to what extent, a specific parameter of a noise-reduction algorithm needs to be modified so as to improve speech intelligibility. Clearly, one factor is related to the fact that we often are not able to estimate accurately the background noise spectrum, which is needed for the implementation of most single-microphone algorithms. While noise tracking or voice-activity detection algorithms have been found to perform well in steady background noise (e.g., car) environments (see Chapter 9), they generally do not perform well in nonstationary types of noise (e.g., multitalker babble). The second factor is that the majority of algorithms introduce distortions, which, in some cases, might be more damaging than the background noise itself [6]. For that reason, several algorithms have been proposed to minimize speech distortion while constraining the amount of noise distortion introduced to fall below a preset value [7,8] or below the auditory masking threshold [9]. Third, nonrelevant stochastic modulations arising from the nonlinear noise-speech interaction can contribute to reduction in speech intelligibility and, in some cases, more so than the deterministic modulation reduction [10]. The study in [5] assessed the effects of noise on speech intelligibility and has shown that the systematic envelope lift (equal to the mean noise intensity) implemented in spectral subtractive algorithms had the most detrimental effects on speech intelligibility. The corruption of the fine structure and introduction of stochastic envelope fluctuations associated with the inaccurate estimates of the noise intensity and nonlinear processing of the mixture envelopes further diminished speech intelligibility. It was argued that it was these stochastic effects that prevented spectral subtractive algorithms from improving speech perception in noise [5]. Next, we discuss some of the earlier factors in more detail and introduce another important factor that has been largely overlooked.

13.1.1 Influence of Speech Distortions

Clearly, the choice of the frequency-specific gain function is critical to the success of the noise-reduction algorithm. The frequency-specific gain function applied to the noisy speech spectrum is far from perfect as it depends on the estimated signal-to-noise ratio (SNR) and estimated noise spectrum. Although the intention (and hope) is to apply a small gain (near 0) only when the masker is present and a high gain (near 1) only when the target is present, that is not feasible since the target and masker signals spectrally overlap. Consequently, the target signal may in some instances be overattenuated (to the point of being eliminated) while in other instances, it may be overamplified. Despite the fact that the gain function is typically bounded between zero and one, the target signal may be overamplified because the soft gain function is applied to the noisy speech spectrum. In brief, there are two types of spectral distortions that can be introduced by the gain functions used in most noise-reduction algorithms: amplification distortion occurring when the target signal is overestimated (e.g., if the true value of the target envelope is say A, and the estimated envelope is $A + \Delta A$, for some positive increment ΔA), and attenuation distortion occurring when the target signal is underestimated (e.g., the estimated envelope is $A - \Delta A$). These distortions may be introduced by any gain function independent of whether the gain is determined by the modulation rate, modulation depth, or SNR. The perceptual effect of these two distortions on speech intelligibility cannot be assumed to be equivalent, and in practice, there has to be the right balance between these two distortions.

To analyze the impact of gain-induced distortions introduced by noise-reduction algorithms on speech intelligibility, one needs to establish a relationship between distortion and intelligibility or alternatively develop an appropriate intelligibility measure. Such a measure could provide valuable insights as to whether we ought to design algorithms that would minimize the attenuation distortion, the amplification distortion, or both, and to what degree. In [11], the fwSNRseg measure (see Chapter 11) was chosen since it has been found in [12] to correlate highly ($r = 0.81$) with the intelligibility of noise-suppressed speech:

$$\text{fwSNRseg} = \frac{10}{M} \sum_{t=0}^{M-1} \frac{\sum_{k=1}^{K} W(k,t) \log_{10} \text{SNR}_{\text{ESI}}(k,t)}{\sum_{k=1}^{K} W(k,t)} \tag{13.1}$$

where $W(k,t)$ is the band-importance function, $X(k,t)$ denotes the clean magnitude spectrum at time frame t, $\hat{X}(k,t)$ denotes the enhanced magnitude spectrum, and $\text{SNR}_{\text{ESI}}(k,t)$ is given by

$$\text{SNR}_{\text{ESI}}(k,t) = \frac{X^2(k,t)}{(X(k,t) - \hat{X}(k,t))^2} \quad (13.2)$$

Dividing both numerator and denominator by $X(k,t)$, we get

$$\text{SNR}_{\text{ESI}}(k,t) = \frac{1}{\left(1 - \frac{\hat{X}(k,t)}{X(k,t)}\right)^2} \quad (13.3)$$

Figure 13.1 provides important insights into the contributions of the two distortions to $\text{SNR}_{\text{ESI}}(k)$, and, for convenience, we divide the figure into multiple regions according to the distortions introduced:

Region I: In this region, $\hat{X}(k,t) \leq X(k,t)$, suggesting only attenuation distortion.

Region II: In this region, $X(k,t) < \hat{X}(k,t) \leq 2 \cdot X(k,t)$, suggesting amplification distortion up to 6.02 dB.

Region III: In this region, $\hat{X}(k,t) > 2 \cdot X(k,t)$, suggesting amplification distortion of 6.02 dB or greater.

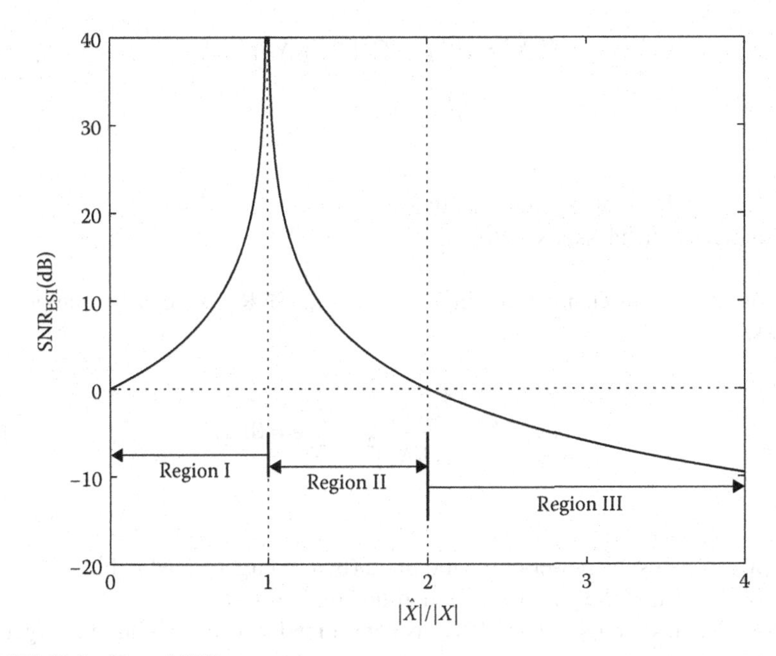

FIGURE 13.1 Plot of SNR_{ESI} metric.

From the earlier regions, we can deduce that in the union of Regions I and II, which we denote as Region I + II, we have the following constraint:

$$\hat{X}(k,t) \leq 2 \cdot X(k,t) \tag{13.4}$$

It is clear from the earlier definitions of these three regions that in order to ensure that $SNR_{ESI} > 1$ (and potentially maximize the fwSNRseg measure and speech intelligibility), the estimated magnitude spectra $\hat{X}(k,t)$ need to be contained in Regions I and II (note that a trivial, but not useful, solution that maximizes SNR_{ESI} is $\hat{X}(k,t) = X(k,t)$). Intelligibility listening tests were conducted in [11,13] and confirmed the earlier hypothesis (more on this in Section 13.4.1). Speech synthesized from Region I + II was found to be perfectly (near 100% correct) intelligible even at extremely low-SNR levels (e.g., SNR = −10dB). Hence, controlling the distortions introduced by noise-reduction algorithms is one method that can be utilized for improving speech intelligibility.

13.1.2 Lack of Effective SNR Increase

Most of the algorithms described in this book make use of a soft gain function G_k for suppressing noise. The fact that the gain function is soft bears its limitations in as far as its ability to improve intelligibility. Consider the corrupted (mixture) spectrum Y_k in frequency bin (or channel) k being processed by a noise-reduction algorithm specified by the gain function G_k. Since the masker is additive, the gain function is applied to both the target spectrum X_k and the masker spectrum N_k. To see this, we can express the magnitude-squared spectrum of the enhanced signal, that is, $\hat{X}_k^2$, as follows:

$$\begin{aligned}\hat{X}_k^2 &= G_k^2 Y_k^2 = G_k^2\left(X_k^2 + N_k^2\right)\\ &= G_k^2 X_k^2 + G_k^2 N_k^2\end{aligned} \tag{13.5}$$

where

X_k denotes the clean signal magnitude spectrum
N_k indicates the masker spectrum

The output SNR in channel or bin k, denoted as $SNR_{out}(k)$, can be computed as follows:

$$SNR_{out}(k) = \frac{(G_k X_k)^2}{(G_k N_k)^2} = \frac{X_k^2}{N_k^2} = SNR_k \tag{13.6}$$

where

$(G_k X_k)^2$ denotes the power of the modified (by G_k) target signal in bin k
$(G_k N_k)^2$ indicates the power of the modified masker signal
SNR_k denotes the input band SNR as determined prior to mixing the target and masker

According to the earlier equation, the *output band SNR cannot be improved by any choice of G_k beyond the value of the input band SNR_k*. From AI theory (see Equation 11.72), we know that intelligibility is proportional to the (weighted) sum of SNRs across all bands. Hence, if the output SNR (following noise reduction) is the same as the input SNR (prior to noise reduction), then we should not expect any improvement in intelligibility. Indeed, this observation is consistent with the lack of intelligibility with existing noise-reduction algorithms by NH listeners [6] (see Chapter 12) and HI listeners [2], at least for algorithms that make use of (soft) gain functions to suppress the background noise. It should be noted that the overall SNR (computed across all bands) and the output band SNR (computed for a specific band as per Equation 13.6) are different. As we will show later, the overall SNR *can* be improved but the band SNR cannot be improved. Based on AI theory (see Section 11.4.1), we can conclude that *only algorithms that can improve the overall SNR (computed across all bands) can improve speech intelligibility*. One strategy for improving the overall SNR (defined as the weighted sum of SNRs across all bands) is to discard bands with unfavorable (extremely low) SNRs while retaining bands with favorable SNR (see proof in [13]). The details and motivation for such strategy are described next.

To summarize, there are two potential methods that can be used to improve speech intelligibility: (1) control the distortions introduced by noise-reduction algorithms and (2) increase the overall band SNR so as to improve the AI. As we will show later, the first method already fulfills the requirements of the second method. Hence, overall, in order to improve speech intelligibility, the AI needs to be improved and that requires the overall band SNR to be improved.

13.2 ALGORITHMS BASED ON CHANNEL SELECTION: A DIFFERENT PARADIGM FOR NOISE REDUCTION

Gain functions (e.g., Wiener, MMSE) aim to attenuate the signal when speech is absent (or the *estimated* SNR is low) and retain the signal when speech is present (or the *estimated* SNR is high). For this approach to work effectively, however, access to accurate SNR estimates (and estimate of the background noise spectrum) is needed. In extremely low-SNR conditions (e.g., SNR < -5 dB), the aforementioned aim is likely not attainable. This is based on past studies (e.g., [6]), showing that state-of-the-art algorithms are not capable of obtaining SNR estimates accurate enough to improve intelligibility even at positive SNR levels (SNR $= 5$ dB). Hence, a different approach is needed that does not require accurate estimates of the SNR.

Given the lack of intelligibility improvement with the speech enhancement algorithms proposed in the last three decades (and described in this book), it is becoming clear that a paradigm shift is needed in the noise-reduction field. The last two subsections provided important insights that can assist us in developing a new paradigm for noise reduction. First, if we somehow control the type of speech distortions that pass through, then we may observe improvement in intelligibility. This suggests that only a subset of available bins (or channels) be allowed through the system (with the remaining channels being discarded). We henceforth use the general term channel to represent the auditory channels at the output of the peripheral stage of the auditory pathway. In the context of speech processing, channels could represent the filter-bank outputs (assuming processing using a bank of bandpass filters) or spectral components corresponding to specific frequency bins (assuming processing using the FFT). Second, the *use of any type of soft gain function estimated from the corrupted speech is unlikely to yield any intelligibility benefits as they are incapable of increasing the overall band SNR* (see Equation 13.6), relative to the input overall band SNR, and consequently the AI. The latter suggests that the use of soft gain functions (e.g., MMSE gain function) *ought to be abandoned* and binary gain functions ought to be adopted. This is not to say that binary gain functions estimated from corrupted speech always improve speech intelligibility [14]. Even if the binary gain functions are estimated optimally (e.g., in the MMSE sense), but the decisions about keeping/discarding TF units are not made with sufficient accuracy, we will not observe improvements in speech intelligibility [14]. (For more information about how accurate the binary mask needs to be computed, see Section 13.6.) As a secondary example, consider the basic form of spectral subtraction. The output spectrum is set to zero whenever the difference between the noisy spectrum and estimated spectrum is negative. That is, a binary gain function is applied to the noisy speech spectrum, yet spectral subtractive algorithms do not improve speech intelligibility [6].

It is reasonable to ask: Under what circumstances, would a soft gain function improve speech intelligibility? Suppose we had a way of estimating the soft gain function very accurately, would that be enough? Or, taking the extreme scenario, suppose that we apply the *ideal* Wiener gain function (i.e., we assume access to the true instantaneous SNR) to the corrupted speech. Would that improve speech intelligibility? The answer is yes, but careful analysis conducted in [15, Fig. 14] showed that the distribution of the values of the Wiener gain function is for the most part bimodal, with one mode located at a gain of 0 and the other at a gain of 1. More precisely, the highest percentage of gain values was found at either 0 dB or below −27 dB [15, Fig. 14]. This suggests that the ideal Wiener gain function is no longer soft but binary. As the number of interfering speakers increased (from 1 to 4), a smaller number of gain values were observed at 0 dB (i.e., a small number of channels was retained), but the number of gain values at −27 dB (or below) remained high (i.e., a large number of channels were discarded) [15]. This suggests that soft gain functions can improve speech intelligibility provided that they are computed with high accuracy (a formidable task at extremely low-SNR conditions, given our inability to compute the gain functions accurately even at positive SNR levels [6]). Soft gain functions computed accurately become binary and discard a large number of unfavorable channels [15]. This in turn improves the overall band SNR and subsequently, the AI, leading to improvement in intelligibility. It should be noted that soft gain functions in general offer the advantage of providing better speech quality compared to the binary gain functions. However, they are more difficult to estimate compared to the binary gain functions.

Historically, binary gain functions have been used in computational auditory scene analysis (CASA) [16] and speech recognition applications [17], but not in the noise-reduction field (more on this later). The direct consequence of applying binary gain functions to the noisy speech spectrum is that certain channels are retained (multiplied by a gain of 1) while other channels are discarded (multiplied by a gain of 0). Such functions can be used, for instance, to retain channels containing attenuation distortions and discard channels containing amplification distortions. Unlike the soft gain functions, which are derived using rigorous minimization techniques and are dependent on several parameters (which need to be estimated from corrupted speech), the binary gain functions are much simpler as they only take values of 0 and 1. The only thing that needs to be determined is the set of channels that needs to be selected out of the set of available channels.

In brief, design criteria are needed that can aid us in the selection of channels from the noisy speech observations. If the SNR_{ESI} metric (Equation 13.2) is used, for instance, as the design criterion and we require that $SNR_{ESI} > 1$, then the set of channels that satisfy this criterion are the ones containing primarily attenuation distortions (with limited, < 3 dB, amplification distortion). Selecting these channels has proven to yield substantial improvements in intelligibility [11,13].

Alternatively, one can use the AI as the design criterion and determine the set of channels that maximize the AI. More precisely, suppose that the noisy speech signal is decomposed (via a filterbank or an FFT) into N channels (or N frequency bins using a $2N$-point FFT). It is reasonable to ask the question: which of the N channels (or frequency bins) should be selected for synthesis such that AI is maximized? To answer this question, we consider the following weighted sum of SNRs computed across N channels as an approximation to the AI:

$$F = \sum_{j=1}^{N} I_j \cdot \text{SNR}(j) \tag{13.7}$$

where

$\text{SNR}(j) = 10\log_{10}(X^2(j)/N^2(j))$ is the SNR in channel j

I_j are the gains or weights ($0 \leq I_j \leq 1$) applied to each channel

Next, we consider the following question: How should the weights I_j be chosen such that the overall SNR (i.e., F) given in Equation 13.7 is maximized? The optimal weights I_j that maximize F in Equation 13.7 are given by [13]

$$I_j^* = \begin{cases} 1 & \text{if SNR}(j) > 0 \\ 0 & \text{if SNR}(j) \leq 0 \end{cases} \tag{13.8}$$

To see why the aforesaid weights are optimal, we can consider two extreme cases in which either $\text{SNR}(j) \leq 0$ or $\text{SNR}(j) \geq 0$ in all frequency bins (or channels). If $\text{SNR}(j) \leq 0$ in all bins, then we have the following upper bound on the value of F:

$$\sum_{j=1}^{N} I_j \cdot \text{SNR}(j) \leq 0 \tag{13.9}$$

Similarly, if SNR(j) ≥ 0 in all bins, then we have the following upper bound:

$$\sum_{j=1}^{N} I_j \cdot \text{SNR}(j) \leq \sum_{j=1}^{N} \text{SNR}(j) \tag{13.10}$$

Both upper bounds (maxima) in Equations 13.9 and 13.10 are attained with the optimal weights given in Equation 13.8. That is, the maximum in Equation 13.9 is attained with $I_j = 0$ (for all j), while the maximum in Equation 13.10 is attained with $I_j = 1$ (for all j). In brief, the main motivation behind maximizing F in Equation 13.7 is to maximize the AI and consequently maximize the amount of retained information contributing to speech intelligibility.

To illustrate the aforesaid concept of channel selection, we show in Figure 13.2 example 1/3-octave spectra of the vowel/iy/before and after channel selection. For this example, the vowel was embedded in speech-shaped noise at 0 dB SNR. The formant frequencies of the clean vowel/iy/ were $F1 = 328$ Hz and $F2 = 2281$ Hz. Clearly, as can be seen from panel (c) of Figure 13.2, the F2 formant is completely masked by noise rendering the vowel difficult to identify. Panel (b) shows the true SNR in each band, and panel (d) shows the selected channels corresponding to SNR > 0 dB. More precisely, panel (d) shows the channels selected from the *noisy* (1/3-octave) vowel spectra (panel (c)), satisfying the SNR > 0 dB criterion. Following the channel

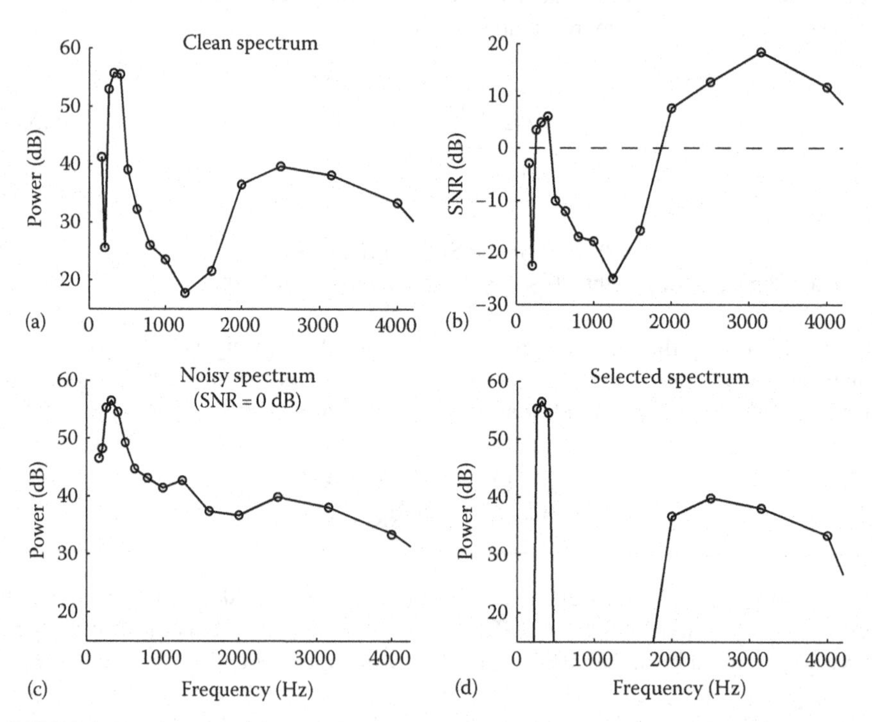

FIGURE 13.2 Spectra of the vowel/iy/excised from the word "heed." (a) Clean spectrum of vowel /iy/; (b) true SNR in each band; (c) spectrum of vowel /iy/ corrupted by speech-shaped noise at 0 dB SNR; and (d) spectrum of corrupted vowel /iy/ after channel selection.

selection, the spectral valley between $F1$ and $F2$ becomes more evident along with the presence of $F2$. The overall (across all bands) SNR of the noisy vowel spectra was −91.2 dB. Following channel selection, the overall SNR increased to 65.2 dB. If we map the individual band SNRs within the range of 0–1, as per the AI procedure (see Equation 11.70), then the AI of the noisy vowel signal is computed to be 0.38 (no band-importance functions were used for this example). The resulting AI after channel selection increases to 0.61, suggesting an improvement in intelligibility. Suppose now that we change the SNR threshold used in Equation 13.8 from 0 to −6 dB. If we select from the noisy spectra only channels with SNR > −6 dB, the resulting AI value becomes 0.60 (overall SNR is 57.8 dB). Hence, the AI increased from 0.38 to 0.60 suggesting again an improvement in intelligibility. This simple example demonstrates that the SNR threshold used in channel selection is not necessarily unique in that other choices of threshold values can yield equitable intelligibility improvement (more on this in Section 13.4.1). This is also evident in the AI-to-intelligibility mapping functions shown in Figure 11.23. For sentence materials, for instance, AI values greater than 0.5 all yield near 100% correct.

Figure 13.3 shows a similar example of channel selection for the fricative/sh/ (taken from the syllable "asha"). The fricative was embedded in speech-shaped noise at −5 dB SNR. The high-frequency ($f > 2$ kHz) spectral dominance, characteristic of/sh/, is present in the clean spectrum but not in the noisy spectrum (panel (c)).

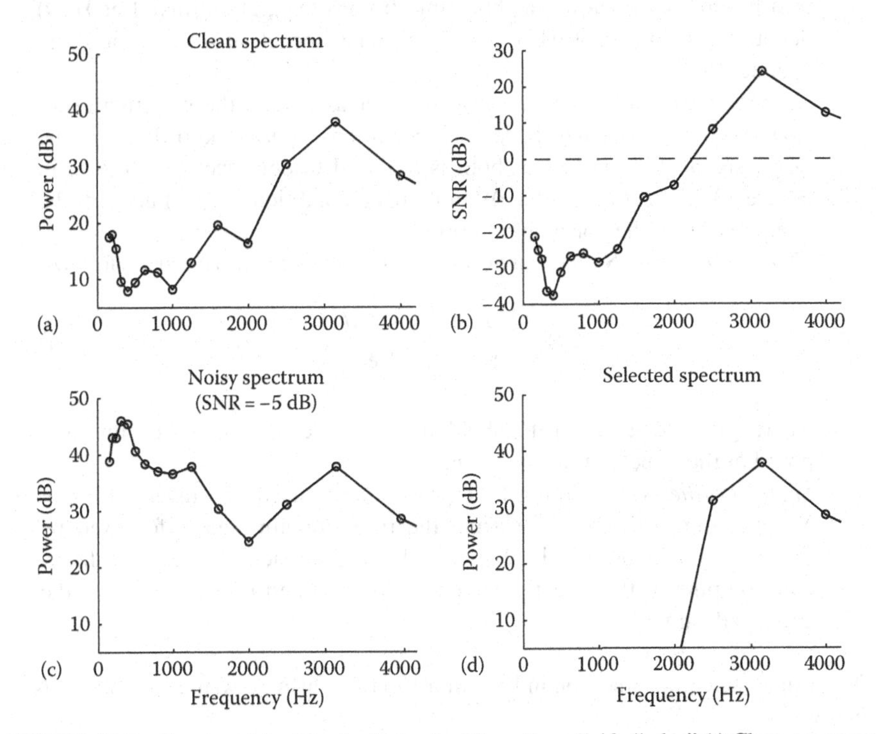

FIGURE 13.3 Spectra of the fricative/sh/excised from the syllable "asha." (a) Clean spectrum of fricative /sh/; (b) true SNR in each band; (c) spectrum of fricative /sh/ corrupted by speech-shaped noise at −5 dB SNR; and (d) spectrum of corrupted fricative /sh/ after channel selection.

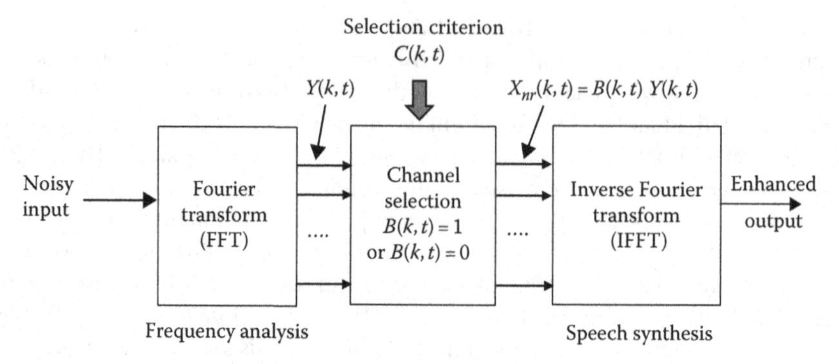

FIGURE 13.4 Block diagram of channel-selection algorithms.

Following channel selection, the high-frequency dominance in the spectrum becomes evident. The AI value before channel selection was computed to be 0.23 and increased to 0.58 after channel selection.

The general steps of channel-selection-based algorithms are outlined next and are also shown in Figure 13.4:

1. *Frequency decomposition:* Perform frequency analysis using either an FFT or a filterbank operating in short-time frames (e.g., 20–30 ms). Let $Y(k, t)$ denote the (complex) FFT spectrum of noisy speech at time frame t and channel k.
2. *Construct channel-selection criterion:* Let us denote the selection criterion for channel k as $C(k, t)$. In ideal conditions, *a priori* knowledge of the target signal, the masker, or both is required to construct $C(k, t)$ (e.g., in Figure 13.2, $C(k, t) = \text{SNR}(k, t)$). In realistic conditions, $C(k, t)$ needs to be computed from the noisy observations.
3. *Channel selection:* Select channels satisfying a prescribed criterion as follows:

$$\hat{X}(k,t) = \begin{cases} Y(k,t) & \text{if } C(k,t) > \gamma \\ 0 & \text{else} \end{cases} \tag{13.11}$$

   where γ denotes a preset threshold and $\hat{X}(k, t)$ denotes the spectrum composed of the selected bins or channels.
4. *Signal synthesis:* Assuming FFT processing is used, the inverse FFT of $\hat{X}(k, t)$ is computed to reconstruct the time-domain signal, followed by the overlap-add procedure. If a filterbank approach is used, the filterbank outputs of the selected channels are summed up to synthesize the enhanced signal.

The channel-selection equation in Equation 13.11 can also be written as follows (see Figure 13.4):

$$\hat{X}(k,t) = B(k,t) \cdot Y(k,t) \tag{13.12}$$

where $B(k,t)$ is the binary gain function defined as

$$B(k,t) = \begin{cases} 1 & \text{if } C(k,t) > \gamma \\ 0 & \text{else} \end{cases} \qquad (13.13)$$

Hence, the conventional soft gain function used in noise reduction is replaced with the binary function specified in Equation 13.13. This binary function is often called the *binary mask* and in ideal conditions (where there is *a priori* knowledge of the clean and masker signals), it is called the *ideal binary mask.* Note that the word mask* is deceiving as the approach itself is not motivated by any type of auditory masking (e.g., simultaneous masking and forward masking).

An FFT implementation of channel-selection-based algorithms was described earlier. Uniform spectral resolution across the signal bandwidth is maintained with the use of the FFT. Brungart et al. [18] used a bank of 128 fourth-order gammatone filters with overlapping passbands with center frequencies allocated on an approximately logarithmic scale. Despite the difference in implementations, the outcomes from the study in [19] that used the FFT and the study in [18] that used the gammatone filters were the same. In both studies, a large number of bands were used for frequency decomposition. The studies in [20,21] demonstrated that high intelligibility can be maintained even with as few as 16–24 bands.

As reported in [22], channel selection can also be implemented in the modulation domain. Speech is first processed framewise using short-time Fourier analysis (FFT). Time trajectories of the FFT magnitude spectrum (for fixed acoustic frequencies) are accumulated over a finite interval of R seconds (e.g., 256 ms) and subjected to a second short-time Fourier analysis to produce the modulation spectrum [23]. The SNR in the short-time modulation spectral domain, denoted as $(S/N)_{mod}$, is constructed, and modulation spectrum components with $(S/N)_{mod}$ greater than a threshold are selected while the remaining components are discarded. Channel selection performed within a 0–18 Hz modulation frequency range was found to yield substantial gains (13 dB improvement in SNR relative to the unprocessed stimuli) in intelligibility [22].

13.3 CHANNEL-SELECTION CRITERIA

In the previous section, we described briefly a channel-selection criterion based on the SNR of each band. This criterion was motivated by AI theory (see Section 13.2). The SNR criterion is not, however, the only criterion that can be used to improve speech intelligibility in noise. Furthermore, while the SNR criterion is appropriate in situations wherein the masker is additive, it is not appropriate in situations where reverberation (and noise) is present. A review of a number of channel-selection criteria (i.e., different forms of $C(k,t)$ in Equation 13.11) that have been shown to yield improvements in intelligibility is given next.

* The term mask is used in semiconductor device fabrication. The photomask, for instance, is used to produce an image on the wafer. The photomask allows the light to pass through in some areas and blocks it in others.

13.3.1 SNR Criterion

Following the steps outlined in Section 13.2 (see also Figure 13.4), channel selection according to the SNR criterion can be implemented by computing the FFT of the noisy signal, and from it, select only the bins (channels) satisfying the following:

$$X_S(k,t) = \begin{cases} Y(k,t) & \text{if } \mathrm{SNR}_I(k,t) > \gamma \\ 0 & \text{else} \end{cases} \tag{13.14}$$

where $\mathrm{SNR}_I(k,t)$ denotes the *instantaneous* SNR (in dB) at time frequency (TF) unit (k,t) computed as

$$\mathrm{SNR}_I(k,t) = 10\log_{10}\frac{|X(k,t)|^2}{|N(k,t)|^2} \tag{13.15}$$

where $X(k,t)$ and $N(k,t)$ denote the (complex) spectra of the target and masker signals, respectively. Typical values for the threshold γ in (13.14) include 0, −3, or −6 dB. Within a finite range of input SNR levels (e.g., −10 to 5 dB), the choice of threshold value does not seem to affect the intelligibility scores (more on this in Section 13.4.1). The aforementioned criterion has been used extensively in CASA studies [16], and in [24], it has been proposed as a computational goal for CASA algorithms. Equation 13.14 forms the basis of the ideal binary mask and has also been referred to in the literature as *a priori* mask [17,25] or as ideal TF segregation [18]. Wang [24] was the first to propose Equation 13.14 for constructing the ideal binary mask [24]. For a more detailed historical overview of the ideal binary mask, the reader is referred to the reviews given in [16, Chap. 1] [26]. It should be noted that, generally, the term binary mask refers to the application of a binary (rather than soft) gain function to the noisy speech spectra, that is, see Equations 13.12 and 13.13. As such, it does not reflect the underlying process of channel selection, that is, the process by which channels that satisfy a certain criterion are retained while channels that do not are discarded (zeroed out). In order to distinguish the original binary mask from the other masks (to be described in the next sections), we will henceforth use the more general term *ideal channel selection*, where the term ideal is used to indicate that *a priori* knowledge (about the target, masker, etc.) is assumed. We will refer to these algorithms as *ideal channel-selection algorithms*.

Channel selection based on the SNR criterion has been shown to be optimal in a number of ways [13,27,28]:

1. It maximizes the time-domain SNR, provided the frequency decomposition is orthonormal [27].
2. It maximizes the $\mathrm{SNR}_{\mathrm{ESI}}$ metric given in Equation 13.2 [27].
3. It maximizes the AI (Equation 13.7) [13].

4. It maximizes the *a posterior* density $f\left(X_k^2 \mid Y_k^2\right)$, where X_k^2 and Y_k^2 denote the DFT magnitude-squared spectra of the target and noisy signals, respectively [28]. That is, it yields the maximum *a posterior* (MAP) estimator of the magnitude-squared spectrum of the target signal. More precisely, assuming that the real and imaginary parts of the DFT coefficients are modeled as independent Gaussian random variables with equal variance (see Section 7.3), then the MAP estimator of the magnitude-squared spectrum of the target signal is given by [28]

$$\hat{X}_k^2 = \arg\max_{X_k^2} f\left(X_k^2 \mid Y_k^2\right)$$

$$= \begin{cases} Y_k^2 & \text{if } \sigma_X^2(k) > \sigma_N^2(k) \\ 0 & \text{else} \end{cases}$$

$$= \begin{cases} Y_k^2 & \text{if } \mathrm{SNR}_A(k) > 1 \\ 0 & \text{else} \end{cases} \tag{13.16}$$

where $\sigma_X^2(k)$ and $\sigma_N^2(k)$ denote the variances of the target and masker signals, respectively, and $\mathrm{SNR}_A(k) \triangleq \sigma_X^2(k)/\sigma_N^2(k)$ denotes the *a priori* SNR. Note the similarity between Equations 13.14 and 13.16. The only difference is that in Equation 13.14, the instantaneous SNR (computed at each frame) is used whereas in Equation 13.16, the statistically averaged SNR is used.

Clearly, from the intelligibility standpoint, the most meaningful metric is the AI, and the SNR criterion maximizes the AI [13].

Figure 13.5 shows an example of spectrograms of a sentence processed via the ideal channel-selection algorithm based on the SNR criterion. The SNR term in Equation 13.15 was computed assuming *a priori* knowledge of the target and masker signals, and the threshold γ in Equation 13.14 was set to $\gamma = -5$ dB. Panel (b) shows the sentence corrupted by speech-shaped noise at −5 dB SNR. It is clear that many of the important phonetic cues, such as $F1$ and $F2$ formants, are absent from the spectrogram, rendering the sentence unintelligible. Panel (c) shows the binary decisions made for each TF unit (k, t), with the black pixels indicating that the corresponding channel was retained and white pixels indicating that the channel was discarded. As mentioned earlier, this set of binary decisions is called the binary mask. Panel (d) shows the spectrogram of the signal synthesized according to Equation 13.14. Mathematically, as indicated by Equations 13.12 and 13.13, panel (d) is obtained by multiplying (element wise) panel (c) with panel (b). As can be seen, the recovered signal resembles much of the input signal. Intelligibility studies (see Section 13.4.1) have confirmed that the synthesized signal is as intelligible as the clean signal [18,19].

Figure 13.6 shows the same sentence processed using different SNR thresholds ranging from $\gamma = -30$ to 15 dB. Clearly, the lower the threshold is the larger the

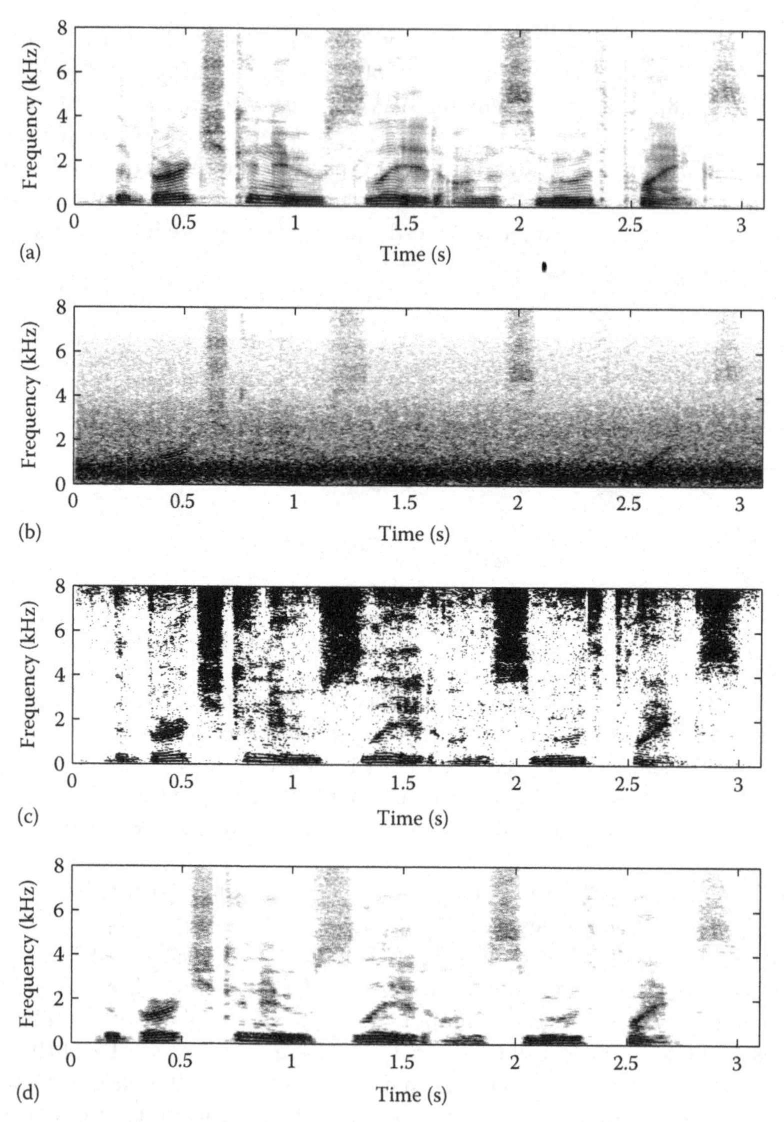

FIGURE 13.5 Spectrograms of the sentence "The birch canoe slid on the smooth planks" processed via the ideal channel-selection algorithm based on SNR criterion. (a) Spectrogram of clean sentence; (b) spectrogram of sentence corrupted by speech-shaped noise at −5 dB SNR; (c) binary mask for corrupted sentence; and (d) spectrogram of the signal synthesized according to Equation 13.14.

number of TF units retained, and the extreme value of $\gamma = -\infty$ dB corresponds to the noisy (unprocessed) signal. As the threshold increases, fewer TF units are retained rendering the synthesized signal quite sparse (see bottom panel). Within the two extremes, there exists an "optimal" set of threshold values that yields the highest intelligibility scores (more on this in Section 13.4.1).

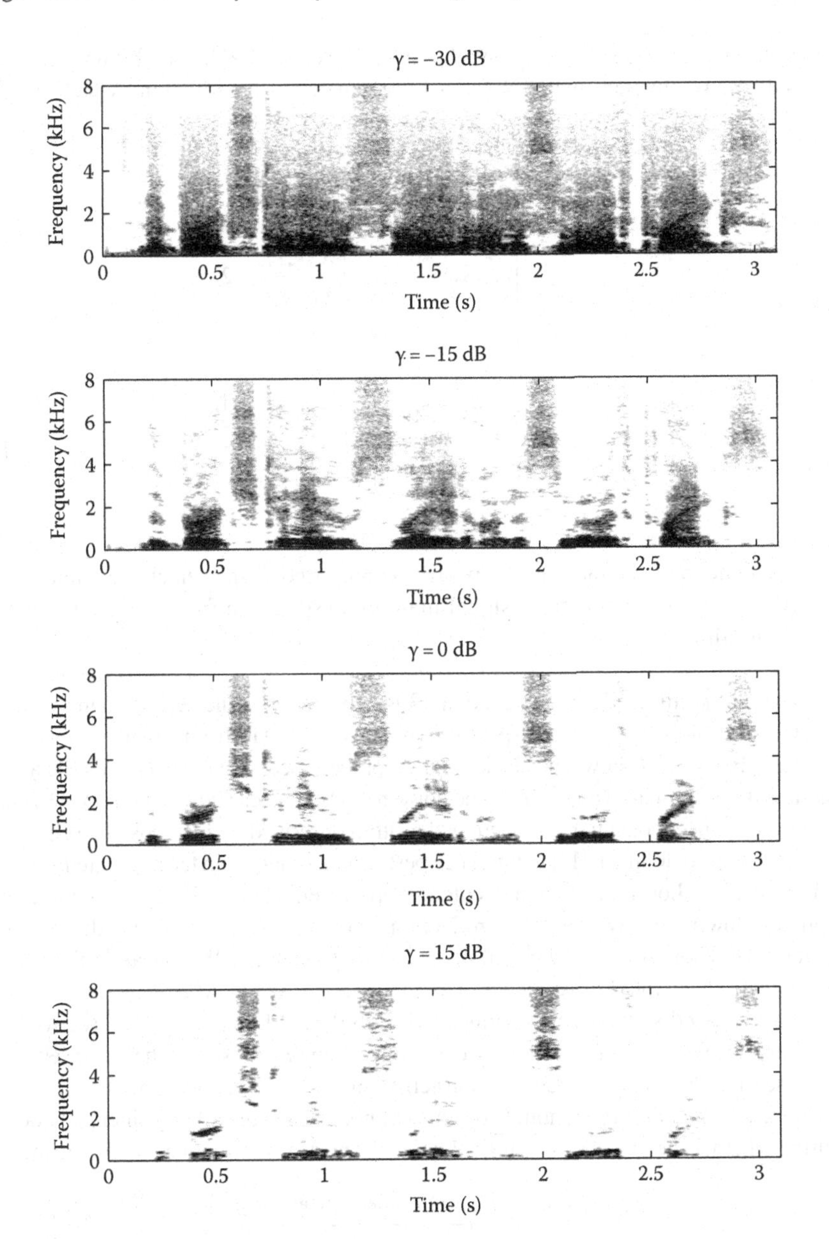

FIGURE 13.6 Sentence processed using different SNR thresholds.

13.3.2 SNR_{ESI} Selection Criterion

As discussed in Section 13.1.1, if we somehow control the type of speech distortions introduced by noise reduction, we can improve speech intelligibility. More precisely, if we use the SNR_{ESI} metric and require that only channels with $SNR_{ESI} > 1$ are allowed to pass through, we can eliminate the large amplification distortions (>6 dB), which have been found in [13] to be quite detrimental to speech intelligibility.

If we thus want to ensure that only channels in Region I + II (see Figure 13.1) are allowed, that is, channels with $SNR_{ESI} > 1$, we can devise the following selection rule:

$$
\begin{aligned}
|X_C(k,t)| &= \begin{cases} |\hat{X}(k,t)| & \text{if } \ SNR_{ESI}(k,t) > 1 \\ 0 & \text{else} \end{cases} \\
&= \begin{cases} |\hat{X}(k,t)| & \text{if } \ \dfrac{|\hat{X}(k,t)|}{|X(k,t)|} < 2 \\ 0 & \text{else} \end{cases} \\
&= \begin{cases} |\hat{X}(k,t)| & \text{if } \ \dfrac{|X(k,t)|}{|\hat{X}(k,t)|} > \dfrac{1}{2} \\ 0 & \text{else} \end{cases}
\end{aligned}
\tag{13.17}
$$

where

$|X_C(k,t)|$ denotes the magnitude spectrum composed of the selected channels

$|\hat{X}(k,t)|$ denotes the enhanced signal magnitude spectrum from a noise-reduction algorithm

Note that unlike the SNR rule (Equation 13.14), the SNR_{ESI} rule selects channels from the enhanced (noise-suppressed) spectrum $|\hat{X}(k,t)|$ rather than from the noise-corrupted spectrum. Figure 13.7 shows the block diagram of the processing involved with the aforementioned SNR_{ESI}-based algorithm. The noise-reduction block shown in Figure 13.7 may include any conventional noise-reduction algorithm described in this book. The choice of algorithm was not found in [13] to influence performance, at least in terms of intelligibility.

Figure 13.8 shows an example sentence processed via the SNR_{ESI} selection rule applied following the Wiener noise-reduction algorithm. Panel (b) shows the spectrogram of the Wiener-processed signal. It is clear that the use of Wiener algorithm alone fails to reconstruct intelligible speech at an input SNR = −5 dB. After selecting from the Wiener-processed spectra only channels with $SNR_{ESI} > 1$, we are able to recover the input target signal (see panel c) with great fidelity. Figure 13.9 shows the same sentence processed now via a basic spectral subtractive algorithm. This was intentionally chosen since it produces large amounts of musical noise (see panel b). Of interest is determining whether the presence of musical noise in spectral subtractive processed speech

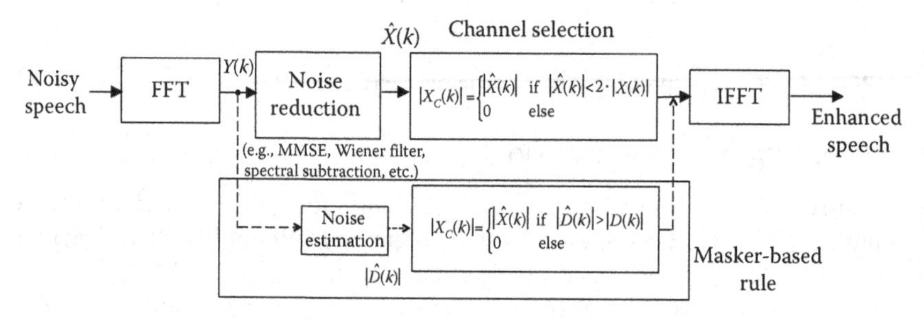

FIGURE 13.7 Block diagram of two different channel-selection algorithms.

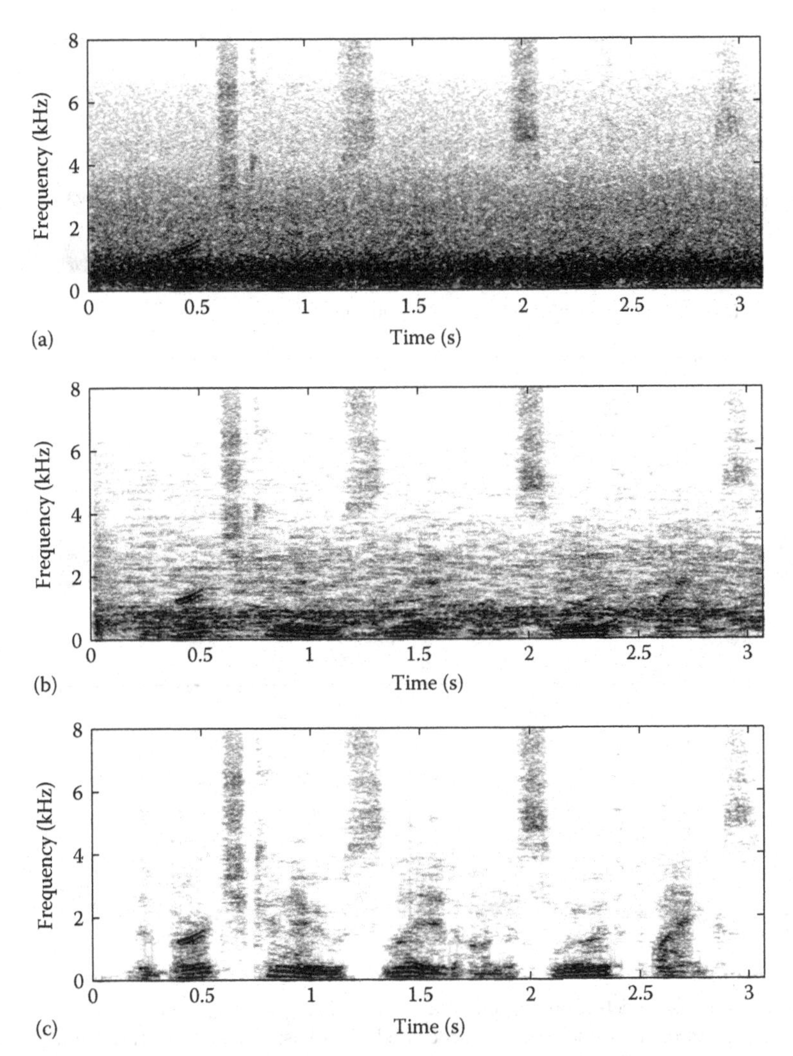

FIGURE 13.8 (a) Spectrogram of sentence corrupted by speech-shaped noise at −5 dB SNR; (b) spectrogram of Wiener-processed signal; and (c) spectrogram of sentence processed via the constraint-magnitude spectrum selection rule using the Wiener algorithm as the noise-reduction algorithm.

would influence the performance of the SNR_{ESI}-based algorithm. As shown in panel (c), following channel selection, some of this musical noise is retained at the output, yet according to [13] that was not enough to impair intelligibility. Acoustic cues, such as *F*1 and *F*2 formant movements and presence of onsets/offsets signaling syllable or word boundaries, were preserved following channel selection.

Why should we expect improvement in intelligibility with the aforementioned SNR_{ESI} selection criterion? The reason is that the overall SNR of the selected channels is always larger (better) than the SNR of the unprocessed signal. This was accomplished by eliminating a large portion of channels with unfavorable SNR.

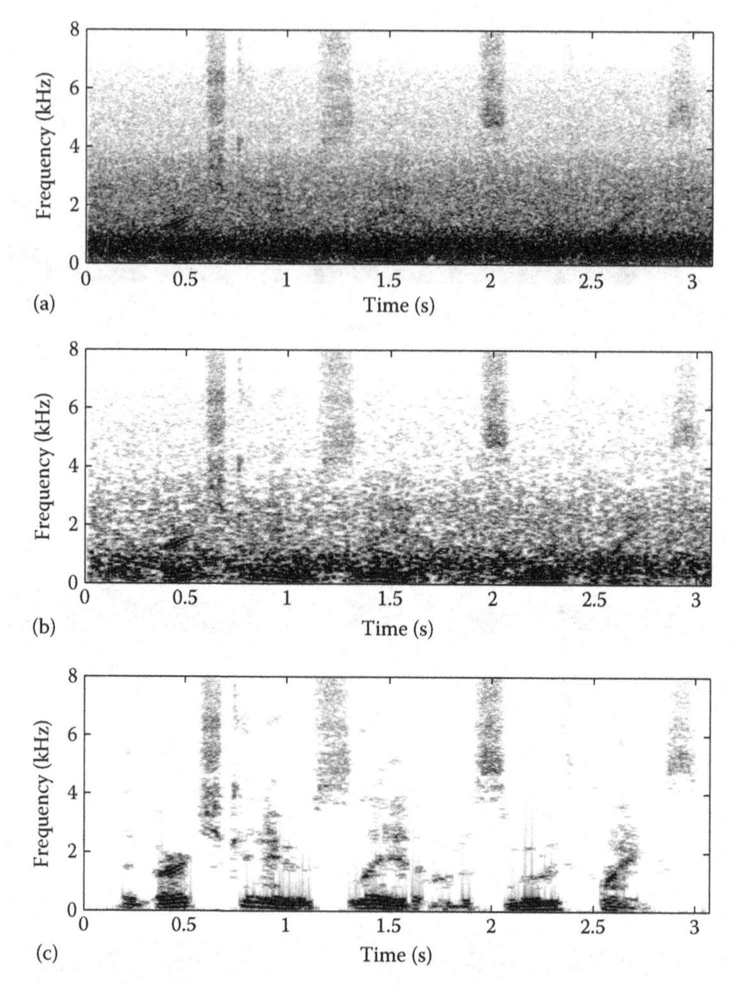

FIGURE 13.9 (a) Spectrogram of sentence corrupted by speech-shaped noise at −5 dB SNR; (b) spectrogram of the same sentence processed via a basic spectral subtractive algorithm; and (c) spectrogram of sentence processed via the constraint-magnitude spectrum selection rule using a basic spectral subtractive algorithm as the noise-reduction algorithm.

Indeed, this is accomplished by selecting only channels in Region I + II (Figure 13.1), that is, channels with $SNR_{ESI} > 1$. The SNR of channels falling in Region III is always negative. In fact, it can be proven analytically that [11]

$$|\hat{X}(k,t)| > 2 \cdot |X(k,t)| \rightarrow SNR_{ESI}(k,t) < 1 \rightarrow SNR(k,t) < 1 \tag{13.18}$$

That is, channels falling in Region III have *always* a negative SNR, that is, they are always masked by noise. This is also evident by the relationship between SNR_{ESI} and SNR displayed in Figure 11.42. Whenever $SNR_{ESI} < 1$, SNR is smaller than 1. On the other hand, $SNR_{ESI} > 1$ does not imply that SNR > 1 (i.e., >0dB). That is, the SNR_{ESI} selection rule does not guarantee that it will retain only the positive SNR TF units. Figure 13.10 shows,

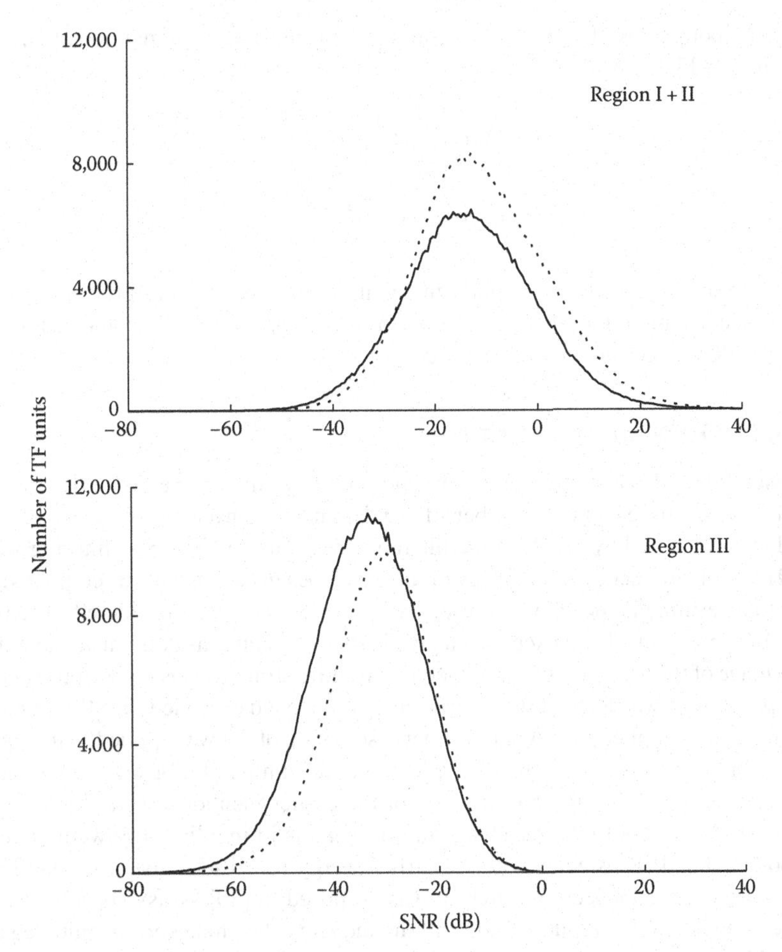

FIGURE 13.10 Histogram of TF units falling in Region I + II ($SNR_{ESI} > 1$) and Region III ($SNR_{ESI} < 1$).

for instance, the histograms of SNRs of TF units falling in Regions I + II and III (histogram was computed based on data from 20 IEEE sentences). As can be seen, the SNRs of TF units falling in Region I + II ($SNR_{ESI} > 1$) are not necessarily positive. On the other hand, the SNRs of all TF units in Region III ($SNR_{ESI} < 1$) were always negative. Hence, eliminating those unfavorable channels can yield substantial benefits in intelligibility. Further analysis in [11] indicated that the percentage of TF units falling in Region III could be quite large, at least for steady noise. More specifically, this percentage varied from 70% at input SNR = −10 dB to 50% at input SNR = 0 dB. In brief, the SNR_{ESI} selection rule eliminates a large number of TF units with unfavorable SNR.

It is interesting to note that the SNR_{ESI} selection rule reduces to the SNR selection rule when the noisy signal is not processed by an enhancement algorithm, that is, when $\hat{X}(k,t) = Y(k,t)$, where $Y(k,t)$ is the noise-corrupted spectrum. In that case, we have

$$|\hat{X}(k,t)|^2 = |Y(k,t)|^2 = |X(k,t)|^2 + |D(k,t)|^2 \quad (13.19)$$

Squaring both sides of Equation 13.4 and substituting the aforementioned equation in Equation 13.4, we get

$$|X(k,t)|^2 \geq \frac{1}{3}|D(k,t)|^2$$

$$\mathrm{SNR}(k,t) \geq \frac{1}{3} \qquad (13.20)$$

Hence, in the absence of any enhancement algorithm or nonlinear processing of the noisy speech signal, the $\mathrm{SNR}_{\mathrm{ESI}} > 1$ rule for retaining channels becomes equivalent to the SNR > 0.33 rule with the SNR criterion.

13.3.3 Other Selection Criteria

An energy-based selection criterion was proposed by Anzalone et al. [29]. The clean stimuli were filtered into a number of bands, and the envelope of each frequency band was computed by squaring the filtered waveforms and low-pass filtering with a 300 Hz cutoff frequency. The energy of the envelopes in each band was computed and used to determine if speech was present or absent. Speech was considered to be present if the energy in a band exceeded a given criterion. This was done such that a fixed percentage of the total energy contained in the entire stimulus was above the criterion. This percentage was fixed at 99%. If the energy in a band exceeded the 99% criterion, a gain of 1 was applied to that band. Otherwise, a gain of 0.2 was applied. After applying the binary gains to each band, the bands were summed to form the final output. It should be noted that the construction of the earlier mentioned selection criterion requires only access to the clean signal. Large gains in intelligibility were obtained for both NH and HI listeners with the earlier energy-based selection criterion [29].

A masker-based selection criterion was proposed in [30]. Noisy speech was first processed via a noise-reduction algorithm, and from the enhanced magnitude spectrum, bins were selected that satisfied the following criterion:

$$|X_M(k,t)| = \begin{cases} |\hat{X}(k,t)| & \text{if } |\hat{D}(k,t)| > |D(k,t)| \\ 0 & \text{else} \end{cases}$$

$$= \begin{cases} |\hat{X}(k,t)| & \text{if } \dfrac{|D(k,t)|}{|\hat{D}(k,t)|} < 1 \\ 0 & \text{else} \end{cases} \qquad (13.21)$$

where

$|\hat{X}(k,t)|$ denotes the enhanced spectrum (i.e., output of noise-reduction algorithm)
$|\hat{D}(k,t)|$ denotes the estimated masker spectrum
$|D(k,t)|$ denotes the true-masker magnitude spectrum

Note that the aforementioned criterion does not require access to the clean input signal, only the masker. Large intelligibility gains were observed relative to unprocessed speech when the aforementioned criterion was applied to speech corrupted by multitalker babble at input SNRs ranging from −10 to 0 dB [30].

Further analysis was done in [30] to better understand the benefit of the aforesaid selection criterion. SNR histograms of frequency bins falling in the overestimated region (as per Equation 13.21) were compared against SNR histograms of frequency bins falling in the underestimated region. It was clear from these histograms (see [30, Fig. 4]) that the SNRs of the noise-underestimated frequency bins were for the most part negative, thus explaining the poor performance (near 0% correct) obtained when bins were selected with the noise spectrum underestimated. In contrast, the SNRs of the noise-overestimated frequency bins were more favorable and were distributed across both positive and negative SNR regions. In brief, the improvement in intelligibility obtained by the masker criterion (Equation 13.21) can be attributed to the overall increase in SNR relative to the SNR of the unprocessed stimuli. The study in [31] further demonstrated that noise spectrum underestimation leads to SNR overestimation errors. Listening tests indicated that SNR overestimation errors severely compromised speech intelligibility [31], consistent with the low SNR of the noise underestimated frequency bins. In contrast, SNR underestimation errors did not degrade intelligibility.

13.3.4 Channel-Selection Criteria for Reverberation

These selection criteria are not applicable in reverberation, as they only take into account additive noise. A number of reverberation-specific channel-selection criteria have been proposed [32–34]. Some require access to the room impulse response (RIR) [32,34], while others do not [33]. In [32], for instance, several reverberant-specific criteria were constructed based on the ratio of the desirable energy (e.g., direct path energy) to undesirable energy (e.g., late reverberation energy). To construct such a criterion, the reverberated signal was decomposed into its direct path, early echo, and reverberant portions by convolving different segments of the impulse response with the anechoic signal. To compute, for instance, the direct path portion of the impulse response, only the initial 9.6 ms of the impulse response was kept (remaining portion was set to 0). Criteria that included the energy from the direct path as desirable yielded good performance, in terms of both intelligibility and automatic speech recognition (ASR) scores. Similar criteria were constructed and tested in [34].

The computation of the aforementioned criteria requires access to the RIR. This presents a great challenge in estimating such criteria in nonideal scenarios, where we only have access to the reverberant signal, as it would require estimation of the RIR. A simpler reverberant criterion that required no access to the room impulse was proposed in [33]. It was constructed based on the ratio of the energies of the anechoic signal and reverberant signal at each TF unit, that is,

$$\mathrm{SRR}(k,t) = \frac{|X(k,t)|^2}{|X_R(k,t)|^2} \tag{13.22}$$

where

$|X(k,t)|$ denotes the anechoic signal spectrum

$|X_R(k,t)|$ denotes the reverberant signal spectrum and signal-to-reverberant ratio (SRR)

TF units with SRR greater than a threshold were retained, while TF units with SRR smaller than a threshold were zeroed out, as follows:

$$|X_M(k,t)| = \begin{cases} |X_R(k,t)| & \text{if } \ \text{SRR}(k,t) > T \\ 0 & \text{else} \end{cases} \tag{13.23}$$

where T denotes a preset threshold. The aforementioned selection rule yielded high intelligibility gains for both NH listeners [35] and HI listeners [33].

Further analysis was conducted in [33] to better understand as to why the aforementioned SRR criterion improves speech intelligibility in reverberant conditions. Figure 13.11c plots the instantaneous SRR values as well as the clean (see Figure 13.11a) and reverberant (see Figure 13.11) signals bandpass filtered at a center frequency of $f = 500$ Hz. Figure 13.11d plots the synthesized time-domain waveforms of the same IEEE sentence processed with threshold $T = -5$ dB. Figure 13.11e shows the same output processed with the threshold set to $T = +5$ dB. The waveforms depicted in Figure 13.11d and e were obtained by retaining the reverberant signal corresponding to SRR > T, while discarding (zeroing out) the reverberant signal when SRR < T.

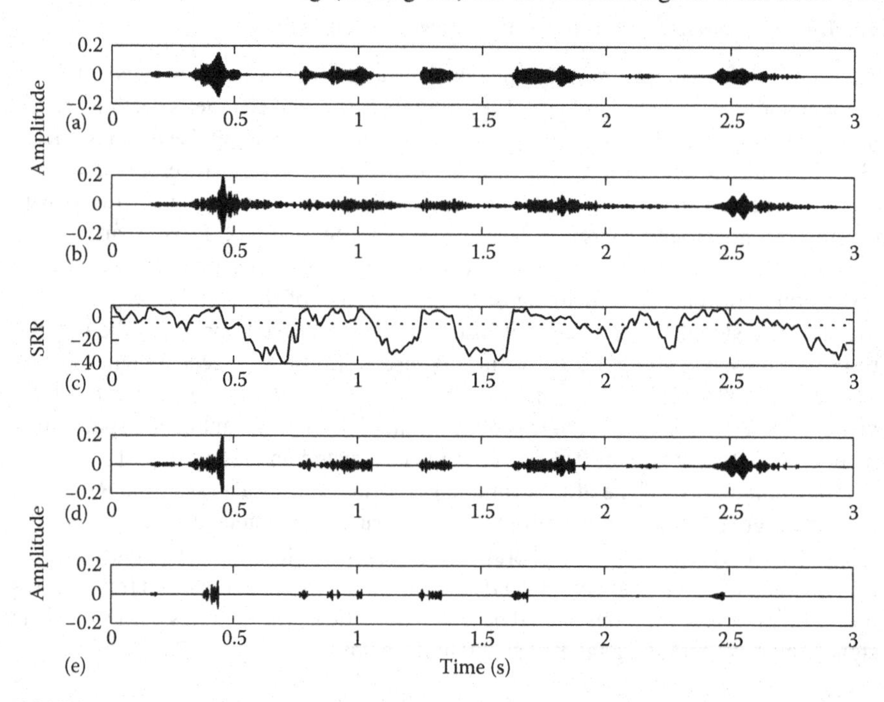

FIGURE 13.11 Example illustrating the bandpass-filtered IEEE sentence "The urge to write short stories is rare" extracted at the center frequency of 500 Hz. (a) Unmodified (uncorrupted) sentence, (b) sentence corrupted with reverberation equal to $T_{60} = 1.0$ s, (c) instantaneous SRR values (dB) along with threshold value fixed at $T = -5$ dB (dashed line), (d) reverberant sentence processed by the ideal SRR selection algorithm with the threshold set to −5 dB, and (e) reverberant sentence processed by the ideal SRR selection algorithm with the threshold set to +5 dB.

For the example shown with $T = -5$ dB, we observe that the reverberant energy residing in the gaps is eliminated (compare Figure 13.11b against Figure 13.11d. As shown in Figure 13.11a and b, during the segments in which the SRR is less than −5 dB, the energy of the reverberant signal is more dominant than the energy of the clean (anechoic) speech signal. Thus, a negative threshold value (e.g., $T = -5$ dB) seems to be appropriate for suppressing the reverberation present in the gaps. In contrast, as shown in Figure 13.11e, when the threshold value is set to $T = +5$ dB, the selection process seems to be too aggressive, since apart from discarding the corrupted unvoiced segments and associated gaps, it also zeroes out (eliminates) useful speech information present in the high-energy voiced frames.

Based on the example shown in Figure 13.11, we can infer that a large SRR value would suggest that the energy from the direct path (and early reflections) dominates, as is often the case during the voiced segments (e.g., vowels) of the utterance. In contrast, a small SRR value would suggest that the reverberant energy, composed of the sum of the energies from the early and late reflections, dominates. This happens primarily during the gaps and is caused primarily by overlap-masking. The example shown in Figure 13.11 illustrates the importance of preserving the voiced/unvoiced gaps, which are typically smeared in reverberation owing to the late reflections. Hence, algorithms that can detect the presence of the voiced/unvoiced gaps, either by estimating the SRR (Equation 13.22) or by other means, ought to improve speech intelligibility in reverberant conditions.

13.3.5 Universal Selection Criterion for All Types of Background Interferers

So far, we described criteria that are appropriate for additive noise (and competing talkers) and other criteria that are appropriate for reverberation. In a realistic implementation of channel-selection algorithms, however, this poses the additional challenge of determining whether a particular listening environment contains reverberation or not. Ideally, we would like to have a selection criterion that can be used for all types of background interferers. Such a criterion exists and is based on the ratio of the target signal power to the corrupted signal power:

$$\text{TCR}(k,t) = \frac{|X(k,t)|^2}{|Y(k,t)|^2} \tag{13.24}$$

where

TCR denotes the target-to-corrupted power ratio

$Y(k,t)$ denotes the corrupted (by noise, reverberation, etc.) spectrum

Channel selection is performed as follows:

$$|X_M(k,t)| = \begin{cases} |Y(k,t)| & \text{if } \text{TCR}(k,t) > T \\ 0 & \text{else} \end{cases} \tag{13.25}$$

It is easy to see that in reverberation (or reverberation + noise conditions), the TCR criterion (Equation 13.24) is the same as the SRR criterion (Equation 13.22), since $Y(k,t) = X_R(k,t)$. In the absence of reverberation, the TCR criterion is the same as the SNR criterion. To see this, we can write the TCR equation as follows:

$$\mathrm{TCR}(k,t) = \frac{|X(k,t)|^2}{|Y(k,t)|^2} = \frac{|X(k,t)|^2}{|X(k,t)|^2 + |D(k,t)|^2} = \frac{\mathrm{SNR}(k,t)}{\mathrm{SNR}(k,t)+1} \tag{13.26}$$

where $D(k,t)$ denotes the spectrum of the masker (e.g., noise, competing talker, etc.). Equation 13.26 is no other than the equation of the short-time Wiener filter. Hence, the channel selection rule in Equation 13.25 is performed by comparing the value of the Wiener gain function against a threshold T. For a given value of T, one can find the corresponding SNR value using Equation 13.26. A value of $T = 0.1368$ ($T_{dB} = -17.3$ dB), for instance, corresponds to SNR = −8 dB (put differently, the Wiener gain for SNR = −8 dB is 0.1368). This was computed by setting the Wiener gain function equal to T and solving for the corresponding SNR using Equation 13.26. Therefore, using $T = 0.1368$ as threshold with the TCR criterion is equivalent to using −8 dB as SNR threshold with the SNR criterion.

In brief, the TCR criterion reduces to the SRR criterion in reverberation and reduces to the SNR criterion in additive noise. On that respect, we refer to the TCR criterion as the universal criterion as it can be used for all types of background interferers.

13.4 INTELLIGIBILITY EVALUATION OF CHANNEL-SELECTION-BASED ALGORITHMS: IDEAL CONDITIONS

A number of studies have tested the aforementioned channel-selection criteria with NH and HI listeners in ideal conditions, that is, in conditions where access to the clean and/or noise signals was assumed. While some might consider these as unrealistic conditions, the outcomes of such experiments are extremely important for several reasons. First and foremost, the outcomes of such experiments provide the upper bound in performance, a bound that might be considered as analogous to the Cramer-Rao bound in estimation theory. In the context of intelligibility scores, the upper bound ought to be near 100% correct. If the performance of the aforementioned ideal channel-selection algorithms is indeed near 100%, that would warrant the effort to design algorithms that would estimate the various criteria described earlier based only on noisy (or reverberant) observations. Second, the outcomes of such ideal (also known as oracle) experiments could provide useful insights as to how humans understand speech in complex listening situations (e.g., restaurant, reverberant rooms). The study in [36], for instance, used the SNR criterion to study how in noisy backgrounds humans are able to "glimpse" segments of speech with favorable SNR and patch or integrate the information contained in those segments ("glimpses") to understand the whole utterance. The study in [18] used the SNR criterion to tease out the effects of energetic and informational masking in competing-talker situations.

Next, we provide a summary of the outcomes of intelligibility studies conducted in ideal conditions using the various criteria described earlier. Given the differences in temporal/spectral characteristics of maskers present in realistic scenarios, we report separately the major findings of these studies in (1) broadband noise conditions (e.g., white noise, multitalker babble, and train noise), (2) competing-talker conditions, and (3) reverberation. These three types of interference cover all listening conditions that can be encountered in real-world situations.

13.4.1 Broadband Noise Conditions

Broadband noise can be stationary (e.g., car noise, speech-shaped noise) or nonstationary (e.g., multitalker babble, restaurant noise). The nonstationary type is particularly challenging for most enhancement algorithms as it is difficult to track the background noise spectrum. A number of studies examined the intelligibility of speech in broadband noise conditions using the SNR criterion. Figure 13.12 (taken from the study in [19]) shows intelligibility scores as a function of the SNR threshold. The masker was multitalker babble, and listeners were tested at input SNRs of −10 and −5 dB. As can be seen, intelligibility is restored (performance at SNR = −10 dB improved from 0% correct to 100% correct) for a range of threshold values (−20 to 0 dB). A similar finding was reported previously in [18] in competing-talker conditions. As can be seen from Figure 13.12, the threshold value used in the

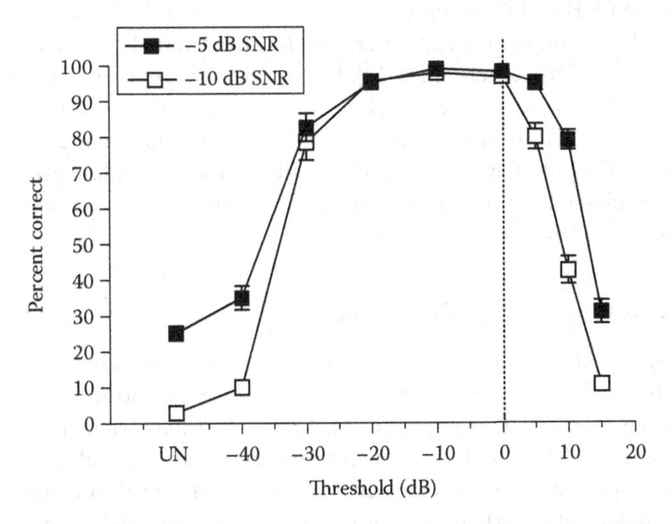

FIGURE 13.12 Mean intelligibility scores obtained by NH listeners with the ideal SNR selection algorithm as a function of the SNR threshold used. The masker was a 20-talker babble. Performance obtained with unprocessed mixtures is indicated as UN. Error bars indicate standard errors of the mean.

SNR criterion did not seem to influence the performance, as long as it fell within the range of −20 to 0 dB. Subsequent studies [37] revealed that the "optimal" threshold value depends on the input SNR. More precisely, the study in [37] demonstrated that the lower the input SNR is, the lower the threshold should be. For instance, if the input SNR is say −40 dB, then the best (in terms of intelligibility scores) to use is −40 dB (or values close to −40 dB). The reason that a low-SNR threshold (e.g., −6 dB) would yield a poor intelligibility score when the input SNR is say −40 dB is because at such a low-input SNR, the number of TF units with SNR > −6 dB is extremely small. Consequently, only a small portion of speech would be retained with the majority set to zero. The study in [37] demonstrated that the SNR criterion can restore speech intelligibility at *any* input SNR level (even at −40 dB), provided that the appropriate threshold is used. In fact, it has been shown [21] that high intelligibility can be obtained even at SNR = −∞. In that study [21], nearly perfect recognition was obtained when the binary gains (mask) obtained from the SNR criterion (see Equation 13.13) were used to modulate noise rather than noisy speech. Speech synthesized with binary-gated noise sounds like whispered speech (i.e., contains no *F*0 information) and is similar to noise-band-vocoded speech [38]. Sixteen binary-gated bands of noise were found in [21] to be sufficient for high intelligibility.

Channel-selection algorithms based on the SNR criterion have also been evaluated with HI listeners [39,40]. The study in [39] reported performance in terms of speech reception threshold (SRT) values (see Section 10.2.4.1), rather than percent correct scores. The measured mean SRT value of HI listeners in cafeteria noise was −20 dB, a 16 dB improvement relative to the SRT obtained with unprocessed stimuli. The performance of NH listeners with the SNR-based selection algorithm was only slightly better (SRT = −22 dB) than that of HI listeners. This outcome suggests that the SNR-based selection algorithm has the potential of eliminating the gap in performance between NH and HI listeners.

Intelligibility with other selection criteria has been found to be as good as that obtained with the SNR criterion [11,30]. Figure 13.13 summarizes the performance obtained with the SNR_{ESI} criterion (Equation 13.17) and the masker-based criterion (Equation 13.21). In those studies [11,30], speech-shaped noise was used as a masker. In brief, all the selection criteria described in Section 13.3 have been shown to restore speech intelligibility in broadband noise conditions, even at extremely low-SNR levels (e.g., SNR = −40 dB).

13.4.2 Competing-Talker Conditions

Handling situations where two or more talkers are speaking simultaneously is extremely challenging for the main reason that we can no longer use VAD or noise-estimation techniques to track the background speaker, since in this scenario, "background noise" is actually a speech produced by another talker. None of the algorithms described in the previous chapters would fare well in competing-talker conditions and would most likely fail. Can the aforementioned channel-selection-based algorithms cope with competing speakers?

The study in [18] used the SNR criterion and demonstrated that this criterion can segregate quite effectively the target speaker from not only a single competing

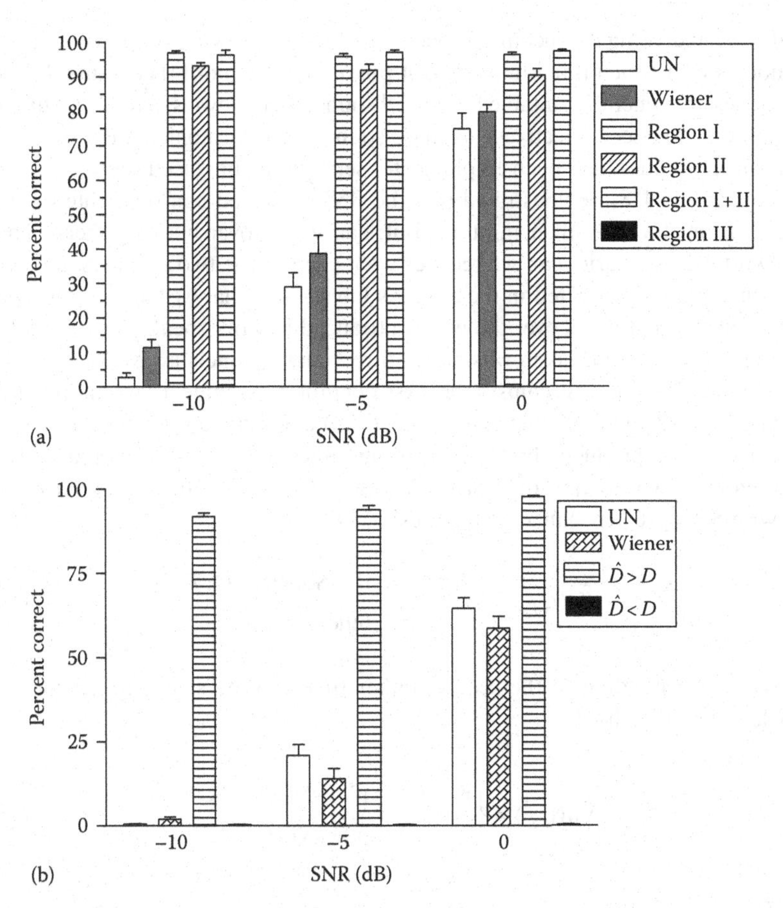

FIGURE 13.13 Mean intelligibility scores obtained by NH listeners with the ideal SNR_{ESI} selection algorithm (a) and ideal masker-based selection algorithm (b). The masker was speech-shaped noise. Intelligibility scores obtained using the Wiener algorithm are superimposed along with those obtained with unprocessed (UN) speech.

speaker but from as many as three background speakers. In their experiments, the input SNR was set to −3 dB, and the SNR threshold varied from a low of −60 dB to a high of 30 dB. Perfect intelligibility scores (100% correct) were obtained when the SNR threshold fell within the range of −10 to 0 dB.

Perhaps, one of the most important findings of the study mentioned earlier is that no F0 information was used to segregate the target speaker from the competing (background) speaker(s), yet the algorithm recovered the target speaker perfectly and restored speech intelligibility. Use of *F*0 information has been the conventional approach for speaker separation. Motivated by perceptual studies [41–43] demonstrating that human listeners can effectively use *F*0 differences to segregate the target speech from concurrent vowels or sentences (see Figure 4.12), a number of algorithms have been proposed in the past for separating two simultaneous voices based on their fundamental frequency (F0) differences (e.g., [42,44,45]). Parsons' [44] approach, for instance, was based on selecting the harmonics of the desired speaker by analyzing the incoming spectrum. Algorithms were proposed to track the harmonics over time taking into account possible overlap of F0 contours. F0-based techniques are generally suitable for voiced sounds (e.g., vowels) but not for unvoiced sounds (e.g., unvoiced fricatives), as these sounds lack harmonicity. For that reason, different techniques have been employed for segregating unvoiced sounds (e.g., [46]).

The study in [18] demonstrated that the SNR criterion can segregate the target speaker from the two-talker mixture. But, can we recover both speakers? That is, in a two-talker scenario, can we recover what each of the two speakers are saying? Listening studies conducted in the author's lab showed that we can indeed separate both speakers, that is, recover the words produced by both speakers in a two-talker mixture. The approach taken was not to throw any channels away, but rather keep them in two separate "streams," the first containing fragments of the phonemes/words produced by the target talker and the second containing fragments of the phonemes/words produced by the competing talker. The two-talker mixture can be separated into two streams: one corresponding to the target talker, by selecting channels with SNR greater than a preset threshold T:

$$\hat{X}_T(t,f) = \begin{cases} Y(t,f) & \text{if} \quad \text{SNR}(t,f) \geq T \\ 0 & \text{otherwise} \end{cases} \tag{13.27}$$

and one corresponding to the second talker (masker), by selecting channels with SNR less than threshold T:

$$\hat{X}_M(t,f) = \begin{cases} Y(t,f) & \text{if} \quad \text{SNR}(t,f) < T \\ 0 & \text{otherwise} \end{cases} \tag{13.28}$$

where

$Y(t,f)$ denotes the mixture magnitude spectrum
$\hat{X}_T(t,f)$ denotes the recovered spectrum of target talker
$\hat{X}_M(t,f)$ denotes the recovered spectrum of the masker talker
T denotes the threshold

After computing the IFFT of $\hat{X}_T(t,f)$ and $\hat{X}_M(t,f)$, two different signals are synthesized, one corresponding to the target (first talker) and one to the masker (second talker). These two signals were presented separately to NH listeners for identification. In some conditions (e.g., mixture at 25 dB SNR), the recovered masker signal will naturally have a low intensity and might not be audible. To rule out audibility effects, the target and masker signals were made equally audible and presented to the listeners at a comfortable level. IEEE sentences (male talker) taken from the DVD of this book were used for testing. The two-talker mixture was generated by adding the masker signal to the target signal at three SNR levels: 0, 15, and 25 dB. Positive SNR levels were chosen to make the task challenging in terms of recovering *both* the masker and target signals, particularly at SNR = 25 dB. A different masker sentence was used to construct each mixture sentence. The masker sentence was produced by the same target male speaker. This was done on purpose to make the task extremely challenging since the $F0$ of the target and masker is identical. In the case that the masker sentence was shorter in duration than the target sentence, the beginning segment of the masker sentence was concatenated (and repeated) at the end of the masker sentence to ensure equal duration. Listening experiments (with 10 NH listeners) were run to find the appropriate threshold T that would recover *both* talkers with high intelligibility.

The mean intelligibility scores are shown in Figure 13.14. The target signal was identified accurately (near 100% correct) for all values of T. This was not surprising given the largely positive input SNR levels (0–25 dB). The recognition of the masker signal (competing talker) depended on both the values of T and input SNR level. Overall, $T = 5$ dB was found to produce consistently high (>80% correct) performance for all the three SNR levels tested. Hence, the masker and target sentences can *both* be identified with high accuracy for a wide range (0–25 dB) of input SNR levels when the SNR segregation threshold is set to 5 dB.

Given that the spectra of the two talkers always overlap, how is it possible to separate them and achieve such high intelligibility scores (Figure 13.14)? The segregation of two-talker mixtures is possible due to the inherent sparsity of speech. More precisely, there exists spectrotemporal sparsity in two-talker mixtures of speech, in that when the mixture is decomposed, through say a cochlear filterbank, into TF units, *only one* of two talkers will be dominant in a given TF unit. This is so because it is

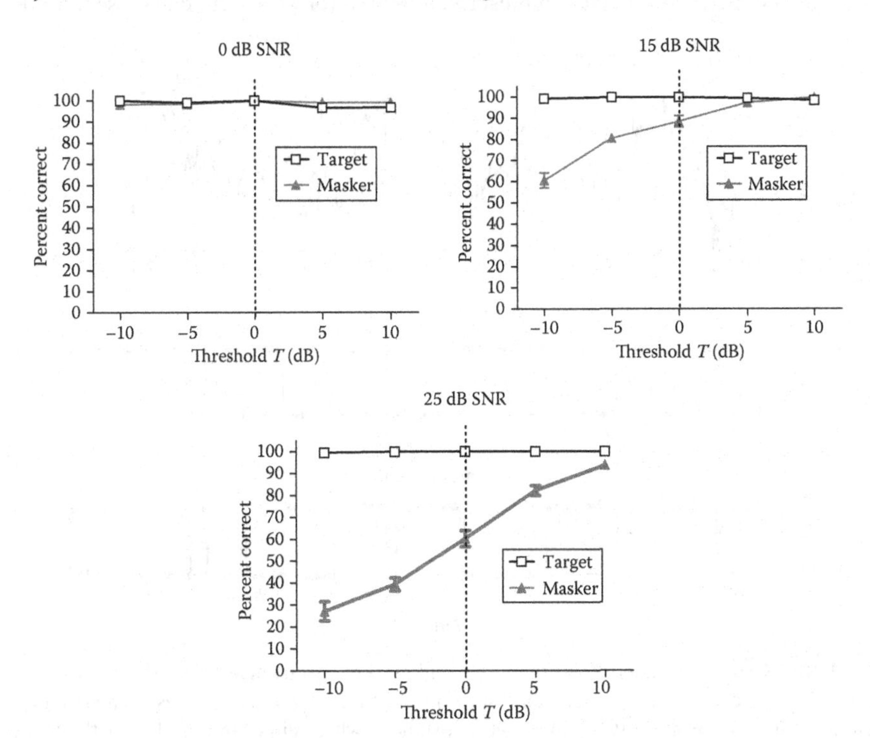

FIGURE 13.14 Mean subject scores obtained for the recognition of target and masker sentences recovered from two-talker mixtures (0–25 dB SNR) using different segregation threshold values T. Error bars indicate standard errors of the mean.

highly unlikely that the spectral components of the two talkers will occupy the same TF unit at the same time. Mathematically, this can be expressed as follows:

$$|Y(k,t)| \approx \max\left(|X_T(k,t)|,|X_M(k,t)|\right) \tag{13.29}$$

where

$|Y(k,t)| = |X_T(k,t) + X_M(k,t)|$ denotes the magnitude spectrum of the two-talker mixture

$|X_T(k,t)|$, $|X_M(k,t)|$ denote, respectively, the magnitude spectra of the target talker and competing talker

Histograms of the difference between the maximum of the two spectra (in dB) and the two-talker mixture spectrum revealed a peak at 0 dB [47], thus confirming the validity of the approximation in Equation 13.29. Analysis in [47] showed that the $|X_T(k,t)|$ and $|X_M(k,t)|$ spectra differ from the maximum by more than 3 dB in fewer than 20% of all TF units present in an utterance.

To illustrate the principle described earlier, we show in Figure 13.15 the magnitude spectrum (at a single frequency bin $f = 950$ Hz) of two talkers plotted over time. The spectra are shown before mixing the two signals at 0 dB SNR and after scaling the masker signal to achieve the prescribed SNR level (0 dB). As can be seen in the

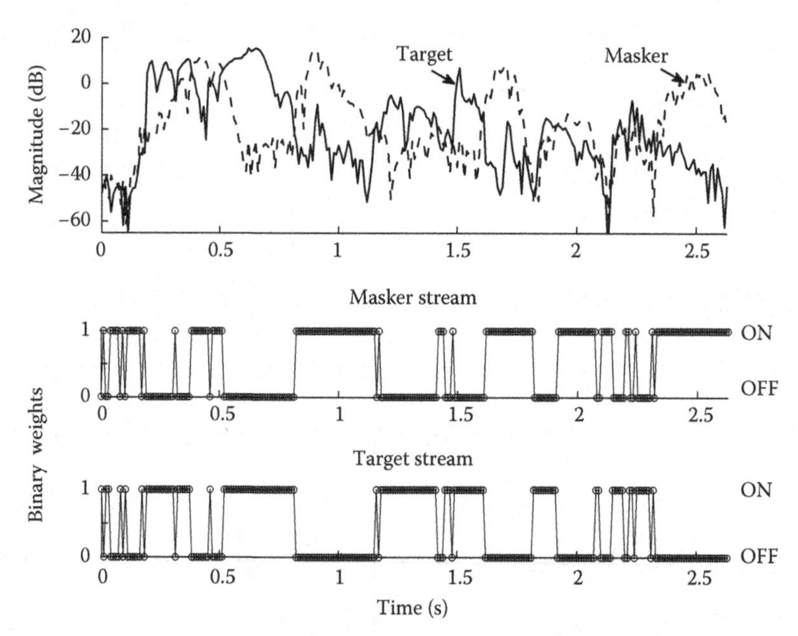

FIGURE 13.15 Top panel shows the target and masker spectrum at $f = 950$ Hz plotted over time. The target and masker spectra are shown prior to mixing the sentences of the two talkers at 0 dB SNR. Bottom two panels show instances where either the masker or the target speaker was spectrally dominant. The mixture component was assigned to the target stream if the target was stronger than the masker (i.e., $T = 0$ dB). Similarly, the mixture component was assigned to the masker stream if the masker was stronger than the target.

top panel, the time instances during which both talkers have the same magnitude are very few and rare. Speech sparsity exists for a wide range of SNR levels spanning from −20 to 20 dB and persists for mixtures [48] consisting of multiple speakers. Keeping track of which speaker is spectrally dominant provides a means to separate a two-talker mixture into two auditory streams corresponding to the speech of the two talkers (see bottom two panels of Figure 13.15). This simple principle uses no primitive grouping cues, such as $F0$ differences or common onsets/offsets, requires no explicit voiced/unvoiced segmentation, and does not rely on any schema-based processes for grouping [49]. The spectrotemporal sparsity of speech has been known for some time, and, in fact, it has been used extensively in ASR algorithms [24,25,50].

In the study by Brungart et al. [18], the SNR criterion yielded high intelligibility gains for input SNR of −3 dB but was not tested at lower SNR levels. The SNR_{ESI} criterion was tested in [11] at SNR = −10 dB with competing talkers and recovered the target sentence perfectly (100% correct). In brief, both the SNR and SNR_{ESI} criteria can cope with competing-talker scenarios.

13.4.3 Reverberant Conditions

The SRR criterion (Equation 13.23) has been shown to yield high intelligibility scores for a range of T_{60} values (T_{60} = 0.3–1.0 s) for both NH [35] and HI listeners [33]. Good performance was observed not only in reverberation-alone conditions but also in conditions where both reverberation and additive noise were present [35]. When NH listeners were tested, for instance, on a consonant (/aCa/) identification task, scores improved from 50% correct in the 0 dB reverberation + noise condition (T_{60} = 1 s) to 95% correct [35].

The criteria used in [34] based on the direct path and early reflections also yielded high intelligibility gains in a number of conditions involving reverberation, noise, and competing talkers. In that study, intelligibility was assessed using SRTs to avoid ceiling effects. That is, an adaptive procedure was used to obtain the SNR required to obtain 50% intelligibility (see Section 10.2.4.1). In reverberation + noise (T_{60} = 0.8 s) conditions, intelligibility improved by nearly 8 dB [34]. Even larger improvements (nearly 12 dB) in intelligibility were observed in conditions that involved reverberation and competing talkers [34].

In summary, all the reverberation-specific criteria discussed in Section 13.3.4 yielded near-perfect (100%) intelligibility scores in reverberation for a wide range of T_{60} values. In terms of estimating the aforementioned criteria or equivalently estimating the binary mask from reverberant signals alone, the SRR criterion offers the advantage that it does not require access to the RIR.

13.5 IMPLEMENTATION OF CHANNEL-SELECTION-BASED ALGORITHMS IN REALISTIC CONDITIONS

So far, we talked about the huge potential of channel-selection algorithms for improving speech intelligibility under ideal conditions, that is, assuming *a priori* knowledge about the target and/or masker signals. The main conclusion that can be drawn from Section 13.4 is that *ideal* channel-selection algorithms can improve speech intelligibility *at any input SNR level* (even at SNR = −40 dB [37]) and for *any type of background interference* including reverberation and competing talker(s).

This raises the practical question: Are the *ideal* channel-selection algorithms feasible, that is, can they be realized in realistic scenarios where we only have access to the corrupted signal? The answer is yes, and this section presents a few realistic implementations of channel-selection algorithms that have been shown to improve speech intelligibility.

Before discussing such algorithms, it is important to note that there exists a huge body literature of algorithms that estimate the binary mask (i.e., channel-selection decisions), but these algorithms have been developed and tested primarily for ASR applications and have not been evaluated with formal intelligibility listening tests. Some of these algorithms make use of speech-specific features and classifiers [5], some use pitch continuity information [2], some use sound localization cues [6], and others use estimates of the posterior SNR [7], just to name a few. Thorough reviews of binary mask estimation algorithms for additive noise can be found in [16,26] and for reverberation in [51].

13.5.1 Simple, But Ineffective, Algorithms for Binary Mask Estimation

The SNR-based channel-selection algorithm (Section 13.3.1) requires an estimation of the instantaneous SNR for making binary decisions (i.e., for constructing the binary mask) as to whether to retain or discard a particular channel. A common method for estimating the SNR is the decision-directed approach (see Section 7.3.3.2). More precisely, the so-called *a priori* SNR (denoted as ξ) at frame m for frequency bin k is estimated as follows [52]:

$$\hat{\xi}_k(m) = a\frac{\left(G(k,m-1)Y_k(m-1)\right)^2}{\hat{D}_k^2(k,m-1)} + (1-a)\max[\gamma_k(m)-1,0] \qquad (13.30)$$

where

$\alpha = 0.98$
$G(k, m-1)$ is the gain function of frame $m-1$ at frequency bin k
$\hat{D}_k$ is the estimate of the noise magnitude spectrum
Y_k is the noisy-speech magnitude spectrum
$\gamma_k = Y_k^2/\hat{D}_k^2$ is the *posterior* SNR

It is clear from the aforementioned equation that the accuracy of the SNR estimate depends on the estimate of the gain function ($G(k, m)$) and the estimate of the noise spectrum ($\hat{D}_k$). For that reason, the study in [53] investigated the performance (in terms of accuracy of the estimated binary mask) of six different gain functions (e.g., MMSE and logMMSE) and three different methods for noise spectrum estimation.

Based on Equation 13.30, we can declare a TF unit as being target dominated if $\xi > 1$ (i.e., local SNR > 0 dB) and masker-dominated if $\xi \leq 1$. Aside from using the SNR value ξ from Equation 13.1 as a criterion, four other criteria were also considered in [53]. These criteria included among others the *posterior* SNR(γ), combined γ and ξ, and the conditional probability of speech-presence, $p(H_1|Y(\omega_k))$ (see Section 7.13), where $Y(\omega_k)$ denotes the complex noisy speech spectrum.

The accuracy of the estimated binary mask was assessed using two probability values: probability of correct detection (HIT) (i.e., hit rate) and probability of false alarm (FA). HIT measures the accuracy in classifying correctly target-dominated TF units, while the FA measures the probability that a masker-dominated TF unit was wrongly classified as target-dominated TF unit. Clearly, we would like the FA to be low (close to 0) and the HIT rate to be high (close to 1).

Overall, results in [53] indicated that the estimation of the binary mask was very poor with all six gain functions examined, all three noise-estimation algorithms, and all five criteria used. In most cases, HIT < 0.3, while FA was as high as 0.45. The low rate (0.3) of detecting TF units as being target dominated is clearly unsatisfactory and insufficient to improve speech intelligibility. One could alternatively increase the detection rate by lowering the thresholds used in the criteria, but that would have raised significantly the FA rate, thus resulting in no net benefit. The important conclusion that can be drawn from the study in [53] is that the estimation accuracy of the instantaneous SNR, via the decision-directed approach (Equation 13.30), using existing gain functions (e.g., MMSE) and noise-estimation algorithms, is quite poor and inadequate for binary mask estimation. The challenge in estimating accurately the instantaneous SNR via the decision-directed approach is that it requires accurate estimates of the background noise spectrum, a formidable task in highly nonstationary conditions.

Better, and more accurate, SNR estimation algorithms were proposed in [54–56]. In some of those studies, the SNR in each channel was estimated using neural network classifiers trained using a large corpus of speech and noise sources. The SNR estimate was subsequently used in a Wiener gain function in [55] and a log-MMSE gain function among others in [54], for speech enhancement applications. Objective results indicated significant improvements in speech quality. No intelligibility tests were conducted, however, with NH listeners; hence it remains unclear whether the use of improved SNR estimates (obtained from the neural network classifiers) would improve speech intelligibility.

13.5.2 Effective Channel-Selection Algorithms Based on Binary Classifiers

The data-driven methods proposed in [54–56] used classifiers to estimate the SNR in each frequency bin. The aim of those studies was to obtain accurate estimates of SNR in order to get in turn accurate estimates of the gain function for noise suppression. But, in the context of channel-selection algorithms discussed in Section 13.3, it is not necessary to get accurate estimates of the SNR. This is because all selection criteria discussed in Section 13.3 are binary in nature. Taking the SNR criterion as an example, and assuming a threshold T, what is most important is that the SNR estimate falls in the right region, that is, it falls in the $> T$ region when the true SNR $> T$ or in the $<T$ region when the true SNR $< T$. Suppose, for instance, that $T = 0$ dB and that the true SNR in a particular channel is 10 dB, the estimated SNR is 20 dB. Despite the large deviation (10 dB) between the true and estimated SNR values, a correct decision is made in retaining the channel, since 20 dB > 0 dB. Hence, what matters the most is that the estimated SNR falls in the correct region rather than whether it is estimated with high accuracy. This simplifies the noise-reduction problem a great deal as it reduces the challenging problem of estimating accurately the SNR to that of classifying the region it belongs to.

A number of studies proposed the use of classifiers for estimating the binary mask. The study in [57] used classifiers to estimate the binary mask in binaural listening conditions. Estimates of the ITD and ILD were fed as input to the classifier. High intelligibility benefits were observed with the proposed algorithm. The study in [58] used a two-class (binary) classifier to estimate the binary mask for missing-feature speech-recognition applications. Features were selected such that they were speech-specific (or speech-appropriate) and lacked any common characteristics with features extracted in background noise. Different features were used for voiced and unvoiced segments and included among others, the autocorrelation peak ratio, sub-band energy to full-band energy ratio, and the comb-filter ratio, which captured the harmonic nature of voiced speech. Binary mask estimation using the aforementioned Bayes' classifier trained with speech-specific features was found to be more accurate than other techniques and was shown in [58] to yield consistently higher speech recognition scores than other binary mask estimation algorithms.

Unlike the classifiers used in the aforementioned binary mask estimation studies, the study in [59] computed (during the training stage) the true band SNR values and divided them into two sets: one with SNR > T and one with SNR < T. Two Gaussian mixture models (GMMs) were subsequently trained, one for each set. Figure 13.16 shows the block diagram of the algorithm proposed in [59], consisting of a training stage (top panel) and an intelligibility enhancement stage (bottom panel). In the training stage, amplitude modulation spectrogram (AMS) features were extracted (as per [55]) from a large speech corpus and then used to train two GMMs representing two feature classes: target speech dominating the masker and masker dominating target speech. The two classes were determined by the computation of the true band SNRs, with SNR > 0 dB, for instance, representing the target speech dominating the masker. In the enhancement stage, a Bayesian classifier is used to classify the TF units of the noise-masked signal into two classes: target-dominated and masker-dominated. More precisely, TF units were classified as λ_0 (masker-dominated) or λ_1 (target-dominated) by comparing two *a posteriori* probabilities, $P(\lambda_0|\mathbf{A}_Y(t, k))$ and $P(\lambda_1|\mathbf{A}_Y(t, k))$, where $\mathbf{A}_Y(t, k)$ denotes the 45-dimensional AMS feature vector. This comparison produced an estimate of the binary mask, $B(t,k)$, as follows:

$$B(t,k) = \begin{cases} 0 & \text{if} \quad P(\lambda_0 \mid \mathbf{A}_Y(t,k)) > P(\lambda_1 \mid \mathbf{A}_Y(\tau,k)) \\ 1 & \text{otherwise} \end{cases} \tag{13.31}$$

Individual TF units of the noise-masked signal are retained if classified as target-dominated or eliminated if classified as masker-dominated and subsequently used to reconstruct the enhanced speech waveform.

The aforementioned algorithm was tested with NH listeners using IEEE sentences corrupted by three types of maskers (babble, factory noise, and speech-shaped noise)

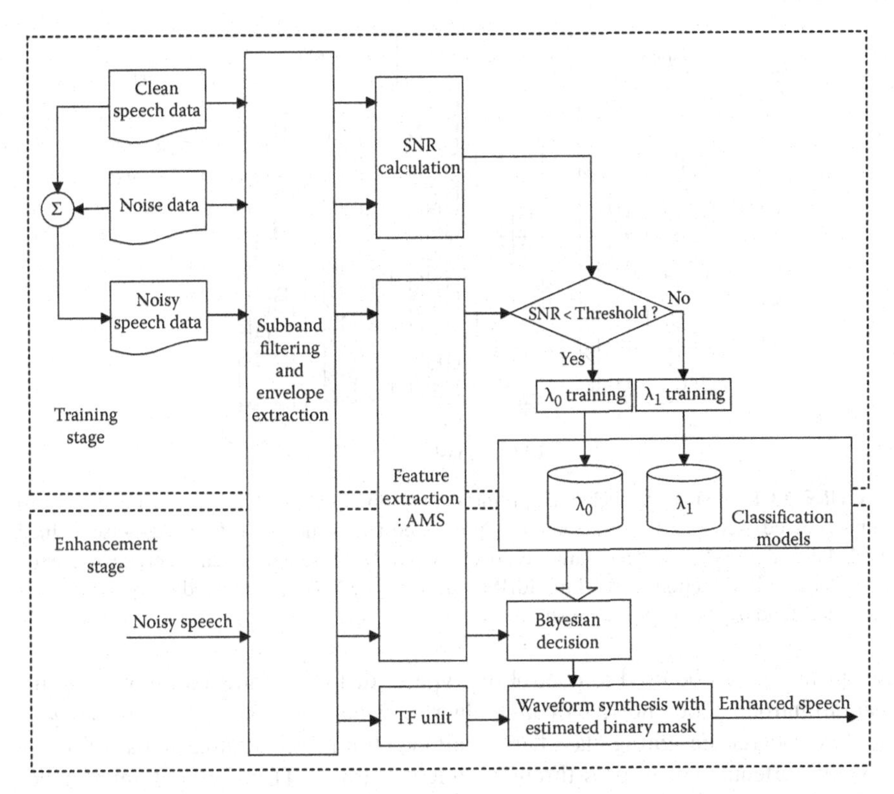

FIGURE 13.16 Block diagram of the training and enhancement stages of the noise-reduction algorithm that uses binary classifiers (GMMs) to determine whether a particular TF unit is masker or target dominated.

at two SNR levels (−5 and 0 dB). Two types of GMM models were trained as classifiers: (1) a single-noise GMM model, denoted as sGMM, trained only on a single type of noise and tested with the same type of noise and (2) a multinoise GMM model, denoted as mGMM, trained on all three types of noise and tested with one of the three types of noise. The latter model (mGMM) was used to assess the performance and robustness of a single GMM model in multiple-noise environments. It should be noted that a limited number (320) of IEEE sentences were used for GMM training. The remaining sentences were used for testing.

Figure 13.17 shows the mean intelligibility scores, computed in terms of percentage of words identified correctly by NH listeners. A substantial improvement in intelligibility was obtained [59] using both sGMM and mGMM models, compared to that attained by human listeners with unprocessed (corrupted) speech. The improvement (over 60% points in some cases) was more evident at −5 dB SNR levels for all three maskers tested.

The aforementioned algorithm (Figure 13.16) used the SNR criterion to train two GMM models, one for classifying target-dominated units (SNR > T) and one for classifying masker-dominated (SNR < T) units. Alternatively, other channel-selection criteria described in Section 13.3 could be used. The $\mathrm{SNR}_{\mathrm{ESI}}$ criterion,

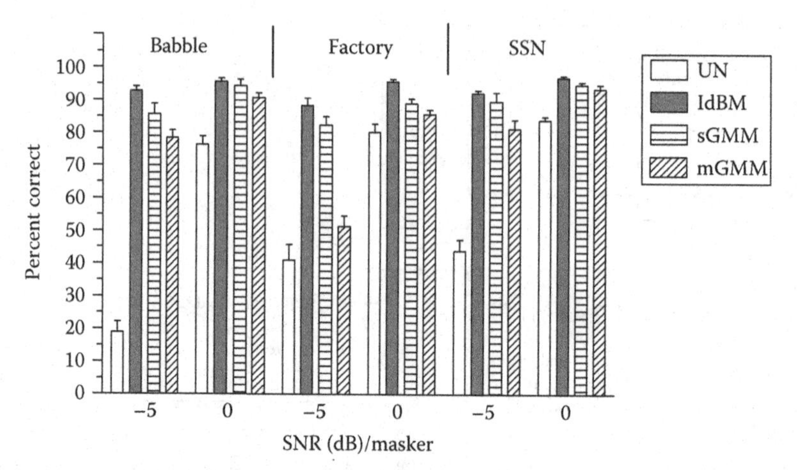

FIGURE 13.17 Mean speech recognition scores obtained by 17 listeners for corrupted (unprocessed) sentences (UN), sentences processed using the sGMM (single-noise trained GMMs), and mGMM models (multiple-noise trained) GMMs, and sentences processed using the ideal SNR selection algorithm (IdBM) in various SNR/masker conditions. Error bars indicate standard errors of the mean.

for instance, can be used to control the type of distortion (attenuation vs. amplification) introduced by noise-reduction algorithms (see Section 13.1.1). The study in [60] considered designing classifiers to allow TF units containing unharmful distortions (attenuation) to pass through while discarding TF units containing undesirable distortions (amplification). The overall algorithm had the same form and structure as shown in Figure 13.16. The main difference was that during training, the $|\hat{X}(k,t)|/|X(k,t)|$ ratio was used in the place of the SNR. When tested with NH listeners in three different masker conditions (babble, airport noise, and speech-shaped noise) and two SNR levels (−5 and 0 dB), the SNR_{ESI}-based algorithm [60] yielded large gains in intelligibility. Intelligibility scores improved from 30% correct obtained with unprocessed (noisy) speech at SNR = −5 dB (multitalker babble) to nearly 75% correct with the SNR_{ESI} algorithm. Further analysis in [60] compared the quality of speech produced by the algorithm based on the SNR criterion [59] to that based on the SNR_{ESI} criterion. PESQ scores indicated that the quality of speech synthesized using the SNR_{ESI} criterion was higher than that produced by the SNR criterion. This was attributed to the fact that better noise suppression was achieved with the SNR_{ESI} approach since the Wiener gain function was applied to the noisy signal first before applying binary masking. That is, the retained channels were already noise-suppressed by the Wiener gain function. In contrast, the SNR approach retains the *corrupted* (and unprocessed) channels with SNR > T.

Highest performance was obtained in [59,60], when the GMM classifier was trained and tested in the same noise environment. Optimizing noise reduction for a particular noise environment [61,62] can find use in many applications including cell phones and hearing aids. Modern hearing aids, for instance, use sound classification algorithms (e.g., [63]) to identify different listening situations and adjust accordingly hearing aid processing parameters. Sound classification algorithms can be implemented in real time in mobile devices (e.g., [64]). Since mobile devices are powered by a digital signal processor chip, the training can take place at the command of the user whenever in a new listening environment. Following the training stage, the user can initiate the noise-specific algorithm to enhance speech intelligibility in extremely noisy environments, for example, restaurants. As shown in Figure 13.17a, single GMM trained on multiple types of noise (mGMM) can also yield high performance; however, a user might encounter a new type of noise not included in the training set. In such circumstances, either new training needs to be initiated or perhaps adaptation techniques can be used to adapt the parameters of existing GMM models to the new data (e.g., [65]). Such adaptation techniques are described briefly next in the context of noise reduction.

13.5.3 Adapting to New Noise Environments

As mentioned earlier, the GMM classifiers used in [59,60] performed the best in the noise environments they were trained. In realistic scenarios, however, the noise characteristics or the type of noise itself might be changing and that will likely degrade the performance of the classifier. Hence, training techniques are needed that will adapt fast to new incoming noise data without the need to retrain the classifier using all the data accumulated. Fortunately, there exist a large number of such techniques that have been used in ASR for speaker adaptation applications (e.g., [65]). GMM classifiers offer the additional advantage that only the model parameters (e.g., means, mixture weights, covariance matrix) need to be updated for fast adaptation to new acoustic environments.

An incremental training approach [66] taken from ASR was adopted in [67] as a means of coping with changing noise environments and/or characteristics. This approach starts from an initial model trained with a small amount of data and updates the model parameters as more data become available. Unlike conventional classifiers (e.g., neural networks) that use a batch-training approach that requires access to the whole data set, the incremental training approach continuously adapts the model parameters as new data arrive. Consequently, the computational load of the incremental approach is smaller than the load of the batch-training approach.

In [67], access to a small amount of speech data recorded in quiet was assumed for the training of the initial model. Such data can be stored in memory. In a new listening environment, noise-only data are collected and mixed with a small number of sentences (10–20 were used in [67]) of clean speech (stored in memory) at various SNR levels. The new GMM model parameters (e.g., means, variances) can be adapted using the new noise-only data and the parameters of the initial model. As more noise-only data are collected, the GMM model is adapted based on new information and parameters of the last GMM model.

The effectiveness of the aforementioned incremental training approach was evaluated in [67] with NH listeners in babble, factory noise, and train noise. GMMs trained with only 20, 40, 80, 140, and 200 sentences were used to classify target-dominated and masker-dominated TF units. Synthesized speech was presented to NH listeners for identification. Figure 13.18 shows the intelligibility scores for the −5 dB SNR babble condition as a function of the amount of training data used (i.e., accumulated

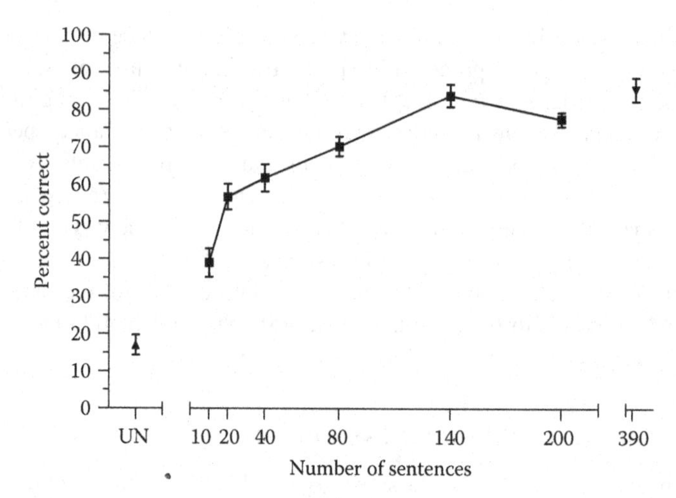

FIGURE 13.18 Mean intelligibility scores obtained by normal-hearing listeners for corrupted (unprocessed) sentences (denoted as Unproc) and sentences synthesized using incrementally updated models as a function of the number of accumulated sentences used in training. The masker was multitalker babble (SNR = −5 dB). The intelligibility scores obtained with batch-trained models based on 390 sentences are also shown for comparison [19]. Error bars indicate standard errors of the mean.

number of sentences used in each model). As expected, word identification accuracy improved as more training data were included. Performance improved substantially from 15% correct obtained with unprocessed sentences to 55% correct with 20-sentence models and to 80% correct with 140-sentence models. Large improvement in intelligibility was also noted with factory noise, when 80 or more sentences were used to train the GMMs. For comparison, Figure 13.18 also shows performance obtained with 390-sentence models [59], trained in batch mode. The difference in performance between the 140-sentence models (or 200-sentence models) and the 390-sentence models is smaller than 10% points.

The outcomes from the aforementioned incremental training approach used in [67] showed a great deal of promise for the deployment of binary SNR classifiers in a number of realistic background environments and applications involving mobile devices and hearing devices (hearing aids and cochlear implants). The adaptation of the GMM classifier parameters is absolutely necessary, since in the majority of real-world listening situations, noise is not stationary.

13.6 EVALUATING BINARY MASK ESTIMATION ALGORITHMS

A two-class GMM classifier was used in the last section to estimate the binary mask at each TF unit. Clearly, other types of classifiers (e.g., SVMs [68]) can be used to estimate the binary mask. But, how can we compare the performance of different classifiers or different mask estimation algorithms without necessarily synthesizing the signal and conducting listening tests? Taking the ideal binary mask as the ground truth, the problem amounts to comparing two $M \times N$ matrices (estimated and ideal) consisting of 0 and 1 s, where M denotes the number of channels and N the number of frames. Such a comparison will produce two types of errors: miss error (ME) and FA. A ME occurs when a 1 (target ON) is misclassified as a 0 (target OFF). The hit rate (HIT) is computed as HIT = 1 – ME and represents the number of times the target (1) was correctly detected. An FA occurs when a 0 (target OFF) is misclassified as a 1 (target ON). That is, TF units that should have been discarded were retained.

Which of the two binary mask errors affects intelligibility the most? The listening study in [19] demonstrated that FA errors produced larger decrements in intelligibility relative to the ME errors, suggesting that when designing two-class classifiers, the FA errors need to be kept to a minimum. This is not to say, however, that the ME errors can be ignored. Both HIT (=1 – ME) and FA need to be taken into account when evaluating binary mask estimation algorithms. A simple difference metric, d, was proposed in [59] for evaluating the performance of binary mask estimation algorithms by taking both errors into account:

$$d = \text{HIT} - \text{FA} \tag{13.32}$$

A large value of d would suggest high performance, while a small value of d would suggest poor performance. Highest performance is obtained with d = 1 (HIT = 1, FA = 0).

It is important to note that the metric d is a simplified form of the sensitivity (or discriminability) index, d', used in psychoacoustics [69,70]. The d' index is often used in psychoacoustics to assess performance (discriminability) in "yes/no" single-interval tasks, two-alternative two-interval forced choice tasks, etc. In a "yes/no" single-interval task, for instance, the listener is presented with a stimulus that may contain a signal (target present) or that may contain noise alone (masker present). For "yes/no" tasks, the d' is defined as [69]

$$d' = \Phi^{-1}(\text{HIT}) - \Phi^{-1}(\text{FA}) \tag{13.33}$$

where Φ^{-1} denotes the inverse cumulative Gaussian function. High values of d' suggest high performance with d' = 1 corresponding to 76% correct and d' = 0%–50% correct (i.e., chance).

To better understand the relationship between the two indices, d and d', we plotted the isosensitivity curves of d' and d, as a function of HIT and FA (see Figure 13.19). The isosensitivity curves of d' were computed by solving Equation 13.33 for HIT. All points in these curves have the same sensitivity d'. The superimposed isodifference curves of d are shown for two fixed values (all points in these curves have the same HIT-FA value). It is clear from Figure 13.19 that for the most part, a value of d = 66% corresponds to d' = 2 or better, a d' value that is considered to be an excellent discriminability score (~90% correct). From this, we can infer that binary mask estimation algorithms capable of yielding d > 68% ought to perform very well and are likely to improve speech intelligibility. Indeed, this was confirmed by listening studies [59,67]. The Bayesian classifiers used by Kim et al. [59], for instance, produced values of d > 68% in nearly all conditions and for all four types of maskers.

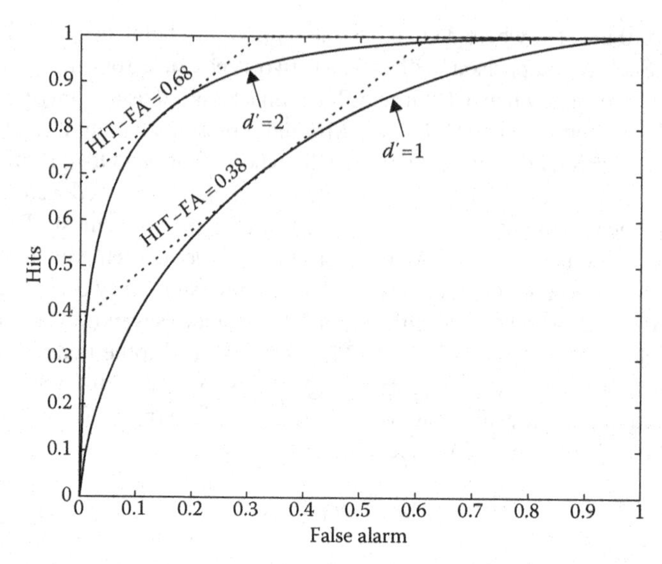

FIGURE 13.19 Isosensitivity plots for $d' = 1$ and $d' = 2$, superimposed to isodifference curves of HIT-FA.

Substantial improvements in intelligibility were obtained by NH listeners [59] when the Bayesian classifiers were used to select target-dominated TF units and discard masker-dominated TF units. Correlation analysis was run in [59,67] between values of d and intelligibility scores. High correlation coefficients ($r = 0.8$–0.97) were obtained with the difference metric d, suggesting that this metric can be used to predict reliably speech intelligibility by binary mask estimation algorithms.

A number of other metrics have been proposed to assess the performance of binary mask algorithms [71,72]. Hu and Wang [71] promoted the use of a modified time-domain SNR measure where the target synthesized from the ideal binary mask was used as the ground truth, that is,

$$\mathrm{SINR} = 10\log 10 \frac{\sum_n x_{IBM}^2(n)}{\sum_n [\hat{x}(n) - x_{IBM}(n)]^2} \tag{13.34}$$

where

SINR denotes the signal-to-ideal-noise ratio
$x_{IBM}(n)$ denotes the time-domain signal synthesized using the ideal binary mask
$\hat{x}(n)$ denotes the estimated target signal

SNR measures similar to Equation 13.34 were also proposed for reverberant conditions, with the main difference being that the reverberated target was used as the ground truth. Experiments conducted in [72] demonstrated that metrics based on SNR (e.g., Equation 13.34) were unable to provide a consistent score for a given binary mask when convolutional distortions were introduced. A metric that did not rely on the resynthesized output was proposed in [72] and found to provide more consistent scores than the SNR-based metrics in most acoustic conditions. This measure, called ideal binary mask ratio (IBMR), was computed as

$$\text{IBMR} = \frac{\text{HIT}}{\text{FA}+1} \tag{13.35}$$

While the IBMR and SNR-based metrics were tested in a number of anechoic and reverberant conditions in [72], no listening tests were conducted to assess if these metrics correlate highly with intelligibility. Without such correlation analysis, the IBMR and SNR-based metrics need to be used with caution.

13.7 CHANNEL SELECTION AND AUDITORY SCENE ANALYSIS

There are a number of competing theories describing how listeners analyze a complex auditory scene to segregate the target speaker amid the presence of multiple noise sources (e.g., [49,73]). How does channel selection fit into those theories? What is the underlying process of (auditory) channel selection and is it physiologically plausible?

Auditory channel-selection models have been pursued for some time in the speech perception literature (see review in [74]), although not in the same manner described in this chapter. A number of models of concurrent vowel identification were based on channel selection (e.g., [75,76]). In those models, only channels dominated by the periodicity of the stronger voice [75,76] were selected. In models of auditory streaming of alternating-tone sequences, the "gain" on each channel determined the strength of the perceptual foreground and background [77,78]. The earlier auditory models were limited to additive noise, concurrent vowel identification, and streaming of AB alternating-tone sequences and did not tackle the more complex problem of speech recognition in noise.

A more general auditory channel-selection model is presented next. Figure 13.20 shows the different stages of the conceptual model. The first stage models the auditory periphery, which decomposes the mixture to an array of individual TF units, with each unit representing the acoustic signal occurring at a particular instance in time and frequency, and with the size (e.g., bandwidth and duration) of each unit representing the smallest auditory event that can be resolved. The first stage thus produces a spectrotemporal representation of the signal. The second stage involves figure/ground analysis, also known as foreground/background analysis. The aim is to determine from the mixtures' spectrotemporal pattern what is foreground (e.g., most likely belonging to the target) and what is background (e.g., not belonging to the target). We define foreground here as the relatively undistorted or unmasked segments (e.g., glimpses of the target) of the mixture. Similarly, we define background as the distorted, noise-masked, or perceptually unreliable segments of the mixture bearing no "resemblance" (i.e., sharing no common attributes) to the target. The figure/ground analysis produces two streams, one belonging to the foreground and one to the background.

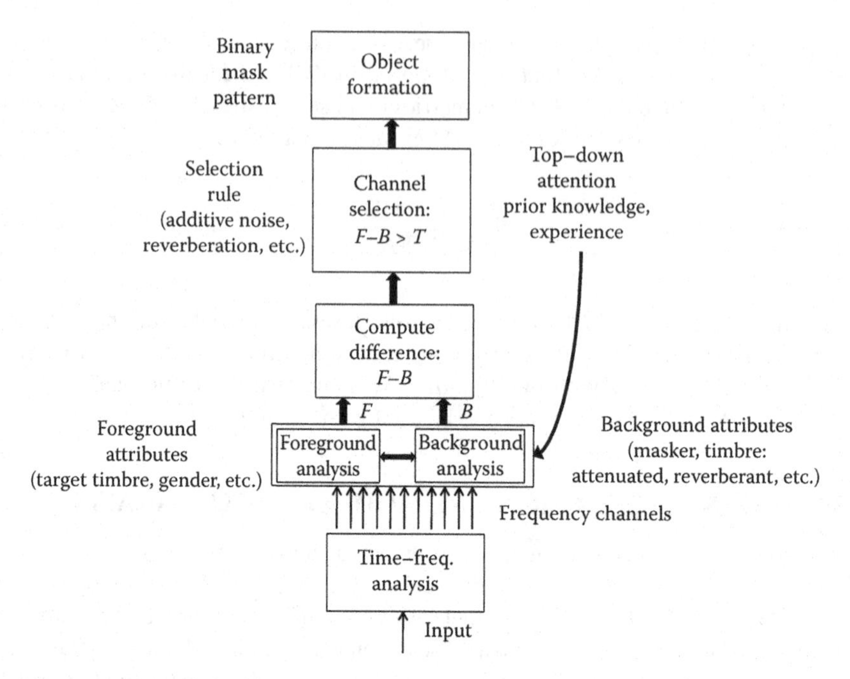

FIGURE 13.20 Conceptual model of auditory channel selection.

But, what cues can listeners use to distinguish the foreground from the background? Among others, learned patterns, prior experience, and *a priori* knowledge of attributes of speech and background noise can provide the major clues. For instance, making use of prior experience, listeners can easily discriminate between speech that is naturally produced and speech that has been processed by say a noise-reduction algorithm or compression algorithms, such as those used in cell phones. Listeners can easily discriminate between muffled (low-pass-filtered) speech and natural speech. Listeners can easily discriminate between natural speech and speech-containing reverberation or echoes. That is, schema-based processes play a major role in the formation of the foreground and background streams. Forming the foreground and background streams, however, is not sufficient. Based on information gathered from each TF unit from the two streams, it is left to be determined whether to retain or discard a particular TF unit.

A criterion or selection rule is thus needed that will select the TF units from the mixture's spectrotemporal pattern that likely belongs to the target (foreground) and turn off (discard) the TF units that likely belong to the masker(s) (background). A number of selection rules were presented in Section 13.3. As described in Section 13.3, the criteria are not based on complex equations or complex algorithms. These criteria are simple and are based, in the linear domain, on the ratio of two numbers or in the log domain on the *relative difference of two numbers* or two attributes of the signal. In our case, the two quantities correspond to some (measurable) attributes of the foreground and background streams. In the third stage of the model, the difference is computed between an attribute of the foreground and an attribute of the background. The foreground and background attributes can be measured or quantified in terms of their strength or power. In additive noise conditions, for instance, this difference would correspond to a crude estimate of the SNR in dB. This is so because the SNR is by definition the difference in dB of the foreground (target) power and the background (masker) power. Similarly, in reverberant conditions, the difference between the foreground power and the power of the reverberant signal would provide a crude estimate of the SRR (see Equation 13.22). In conditions where the speech signal is subjected to nonlinear processing or noise suppression, the difference between the foreground power and the power of the processed signal (background) would provide a crude estimate of the SNR_{ESI} (Equation 13.17).

Finally, in the fourth stage of the model, a decision needs to be made based on the difference between the strengths (powers) of the foreground and the background. If the difference in strengths (powers) between the foreground and background at a particular TF unit is beyond a certain threshold (e.g., 0 dB), then the corresponding output of the auditory channel of that TF unit is allowed to pass through the higher stages of the auditory pathway; otherwise, it is turned off. In the simplest case, a threshold of 0 dB would suggest a dominant selection mechanism that always selects the stronger of the two (foreground vs. background). The binary decisions (1 to retain and 0 to discard) made along the way for all TF units constitute the most important output of the model, since the decisions themselves (collectively) carry information about the target. More precisely, the decisions provide information about "where" (in frequency) and "when" (in time) is the target present in the mixture's spectrotemporal pattern (i.e., the TF plane). Neurophysiologically, these binary decisions would create a spectrotemporal pattern of on/off neural activity along the auditory pathway. Plotted on a TF plane, this is no other than the binary mask pattern (see example in Figure 13.5c). It is clear from Figure 13.5 that the binary mask pattern resembles the target spectrogram. But, in the context of auditory scene analysis, what does the binary mask pattern represent? The *binary mask pattern represents the target auditory object*. The binary mask pattern can be modulated by the mixture itself or by noise to produce intelligible speech. In fact, it can be modulated by music, street noise, car noise, etc., and still produces intelligible speech.

There is at least one fundamental difference between the aforesaid model (Figure 13.20) and other channel-selection models [76–78]. The aforesaid model does not rely on the use of primitive cues (e.g., common onsets and offsets, amplitude and frequency modulations, and common periodicity) but rather on schema-based cues. One might argue that the primitive cues are potentially used in the foreground/background analysis, but those must be weak compared to the top-down and schema-driven cues. Evidence in support of the fact that primitive cues are not necessary for the aforementioned channel-selection model to work was provided in [59] where an SNR-based channel-selection algorithm was implemented using GMM classifiers. The AMS features used in the classifier captured primarily low-frequency envelope modulations and did not explicitly track common onsets or offsets of speech or across frequency modulations. In fact, binary decisions were made independently for each channel. Finally, unlike previous channel-selection models, the model shown in Figure 13.20 is applicable to all types of background interferer(s) including additive broadband noise (e.g., multitalker babble), competing talker(s), and reverberation.

13.8 SUMMARY

A new family of algorithms was described in this chapter. Unlike those presented in Chapters 5 through 8, these algorithms make use of binary gain functions. It was argued that conventional soft gain functions are unlikely (if not impossible) to improve speech intelligibility as they do not improve the overall (across all bands) SNR. According to AI theory (Section 11.4.1), no improvement in intelligibility is to be expected if the overall SNR is not improved. The underlying process of applying binary gain functions was referred to as channel selection, since, in effect, the algorithms retain channels (bands/frequency bins) that satisfy a certain criterion (e.g., SNR > 0 dB) and discard channels not satisfying the criterion. The SNR criterion, in particular, has been used extensively in CASA and ASR applications, but it was not until recently that has been applied to noise reduction. The SNR criterion has been proven to maximize the AI and consequently speech intelligibility. A number of other channel-selection criteria were described, some of which were appropriate for reverberant environments. Data from oracle (i.e., assuming *a priori* knowledge of the target and/or masker signals) intelligibility listening studies were presented showing that ideal channel-selection-based algorithms can improve (and, in some cases, restore) speech intelligibility at *any SNR level* (even at SNR = −40 dB or lower) and for *any form of background interference, including reverberation*. Realistic implementations of channel-selection algorithms, based on binary classifiers, were presented. These algorithms have been found to yield substantial improvements in intelligibility, even at negative SNR levels (−5 dB). A channel-selection model for auditory scene analysis was also presented in this chapter. Overall, channel-selection algorithms convert the complex target segregation problem to a binary classification problem, a much easier task. As such, they are more likely to be deployed in real-world applications, such as mobile devices and hearing devices (e.g., hearing aids) to improve speech intelligibility in noise.

REFERENCES

1. Levitt, H. (1997), Digital hearing aids: Past, present and future, in Tobin, H. (Ed.), *Practical Hearing Aid Selection and Fitting*, Washington, DC: Department of Veteran Affairs, pp. xi–xxiii.
2. Bentler, R., Wu, Y., Kettel, J., and Hurtig, R. (2008), Digital noise reduction: Outcomes from laboratory and field studies, *Int. J. Audiol.*, 47, 447–460.
3. Luts, H., Eneman, K., Wouters, J., Schulte, M. et al. (2010), Multicenter evaluation of signal enhancement algorithms for hearing aids, *J. Acoust. Soc. Am.*, 123, 1491–1505.
4. Weiss, M. and Neuman, A. (1993), Noise reduction in hearing aids, in Studebaker, G. (Ed.), *Acoustical Factors Affecting Hearing Aid Performance*, Needham Heights, MA: Allyn and Bacon, pp. 337–352.
5. Dubbelboer, F. and Houtgast, T. (2007), A detailed study on the effects of noise on speech intelligibility, *J. Acoust. Soc. Am.*, 122, 2865–2871.
6. Hu, Y. and Loizou, P. (2007), A comparative intelligibility study of single-microphone noise reduction algorithms, *J. Acoust. Soc. Am.*, 122(3), 1777–1786.
7. Ephraim, Y. and Van Trees, H.L. (1995), A signal subspace approach for speech enhancement, *IEEE Trans. Speech Audio Process.*, 3(4), 251–266.

8. Chen, J., Benesty, J., Huang, Y., and Doclo, S. (2006), New insights into the noise reduction Wiener filter, *IEEE Trans. Audio Speech Lang. Process.*, 14, 1218–1234.
9. Hu, Y. and Loizou, P. (2004), Incorporating a psychoacoustical model in frequency domain speech enhancement, *IEEE Signal Process. Lett.*, 11(2), 270–273.
10. Noordhoek, I. and Drullman, R. (1997), Effect of reducing temporal intensity modulations on sentence intelligibility. *J. Acoust. Soc. Am.*, 101, 498–502.
11. Kim, G. and Loizou, P. (2011), Gain-induced speech distortions and the absence of intelligibility benefit with existing noise-reduction algorithms, *J. Acoust. Soc. Am.*, 130(3), 1581–1596.
12. Ma, J., Hu, Y., and Loizou, P. (2009), Objective measures for predicting speech intelligibility in noisy conditions based on new band-importance functions, *J. Acoust. Soc. Am.*, 125(5), 3387–3405.
13. Loizou, P. and Kim, G. (2011), Reasons why current speech-enhancement algorithms do not improve speech intelligibility and suggested solutions, *IEEE Trans. Audio Speech Lang. Process.*, 19(1), 47–56.
14. Jensen, J. and Hendriks, R. (2012), Spectral magnitude minimum mean-square error estimation using binary and continuous gain functions, *IEEE Trans. Audio Speech Lang. Process.*, 20(1), 92–102.
15. Boldt, J. (2011), Binary masking and speech intelligibility, PhD dissertation, Department of Electronic Systems, Aalborg University, Esbjerg, Denmark.
16. Wang, D. and Brown, G. (2006), *Computational Auditory Scene Analysis: Principles, Algorithms, and Applications*, New York: Wiley/IEEE Press.
17. Cooke, M., Green, P., Josifovski, L., and Vizinho, A. (2001), Robust automatic speech recognition with missing and uncertain acoustic data, *Speech Commun.*, 34, 267–285.
18. Brungart, D., Chang, P., Simpson, B., and Wang, D. (2006), Isolating the energetic component of speech-on-speech masking with ideal time-frequency segregation. *J. Acoust. Soc. Am.*, 120, 4007–4018.
19. Li, N. and Loizou, P. (2008), Factors influencing intelligibility of ideal binary-masked speech: Implications for noise reduction, *J. Acoust. Soc. Am.*, 123, 1673–1682.
20. Li, N. and Loizou, P. (2008), Effect of spectral resolution on the intelligibility of ideal binary masked speech, *J. Acoust. Soc. Am.*, 123(4), EL59–EL64.
21. Wang, D., Kjems, U., Pedersen, M., Boldt, J., and Lunner, T. (2008), Speech perception of noise with binary gains, *J. Acoust. Soc. Am.*, 124, 2303–2307.
22. Wojcicki, K. and Loizou, P. (2012), Channel selection in the modulation domain for improved speech intelligibility in noise, *J. Acoust. Soc. Am.*, 131(4), 2904–2913.
23. Paliwal, K., Wojcicki, K., and Schwerin, B. (2010), Single-channel speech enhancement using spectral subtraction in the short-time modulation domain, *Speech Commun.*, 52, 450–475.
24. Wang, D. (2005), On ideal binary mask as the computational goal of auditory scene analysis, in Divenyi, P. (Ed.), *Speech Separation by Humans and Machines*, Dordrecht, the Netherlands: Kluwer Academic, pp. 181–187.
25. Brown, G. and Cooke, M. (1994), Computational auditory scene analysis, *Comp. Speech Lang.*, 8, 297–336.
26. Wang, D. (2008), Time-frequency masking for speech separation and its potential for hearing aid design, *Trends Amplif.*, 12, 332–353.
27. Li, Y. and Wang, D. (2009), On the optimality of ideal binary time-frequency masks, *Speech Commun.*, 51, 230–239.
28. Lu, Y. and Loizou, P. (2011), Estimators of the magnitude-squared spectrum and methods for incorporating SNR uncertainty, *IEEE Trans. Audio Speech Lang. Process.*, 19, 1123–1137.
29. Anzalone, M., Calandruccio, L., Doherty, K., and Carney, L. (2006), Determination of the potential benefit of time-frequency gain manipulation, *Ear Hear.*, 27, 480–492.

30. Kim, G. and Loizou, P. (2010), A new binary mask based on noise constraints for improved speech intelligibility, *Proc. Interspeech*, 1632–1635.
31. Chen, F. and Loizou, P. (2012), Impact of SNR and gain-function over- and under-estimation on speech intelligibility, *Speech Commun.*, 54, 272–281.
32. Mandel, M., Bressler, S., Shinn-Cunningham, B., and Ellis, D. (2010), Evaluating source separation algorithms with reverberant speech, *IEEE Trans. Audio Speech Lang. Process.*, 18, 1872–1883.
33. Kokkinakis, K., Hazrati, O., and Loizou, P. (2011), A channel-selection criterion for suppressing reverberation in cochlear implants, *J. Acoust. Soc. Am.*, 129(5), 3221–3232.
34. Roman, N. and Woodruff, J. (2011), Intelligibility of reverberant noisy speech with ideal binary masking, *J. Acoust. Soc. Am.*, 130, 2153–2161.
35. Hazrati, O. and Loizou, P. (2012), Tackling the combined effects of reverberation and masking noise using ideal channel selection, *J. Speech Lang. Hear. Res.*, 55, 500–510.
36. Li, N. and Loizou, P. (2007), Factors influencing glimpsing of speech in noise. *J. Acoust. Soc. Am.*, 122(2), 1165–1172.
37. Kjems, U., Boldt, J., and Pedersen, M. (2012), Role of mask pattern in intelligibility of ideal binary-masked noisy speech, *J. Acoust. Soc. Am.*, 126, 1415–1426.
38. Shannon, R., Zeng, F.-G., Kamath, V., Wygonski, J., and Ekelid, M. (1995), Speech recognition with primarily temporal cues, *Science*, 270, 303–304.
39. Wang, D., Kjems, U., Pedersen, M., Boldt, J., and Lunner, T. (2009), Speech intelligibility in background noise with ideal binary time-frequency masking, *J. Acoust. Soc. Am.*, 125, 2336–2347.
40. Hu, Y. and Loizou, P. (2008), A new sound coding strategy for suppressing noise in cochlear implants, *J. Acoust. Soc. Am.*, 124, 498–509.
41. Brokx, J. and Nooteboom, S. (1982), Intonation and perception of simultaneous voices, *J. Phonet.*, 10, 23–26.
42. Scheffers, M. (1983), Sifting vowels: Auditory pitch analysis and sound segregation, PhD thesis, Rijksuniversiteit te Groningen, Groningen, the Netherlands.
43. Culling, J. and Darwin, C. (1993), Perceptual separation of simultaneous vowels: Within and across-formant grouping by F0, *J. Acoust. Soc. Am.*, 93, 3454–3467.
44. Parsons, T.W. (1976), Separation of speech from interfering speaker by mean of harmonic selection, *J. Acoust. Soc. Am.*, 60(4), 918.
45. Stubbs, R. and Summerfield, Q. (1988), Evaluation of two voice-separation algorithms using normal-hearing and hearing-impaired listeners, *J. Acoust. Soc. Am.*, 84(4), 1238–1249.
46. Hu, G. and Wang, D. (2008), Segregation of unvoiced speech from nonspeech interference, *J. Acoust. Soc. Am.*, 124(2), 1306–1319.
47. Ellis, D. (2006), Model-based scene analysis, in Wang, D. and Brown, G. (Ed.), *Computational Auditory Scene Analysis*, Hoboken, NJ: IEEE Press/John Wiley & Sons, pp. 115–146.
48. Yilmaz, O. and Rickard, S. (2004), Blind separation of speech mixtures via time-frequency masking, *IEEE Trans. Signal Process.*, 52, 1830–1847.
49. Bregman, A. (1990), *Auditory Scene Analysis*, Cambridge, MA: MIT Press.
50. Nadas, M., Nahamoo, D., and Picheny, M. (1989), Speech recognition using noise-adaptive prototypes, *IEEE Trans. Speech Audio Process.*, 37, 1495–1503.
51. Brown, G. and Palomaki, K. (2006), Reverberation, in Wang, D. and Brown, G. (Ed.), *Computational Auditory Scene Analysis*, Hoboken, NJ: IEEE Press/John Wiley & Sons, pp. 209–250.
52. Ephraim, Y. and Malah, D. (1984), Speech enhancement using a minimum mean-square error short-time spectral amplitude estimator, *IEEE Trans. Acoust. Speech Signal Process.*, ASSP-32(6), 1109–1121.

53. Hu, Y. and Loizou, P. (2008), Techniques for estimating the ideal binary mask, *Proceedings of the 11th International Workshop on Acoustic Echo and Noise Control*, Seattle, WA.
54. Suhadi, S., Last, C., and Fingscheidt, T. (2011), A data-driven approach to *a priori* SNR estimation, *IEEE Trans. Audio Speech Lang. Process.*, 19, 186–195.
55. Tchorz, J. and Kollmeier, B. (2003), SNR estimation based on amplitude modulation analysis with applications to noise suppression, *IEEE Trans. Speech Audio Process.*, 11, 184–192.
56. Kim, G. and Loizou, P. (2009), A data-driven approach for estimating the time-frequency binary mask, *Proc. Interspeech*, 844–847.
57. Roman, N., Wang, D., and Brown, G. (2003), Speech segregation based on sound localization, *J. Acoust. Soc. Am.*, 114, 2236–2252.
58. Seltzer, M., Raj, B., and Stern, R. (2004), A Bayesian classifier for spectrographic mask estimation for missing feature speech recognition, *Speech Commun.*, 43, 379–393.
59. Kim, G., Lu, Y., Hu, Y., and Loizou, P. (2009), An algorithm that improves speech intelligibility in noise for normal-hearing listeners, *J. Acoust. Soc. Am.*, 126(3), 1486–1494.
60. Kim, G. and Loizou, P. (2010), Improving speech intelligibility in noise using a binary mask that is based on magnitude spectrum constraints, *IEEE Signal Process. Lett.*, 17(2), 1010–1013.
61. Erkelens, J., Jensen, J., and Heusdens, R. (2007), A data-driven approach to optimizing spectral speech enhancement methods for various error criteria, *Speech Commun.*, 49, 530–541.
62. Fingscheidt, T., Suhadi, S., and Stan, S. (2008), Environment-optimized speech enhancement, *IEEE Trans. Audio Speech Lang. Process.*, 16, 825–834.
63. Nordqvist, P. and Leijon, A. (2004), An efficient robust sound classification algorithm for hearing aids, *J. Acoust. Soc. Am.*, 115, 3033–3041.
64. Gopalakrishna, V., Kehtarnavaz, N., Mirzahasanloo, T., and Loizou, P. (2012), Real-time automatic tuning of noise suppression algorithms for cochlear implant applications, *IEEE Trans. Biomed. Eng.*, 59(6), 1691–1700.
65. Reynolds, D., Quatieri, T., and Dunn, R. (2000). Speaker verification using adapted Gaussian mixture models, *Digital Signal Process.*, 10, 19–41.
66. Huo, Q. and Lee, C.-H. (1997). On-line adaptive learning of the continuous density hidden Markov model based on approximate recursive Bayes estimate. *IEEE Trans. Speech Audio Process.*, 5, 161–172.
67. Kim, G. and Loizou, P. (2010). Improving speech intelligibility in noise using environment-optimized algorithms, *IEEE Trans. Audio Speech Lang. Process.*, 18(8), 2080–2090.
68. Han, K. and Wang, D. (2011), An SVM based classification approach to speech separation, *Proceedings of the IEEE International Conference on Acoustics, Speech, and Signal Processing*, Prague, Czech Republic, pp. 5212–5215.
69. Macmillan, N. and Creelman, C. (2005), *Detection Theory*, New York: Lawrence Erlbaum Associates.
70. Green, D. and Swets, J. (1988), *Signal Detection Theory and Psychophysics*, Los Altos Hills, CA: Peninsula Publishing.
71. Hu, G. and Wang, D. (2004), Monaural speech segregation based on pitch tracking and amplitude modulation, *IEEE Trans. Neural Netw.*, 15, 1135–1150.
72. Hummersone, C., Nasin, R., and Brookes, T. (2011), Ideal binary mask ratio: A novel metric for assessing binary-mask-based sound source separation algorithms, *IEEE Trans. Audio Speech Lang. Process.*, 19, 2039–2045.
73. Shinn-Cunningham, B. and Best, V. (2008), Selective attention in normal and impaired hearing, *Trends Amplif.*, 12(4), 283–299.

74. Brown, G. (2010), Physiological models of auditory scene analysis, in Meddis, R., Lopez-Poveda, E., Popper, A., and Fay, R. (Eds.), *Computational Models of the Auditory System*, New York: Springer Verlag, pp. 203–236.
75. Weintraub, M. (1985), A theory and computational model of auditory monaural sound separation, PhD dissertation, Stanford University, Stanford, CA.
76. Meddis, R. and Hewitt, M. (1992), Modeling the identification of vowels with different fundamental frequencies, *J. Acoust. Soc. Am.*, 91, 233–245.
77. Beauvois, M. and Meddis, R. (1996), Computer simulation of auditory stream segregation in alternating-tone sequences, *J. Acoust. Soc. Am.*, 99(4), 2270–2280.
78. McCabe, S. and Denham, M. (1997), A model of auditory streaming, *J. Acoust. Soc. Am.*, 101(3), 1611–1621.

Appendix A: Special Functions and Integrals

In this appendix, we provide the special functions and integral relationships used in Chapter 7. These functions were taken from [1,2].

A.1 BESSEL FUNCTIONS

The Bessel functions are solutions to the following differential equation of order ν [3, ch. 10]:

$$x^2 y'' + x\,y' + (x^2 - \nu^2)y = 0 \tag{A.1}$$

The preceding differential equation has many solutions, most of which can be expressed in terms of the Bessel function of the first kind. Different symbols are used to discriminate between the different types of Bessel functions. The Bessel function of the first kind of order ν is denoted by the symbol $J_\nu(x)$ and is given by

$$J_\nu(x) = \sum_{m=0}^{\infty} \frac{(-1)^m x^{\nu+2m}}{2^{\nu+2m} m!\Gamma(\nu+m+1)} \tag{A.2}$$

where Γ(.) denotes the gamma function. Graphs of $J_0(x)$ and $J_1(x)$ are shown in Figure A.1a. It is interesting to note that these two functions resemble the cos(x) and sin(x) functions.

The *modified* Bessel function of the first kind of order ν is denoted by the symbol $I_\nu(x)$ and is obtained (within a constant) by evaluating $J_\nu(x)$ at jx, where j denotes the complex number. Note that

$$J_\nu(jx) = j^\nu \sum_{m=0}^{\infty} \frac{x^{\nu+2m}}{2^{\nu+2m} m!\Gamma(\nu+m+1)} \tag{A.3}$$

and after multiplying both sides by $(j)^{-\nu}$ we get $I_\nu(x)$

$$I_\nu(x) \triangleq j^{-\nu} J_\nu(jx) = \sum_{m=0}^{\infty} \frac{x^{\nu+2m}}{2^{\nu+2m} m!\Gamma(\nu+m+1)} \tag{A.4}$$

In general, the following relationship holds between $I_\nu(x)$ and $J_\nu(x)$

$$I_\nu(x) = j^{-\nu} J_\nu(jx) \tag{A.5}$$

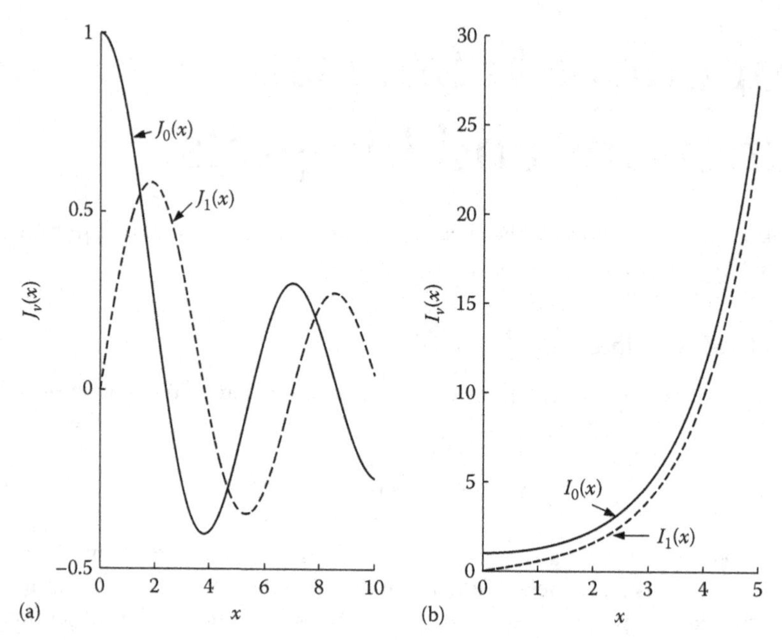

FIGURE A.1 Plots of Bessel functions of the first kind (a) and modified Bessel functions of the first kind (b).

For $\nu = 0$, we have

$$I_0(x) = J_0(jx) \tag{A.6}$$

Plots of $I_0(x)$ and $I_1(x)$ are shown in Figure A.1b. These two functions resemble the exponential function. In fact, the function $I_0(x)$ can be approximated as

$$I_0(x) \approx \begin{cases} e^{x^2/4} & x^2 \ll 1 \\ \dfrac{e^x}{\sqrt{2\pi x}} & x \gg 1 \end{cases} \tag{A.7}$$

Some useful integral relationships of the Bessel functions include

$$J_n(x) = \frac{1}{\pi}\int_0^{\pi} \cos(n\varphi - x\sin\phi)d\phi, \quad n \text{ integer} \tag{A.8}$$

$$J_0(x) = \frac{1}{\pi}\int_0^{\pi} \cos(x\sin\phi)d\phi = \frac{1}{2\pi}\int_0^{2\pi} e^{\pm jx\cos\phi}d\phi \tag{A.9}$$

$$I_0(x) = \frac{1}{2\pi}\int_0^{2\pi} e^{x\cos\phi}d\phi = \frac{1}{2\pi}\int_0^{2\pi} e^{x\sin\phi}d\phi \tag{A.10}$$

A.2 CONFLUENT HYPERGEOMETRIC FUNCTIONS

The confluent hypergeometric function $\Phi(a, b; z)$ is defined as

$$\Phi(a,b;z) = 1+\frac{a}{b}\frac{z}{1!}+\frac{a(a+1)}{b(b+1)}\frac{z}{2!}+\frac{a(a+1)(a+2)}{b(b+1)(b+2)}\frac{z}{3!}+\cdots \tag{A.11}$$

The function $\Phi(a, b; z)$ is also denoted as ${}_1F_1(a; b; z)$ in some textbooks. Some useful relationships of the confluent hypergeometric function include

$$\Phi(a,b;z) = e^{z}\Phi(b-a,b;-z) \tag{A.12}$$

$$\Phi(a,a;z) = e^{z} \tag{A.13}$$

$$\Phi(-0.5,1;-z) = e^{-z/2}\left[(1+z)I_0(z/2)+zI_1(z/2)\right] \tag{A.14}$$

Other relationships of the confluent hypergeometric function can be found in [1, p. 1013] and in [2, app. 1].

A.3 INTEGRALS

The following integral equation is used in the derivation of the MMSE estimator in Appendix B:

$$\int_0^\infty x^c e^{-ax^2} J_\nu(bx)dx = \frac{b^\nu \Gamma(0.5\nu+0.5c+0.5)}{2^{\nu+1}a^{\frac{1}{2}(c+\nu+1)}\Gamma(\nu+1)}\Phi\left(\frac{c+\nu+1}{2},\nu+1;-\frac{b^2}{4a}\right) \tag{A.15}$$

where $\text{Re}\{a\} > 0$ and $\text{Re}\{c + \nu\} > -1$. $\Gamma(.)$ denotes the gamma function, $J_\nu(.)$ the Bessel function of the νth kind, and $\Phi(a, b; z)$ denotes the confluent hypergeometric function (Equation A.11). Note that if the integral of interest involves the modified Bessel function $I_\nu(x)$ rather than $J_\nu(x)$, we need to make use of the relationship given in Equation A.5. So, when $I_0(x)$ is involved (i.e., $\nu = 0$), the preceding integral simplifies to

$$\int_0^\infty x^c e^{-ax^2} I_0(bx)dx = \frac{\Gamma(0.5c+0.5)}{2a^{\frac{1}{2}(c+1)}}\Phi\left(\frac{c+1}{2},1;\frac{b^2}{4a}\right) \tag{A.16}$$

REFERENCES

1. Gradshteyn, I. and Ryzhik, I. (2000), *Table of Integrals, Series and Products*, 6th ed., San Diego, CA: Academic Press.
2. Middleton, D. (1996), *An Introduction to Statistical Communication Theory*, New York: IEEE Press.
3. Wylie, C.R. and Barrett, L. (1982), *Advanced Engineering Mathematics*, 5th ed., New York: McGraw-Hill.

Appendix B: Derivation of the MMSE Estimator

In this appendix, we derive the MMSE estimator given in Equation 7.37. We start from Equation 7.28

$$\hat{X}_k = \frac{\int_0^{\infty}\int_0^{2\pi} x_k p\left(Y(\omega_k) \mid x_k,\theta_x\right) p(x_k,\theta_x) d\theta_x dx_k}{\int_0^{\infty}\int_0^{2\pi} p\left(Y(\omega_k) \mid x_k,\theta_x\right) p(x_k,\theta_x) d\theta_x dx_k} \tag{B.1}$$

The $p(Y(\omega_k)|x_k,\theta_x)$ and $p(x_k, \theta_x)$ probability density functions (pdfs) were derived in Equations 7.30 and 7.31 and are as follows:

$$p\left(Y(\omega_k) \mid x_k,\theta_x\right) = \frac{1}{\pi\lambda_d(k)} \exp\left\{-\frac{1}{\lambda_d(k)} \mid Y(\omega_k) - X(\omega_k) \mid^2\right\} \tag{B.2}$$

$$p(x_k,\theta_x) = \frac{x_k}{\pi\lambda_x(k)} \exp\left\{-\frac{x_k^2}{\lambda_x(k)}\right\} \tag{B.3}$$

Substituting Equations B.2 and B.3 into Equation B.1, we get

$$\begin{aligned}
\hat{X}_k &= \frac{\int_0^{\infty}\int_0^{2\pi} x_k^2 \exp\left[-\frac{Y_k^2 - 2x_k \mathrm{Re}\{e^{-j\theta_x} Y(\omega_k)\} + x_k^2}{\lambda_d(k)} - \frac{x_k^2}{\lambda_x(k)}\right] d\theta_x dx_k}{\int_0^{\infty}\int_0^{2\pi} x_k \exp\left[-\frac{Y_k^2 - 2x_k \mathrm{Re}\{e^{-j\theta_x} Y(\omega_k)\} + x_k^2}{\lambda_d(k)} - \frac{x_k^2}{\lambda_x(k)}\right] d\theta_x dx_k} \\
&= \frac{\int_0^{\infty} x_k^2 \exp\left[-\frac{x_k^2}{\lambda_k}\right] \int_0^{2\pi} \exp\left[\frac{2x_k \mathrm{Re}\{e^{-j\theta_x} Y(\omega_k)\}}{\lambda_d(k)}\right] d\theta_x dx_k}{\int_0^{\infty} x_k \exp\left[-\frac{x_k^2}{\lambda_k}\right] \int_0^{2\pi} \exp\left[\frac{2x_k \mathrm{Re}\{e^{-j\theta_x} Y(\omega_k)\}}{\lambda_d(k)}\right] d\theta_x dx_k}
\end{aligned} \tag{B.4}$$

where

$$\frac{1}{\lambda_k} = \frac{1}{\lambda_d(k)} + \frac{1}{\lambda_x(k)} \tag{B.5}$$

Note that λ_k can also be expressed as

$$\lambda_k = \frac{\lambda_x(k)\lambda_d(k)}{\lambda_x(k)+\lambda_d(k)} = \frac{\lambda_x(k)}{1+\xi_k} \tag{B.6}$$

The inner integral in Equation B.4 is the modified Bessel function of the first kind, and has the following form:

$$I_0(|z|) = \frac{1}{2\pi}\int_0^{2\pi} \exp\left[\mathrm{Re}(z e^{-j\theta_x})\right] d\theta_x \tag{B.7}$$

where $z = 2x_k Y(\omega_k)/\lambda_d(k)$. Using the preceding integral relationship of the Bessel function in Equation B.4, we get

$$\hat{X}_k = \frac{\int_0^\infty x_k^2 \exp\left[-\frac{x_k^2}{\lambda_k}\right] I_0\left(2x_k Y_k / \lambda_d(k)\right) dx_k}{\int_0^\infty x_k \exp\left[-\frac{x_k^2}{\lambda_k}\right] I_0\left(2x_k Y_k / \lambda_d(k)\right) dx_k} \tag{B.8}$$

The ratio $Y_k/\lambda_d(k)$ in the preceding equation can be expressed in terms of λ_k (Equation B.6) as follows:

$$\begin{aligned}
\frac{Y_k}{\lambda_d(k)} &= \sqrt{\frac{Y_k^2}{\lambda_d(k)}\frac{\lambda_x(k)}{\lambda_d(k)}\frac{1}{\lambda_x(k)}} \\
&= \sqrt{\frac{\gamma_k \xi_k}{\lambda_x(k)}} = \sqrt{\frac{\frac{\gamma_k}{\xi_k+1}\xi_k}{\frac{\lambda_x(k)}{\xi_k+1}}} \\
&= \sqrt{\frac{v_k}{\lambda_k}}
\end{aligned} \tag{B.9}$$

and Equation B.4 reduces to

$$\hat{X}_k = \frac{\int_0^\infty x_k^2 \exp\left[-\frac{x_k^2}{\lambda_k}\right] I_0\left(2x_k\sqrt{\frac{v_k}{\lambda_k}}\right) dx_k}{\int_0^\infty x_k \exp\left[-\frac{x_k^2}{\lambda_k}\right] I_0\left(2x_k\sqrt{\frac{v_k}{\lambda_k}}\right) dx_k} \tag{B.10}$$

We can evaluate the preceding integral using Equation A.16

$$\hat{X}_k = \frac{\Gamma(1.5)(\lambda_k)^{3/2}\Phi\left(\frac{3}{2},1;v_k\right)}{\lambda_k\,\Phi(1,1;v_k)}$$
$$= \Gamma(1.5)\sqrt{\lambda_k}\,\frac{\Phi\left(\frac{3}{2},1;v_k\right)}{\Phi(1,1;v_k)} \tag{B.11}$$

where $\Phi(a, b; z)$ is the confluent hypergeometric function defined in Equation A.11, and $\Gamma(1.5) = \sqrt{\pi}/2$. Using the hypergeometric relationship given in Equation A.12 for the numerator and the relationship given in Equation A.13 for the denominator, the preceding estimator finally simplifies to

$$\hat{X}_k = \Gamma(1.5)\sqrt{\lambda_k}\,\frac{e^{v_k}\Phi(-0.5;1;-v_k)}{e^{v_k}}$$
$$= \Gamma(1.5)\sqrt{\lambda_k}\,\Phi(-0.5;1;-v_k) \tag{B.12}$$

Using Equation A.14, we can alternatively write the preceding estimator in terms of Bessel functions:

$$\hat{X}_k = \frac{\sqrt{\pi}}{2}\sqrt{\lambda_k}\exp\left(-\frac{v_k}{2}\right)\left[(1+v_k)\,I_o\left(\frac{v_k}{2}\right)+v_k I_1\left(\frac{v_k}{2}\right)\right] \tag{B.13}$$

where $I_0(\cdot)$ and $I_1(\cdot)$ denote the modified Bessel functions of zero and first order, respectively (see Appendix A for definitions).

Appendix C: MATLAB® Code and Speech/Noise Databases

This appendix describes the contents of the DVD-ROM included with the book. The DVD-ROM was updated from the first edition and organized into three main folders. The first folder contains speech files recorded in our lab along with real-world noise recordings. These files can be used to evaluate the quality and intelligibility of speech processed by noise suppression algorithms. The second folder contains MATLAB® code for the implementation of major speech enhancement algorithms taken from each chapter of the book. The third folder contains C/C++ code for training binary SNR classifiers using GMMs and enhancing speech based on the trained GMM models (see Section 13.5.2). The folder organization of the DVD-ROM contents is shown in Figure C.1.

C.1 NOISE AND SPEECH DATABASES

The `Noise Recordings` folder contains 19 real-world recordings taken from various environments which include (a) construction site, (b) train, (c) street, (d) cafeteria, (e) commercial airplane, (f) car, and (g) office. Files were recorded at a 44 kHz sampling frequency. In addition, the folder contains speech-shaped noise which was created such that the long-term average spectrum of the speech-shaped noise matches the long-term average spectrum of the male talker of the IEEE corpus included in the DVD-ROM. The long-term average spectrum of the speech-shaped noise is shown in Figure C.2.

The `Speech` Database folder (Figure C.1) contains three sub-folders, each containing a different set of speech materials. The NOIZEUS folder contains clean and noisy speech files corrupted in various noise environments at different SNR levels (see Chapter 12 for more details). The NOIZEUS/clean sub-folder contains the 30 sentences recorded in quiet as well as the phonetic transcriptions files of these sentences. The transcription files have the extension.phn and have the same format as the files found in the TIMIT database. For example, the first five lines of the transcription file 'sp01.phn' corresponding to the file 'sp01.wav' are given next.

```
0 1301 sil
1301 1425 f
1425 1813 v
1813 2231 cl
2231 2340 s
......
```

where the first column of numbers indicates the starting sample number of a phonetic segment, the second column the end sample number, and the last column of strings

```
Databases
        - Noise Recordings
        - Speech
                - Consonants
                         - Narrowband
                         - Wideband
                - IEEE corpus
                         - Narrowband
                         - Wideband
                - NOIZEUS
                         - Airport
                             - 0dB
                             - 5dB
                             - 10dB
                             - 15dB
                         + Babble
                         + Car
                         + Clean
                         + Exhibition
                         + Restaurant
                         + Station
                         + Street
                         + Train
+ GMM SNR classifier (C/C++ code)
MATLAB code
        - Ideal_channel_selection
        - Noise_estimation
        - Objective_measures
                - Intelligibility
                - Quality
        - Spectral subtractive
        - Statistical_based
        - Subspace
```

FIGURE C.1 Directory structure of the contents of the DVD-ROM.

indicates the corresponding broad phonetic class. Silence and closure segments were indicated by 'sil' and 'cl,' respectively. The NOIZEUS files were phonetically segmented into the following six broad classes of sounds: vowels ('v'), fricatives ('f'), stops ('s'), affricates ('a'), nasals ('n'), and semivowels ('g'). The original recordings (sampled at 25 kHz) of the NOIZEUS database can be found in the folder NOIZEUS/clean/wideband.

The NOIZEUS corpus was designed to facilitate comparisons of speech enhancement algorithms among research groups. It can be used primarily for subjective quality assessment and objective evaluation of speech enhancement algorithms [1,2].

The other two folders contain speech material appropriate for evaluation of the intelligibility of processed speech. The consonants sub-folder contains 20 consonants recorded in/aa C aa/context, where C indicates the consonant. The following consonants were recorded:/p, t, k, b, d, g, m, n, ch, dh, w, l, r, y, f, v, s, z, sh, jh/. Example tokens in the consonants folder include/aa p aa/,/aa t aa/,/aa m aa/, etc.

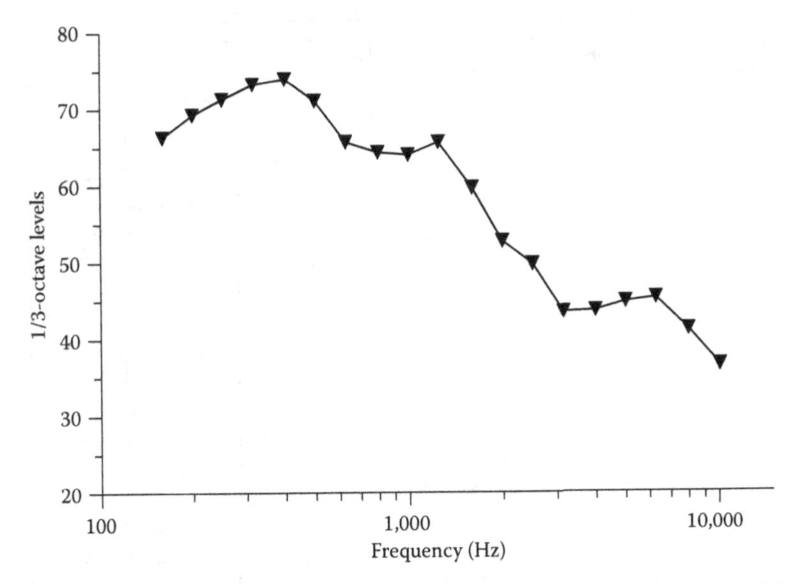

FIGURE C.2 Long-term average spectrum of the speech-shaped noise (SSN_IEEE.wav) included in the DVD-ROM.

The original wideband recordings, sampled at 24.4 kHz, as well as the narrowband (down-sampled to 8 kHz) files are available in separate sub-folders. All consonants were produced by a female speaker.

The IEEE-corpus folder contains 720 sentences taken from the IEEE-Harvard corpus [3]. The sentences were produced by a male talker. The original wideband recordings, sampled at 25 kHz, as well as the narrowband (down-sampled to 8 kHz) files are available in separate sub-folders. The narrowband files were produced by first bandpass-filtering the wideband recordings with a 300–3200 Hz bandpass filter (see Section 11.1 for more details) to simulate the telephone bandwidth and then down-sampling the recordings to 8 kHz.

The speech recordings were done in a double-walled sound-proof room using Tucker-Davis Technologies (TDT) recording equipment. The recording setup is shown in Figure C.3. A dual microphone preamplifier (model SX202) was first used to pre-amplify the signal picked up by the microphone. The signal was then sent to the TDT equipment (System 3), comprising of a programmable attenuator (PA5), A/D converters, D/A converters, and a DSP processor. A 50 MHz Sharc DSP processor is used in the TDT (system 3) equipment. In our application, the DSP processor was merely used to buffer the recorded data and send the data to the PC. The TDT hardware is connected to the PC via a USB cable. A Shure microphone (model SM94) was used for all recordings. This microphone is a unidirectional electret condenser microphone with a flat frequency response in the range of 40–16 kHz.

A total of seven speakers were recruited for the recordings of the three speech databases, NOIZEUS, IEEE corpus, and consonants. All were native speakers of American English and ranged in age from 18 to 26 years old. Speakers were raised in different states of the United States which included Texas, Kentucky, California,

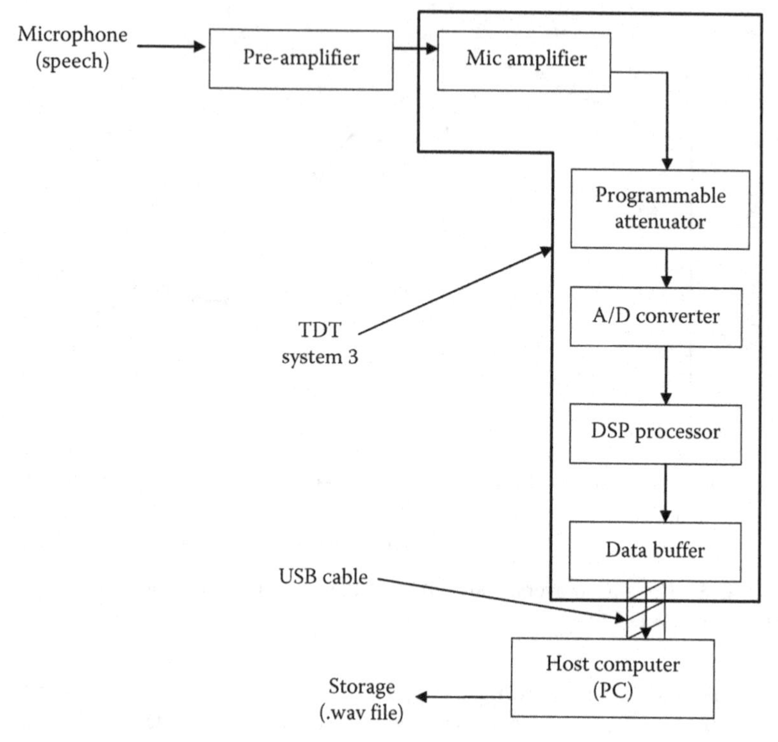

FIGURE C.3 Recording setup.

and North Carolina. Three male and three female speakers were recruited for the NOIZEUS database. One male speaker produced all 720 sentences of the IEEE-Harvard corpus, while the others produced only a subset. One additional female speaker was recruited for the consonant recordings. The speaker characteristics are given in Table C.1. The table also lists the NOIZEUS sentences recorded by each speaker.

TABLE C.1
Speaker Characteristics

Speaker	Age	State Raised	Gender	F0 (Hz)	NOIZEUS Sentences	Database
CH	21	Texas	M	135	sp01–sp05	NOIZEUS
DE	20	California	M	134	sp06–sp10	NOIZEUS
SI	20	Texas and Kentucky	M	144	sp21–sp25	NOIZEUS, IEEE
JE	19	North Carolina and Texas	F	225	sp11–sp15	NOIZEUS
KI	22	Texas	F	245	sp16–sp20	NOIZEUS
TI	22	Texas	F	225	sp26–sp30	NOIZEUS
JD	23	Texas	F	225	—	Consonants

C.2 MATLAB® CODE

The following basic system requirements are needed to run the MATLAB code included in the DVD-ROM:

1. MATLAB® (tested with version 7.12)
2. MATLAB's Signal Processing Toolbox (tested with version 6.15)
3. 4 MB of storage
4. 512 MB of RAM

The MATLAB code was run and tested in Windows XP and Windows 7 operating systems, and was not fully tested in the UNIX environment. To run the code, first copy the contents of the folder MATLAB_code (~4 MB) to the local hard drive. Instructions with examples for running individual algorithms are given next.

Representative speech enhancement algorithms taken from each chapter of the book are included in the DVD-ROM. As shown in Figure C.1, the algorithms are organized in different sub-folders. The algorithms included in each sub-folder are shown in Table C.2. The majority of the speech enhancement algorithms take two input arguments: the filename of the noisy speech signal (in Microsoft Windows.wav format) and the name of the output file containing the enhanced speech signal. Example noisy files from the NOIZEUS corpus are included in each sub-folder.

To run a spectral-subtractive algorithm, for instance, take the following steps (after copying the contents of the DVD-ROM to the local hard-drive):

- *Step 1:* Run MATLAB (all algorithms were tested using MATLAB version 7.0.1)
- *Step 2:* Change to the folder containing the spectral-subtractive algorithms by typing in MATLAB:

```
>> cd c:\MATLAB_code\spectral_subtractive
```

- *Step 3:* Select a spectral subtraction algorithm (see list in Table C.2) and execute it. To enhance, for instance, the noisy file `sp04 _ babble _ sn10.wav` (included in this folder) using the basic spectral subtraction algorithm [4], simply type the following in the MATLAB prompt:

```
>> specsub('sp04_babble_sn10.wav','out_spec_sub.wav')
where out_spec_sub.wav is the file containing the
  enhanced signal.
```

Any audio program (e.g., Windows Media player, Adobe Audition, etc.) supporting the.wav sound format can be used to listen to the enhanced signals. The MATLAB speech analysis toolbox (COLEA) developed in our lab and available from the author or online [5] can also be used.

The majority of algorithms assume the presence of speech-absent segments in the beginning of each sentence. These speech-absent segments (lasting for about 120 ms) are used to estimate the noise spectrum. Some of the algorithms

TABLE C.2
Filenames, Descriptions, and References for the MATLAB® Algorithms Included in the DVD-ROM

Folder	Filename	Algorithm	Ref.
spectral_subtractive	specsub.m	Basic spectral subtraction algorithm	[4]
	mband.m	Multi-band spectral subtraction	[13]
	ss_rdc.m	Spectral subtraction with adaptive gain averaging and reduced delay convolution	[14]
statistical_based	wiener_iter.m	Iterative Wiener algorithm based on all-pole speech production model	[15]
	wiener_as.m	Wiener algorithm based on *a priori* SNR estimation	[16]
	wiener_wt.m	Wiener algorithm based on wavelet thresholding multi-taper spectra	[17]
	mt_mask.m	Psychoacoustically motivated algorithm	[18]
	audnoise.m	Audible noise suppression algorithm	[19]
	mmse.m	MMSE algorithm with and without speech-presence uncertainty	[20]
	logmmse.m	LogMMSE algorithm	[21]
	logmmse_SPU	LogMMSE algorithm incorporating speech-presence uncertainty	[22]
	stsa_weuclid.m	Bayesian estimator based on weighted-Euclidean distortion measure	[23]
	stsa_wcosh.m	Bayesian estimator based on weighted-cosh distortion measure	[23]
	stsa_wlr.m	Bayesian estimator based on weighted-likelihood ratio distortion measure	[23]
	stsa_mis.m	Bayesian estimator based on modified Itakura-Saito distortion measure	[23]
subspace	klt.m	Subspace algorithm with embedded pre-whitening	[24]
	pklt.m	Perceptually motivated subspace algorithm	[25]
noise_estimation	specsub_ns.m	Basic spectral subtraction algorithm implemented with different noise estimation algorithms:	
	martin_estimation.m	1. Martin's minimum tracking	[7]
	mcra_estimation.m	2. MCRA algorithm	[26]
	mcra2_estimation.m	3. MCRA-2 algorithm	[8]

	imcra_estimation.m	4. IMCRA algorithm	[27]
	doblinger_estimation.m	5. Continuous minimal tracking	[28]
	hirsch_estimation.m	6. Weighted spectral average	[29]
	connfreq_estimation.m	7. Connected time-frequency regions	[30]
objective_measures\quality	comp_snr.m	Computes the overall and segmental SNR	[31]
	comp_wss.m	Computes the weighted-spectral slope metric	[32]
	comp_llr.m	Computes the likelihood-ratio measure	[33]
	comp_is.m	Computes the Itakura-Saito measure	[33]
	comp_cep.m	Computes the cepstrum distance measure	[34]
	comp_fwseg	Computes the frequency-weighted segmental SNR (fwSNRseg)	[35]
	comp_fwseg_variant	Computes the frequency-variant fwSNRseg measure	Chapter 11, Equation 11.5
	comp_fwseg_mars	Computes the frequency variant fwSNRseg measure based on MARS analysis	Chapter 11, Equation 11.37
	pesq.m	Computes the narrowband and wideband PESQ values	[9–11]
	composite.m	Computes a composite measure	[2]
	addnoise_asl.m	Adds noise to the clean signal at a specified SNR level based on active speech level	[36]
objective_measures\ intelligibility	sii.m	Computes the SII measure	[37]
	ncm.m	Computes the NCM measure	[38]
	csii.m	Computes the CSII measure	[39]
ideal_channel_selection	ics.m	SNR-based channel selection (ideal binary mask)	[40]
	ics_constr_rule.m	Channel selection based on the SNR_{ESI} rule	[41,42]
	ics_masker_rule.m	Channel selection based on masker constraints	[43]
	ics_reverb_rule.m	Channel selection based on the SRR rule	[44]
GMM SNR classifier\[code in C/C++ and MATLAB]		AMS feature extraction, GMM training, Bayes' classification, speech synthesis	Chapter 13

included in the DVD-ROM use a voice-activity algorithm (VAD) [6] to estimate and update the noise spectrum. Alternative, noise-estimation algorithms can be used in place of the VAD algorithm to continuously update/estimate the noise spectrum. The sub-folder `noise _ estimation` contains several noise-estimation algorithms which can be used in lieu of the VAD algorithms to continuously update and estimate the noise spectra. A total of seven different noise estimation algorithms were implemented. These algorithms can be easily integrated in your own code by simply inserting the following five lines of code as shown in the example next:

```
for t = 1:Numberframes
  %– – - compute spectrum of windowed signal– – – – – – – – –
    – – – –
  %
  win_x = win.*x(k:k+len-1); %Window input signal x(.) with
    window win(.)
  X = fft(win_x,nFFT); %compute the Discrete Fourier Transform
  Px = abs(spec).^2; % compute the power spectrum
  %– - use a noise-estimation algorithm to estimate/update
    noise spectrum –
  %
  if t = = 1
   parameters = initialise_parameters(Px, SamplingFreq,
      method);
  else
   parameters = noise_estimation(Px, method, parameters);
  end
  noise_PSD = parameters.noise_ps; % the estimated power
    spectrum of noise
    (insert your algorithm here)
end
```

The string "method" in the aforementioned code specifies the noise-estimation algorithm. The list of noise estimation algorithms included in the DVD-ROM is shown in Table C.2. The sub-folder noise_estimation contains as an example the basic spectral subtraction algorithm [4] (specsub_ns.m) implemented with noise estimation. To execute the spectral subtraction algorithm, for instance, using Martin's [7] noise estimation algorithm, type the following in MATLAB:

```
>> specsub_ns('sp04_babble_sn10.wav','martin','out_martin.wav');
```

where `sp04 _ babble _ sn10`.wav is the noisy speech file and out_martin.wav is the name of the file containing the enhanced signal. Similarly, to execute the spectral subtraction algorithm using the MCRA-2 algorithm [8], type the following in MATLAB:

```
>> specsub_ns('sp04_babble_sn10.wav','mcra2','out_mcra2.wav');
```

The code for objective evaluation of speech enhancement algorithms is contained in two separate folders, one for quality evaluation and one for intelligibility evaluation (see Table C.2). The majority of the objective quality evaluation algorithms takes two input arguments and produces one output value, the value of the objective measure. The two input arguments consist of the filenames of the clean speech (reference) signal and enhanced (or degraded) signal, respectively. To compute, for instance, the PESQ score of the enhanced file enhanced.wav, type in MATLAB the following:

```
>> pesq_score = pesq (cleanfile.wav, enhanced.wav)
```

where `pesq _ score` is the returned PESQ score. If the detected sampling frequency is 8 kHz, then it returns 2 PESQ scores, the raw PESQ score according to ITU P.862 [9] and the MOS-mapped score according to ITU P.862.1[10]. If the detected sampling frequency is 16 kHz, then it returns the MOS-mapped score according to ITU P.862.2 [11], which covers the wideband implementation of the PESQ measure.

The 'composite.m' file contains an implementation of the composite measures proposed in [2] (see also Chapter 11) and returns three output values, one for the rating of the signal distortion, one for the rating of background intrusiveness, and one for the rating of overall quality. The usage of 'composite.m' is given as follows:

```
>> [sig, bak, ovrl] = composite(cleanfile.wav,enhanced.wav)
```

where the `sig`, `bak`, and `ovrl` are the predicted ratings (on a 5-point scale) of signal distortion, background distortion, and overall quality respectively. The frequency variant measures based on multiple linear regression (comp_fwseg_variant.m) and MARS analysis (comp_fwseg_mars.m) also return three output values corresponding to the ratings of signal distortion, background distortion, and overall quality.

Each sub-folder in MATLAB_code contains a reamde.txt text file (and a readme.pdf file) providing usage information for all MATLAB files.

C.3 GMM SNR CLASSIFIER (C/C++ CODE)

The folder `GMM SNR classifier` contains C/C++ code with the implementation of the SNR-based channel selection (binary mask) algorithm presented in [9]. This binary mask algorithm does not operate in ideal conditions (i.e., does not assume *a priori* access to the clean and noise signals), but rather takes as input corrupted speech. This algorithm has been shown to improve substantially speech intelligibility by normal-hearing listeners (for more details, see Section 13.5.2) in various backgrounds at input SNR levels of −5 and 0 dB [12]. The code was tested under Ubuntu 11.10 Linux OS. Basic requirements to run the code include MATLAB R2012a for feature extraction, GNU GCC compiler version 4.6.1 for compilation of C/C++ sources of GMM tools, Bash shell for execution of shell scripts and 2.5 GB of disk space. The experiment cannot be run from the DVD-ROM. Instead, the root directory of the experiment has to be copied on to the hard drive. Then, read and write permissions have to be set for the files and folders prior to execution of the demo.

The bash script "demo.sh", contained in the root directory, performs the following: (a) AMS feature extraction, (b) GMM training, (c) GMM testing, and (d) enhancement of speech corrupted by speech-shaped noise at input SNR of −5 dB. After the "demo.sh" script completes, the enhanced speech files along with spectrograms (in PDF format), can be found in the "feature-extraction" sub-folder. The training and testing settings, including the GMM parameters (e.g., number of mixtures, number of EM iterations, etc.) are set to match those used in [9]. The files containing the settings ("train.txt" and "test.txt", respectively) are located in the root directory.

Caution should be exercised when using the aforementioned code to enhance speech in other background environments, and particularly in highly non-stationary environments. For demonstration purposes, only limited amount of data was used in the code included in the DVD-ROM to train GMM SNR classifiers for speech-shaped noise. For other background environments, the amount of training data might need to increase substantially and the system parameters (e.g., number of feature dimensions, number of GMM mixtures, number of EM iterations, etc.) might need to be adjusted accordingly. The code provided in this DVD-ROM is only meant to serve as a starting point for other researchers to develop better binary SNR classifiers for binary mask estimation.

Questions, feedback, and bug reports should be sent to the author at loizou@utdallas.edu or pcloizou@gmail.com.

REFERENCES

1. Hu, Y. and Loizou, P. (2006), Subjective comparison of speech enhancement algorithms, *Proc. IEEE Int. Conf. Acoust. Speech Signal Processing*, I, 153–156.
2. Hu, Y. and Loizou, P. (2006), Evaluation of objective measures for speech enhancement. *Proceedings of Interspeech*, Pittsburg, PA, pp. 1447–1450.
3. IEEE Subcommittee (1969), IEEE recommended practice for speech quality measurements, *IEEE Trans. Audio Electroacoust.*, AU-17(3), 225–246.
4. Berouti, M., Schwartz, M., and Makhoul, J. (1979), Enhancement of speech corrupted by acoustic noise, *Proceedings of IEEE International Conference Acoustics, Speech, Signal Processing*, Washington, DC, pp. 208–211.
5. Loizou, P. (2006), COLEA: A MATLAB software tool for speech analysis. Online http://www.utdallas.edu/~loizou/speech/colea. htm]
6. Sohn, J. and Kim, N. (1999), Statistical model-based voice activity detection, *IEEE Signal Process. Lett.*, 6(1), 1–3.
7. Martin, R. (2001), Noise power spectral density estimation based on optimal smoothing and minimum statistics, *IEEE Trans. Speech Audio Process.*, 9(5), 504–512.
8. Rangachari, S. and Loizou, P. (2006), A noise estimation algorithm for highly nonstationary environments, *Speech Commun.*, 28, 220–231.
9. ITU (2000), Perceptual evaluation of speech quality (PESQ), and objective method for end-to-end speech quality assessment of narrowband telephone networks and speech codecs, ITU-T Recommendation P. 862.
10. ITU (2003), Mapping function for transforming P.862 raw result scores to MOS-LQO, ITU-T Recommendation P. 862. 1.
11. ITU (2007), Wideband extension to Recommendation P.862 for the assessment of wideband telephone networks and speech codecs, ITU-T Recommendation P. 862. 2.
12. Kim, G., Lu, Y., Hu, Y., and Loizou, P. (2009), An algorithm that improves speech intelligibility in noise for normal-hearing listeners, *J. Acoust. Soc. Am.*, 126(3), 1486–1494.

13. Kamath, S. and Loizou, P. (2002), A multi-band spectral subtraction method for enhancing speech corrupted by colored noise, *Proceedings of the IEEE International Conference Acoustics Speech, and Signal Processing*, Orlando, FL, Vol. 4, pp. 4160–4164.
14. Gustafsson, H., Nordholm, S., and Claesson, I. (2001), Spectral subtraction using reduced delay convolution and adaptive averaging, *IEEE Trans. Speech Audio Process.*, 9(8), 799–807.
15. Lim, J. and Oppenheim, A.V. (1978), All-pole modeling of degraded speech, *IEEE Trans. Acoust. Speech Signal Proc.*, ASSP-26(3), 197–210.
16. Scalart, P. and Filho, J. (1996), Speech enhancement based on a priori signal to noise estimation, *Proceedings of the IEEE International Conference on Acoustics Speech, and Signal Processing*, Atlanta, GA, pp. 629–632.
17. Hu, Y. and Loizou, P. (2004), Speech enhancement based on wavelet thresholding the multitaper spectrum. *IEEE Trans. Speech Audio Process.*, 12(1), 59–67.
18. Hu, Y. and Loizou, P. (2004), Incorporating a psychoacoustical model in frequency domain speech enhancement. *IEEE Signal Process. Lett.*, 11(2), 270–273.
19. Tsoukalas, D.E., Mourjopoulos, J.N., and Kokkinakis, G. (1997), Speech enhancement based on audible noise suppression. *IEEE Trans. Speech Audio Process.*, 5(6), 497–514.
20. Ephraim, Y. and Malah, D. (1984), Speech enhancement using a minimum mean-square error short-time spectral amplitude estimator, *IEEE Trans. Acoust. Speech, Signal Process.*, ASSP-32(6), 1109–1121.
21. Ephraim, Y. and Malah, D. (1985), Speech enhancement using a minimum mean-square error log-spectral amplitude estimator, *IEEE Trans. Acoust. Speech Signal Process.*, ASSP-23(2), 443–445.
22. Cohen, I. (2002), Optimal speech enhancement under signal presence uncertainty using log-spectra amplitude estimator, *IEEE Signal Process. Lett.*, 9(4), 113–116.
23. Loizou, P. (2005), Speech enhancement based on perceptually motivated Bayesian estimators of the speech magnitude spectrum, *IEEE Trans. Speech Audio Process.*, 13(5), 857–869.
24. Hu, Y. and Loizou, P. (2003), A generalized subspace approach for enhancing speech corrupted by colored noise, *IEEE Trans. Speech Audio Process.*, 11, 334–341.
25. Jabloun, F. and Champagne, B. (2003), Incorporating the human hearing properties in the signal subspace approach for speech enhancement, *IEEE Trans. Speech Audio Process.*, 11(6), 700–708.
26. Cohen, I. (2002), Noise estimation by minima controlled recursive averaging for robust speech enhancement, *IEEE Signal Proc. Lett.*, 9(1), 12–15.
27. Cohen, I. (2003), Noise spectrum estimation in adverse environments: Improved minima controlled recursive averaging, *IEEE Trans. Speech Audio Process.*, 11(5), 466–475.
28. Doblinger, G. (1995), Computationally efficient speech enhancement by spectral minima tracking in subbands, *Proc. Eurospeech*, 2, 1513–1516.
29. Hirsch, H. and Ehrlicher, C. (1995), Noise estimation techniques for robust speech recognition, *Proceedings of the IEEE International Conference Acoustics, Speech, Signal Processing*, Detroit, MI, pp. 153–156.
30. Sorensen, K. and Andersen, S. (2005), Speech enhancement with natural sounding residual noise based on connected time-frequency speech presence regions, *EURASIP J. Appl. Signal Process.*, 18, 2954–2964.
31. Hansen, J. and Pellom, B. (1998), An effective quality evaluation protocol for speech enhancement algorithms, *Proceedings International Conference on Spoken Language Processing*, Sydney, Australia, Vol. 7, pp. 2819–2822.
32. Klatt, D. (1982), Prediction of perceived phonetic distance from critical band spectra, *Proceedings of the IEEE International Conference Acoustics, Speech, Signal Processing*, Paris, France, Vol. 7, pp. 1278–1281.

33. Quackenbush, S., Barnwell, T., and Clements, M. (1988), *Objective Measures of Speech Quality*, Englewood Cliffs, NJ: Prentice-Hall.
34. Kitawaki, N., Nagabuchi, H., and Itoh, K. (1988), Objective quality evaluation for low bit-rate speech coding systems. *IEEE J. Select. Areas Commun.*, 6(2), 262–273.
35. Tribolet, J., Noll, P., McDermott, B., and Crochiere, R.E. (1978), A study of complexity and quality of speech waveform coders. *Proceedings of the IEEE International Conference Acoustics, Speech, Signal Processing*, Tulsa, OK, 586–590.
36. ITU-T (1993), Objective measurement of active speech level, ITU-T Recommendation P. 56.
37. ANSI S3-5 (1997), Methods for calculation of the speech intelligibility index. American National Standards Institute, New York.
38. Goldsworthy, R. and Greenberg, J. (2004), Analysis of speech-based speech transmission index methods with implications for nonlinear operations, *J. Acoust. Soc. Am.*, 116, 3679–3689.
39. Kates, J. and Arehart, K. (2005), Coherence and the speech intelligibility index, *J. Acoust. Soc. Am.*, 117(4), 2224–2237.
40. Li, N. and Loizou, P. (2008), Factors influencing intelligibility of ideal binary-masked speech: Implications for noise reduction, *J. Acoust. Soc. Am.*, 123, 1673–1682.
41. Loizou, P. and Kim, G. (2011), Reasons why current speech-enhancement algorithms do not improve speech intelligibility and suggested solutions, *IEEE Trans. Audio Speech Lang. Process.*, 19(1), 47–56.
42. Kim, G. and Loizou, P. (2011), Gain-induced speech distortions and the absence of intelligibility benefit with existing noise-reduction algorithms, *J. Acoust. Soc. Am.*, 130(3), 1581–1596.
43. Kim, G. and Loizou, P. (2010), A new binary mask based on noise constraints for improved speech intelligibility, *Proc. Interspeech*, 1632–1635.
44. Kokkinakis, K., Hazrati, O., and Loizou, P. (2011), A channel-selection criterion for suppressing reverberation in cochlear implants, *J. Acoust. Soc. Am.*, 129(5), 3221–3232.

Index

D

E

F

G

H

I

K

L

M

P

T

U

V

W

Y